Manual of Pediatric Nephrology

Kishore Phadke • Paul Goodyer
Martin Bitzan
Editors

Manual of Pediatric Nephrology

Springer

Editors
Kishore Phadke
Department of Pediatric Nephrology
Children's Kidney Care Center
St. John's Medical College Hospital
Bangalore, KA
India

Martin Bitzan
Division of Pediatric Nephrology
Montreal Children's Hospital
McGill University
Montreal, QC
Canada

Paul Goodyer
Division of Pediatric Nephrology
Montreal Children's Hospital
McGill University
Montreal, QC
Canada

ISBN 978-3-642-12482-2 ISBN 978-3-642-12483-9 (eBook)
DOI 10.1007/978-3-642-12483-9
Springer Heidelberg New York Dordrecht London

Library of Congress Control Number: 2013948392

Printed on acid-free paper

Springer is part of Springer Science+Business Media (www.springer.com)

Foreword I

The International Society of Nephrology strives to improve access to the best possible kidney care worldwide. An important step is the training of nephrologists and physicians treating patients with renal diseases. These goals form the basis of the ISN "Global Outreach" (GO) programs – to build health equality worldwide and improve kidney care and prevention strategies around the globe by making the knowledge and experience of the developed world accessible to kidney doctors and other specialists in emerging countries.

Children are a particularly vulnerable population. Unacceptable delays in the recognition and treatment of (severe) renal disease due to lack of access to basic and comprehensive care often leads to preventable, acute and chronic adverse effects caused by malfunctioning kidneys. Kidney disease during infancy to adolescence due to (intrauterine) malnutrition, genetic inheritance, nephrotoxic agents or poorly treated primary diseases has devastating, often irreversible, effects on bone health, growth and intellectual development.

Disparities in preventive and curative or supportive care arise from the lack of knowledgeable health care professionals, lack of (public) health care resources and lack of individual financial means to initiate and support therapies that are taken for granted in more affluent countries.

To come to grips with the global challenge of rising numbers of patients with renal diseases, the ISN created the Sister Renal Center program pairing emerging and supporting (established) centers across all continents. As the chair and ardent supporter of our GO programs, I am proud to witness the involvement of dedicated pediatric nephrologists in this endeavor.

This Manual is the collaborative product of one of the few and successful pediatric sister center pairs, the Children's Kidney Care Center at the St. John's Medical College Hospital in Bangalore, India, and the Nephrology Division at the Montreal Children's Hospital in Montreal, Canada. Written in a collaborative spirit, it emphasizes a global perspective.

May it serve health care professionals, trainees, and physicians to improve the diagnosis and treatment of children with renal diseases worldwide.

Paul N. Harden
Professor of Nephrology
Chair, International Society of Nephrology Sister Renal Program
Oxford, UK

Foreword II

Today, kidney issues dramatically impact global health, especially the health of children. In developing countries, millions of people – most of them children – die each year from diseases that are preventable and treatable. For many of these children, kidney problems represent a serious threat to their survival.

Important examples include – but are not limited to – the delayed recognition and treatment for congenital abnormalities of the kidney and urinary tract, which are a major cause of chronic kidney disease and secondary health problems; severe fluid and electrolyte disturbances and acute kidney injury due to diarrhea, the #2 cause of death in children worldwide; infants with low birth weight in low income groups due to malnutrition and lack of prenatal care, with an increased risk of small kidneys, hypertension in adolescence and chronic kidney disease; HIV associated nephropathy, particularly in areas where highly active antiretroviral therapy is not accessible.

A major goal of the International Pediatric Nephrology Association (IPNA) is to reach physicians throughout the world through educational and fellowship programs and enable them to care for children with kidney diseases. This *Manual of Pediatric Nephrology* is designed to give pediatrician and general physicians as well as trainees and other health care professionals a quick and practical approach to the diagnosis and treatment of children with different types of kidney diseases. The well-structured text is easy to read and covers all important areas in the field.

On behalf of IPNA, I welcome this new manual as a valuable resource for practitioners and trainees in (pediatric) nephrology alike. Its appeal lies in the combined perspective provided by experienced nephrologists from different continents that takes into account the realities in emerging countries. It corresponds well to IPNA's goals to "work to disseminate knowledge about kidney disease in children in the areas where care is needed most".

Isidro B, Salusky, M.D.
Secretary General IPNA
Distinguished Professor of Pediatrics
David Geffen School of Medicine at UCLA
Los Angeles, CA, USA

Preface

This manual does not want to replace standard textbooks of nephrology or pediatric nephrology. Rather, it offers a first, quick and practical approach for the care of children with kidney disease. It is meant to serve practitioners, trainees, pediatricians, general physicians, and other health care professionals.

The manual is the product of a long-lasting collaboration between two pediatric nephrology units, the Children's Kidney Care Center at the Saint John's Medical College Hospital (St-John's) in Bangalore, India, and the Division of Nephrology at the Montreal Children's Hospital (MCH) in Montreal, Canada.

The authors approached each chapter with the practical reality in emerging and resource-poor countries in mind. We hope that this concept renders the manual useful and versatile in a variety of settings and diverse medical practices. To this end, we are proud of the manual's endorsement by the International Society of Nephrology Global Outreach initiative and the support by the International Pediatric Nephrology Association.

It is unavoidable in a practically oriented, abbreviated book like ours that topics are missing or only mentioned cursorily. The editors purposefully focused on relatively frequent and clinically important disorders and practical, mainly diagnostic and therapeutic, aspects. Detailed pathological and pathophysiological reviews were omitted to keep the text short and lean. The reader is strongly encouraged to seek in-depth information in more comprehensive textbooks.

The editors appreciate specific suggestions that help improve the utility and ameliorate the shortcomings of this manual. Please, email the editors your comments. We hope that the global pediatric nephrology community will adopt the manual as a dynamic, interactive project with input from trainees and practitioners alike.

The editors have an enduring commitment to research and education in pediatric renal diseases locally and internationally with the ultimate goal of improving children's access to renal care – irrespective of monetary resources, societal status, or geography. They are connected through a long-standing collaboration within the ISN Sister Renal Center program. Kishore Phadke, Professor of Pediatrics and Nephrology, Director of the Children's Kidney Care Center and former Chair of Pediatrics at St-John's was the driving force behind this manual. He established a successful, internationally recognized Pediatric Nephrology Training Program, whose trainees now work across India, and in Sri Lanka, Bangladesh and the Middle

East. Paul R. Goodyer, McGill Professor, former Director of the Division of Nephrology at the MCH, is a successful investigator of kidney development and genetic renal diseases with a number of international collaborations, including St-John's. Martin Bitzan, Associate Professor of Pediatrics and Pediatric Nephrology and current Director of the Division of Nephrology and of the Pediatric Nephrology Training program at the MCH has a focused research and clinical interests in glomerular and systemic renal diseases and international education in pediatric nephrology.

The editors wish to acknowledge their collaborators from the St-John's and the MCH. Their input and contributions were instrumental in the genesis of this manual. Not all of them are named individually. "Thank you" also to the associate/publishing editors and "midwives" of this oeuvre, Sandra Lesny, Rosmarie Unger, Marion Krämer, and Dr. Tobias Kemme from Springer, and project manager Steven Muthu Raj Joe Arun from SPi Global, India, for their patient professionalism. We apologize to our families, particularly our spouses, for enduring long absences and distractions associated with this manual and with our clinical work. Last, but not least, we thank our students and trainees for reminding us of our educational mission, and our patients and their families, who taught us so much and who continue inspiring us.

Bangalore, India	Kishore Phadke
Montreal, Canada	Paul Goodyer
Montreal, Canada	Martin Bitzan

Contents

Abbreviations

μg	Micrograms
ABG	Arterial blood gases
ABPM	Ambulatory blood pressure monitoring
ACE	Angiotensin-converting enzyme
ADH	Anti diuretic hormone
ADH rickets	Autosomal dominant hypophosphatemic rickets
ADPKD	Autosomal dominant polycystic kidney disease
AG	Anion gap
AKI	Acute kidney injury
ANA	Antinuclear antibodies
ANCA	Anti neutrophilic cytoplasmic antibodies
anti-DsDNA	Anti-deoxyribonuclease B
anti-GBM antibodies	Anti glomerular basement antibodies
APLA	Antiphospholipid antibodies
ARB	Angiotensin receptor blocker
ARH rickets	Autosomal recessive hypophosphatemic rickets
ARPKD	Autosomal recessive polycystic kidney disease
ATN	Acute tubular necrosis
ATN	Acute interstitial nephritis
AVP	Arginine vasopressin
BE	Base excess
BMD	Bone mineral density
BP	Blood pressure
BUN	Blood urea nitrogen
BUN	Blood urea nitrogen
CAPD	Continuous ambulatory peritoneal dialysis
CCPD	Continuous cycling peritoneal dialysis
CDI	Central diabetes insipidus
CHD	Coronary heart disease
CKD	Chronic kidney disease
Cl	Chloride
CNI	Calcineurin inhibitors
COX-2	Cyclooxygenase type 2
Cr	Creatinine

Cr	Creatinine clearance
CTA	CT angiography
CVD	Cerebrovascular disease
D5	5 % dextrose
DABP	Diastolic ambulatory blood pressure
DBP	Diastolic blood pressure
DDS	Dialysis equilibrium syndrome
DIC	Disseminated intravascular coagulation
DKA	Diabetic ketoacidosis
DMSA	Dimercaptosuccinic acid
DRCG	Direct nuclide cystography
DXA	Dual-energy X-ray absorptiometry
e GFR	Estimated GFR
e.g.	For example
EKG	Electrocardiogram
ELBW	Eextremely low birth weight
ESRD	End-stage renal disease
ESWL	Extracorporeal lithotripsy
GBM	Glomerular basement membrane
GCD	Glomerulocystic disease
GFR	Glomerular filtration rate
GI	Gastrointestinal
gm	Gram
HAART	Highly active antiretroviral therapy
HBPM	Hemoglobin
HBPM	Home blood pressure monitoring
HCO3	Bicarbonate
HIVAN	HIV-associated nephropathy
HTN	Hypertension
HUS	Hemolytic uremic syndrome
IRIS	Immune reconstitution inflammatory syndrome
kDa	Kilodaltons
kDa	Potassium
KIM-1	Kidney injury molecule –1
LDH	Lactic dehydrogenase
LVH	Left ventricular hypertrophy
m L	Milliliters
MA	Metabolic acidosis
MAG 3	Mercaptoacetyltriglycine 3
MCKD	Multicystic kidney disease
mEq	Milliequivalent
mg	Milligrams
MH	Masked hypertension
MNE	Monosymptomatic enuresis
mosm	Milliosmoles

MRA	MR angiography
MRV	MR venography
Na	Sodium
NDI	Nephrogenic diabetes insipidus
NGAL	Neutrophil gelatinase-associated lipocalin
NHBPEP	National high blood pressure education program
NPHP	Nephronophthisis
NRTI	Nucleoside reverse transcriptase inhibitor
NS	Normal saline
ORS	Oral rehydration solution
PCNL	Percutaneous nephrolithotomy
PCO2	Partial pressure of carbon dioxide
PET	Peritoneal equilibration test
PH	Primary hyperoxaluria
PI	Protease inhibitors
PO2	Partial pressure of oxygen
PRA	Panel reactive antibodies
PRA	Plasma renin activity
RBC	Red blood cell
rhGH	Human recombinant growth hormone
RPGN	Rapidly progressive glomerulonephritis
RTA	Renal tubular acidosis
RTA	Renal tubular acidosis
SABP	Systolic ambulatory blood pressure
SBP	Systolic blood pressure
SIAD	Syndrome of inappropriate antidiuresis
TIN	Tubulointerstitial nephritis
TmP	Renal tubular phosphate threshold maximum
TRP	Tubular reabsorption of phosphate
TTKG	Transtubular potassium gradient
UAG	Urine anion gap
UAG	Urinary anion gap
UOG	Urine osmolal gap
UTI	Urinary tract infection
VACTERL	Vertebral, anorectal, cardiac, tracheoesophageal, renal, limb defects
VATER	Vertebral, anorectal, tracheal, esophageal, renal
VCUG	Voiding cystourethrography
VUR	Vesicoureteral reflux
WBC	White blood cell
XLH rickets	X-linked hypophosphatemic rickets

Evaluation of Renal Disease 1

Paul Goodyer and Kishore Phadke

1.1 History and Physical Examination

The clinical presentation of renal diseases may be nonspecific with paucity of symptoms and signs. The physicians caring for children should be familiar with various modes of presentations of renal diseases. They should have a high index of suspicion and have a sound knowledge of "clues to renal diseases." Manifestations of renal disease may be vague, nonspecific, and subtle and may be related to other systems like gastrointestinal or central nervous system or other systems. Symptoms and signs of renal disease may mimic other systemic diseases. Clinical diversity of renal diseases should be borne in mind. Some guidelines regarding history and physical examination are given below.

- Glomerular versus tubulointerstitial diseases: The two important categories of kidney diseases that present with contrasting clinical scenarios are glomerular diseases and tubulointerstitial diseases. Glomerular diseases often present with edema, oliguria, proteinuria, and/or hematuria with or without hypertension. On the other hand, failure to thrive, short stature, and non-oliguria/polyuria are features of underlying tubular disorders.

P. Goodyer (✉)
Division of Pediatric Nephrology, Montreal Children's Hospital,
McGill University, 2300, rue Tupper, Montreal,
QC H3H 1P3, Canada
e-mail: paul.goodyer@mcgill.ca

K. Phadke
Department of Pediatric Nephrology, Children's Kidney Care Center,
St. John's Medical College Hospital,
Koramangala, Bangalore 560078, KA, India

Department of Pediatrics, Children's Kidney Care Center,
St. John's Medical College Hospital,
Koramangala, Bangalore 560078, KA, India
e-mail: kishorephadke@yahoo.co.in

K. Phadke et al. (eds.), *Manual of Pediatric Nephrology*,
DOI 10.1007/978-3-642-12483-9_1, © Springer-Verlag Berlin Heidelberg 2014

- Acute versus chronic renal disorders: For a clinician, the differentiation whether the child has an acute or a chronic renal problem is critical. In some conditions, prior history of illness is important (e.g., history of sore throat or pyoderma in a child with post-streptococcal nephritis, history of diarrhea in D+HUS). Anemia may be a predominant feature in some cases of acute kidney injury such as hemolytic uremic syndrome and connective tissue disorders or in conditions that are associated with hemolysis or blood loss. Chronic unexplained anemia that is refractory to iron therapy should be considered as a clue to chronic kidney disease. Growth failure and presence of renal osteodystrophy (bony deformities) are other useful pointers to chronicity.
- Transient versus persistent versus recurrent symptoms and/or urinary abnormalities: In day-to-day practice, transient urinary abnormalities may accompany systemic conditions. Febrile illness can present with transient proteinuria, pyuria, or microscopic hematuria. It is important to closely follow up these findings as the child recovers from acute illness. Persistent urinary abnormalities beyond 2–3 months warrant further evaluation, even if the child is asymptomatic. Recurrence of symptoms may be a key in diagnosing some conditions. Recurrent fever without a focus could be a manifestation of recurrent urinary tract infections. Recurrent hematuria may be encountered in IgA nephropathy or idiopathic hypercalciuria. Recurrent edema is characteristic of relapsing nephrotic syndrome. Recurrent vomiting may be seen in renal tubular acidosis.
- Systemic features: Presence of constitutional symptoms and skin and joint involvement suggests possibility of a systemic disease with renal involvement. For details on renal involvement associated with dysmorphic features, syndromic associations, and diseases of other organs, please refer to Sect. 1.2.
- Renal edema is classically described as puffiness of eyelids, more in morning, later progressing to generalized anasarca with pitting edema and weight gain. It is often mistaken as "due to allergy" in early stages. The other causes of generalized edema are cardiac, hepatic conditions, malnutrition, and hypothyroidism. Symptoms and signs of these diseases will be absent in a child with renal disease. The child may have decreased urine output and frothing of urine. The edema is influenced by gravity, may not be uniformly distributed, being more predominant in sacral area or in places where the skin overlying bone is loose (e.g., scalp, submandibular region in some patients). Scrotal/vulvar edema may be bothersome in some children. Puffiness of face is glaring in smaller children. However, in older children, facial edema may sometimes not be so obvious. Edema in acute nephritis and in acute renal failure is due to low glomerular filtration rate and is accompanied by expansion of intravascular volume, with risk of hypertension and pulmonary edema. On the other hand, in nephrotic syndrome, often there is depleted intravascular volume. Assessment of dehydration may be difficult in a child who is obese and is grossly edematous. Evidence of early dehydration such as cooler extremities, tachycardia, tachypnea, increased capillary refill time, and

orthostatic hypotension should be looked for. The stretched overlying skin may look sallow giving a false impression of anemia. One should look for cracks in the skin which may be a source of infection, also for evidence of fungal infection (skin creases, mouth) and striae due to long-term stretching. An edematous child can develop respiratory distress due to tense massive ascites with interference in diaphragmatic movements or due to development of pleural effusion or underlying respiratory infection.

- Fever: Fever without focus should arouse suspicion for urinary tract infection (UTI). Newborns with UTI may be hypothermic. Fever may be suppressed in an immunocompromised child. Fever usually implies underlying infection. However, it can also be a part of clinical spectrum of collagen vascular diseases.
- Urine output: In a child with acute gastroenteritis, it is important to know the duration of oliguria/anuria. It should be borne in mind that renal failure can exist with a normal urine output. One should ask history of polyuria in a child with failure to thrive, short stature, or polydipsia. Polyuria should be differentiated from increased frequency of passing small quantities of urine. Sometimes, history of polyuria may not be available. However, indicators, such as maintenance of fair urine output despite dehydration, dehydration out of proportion to volume losses, presence of antenatal polyhydramnios, and constipation, should arouse suspicion of underlying polyuric states.
- Urinary symptoms: Lower urinary tract symptoms such as ballooning of prepuce, dysuria, straining, urgency, dribbling, precipitancy, frequency, abnormal urinary stream, urinary retention, incontinence, and voiding postures indicate a need for lower urinary tract evaluation. Daytime symptoms should be carefully looked at, while evaluating enuresis.
- Antenatal history, birth history: History of maternal illnesses, oligo-/polyhydramnios, antenatal diagnosis of renal anomalies, and history of birth asphyxia are important in evaluating newborn kidneys. The clues for "renal disease in newborn" are given in Chap. 15.
- Family history, history of consanguinity: A positive history will guide in making a diagnosis in various tubular disorders, genetic forms of nephrotic syndrome, polycystic kidney disease, vesicoureteric reflux, Alport syndrome, etc.
- Drug intake: History of drug intake is often overlooked. Some drugs may require dosage modifications for renal dysfunction. Details of nephrotoxic drugs are given in Chap. 16.
- Hypertension: Childhood hypertension can be asymptomatic. Control of hypertension helps in preserving renal functions. Compared to adults, hypertension in children is often secondary due to renal causes. It is often an incidental finding picked up during routine examination. A regular annual blood pressure recording should be done in all children above 3 years of age.
- Acidotic breathing: Unexplained rapid breathing could be "acidotic breathing."
- Good judgment comes with experience but the best experience comes with bad judgment!

1.2 Dysmorphic Features, Organs, Systems, and Kidney Involvement

- Dysmorphic features and kidneys
- Cardiovascular diseases and kidneys
- Developmental delay and kidneys
- Orofacial disorders and kidneys
- Eyes and kidney
- Hepatic and gastrointestinal diseases and kidneys
- Respiratory system and kidneys
- Skin and kidneys

The conditions are given alphabetically in each above category.

1.2.1 Dysmorphic Features and Kidneys

Dysmorphic disorders	Renal involvement
Aniridia, hemihypertrophy, mental retardation (WAGR syndrome)	Wilms' tumor, renal dysplasia
CHARGE association—eye coloboma, heart defect, choanal atresia, mental retardation, microphallus, ear abnormalities, deafness	Renal dysplasia, vesicoureteric reflux
COACH association—cerebellar vermis hypoplasia, congenital ataxia, ocular coloboma, hepatic fibrosis	Cystic dysplasia
Deformed or low set ears	Renal dysplasia
Down syndrome	Cystic dysplastic kidney
Denys–Drash syndrome	Nephrotic syndrome, renal failure, Wilms' tumor
Edwards' syndrome, Patau syndrome	Cystic dysplastic kidneys, horseshoe kidneys
Marfan syndrome	Cystic dysplastic kidneys
Potter syndrome	Renal agenesis
Prune belly	Megaureters, atonic bladder, VUR, hydronephrosis
Turner syndrome	Horseshoe kidney, coarctation of aorta
VATER or VACTERL association	Renal dysplasia, ectopia, VUR

1.2.2 Cardiovascular Diseases and Kidneys

	Renal involvement
Atrial myxoma	Renal infarction and hematuria
Coarctation of aorta (Turner's syndrome)	Cystic kidneys, horseshoe kidney
Infective endocarditis	Renal abscess, immune complex-mediated glomerulonephritis, renal emboli
Lupus endocarditis	Glomerulonephritis, tubulointerstitial disease, renal vascular thrombosis

	Renal involvement
Myocarditis	HUS, SLE, Churg–Strauss syndrome, amyloidosis
Pericarditis	Uremic pericarditis, lupus pericarditis
Takayasu arteritis	Renovascular hypertension
Tetralogy of Fallot	Hyperfiltration, focal segmental glomerulosclerosis
Williams syndrome (supravalvular aortic stenosis, pulmonary arterial branch stenosis, elfin facies, mental retardation)	Hypercalcemia, nephrocalcinosis

1.2.3 Developmental Delay and Kidneys

	Renal involvement
Bardet–Biedl syndrome—obesity, polysyndactyly, retinopathy (rod-cone dystrophy), hypogonadism	Renal dysplasia, hydronephrosis, duplication, diverticulae, focal segmental glomerulosclerosis, vesicoureteral reflux
Cat-eye syndrome—congenital heart disease, colobomas, anal and digital anomalies	Renal agenesis/hypoplasia, horseshoe/ectopic kidney, polycystic kidneys, renal dysplasia, hydronephrosis, vesicoureteric reflux, ureteral atresia
Cerebro-osteo-nephrodysplasia syndrome—rhizomelic limb shortening, cerebral atrophy, seizures	Renal dysplasia, nephritic and nephrotic presentation, early renal dysfunction
Congenital rubella syndrome—congenital heart disease, deafness, cataract, growth retardation	Renal agenesis, polycystic kidneys, renal dysplasia, duplication
Facio-cardio-renal syndrome—cardiomyopathy, conduction defects, typical facies	Horseshoe kidney, hydronephrosis, ureteral atresia
Fetal alcohol syndrome—IUGR, microcephaly, short palpebral fissure	Renal agenesis, horseshoe kidney, ectopic kidney, renal dysplasia, duplication, hydronephrosis
Galactosemia—failure to thrive, vomiting diarrhea, cataract, hypotonia, hepatomegaly, infections, growth retardation	Renal tubular dysfunction
Hydrocephalus—ventricular peritoneal shunt	Shunt nephritis
Miller–Dieker syndrome—lissencephaly, microgyria, agyria, seizures, typical facies	Renal agenesis, renal dysplasia
Nail–patella syndrome—absent/displaced patella, absent/pitted nails, small nails, nails do not reach the nail border	Renal tubular defects, renal dysplasia, proteinuria, hematuria, nephrotic syndrome
Noonan syndrome—webbed neck, short stature, pulmonary stenosis	Renal cysts, renal dysplasia, unilateral renal ectopia, duplex collection system, hydronephrosis
Oculo-cerebello-renal syndrome—spastic diplegia, choreoathetosis, retinopathy, nystagmus	Infantile polycystic kidneys, interstitial nephritis
Pseudo-Zellweger syndrome—hypotonia, seizures, typical face, failure to thrive, hepatomegaly	Polycystic kidneys, renal dysplasia

	Renal involvement
Rubinstein–Taybi syndrome—short stature, broad thumbs and great toes, typical facies	Renal agenesis, ectopic kidney, renal dysplasia, duplication, urethral atresia, vesicoureteral reflux
Sotos syndrome—overgrowth, typical facies, embryonal tumors, advanced bone age, seizures, congenital heart disease	Urethral atresia, vesicoureteral reflux
Tuberous sclerosis—seizures, cortical tubers, adenoma sebaceum, ash leaf macule, periungual fibromas, shagreen patches, multiple nodular hamartomas	Renal hamartomas, renal cell carcinoma, Wilms' tumor, angiomyolipoma, renal cysts
Von Hippel–Lindau disease—cerebellar and spinal hemangiomas/aneurysms	Renal cysts and tumors—hemangioblastomas

1.2.4 Orofacial Disorders and Kidneys

	Renal involvement
Acro-renal-mandibular hypoplastic mandible syndrome	Unilateral renal agenesis
Branchiootorenal syndrome—preauricular pits, pinhead-sized depression in upper pinna, preauricular tags, bat ears or microtia, malformation of ossicles, hypoplastic cochlea, conductive or sensorineural hearing loss	Renal dysplasia, duplication of collecting system
Hypothyroidism, sensory neural deafness, and renal anomalies (HDR) syndrome—sensorineural hearing loss	Dysplasia
Kallmann syndrome—anosmia/hyposmia, hearing impairment, cleft lip, cleft lip palate	Dysplastic kidney, hydronephrosis, vesicoureteric reflux
Meckel–Gruber syndrome—cleft lip, cleft palate	Dysplastic kidneys, hypospadias
Ochoa syndrome—facial grimacing with lateral displacement of mouth	Duplication, hydronephrosis, hydroureter
Townes–Brocks syndrome/REAR (renal–ear–anal–radial) syndrome, external ear defects, sensory neural hearing loss	Unilateral renal agenesis, dysplasia, hypoplasia

1.2.5 Eyes and Kidneys

	Renal involvement
Acro-renal-ocular syndrome—optic coloboma	Unilateral renal agenesis, ectopic kidney, hypoplasia
Alport syndrome—megalocornea, anterior lenticonus, cataract	Hematuria, proteinuria, nephritis, renal failure
Congenital syphilis—interstitial keratitis and chorioretinitis	Congenital nephrotic syndrome

	Renal involvement
Cytomegalovirus—cotton cheese with ketchup type of peripheral chorioretinitis, uveitis, optic atrophy	Congenital nephrotic syndrome
Cystinosis—refractile polychromatic deposits in cornea	Proximal RTA—polyuria–polydipsia, vitamin D-resistant rickets. May progress to ESRD
Familial hypomagnesemic hypercalciuric syndrome, myopia	Polyuria, hypercalciuria, hypomagnesemia
Goldenhar syndrome—epibulbar dermoid, microphthalmia	Renal dysplasia, duplication, hydronephrosis, reflux
Hypercalcemia—band keratopathy, metastatic crystallization of calcium, phosphate and hydroxyl appetite in conjunctiva	Nephrocalcinosis
Lowe syndrome—cataract, strabismus	Fanconi syndrome, proteinuria
Primary hyperoxaluria type I—changes in retinal pigment epithelium, retinal vascular obstruction, optic nerve atrophy	Recurrent calcium oxalate stones, urolithiasis, nephrocalcinosis, ESRD
Renal coloboma syndrome—coloboma of the optic nerve	Renal hypoplasia, progressive proteinuric renal failure, oligomeganephronia, VUR, multicystic kidneys, PUJ obstruction
Senior–Loken syndrome—retinitis pigmentosa	Nephronophthisis
TINU syndrome—uveitis	Tubulointerstitial nephritis
Toxoplasmosis—central destructive chorioretinitis, optic atrophy, uveitis, cataract, strabismus, nystagmus, visual impairment	Congenital nephrotic syndrome

1.2.6 Hepatic and Gastrointestinal Diseases and Kidneys

	Renal involvement
Liver cysts	ADPKD
Alagille syndrome (arteriohepatic dysplasia)	Renal dysplasia, renal mesangiolipidosis, absent renal peroxisomes, hypospadias
Behcet disease	Renal amyloidosis, glomerulonephritis, renovascular disease (aneurysms), interstitial nephritis, cryoglobulinemia, renal insufficiency
Celiac disease	IgA nephropathy
Chronic intestinal pseudo-obstruction (intestinal neuropathy or myopathy)	Recurrent urinary tract infections, megacystis, obstructive uropathy
Congenital hepatic fibrosis, Caroli's disease	ARPKD, nephronophthisis (rare)
Esophageal atresia and tracheoesophageal fistula (VACTERL)	Renal dysplasia, hypoplasia, ectopia, hydronephrosis, hypospadias
Imperforate anus—associated with inguinal hernias	Fistulas to genitourinary tract, vesicoureteral reflux, renal agenesis, renal dysplasia, ureteral duplication, cryptorchidism, hypospadias
Inflammatory bowel disease—ulcerative colitis, Crohn's disease	Nephrolithiasis, retroperitoneal abscess/fibrosis, ureteral obstruction, fistulas, renal amyloidosis, IgA nephropathy, oxalate and uric acid crystals in urine

	Renal involvement
Intussusception	Henoch–Schonlein purpura
Meckel–Gruber syndrome	Small genitalia, ambiguous genitalia, cryptorchidism, separated vagina, uterine abnormalities, polycystic kidneys, renal agenesis, duplicated ureters, hypoplastic bladder
Renal–hepatic–pancreatic dysplasia (with Dandy–Walker malformation)	Renal dysplasia, renal cysts, enlarged kidneys, decreased number of nephrons, deficient nephron differentiation, glomerular cysts, renal failure
Wilson's disease	Fanconi syndrome, progressive renal failure, elevated urinary copper excretion
Zellweger cerebrohepatorenal syndrome	Renal cortical microcysts, hydronephrosis, absent renal peroxisomes, hypospadias

1.2.7 Respiratory System and Kidneys

	Renal involvement
α-1 antitrypsin deficiency—emphysema	Fibromuscular dysplasia, renal artery stenosis
Chronic pulmonary infections—bronchiectasis, cystic fibrosis, tuberculosis	Amyloidosis, glomerulonephritis, hypercalcemia
Goodpasture syndrome—pulmonary hemorrhage, hemoptysis	Anti-GBM antibody disease
Pneumococcal pneumonia	D-HUS
Relapsing polychondritis—inflammation of ear and nose, larynx, and trachea; ulcers	Vasculitis/crescentic nephritis, autoantibodies against type II collagen
Sarcoidosis—interstitial lung disease	Hypercalcemia, hypercalciuria, renal stones, membranous glomerulonephritis, chronic interstitial nephritis, renal failure with minimal or no proteinuria, aseptic leukocyturia
Thromboembolic lung disease	Deep vein thrombosis in nephrotic syndrome
Wegener's—necrotizing ulcers, sinusitis	Pulmonary renal syndrome, rapidly progressive glomerulonephritis

1.2.8 Skin and Kidneys

	Renal involvement
Bullous pemphigoid lesions	Membranous glomerulopathy
Cholesterol emboli—petechiae, livedo reticularis, blue toes	Renal emboli
Diabetes mellitus—diabetic dermopathy, necrobiosis lipoidica, acanthosis nigricans, eruptive xanthomas, Kyrle disease, scleredema	Diabetic nephropathy
End-stage renal disease—urea frosting, dry scaly skin, muddy brown hyperpigmentation, melanin deposition, half and half nails, purpura, pruritus, metastatic skin calcification, perforating folliculitis, poor primary and secondary dentition	Chronic renal insufficiency
Fabry disease—angiokeratomas	Nephrotic syndrome, hematuria, renal failure

	Renal involvement
Neurofibromatosis	Hypertension
Partial lipodystrophy, angioedema	Membranoproliferative glomerulonephritis, renal failure
Psoriasis	Focal segmental glomerulosclerosis, IgA nephropathy, renal amyloidosis, nephrotic syndrome
Sarcoidosis—erythema nodosum, maculopapular lesions, reddish brown plaques, eczema	Hypercalcemia, nephrolithiasis, nephrocalcinosis, diffuse interstitial nephritis
Subacute bacterial endocarditis—petechiae, purpura, splinter hemorrhages, Osler's nodules, Janeway lesions	Renal emboli, proliferative glomerulonephritis
Syphilis—papular follicular syphilids involving hair follicles; patchy alopecia; mucosal ulcerations; diffuse rashes with sloughing on palms, soles, perianal and perioral regions; parrot lines (linear scars radiating from the orifice of the mouth); Hutchinson teeth; mulberry molars	Congenital nephrotic syndrome, membranous nephropathy

1.3 Urine Analysis

Urine analysis is a simple useful test aiding diagnosis of conditions pertaining to the urinary tract. It can be described as a "window to the urinary tract." Timing of urine collection, its storage, and method of analysis can affect accuracy of results. Different methods of urine collection have been described in details in the Appendix. Urine should be examined fresh, preferably within 1 h of voiding. If delay is anticipated, it can be stored at 4 °C in the refrigerator, adding a few drops of acetic acid.

1.3.1 Standardized Method for Processing Urine

- Centrifugation of 10 ml aliquot of urine for 5 min at 3,000 rpm. Remove 9.5 ml of supernatant urine.
- Gentle but thorough resuspension of sediment by pipette in the remaining 0.5 ml of urine.
- Transfer 50 μl of resuspended urine to a glass slide and cover with a coverslip.
- Examination of the slide at low (160×) and high (400×) power.

1.3.2 Examining the Supernatant

1.3.2.1 Color

- Normally, colorless to clear yellow to amber—depends on the concentration of urochromes.

- To be checked in good light, in a transparent container, against a white background.
- The most common abnormal color observed in clinical practice is red to brown urine:
  - Hematuria is the cause if only the sediment is red color and has red blood cells (RBC), with the supernatant being clear.
  - A red supernatant that is positive for heme (dipstick) with no RBCs in sediment is usually due to myoglobinuria or hemoglobinuria (plasma is pink in hemoglobinuria while it is clear in myoglobinuria).
  - A red supernatant that is negative for heme is due to ingestion of beet root, food dyes, medications like phenazopyridine, and multivitamin syrups and in porphyria.
- The other urine colors seen are:
  - White—phosphaturia, pyuria, chyluria
  - Brown black—alkaptonuria (on prolonged standing), methemoglobin, myoglobin
  - Green—triamterene, amitriptyline, propofol, and pseudomonas infection
  - Blue—methylene blue
  - Brown urine—chloroquine, nitrofurantoin
  - Darkening on standing—imipenam, methyldopa, metronidazole
  - Pink urine—uric acid crystalluria
  - Orange—rifampicin, warfarin
  - Cloudy—usually due to crystal formation on standing, uric acid crystals form in acidic urine, phosphate crystals form in alkaline urine

1.3.2.2 Odor

- Normally, the urine has an aromatic smell but can have a fetid or foul smell due to urinary tract infection.
- Presence of ketones imparts a fruity smell to urine.
- Maple syrup urine disease—urine smells similar to maple syrup.
- Phenylketonuria—urine has a mousy smell.
- Isovaleric acidemia, glutaric acidemia—sweaty smell.
- Tyrosinemia—rancid smell.

1.3.2.3 Relative Density

Specific Gravity

- A measure of urinary concentration (weight of the solution compared with that of an equal volume of distilled water).
- Instrument used—urinometer/hydrometer. Bears a scale from 1.000 to 1.600.
- Disadvantages:
  1. 25 ml urine required
  2. Difficulty in reading meniscus
  3. Device clings to the side of the tube
  4. Requires periodic calibration

- Normal range, 1.010 to 1.030.
  Isosthenuria, fixed specific gravity of 1.010.
  Hyposthenuria, specific gravity ≤1.007.
- A low specific gravity is seen in polydipsia and diabetes insipidus and in conditions affecting renal concentrating ability (e.g., acute tubular necrosis).
- A high specific gravity is seen with inadequate fluid intake, dehydration.
- Changes in specific gravity with relatively little change in osmolality can occur in the presence of large molecules in the urine, such as glucose or radiocontrast media.
- Contamination during collection may give falsely elevated specific gravity.

Osmolality

- Measures number of solute particles per unit volume.
- Normal range, 40–1,500 mOsm/l.
- An early morning urine specimen with osmolality >800 mOsm/l indicates a reasonably normal urinary concentrating ability.
- Measured with an osmometer, by freezing-point depression method.
- This measurement is useful in the diagnosis of patients with hyponatremia, hypernatremia, and polyuria.

Refractometry

- Based on the measurement of refractive index (RI).
- RI depends on weight and size of solutes per unit volume, and it correlates well with osmolality.
- Advantage—requires only one drop of urine.
- It can be used as an indirect indicator of hydration status in patients with acute gastroenteritis with no intrinsic renal failure.

1.3.2.4 pH

- Normal, 4.5–7. It varies with food intake (lower pH with high protein diet).
- Measured by pH meter with a glass electrode (more accurate) or reagent strips.
- Early morning pH <5.5 is an indicator of good acidification.
- pH >7 may suggest defective acidification in absence of infection and prolonged storage.
- Dipsticks can read pH 5–9.They are not accurate when pH <5.5 or >7.5.
- Alkaline urine in a patient with urinary tract infection suggests presence of a urea-splitting organism like *Proteus*.
- Therapeutic urinary alkalinization may be indicated in cystine and urate stones, poisonings (salicylates, methotrexate, and barbiturates), and in rhabdomyolysis.

1.3.2.5 Proteins

- *Normal values*
  - Nil or trace on a dipstick.
  - 24-h urine protein, <4 mg/m^2/h.
  - More than 40 mg/m^2/h or 50 mg/kg/day is considered nephrotic range.

  - Spot urine protein/creatinine ratio.
    - Normal, <0.2 mg/mg (<2 mg/mmol SI units)
    - Nephrotic range, >2 mg/mg (<20 mg/mmol SI units)
  - Microalbuminuria
    - Microalbuminuria precedes presence of overt proteinuria.
    - Microalbuminuria detects 15–300 mg/day albuminuria.
    - Measured by sensitive radioimmunoassay techniques.
    - Urine albumin >30 mg/l or albumin to creatinine ratio 2–30 mg/mmol creatinine (200–300 μg/g creatinine) is considered significant.
    - It may be used in conditions like diabetes mellitus or reflux nephropathy as an early marker of glomerular injury.
- *Methods*
  - Dipstick method
  - Turbidimetric method
    Heat coagulation test
    Sulfosalicylic acid (SSA) test (acid precipitation method)
  - Quantification
    24-h urinary protein estimation
    Spot urine protein/creatinine ratio

Urine Dipstick

- Primarily detects albumin and test is highly specific, but not very sensitive for the detection of proteinuria (protein excretion must be more than 100 mg/day).
- Principle: strips are impregnated with a reagent called tetrabromophenol blue, buffered to an acidic pH of 3, which reacts with albumin in the urine in 30–60 s, forming a chromogen, which yields a color change.
- Color change: pale green → green → blue.
- Correlation: trace, <20 mg/dl; 1+, 30 mg/dl; 2+, 100 mg/dl; 3+, 300 mg/dl; 4+, >2,000 mg/dl.
- False positive in alkaline urine, concentrated urine, pyuria, bacteriuria.
- False negative in dilute urine, low-molecular-weight proteinuria.

Turbidimetric Method

Heat Coagulation Test

Less reliable as a result of many false-positive and false-negative results.

Method: semiquantitative. A test tube containing about 10 ml of urine is heated in the upper part until it boils. The precipitate which does not disappear after addition of three drops of concentrated acetic acid suggests proteinuria.

Sulfosalicylic Acid (SSA) Test

Method: 5 ml or urine +5–10 drops of 20 % SSA → look for turbidity

Interpretation (parentheses represent the approximate protein concentration):

- No or slight turbidity, 0 (0–10 mg/dl)
- Turbidity without granule formation (through which print can be read), 1+ (15–30 mg/dl)

- Turbidity with granule formation (through which heavy black lines on a white background can be seen), 2+ (40–100 mg/dl)
- Turbidity with granule formation and flocculation (through which heavy black lines on a white background cannot be seen), 3+ (150–350 mg/dl)
- Flocculent precipitation, 4+ (>500 mg/dl)
  - False positive—concentrated urine, gross hematuria, contrast media, penicillin, sulfonamides, miconazole, cephalosporins, tolbutamide

Quantification of Protein

- In children with persistent proteinuria, quantitative estimation of the proteinuria is indicated.
- It helps in diagnosis, prognostication, and in assessing response to therapy.
- The ideal method is a 24-h urine measurement; however, collecting these specimens may be cumbersome in small children. Timed 6- or 12-h samples also can be used.
- 24-h urinary creatinine <20 mg/kg in girls and 30 mg/kg in boys indicates inadequate collection.
- An alternative method is to measure protein-to-creatinine ratio on a random urine sample (preferably second morning urine specimen).

1.3.2.6 Glucose

- Glucosuria occurs due to inability of the kidney to reabsorb filtered glucose in the proximal tubule despite normal plasma levels (renal glucosuria) or due to urinary spillage because of abnormally high plasma concentrations.
- Methods—Benedict's test, dipstick method, clinitest tablets, and enzymatic estimation using hexokinase.
- Benedict's test—detects reducing substances. Not specific for glucose.
- Dipsticks—specific for glucose.
  - Based on glucose oxidase–peroxidase method, a double sequential enzymatic method.
  - Glucose in urine reacts with O_2 in the presence of glucose oxidase impregnated on the test strip, which yields H_2O_2, which in turn reacts with the chromogen on the test strip, to form an oxidized chromogen, bringing about the color change.
  - The actual change depends on the chromogen used in the test strip:
    For example, with o-toluidine, pink → purple.
    With potassium iodide, blue → green.
    With aminopropyl-carbazol, yellow → orange brown.
  - Presence of hypochlorite ions or other oxidants may give a false-positive reaction, while large amount of ascorbic acid, ketones, and tetracycline may result in a false-negative reaction.
  - Reducing sugars other than glucose can be identified using an osazone test.

1.3.2.7 Blood

- The dipstick method detects heme (either red blood cells, hemoglobin, or myoglobin).

- False positive occurs with oxidizing agents, alkaline urine (pH >9), presence of bacteria, betadine, and excess ascorbic acid.
- Dipstick is highly sensitive and a negative dipstick reliably excludes hematuria.
- Urine microscopy should be performed whenever dipstick test is positive.

1.3.2.8 Ketones

- Principle: based on a reaction of acetoacetate and acetone with nitroprusside on the strip in the presence of glycine as the nitrogen source
- Does not detect β-hydroxybutyrate
- Positive with ketonemia (e.g., prolonged fasting, DKA, GSD, methylmalonic acidemia, propionic acidemia)
- False positive with ascorbic acid, captopril, acidic and concentrated urine, and in phenylketonuria.

1.3.2.9 Nitrate Reduction Test

- This dipstick test can be used as a screening test for UTI.
- Principle: nitrate-splitting bacteria split nitrates in urine into nitrites which react with an aromatic amine on the test strip, giving a colored diazonium compound (red violet).
- The test is positive with UTI caused by coliforms.
- A negative test does not reliably rule out infection.
- Negative test in the presence of UTI is usually due to non-nitrate-splitting organisms—pseudomonas sp, *Staphylococcus albus*, *Staphylococcus saprophyticus*, *Streptococcus faecalis*.
- Pollakiuria, ureterostomy, low urine nitrates, ascorbic acid, and non-nitrate-reducing bacteria may result in a false-negative test.

1.3.2.10 Leukocyte Esterase Test

- It is another screening test for UTI.
- Principle: depends on the esterase activity of granulocytes. 3-Hydroxy-5-phenylpyrrole esterified with amino acid or an indoxyl carbonic acid ester is used as the substrate. It undergoes hydrolysis by the esterase, releasing 3-hydroxy-5-phenylpyrrole, which reacts with a diazonium salt to form an azo dye (purple color).
- A positive test should be followed by microscopic examination of urine.
- False-positive test is seen in noninfectious inflammatory states.
- False-negative tests occur with excess proteins, ketones, and drugs (cephalexin, cephalothin, nitrofurantoin, gentamicin, tetracycline, tobramycin).
- A negative test in the absence of symptoms rules out UTI.
- In alkaline urine: test would be positive despite negative microscopy as WBCs would be lysed. Hence, both microscopy and leukocyte esterase test are to be done when investigating UTI.
- Correlation: 1+, 10–25 WBCs/mm^3; 2+, >75 WBCs/mm^3; 3+, >500 WBCs/mm^3.
- Less sensitive in presence of glucose or concentrated urine and in newborns.

1.3.3 Examining the Sediment

Figures 1.1–1.14 illustrate findings of "some cells, casts and crystals" seen on microscopic examination of urinary sediment.

1.3.3.1 Cells

The cellular elements found in the urinary sediment include red blood cells (RBCs), white blood cells (WBCs), and epithelial cells.

RBCs

- At least 20 high-power fields (HPF) are examined and the average is reported.
- The color change does not necessarily reflect the degree of blood loss since as little as 1 ml of blood per liter of urine can induce a visible color change.
- Hematuria is defined as presence of more than 5 RBCs/HPF in a centrifuged specimen of urine.
- Evaluation of red cell morphology may be helpful in a patient with hematuria to differentiate between glomerular and non-glomerular causes of hematuria.
- The RBCs appear dysmorphic (blebs, budding, and segmental loss of membrane) in children with glomerular renal lesions while it is normal (typically uniform and round) in extrarenal lesions (e.g., cystitis, urethral trauma, lower urinary tract malignancies). These changes are well appreciated with the use of phase contrast microscopy.

Leukocytes

- Neutrophils are the most common white cells present in urine, and they can be identified by their characteristic granular cytoplasm and multilobed nuclei.
- Leukocyturia is defined as presence of more than 5 cells/HPF in centrifuged urine or >10/mm^3 in uncentrifuged urine.
- Eosinophils may be seen in urine (as in acute interstitial nephritis) and can be identified by Hansel's stain of the sediment.

Epithelial Cells

- Epithelial cells may appear in the urine after being shed from anywhere within the genitourinary tract. Three types of cells are seen:
  1. Renal tubular cells: round/rectangular/polygonal/columnar
  2. Urothelial cells: superficial/deep
  3. Squamous cells: a constant finding, abundant cytoplasm, few granules, small central nucleus, folded edges
- Tubular cell casts are seen in nephrotic syndrome, acute tubular necrosis, and pyelonephritis.
- Superficial urothelial cells seen in mild diseases of urinary tract.
- Deep urothelial cells are seen in moderate or severe diseases of the urinary tract, e.g., urolithiasis and hydronephrosis.
- Squamous cells: normally present or as contamination from vaginal discharge.

1.3.3.2 Lipids

- Seen as droplets—free or clumped within oval fat bodies or casts, round and translucent. Appears as maltese crosses under polarized light

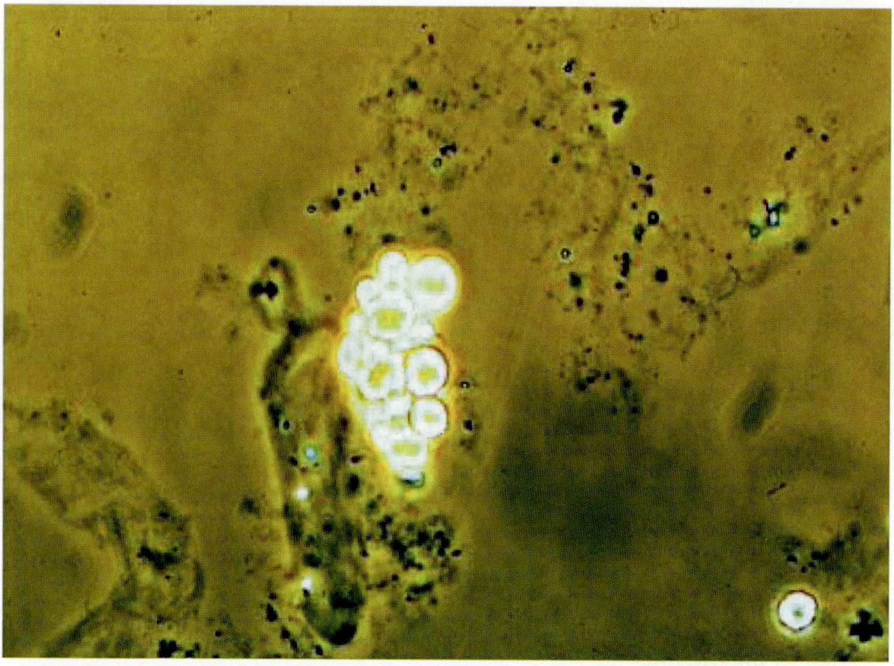

Fig. 1.1 Lipid droplets as seen by phase contrast microscopy

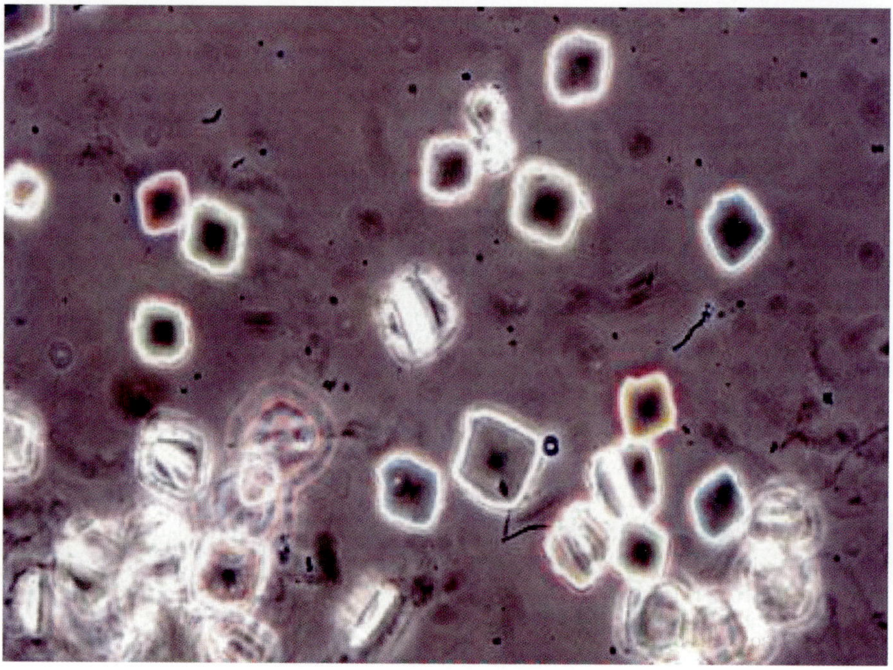

Fig. 1.2 Uric acid crystals as seen by phase contrast microscopy

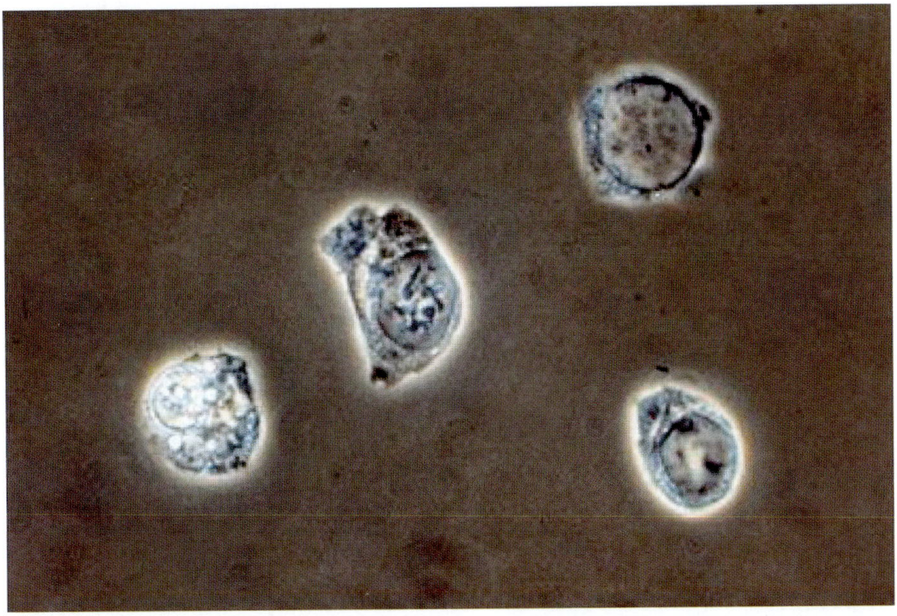

Fig. 1.3 Decoy cells by phase contrast microscopy in Balkan virus nephropathy (enlargement of the nucleus which appears as a ground glass)

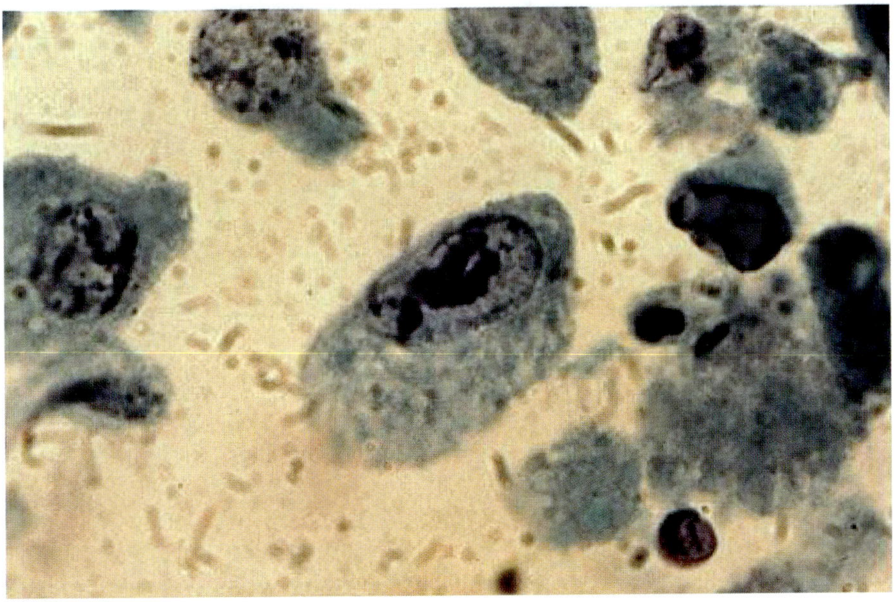

Fig. 1.4 Decoy cells by Papanicolaou staining (inclusion bodies within the nuclei)

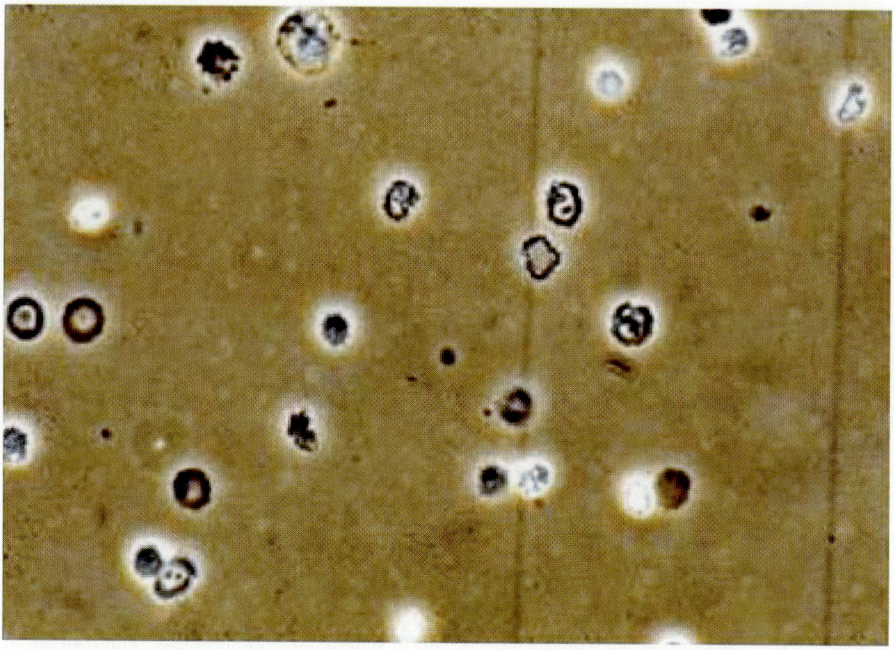

Fig. 1.5 Glomerular hematuria—dysmorphic erythrocytes

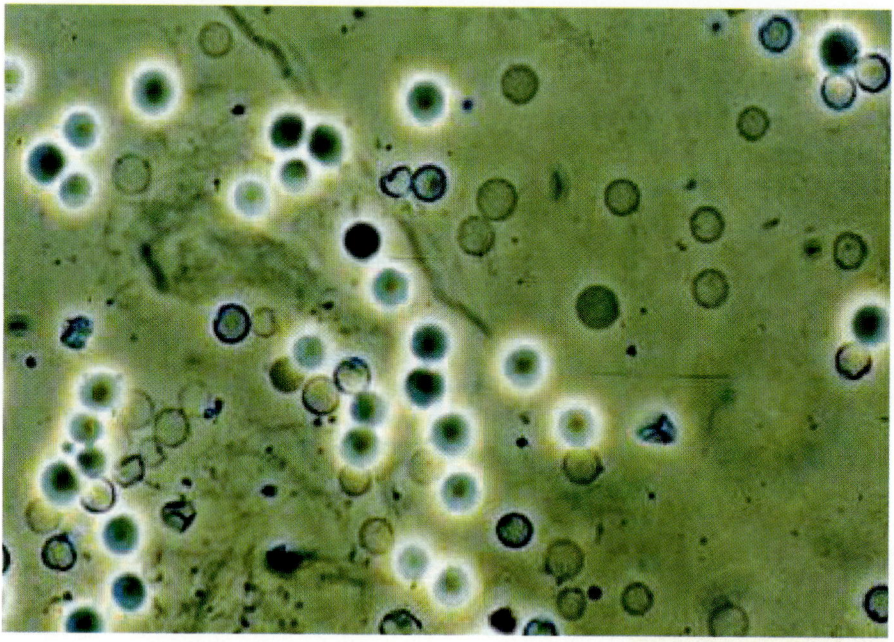

Fig. 1.6 Non-glomerular hematuria—isomorphic erythrocytes

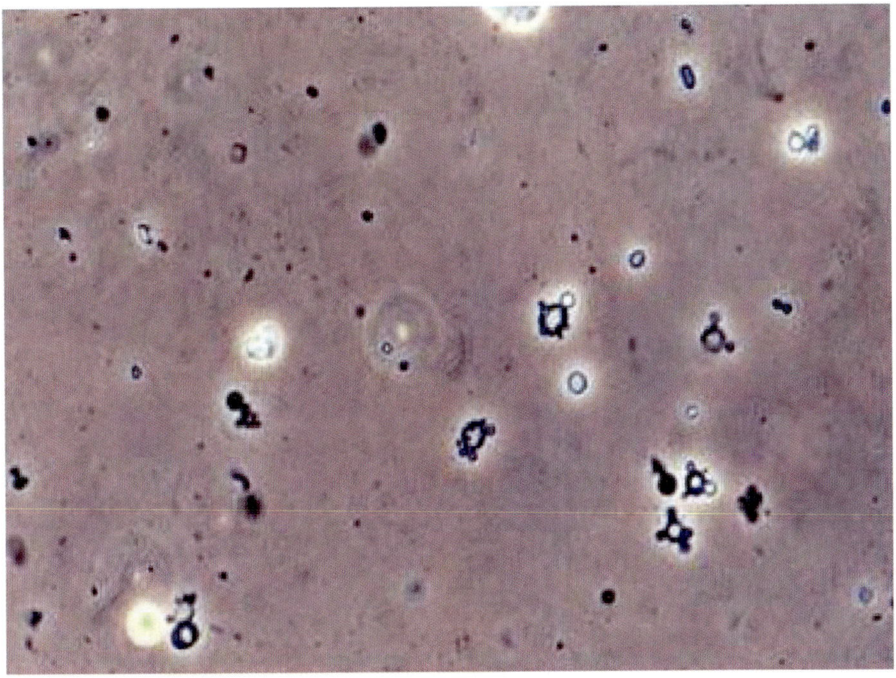

Fig. 1.7 Acanthocytes identified by phase contrast microscopy

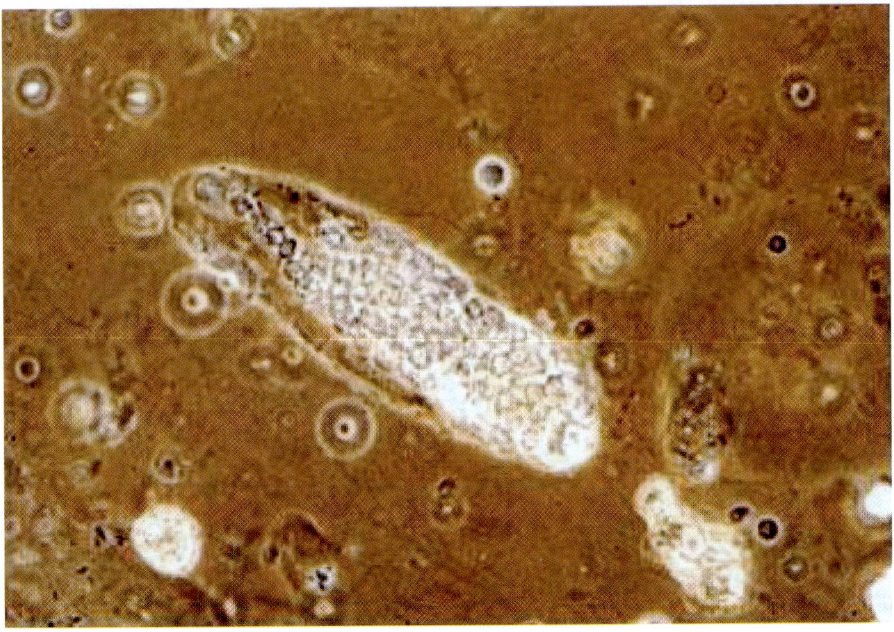

Fig. 1.8 Erythrocyte cast

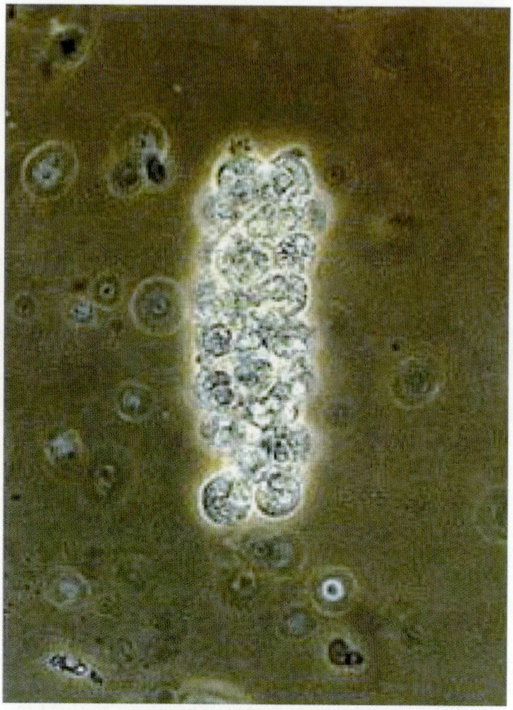

Fig. 1.9 Leukocyte cast

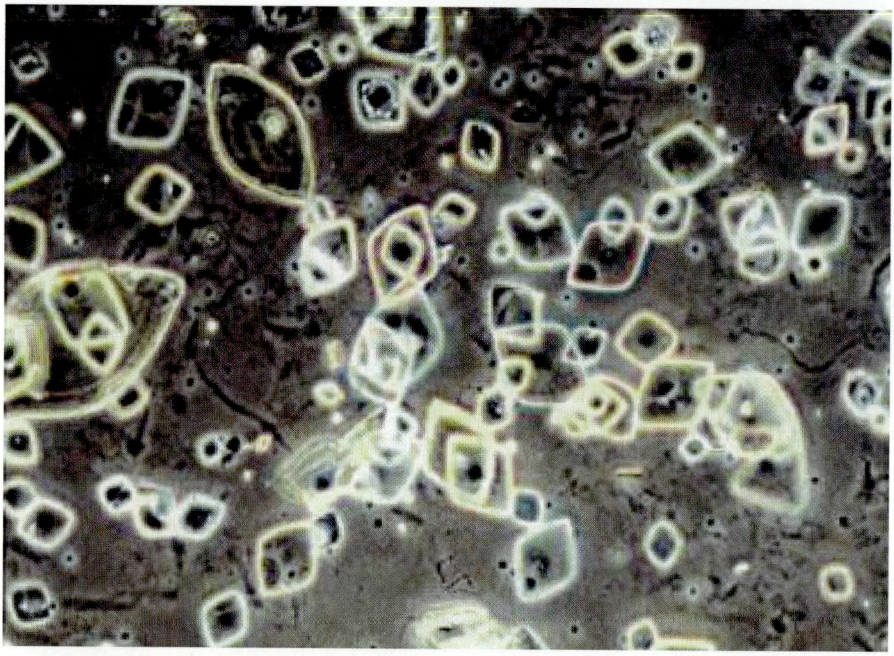

(U–pH ≤5.4)

Fig. 1.10 Uric acid crystals by phase contrast microscopy

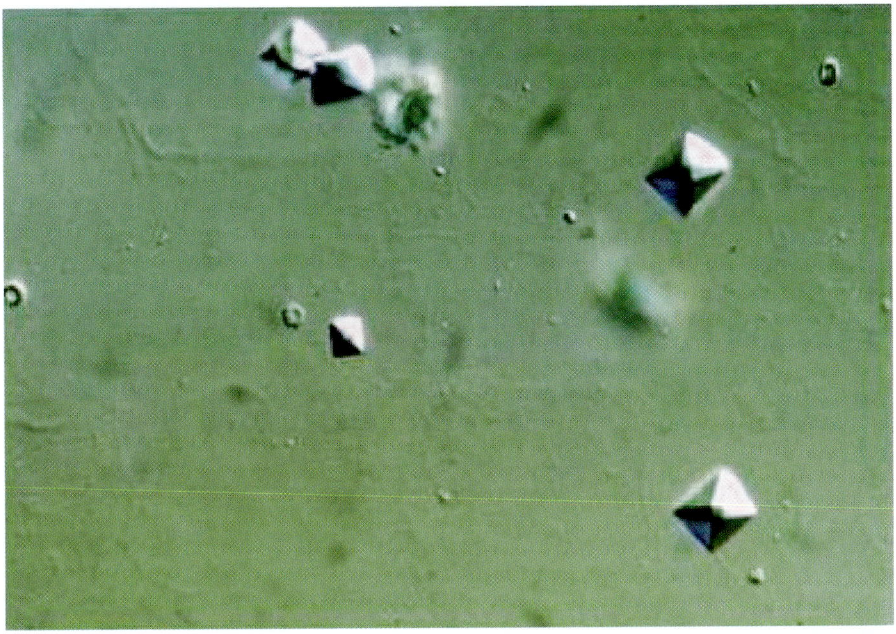

(U–pH <5.4–6.7)

Fig. 1.11 Calcium oxalate crystals

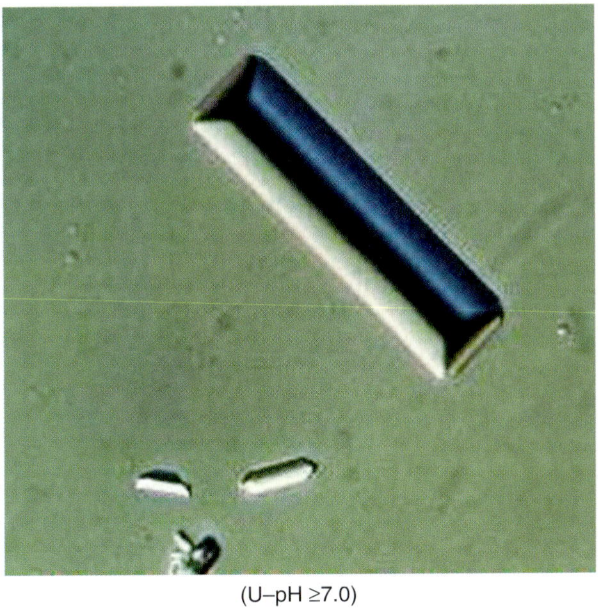

(U–pH ≥7.0)

Fig. 1.12 Triple phosphate crystal

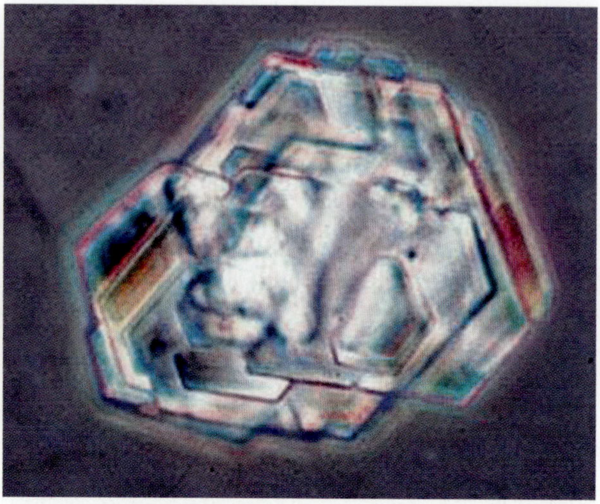

Fig. 1.13 Cystine crystals

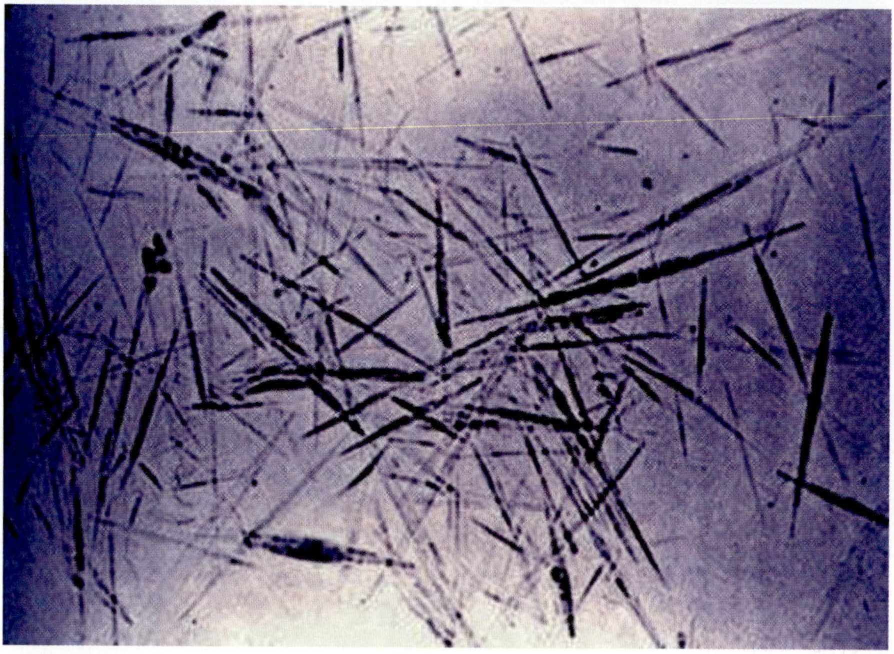

Fig. 1.14 Acyclovir crystals

- May be seen as crystals
- Seen in nephritic syndrome, with heavy proteinuria and in Fabry's disease

1.3.3.3 Casts

Casts are elongated elements with a basic cylindrical shape. They are formed in distal tubule and collecting duct. It consists of a matrix of Tamm–Horsfall protein with or without entrapped cells.

- Hyaline casts—May be normally present and consist of matrix without cells. They are seen in all glomerular diseases which cause proteinuria. They are also seen in patients with fever, after strenuous exercise, while on diuretic therapy and with use of amphotericin B or ethacrynic acid. They dissolve rapidly in alkaline urine.
- Granular casts—They consist of proteins and degenerated tubular cells. They are seen in active glomerulonephritis, pyelonephritis, diabetic nephropathy, lead intoxication, amyloidosis, malignant hypertension, acute allograft rejection, strenuous exercise, fever, and certain drugs like amphotericin B, indomethacin, and kanamycin.
- RBC casts—The presence of even one RBC cast is suggestive of a glomerular pathology. They can be seen in all forms of glomerulonephritis, renal infarction, and in patients with malignant hypertension.
- WBC casts—Their presence is suggestive of tubulointerstitial diseases and acute pyelonephritis. They are also present in lupus nephritis.
- Epithelial casts—Rarest of casts to be reported. They are usually seen in acute tubular necrosis, viral diseases (like CMV), heavy metal poisoning, ethylene glycol or salicylate intoxication, and acute glomerulonephritis. They may be one of the indicators of acute allograft rejection, when detected in significant numbers during early posttransplant period.
- Fatty casts—Consist of fat globules of cholesterol esters and cholesterol within the degenerating epithelial cell casts. They are seen in nephrotic syndrome and in diseases associated with heavy proteinuria.
- Waxy cast—Represents last stage of the degeneration of a granular cast and is large, with clear cut edges, and appears refractive, amorphous looking. Most frequently seen in CKD. Also seen in rapidly progressive renal failure, acute allograft rejection, and amyloidosis.
- Mixed cast—Usually a combination of two more casts (e.g., granular hyaline). Seen commonly in tubulointerstitial diseases.
- Pseudo-cast—It is morphologically similar to casts but is due to crystals and contaminants.

1.3.3.4 Crystals

- Crystals are not always pathological. They are formed due to supersaturation of urine.
- Influenced by metabolic abnormalities, diet, delay in analysis, temp, and pH changes.
- Seen in larger numbers and in aggregated forms in stone formers.

- Cystine, tyrosine, leucine, and cholesterol crystals are always pathological.
- Crystals in acidic urine: uric acid, amorphous urates, calcium oxalate, cystine, leucine, tyrosine.
- Crystals in alkaline urine: calcium phosphate, triple phosphate, amorphous phosphate.

Types of Crystals

- Uric acid: diamond/lozenge/barrel/trapezoid shaped, amber colored, birefringent.

Seen in uricosuric states.

- Calcium oxalate: monohydrate—oval/round discs or dumbbell shaped, birefringent. Dihydrate—pyramid/envelop shaped, not birefringent. Seen in hypercalciuric state, not dependent on pH.
- Magnesium–ammonium phosphate (triple phosphate): coffin shaped, large and birefringent. Occurs in alkaline pH, commonly with urinary tract infection with a urease-producing organism, such as *Proteus* or *Klebsiella.*
- Calcium phosphate: plates with granular surface, not birefringent; needles/prisms in fan-shaped arrangement, birefringent. They form in relative alkaline urine.
- Amorphous phosphates: granular material in clumps.
- Cystine: thin, flat, hexagonal plates—isolated/heaped/clumped, birefringent. They are present in cystinuria.
- Tyrosine: thin needles in bundles/rosette. Seen in acute liver atrophy.
- Leucine: oily-looking spheres with concentric striations. Seen in acute liver atrophy.
- Cholesterol: brownish transparent thin plates, sharp edges. Seen in nephrotic syndrome.
- Crystals due to drugs:
  - Drugs causing crystalluria—sulfadiazine, acyclovir, indinavir, vitamin C, amoxicillin.
  - Drug overdose and dehydration favor crystal formation.
  - Clinical manifestations—asymptomatic, microscopic or gross hematuria, obstructive uropathy.
  - Consider "drug intake" whenever crystals are seen with unusual appearance.

1.3.3.5 Microorganisms

- Bacteria are frequently seen in sediment, often due to contamination. This is significant if leukocytes are also present.
- Urine should be looked for acid-fast bacilli in the setting sterile acid pyuria to diagnose genitourinary Koch's infection.
- Commonly seen fungus is of *Candida* species. It is often due to contamination from external genitalia. It also can be associated with structural urinary tract anomalies, with immunosuppression, indwelling catheters, and prolonged antibiotics.
- *Trichomonas vaginalis*—often a contaminant.

1.4 Assessment of Glomerular Functions

1.4.1 Serum Creatinine (Cr)

It is the most commonly used parameter to assess renal functions.

- When elevation in serum creatinine is seen, it may indicate as much as 50 % loss of renal function.
- Serum creatinine is proportional to the muscle mass and to protein intake.
- Normal serum Cr [mg/dl in conventional (C) units and μmmol/l in SI units] values for term and preterm neonates (mean ± 2 SD in brackets) are given in the below table.

Age (days)	<28 weeks C units	<28 weeks SI units	29–32 weeks C units	29–32 weeks SI units	33–36 weeks C units	33–36 weeks SI units	>37 weeks C units	>37 weeks SI units
7	0.95 (1.31)	83.6 (115.28)	0.94 (1.40)	82.72 (123.2)	0.77 (1.25)	67.76 (110)	0.56 (0.96)	49.28 (84.48)
14	0.81 (1.17)	71.28 (102.96)	0.78 (1.14)	63.36 (100.32)	0.62 (1.02)	54.56 (89.76)	0.43 (0.65)	37.84 (57.2)
28	0.66 (0.94)	58.08 (82.72)	0.59 (0.97)	51.92 (85.36)	0.40 (0.68)	35.2 (59.84)	0.34 (0.54)	29.92 (47.52)

Maternal serum creatinine will influence serum creatinine in the newborn in first 72 h of life

Normal S Cr. values in children

Age (years)	Serum creatinine (mg/dl)	Serum creatinine (μmol/l—SI units)
1–5	0.3–0.5	26.4–44
6–11	0.5–0.7	44–61.6
Girls >11	0.7–0.9	61.6–79.2
Boys >11	0.7–1.2	61.6–105.6

1.4.2 Blood Urea

- Blood urea is generally twice the BUN (blood urea nitrogen) values.
- Normal urea/creatinine ratio is 10:20.
- Disproportionate rise in blood urea compared to serum creatinine is seen in dehydration (prerenal azotemia), upper GI bleed, and hyper-catabolic states (sepsis, burns, crush injuries, patients on steroids).
- Lower blood urea values are seen in starvation, low protein intake, and severe liver disease.

1.4.3 Creatinine Clearance (CrCl)

$$C = \frac{U \times V}{P}$$

where C = Clearance/min (ml/min), U = Urinary concentration (mg/dl), P = Plasma concentration (mg/dl), V = urine volume/min (ml/min)

- If a given substance is freely filtered and neither reabsorbed nor excreted, its clearance rate would accurately reflect true GFR. It should be inert and nontoxic and should not alter renal function. Inulin is one such substance which satisfies all these criteria. Inulin clearance is taken as the gold standard for GFR. However, it cannot be used routinely in clinical practice. The creatinine clearance is often used in clinical practice for estimation of GFR.
- In patients with renal failure, CrCl will overestimate GFR due to tubular secretion of creatinine.
- CrCl can be estimated using cimetidine or trimethoprim which blocks tubular secretion of creatinine.

1.4.4 GFR Estimation

Normal adult values of GFR are reached by 2 years of age:

Neonate—26 ± 2 ml/min/1.73 m^2
1–2 weeks—54 ± 8 ml/min/1.73 m^2
6–12 months—77 ± 14 ml/min/1.73 m^2
1–2 years—96 ± 22 ml/min/1.73 m^2
Adult—118 ± 18 ml/min/1.73 m^2

For practical purposes, plasma creatinine and endogenous creatinine clearance are commonly used as more convenient though less accurate methods for GFR assessment.

Other methods for estimation of GFR are:

A. *Schwartz formula*

Estimation of GFR by using serum creatinine and height values:

$$\text{GFR}\left(\text{ml/min/1.73 m}^2\right) = \frac{K \times \text{height in cm}\left(\text{or length}\right)}{\text{Serum Cr}\left(\text{mg/dl}\right)}$$

K—0.33 low-birth-weight babies (<2.5 kg birth weight) in first year of life
0.45—term, normal infants during first year of life
0.55—children and adolescent girls
0.70—adolescent boys

B. *Other formulae*: In adults, the Cockraft–Gault equation uses serum creatinine, age, and body weight for estimating GFR. The multicentric Chronic Kidney Disease in Children (CKiD) study in North America, in order to overcome the shortcomings of the Schwartz formula in overestimating GFR, has generated formulae such as:

Estimated GFR = 39.1 $[\text{Ht(m)/SCr}]^{0.516}[1.8/\text{CysC}]^{0.294}[30/\text{BUN}]^{0.169}\ [1.099^{\text{male}}]\ [\text{Ht}/1.4]^{0.188}$ or

Estimated GFR = 0.413 × Ht (cm)/SCr

(Ht is height, SCr is serum creatinine, CysC is serum cystatin C, and BUN is blood urea nitrogen)

C. *Radioisotope-based methods*: The technique is based on use of single-injection, plasma disappearance curves to estimate GFR. The radionuclide dye (^{99m}Tc-DTPA or 51Cr-EDTA or ^{125}I- iothalamate) is injected, and the signal from the radiolabelled form is used to obtain measurement. However, this method requires facilities of a gamma camera. Split renal functions can be estimated using this method.

D. *Cystatin C*

- It is a low molecular protein (13 Kd) produced at a constant rate by all nucleated cells.
- It is freely filtered by the glomeruli, not secreted but totally reabsorbed and catabolized by renal tubules.
- It is eliminated from the circulation exclusively by glomerular filtration. There are no sites of extra renal metabolism.
- It is not affected by age, gender, body composition, or muscle mass.
- The reciprocal serum values correlate linearly with GFR.
- The blood levels can be estimated by enzyme immunoassays or immune-turbidimetry.
- Normal adults have circulating levels of approximately 1 mg/l.
- Log_{10} GFR = 1.962 + [1.123 × $\log_{10}$ (1/CysC)] where CysC is the serum cystatin level.

1.5 Assessment of Tubular Functions

1.5.1 Fractional Excretion of Sodium (FeNa)

$$\text{FeNa}\left(\text{expressed in }\%\right)=\frac{U_{\text{Na}}\times P_{\text{Cr}}\times 100}{P_{\text{Na}}\times U_{\text{Cr}}}$$

U_{Na} = Urinary sodium FeNa in preterms <30 weeks, <5 %

S_{Na} = Serum sodium FeNa in term neonates, <2 %

U_{Cr} = Urinary creatinine FeNa in Children, <1 %

P_{Cr} = Serum creatinine

- Most commonly used test for assessment of tubular integrity.
- It must be interpreted in the context of patient's sodium and volume status.
- It is of no value if the child has received diuretics.
- Prerenal failure (renal hypoperfusion) → extracellular volume contraction + normal tubular integrity → FeNa will be low.
- Acute tubular necrosis → tubular integrity lost → FeNa will be elevated.

1.5.2 Tubular Handling of Phosphate

(a) TRP (tubular reabsorption of phosphate) % = (1 − Fractional excretion of phosphate) × 100:

$$TRP\ \% = \left\{ \frac{1 - U_{Ph} \times P_{Cr} \times 100}{P_{Ph} \times U_{Cr}} \right\}$$

(b) TmP (renal tubular phosphate threshold maximum) can be calculated using the formula given below:

$$\mathrm{TmP} = \frac{[P_{\mathrm{Ph}} - (U_{\mathrm{Ph}} \times P_{\mathrm{Cr}})]}{U_{\mathrm{Cr}}}$$

(c) TmP/GFR is the preferred method for assessment of tubular phosphate handling.
   - Usually 85–95 % of phosphate is reabsorbed in the PCT.
   - TRP >85 % is usually considered normal in clinical practice, and <85 % indicates urinary phosphate loss.
   - Low TRP percentage seen in hyperparathyroidism and in proximal tubular disorders.
   - TRP is influenced by changes in GFR and plasma phosphate.
   - TmP/GFR (tubular maximum for phosphate corrected for GFR) is an index for renal threshold for phosphate. It is independent of plasma phosphate and renal functions and can be determined by a nomogram—Walton and Bijvoet index (see the nomogram below). Normally TMP/GFR should be >2.8 mg/dl.

Nomogram for estimation of the rental threshold phosphate concentraction

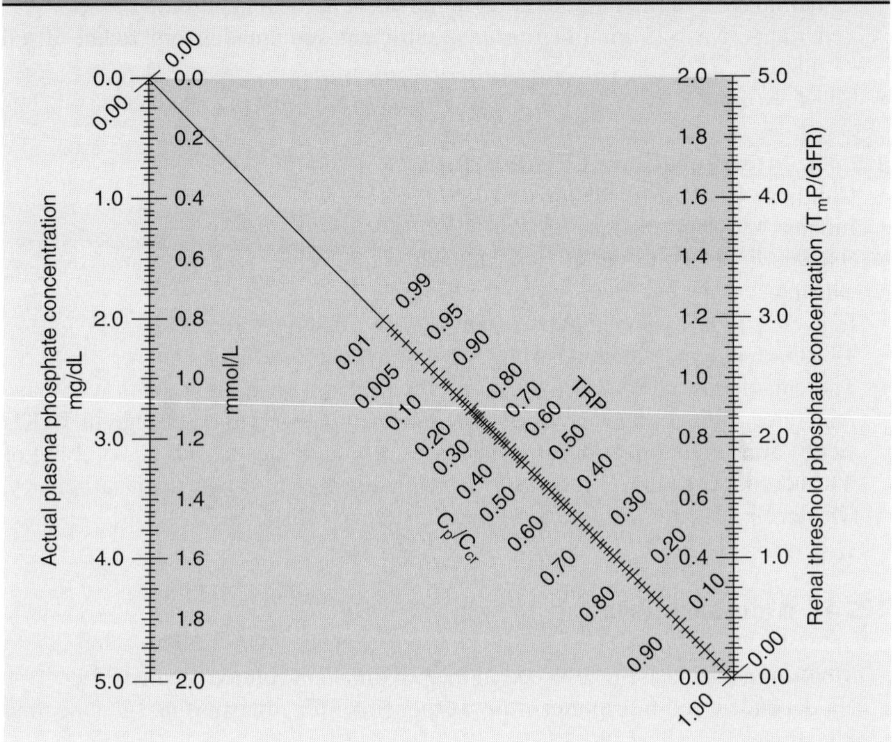

Normal values of TmP/GFR are relatively higher in children (0–1 month, 4–10.7 mg/dl; 1–3 months, 4–9.5 mg/dl; 3–6 months, 4–8.2 mg/dl; 6 months to 5 years, 2.9–4.6 mg/dl; 5–12 years, 2.8–4.4 mg/dl; >12 years, 2.8–4.2 mg/dl). Values lower than 2.8 suggest renal phosphate wasting, while values beyond the upper range suggest hypoparathyroidism.

1.5.3 Transtubular Potassium Gradient (TTKG)

- TTKG is used to assess renal potassium excretion by the cortical collecting duct.
- It indirectly estimates the degree of aldosterone activity by measuring tubular fluid K^+ concentration at the end of the cortical collecting duct.

- Prerequisites:
  - Urine osmolality should be greater than serum osmolality (vasopressin is required for optimal *K* excretion in the distal cortical nephron).
  - Urinary Na >25 mmol/l (ensures sufficient sodium delivery to the distal tubule).
- TTKG = (urine $K \times$ plasma osmolality)/(plasma $K \times$ urine osmolality).

1.5.3.1 Interpretation of TTKG Values

- Children: 4.1–10.5 (median 6.0).
- Infants: 4.9–15.5 (median 7.8).
- Expected TTKG value in hypokalemia <2.5, value >2.5 indicates renal *K* wasting.
- Expected TTKG value in hyperkalemia ≥7 (normal *K* excretion).
- TTKG <5 in hyperkalemia is suggestive of hypoaldosteronism.
- The calculation of TTKG may be useful in distinguishing patients who have mineralocorticoid deficiency versus resistance by observing a change in TTKG values after giving pharmacological doses of mineralocorticoids (0.05–2 mg of fludrocortisone). TTKG increases to >6 within 2–4 h in adrenal insufficiency, whereas it does not increase to >6 in aldosterone resistance.

1.5.4 Aminoaciduria

- Most amino acids are reabsorbed in the proximal convoluted tubule (PCT).
- Na-dependent co-transporters are responsible for transporting glycine and glutamine.
- Na-independent co-transporters are responsible for transportation of leucine, isoleucine, phenylalanine, cystine, arginine, ornithine, and lysine.
- Cyanide nitroprusside test is an easy way to detect urinary amino acids. The test can detect presence of cystine, cysteine, homocystine, and homocysteine.
- Cyanide nitroprusside test should be performed in evaluation of nephrolithiasis.
- Generalized aminoaciduria is associated with Fanconi syndrome.

1.5.5 Measurement of Urinary Ammonium Excretion

Measurement of the urine anion gap (UAG) and urine osmolar gap (UOG) may be helpful in the evaluation of patients with a normal anion gap (AG) metabolic acidosis by providing an indirect estimate of urinary ammonium excretion.

1.5.5.1 Urine Anion Gap

- Indirect measurement of ammonium production by the distal nephron.
- Principle: If ammonium is present in urine, the sum of sodium and potassium will be less than the chloride since ammonium is an unmeasured cation and chloride is the predominant anion in urine.

- Urine anion gap = $(U_{Na} + U_K) - U_{Cl}$.
- In normal subjects, the urine anion gap is usually near zero or is positive.
- In distal renal tubular acidosis (RTA), ammonium excretion is low and urine anion gap is positive, whereas urinary ammonium excretion is high in gastrointestinal losses and urine anion gap is negative.
- Limitations: Urinary anion gap cannot be interpreted in volume-depleted states ($U_{Na} < 25$ mmol/l) and in conditions associated with increased excretion of unmeasured anions (e.g., keto acids in DKA, hippurate in toluene ingestion).

1.5.5.2 Urine Osmolar Gap

- Osmolar gap is the difference between calculated and measured osmolality.
- Sodium (Na^+), chloride (Cl^-), HCO_3^-, urea (BUN), and glucose are major determinants of plasma osmolarity, and these parameters are used to calculate serum osmolality. Serum osmolarity can also be measured directly by freezing-point depression.
- The contribution of Cl^- and HCO_3 to osmolality is estimated by doubling the Na^+ concentration as both are bound to Na^+.
- Calculated plasma osmolality = 2(Na^+) + [Glucose/18] + [BUN/2.8].
- Osmolar gap = Measured plasma osmolality − Calculated serum osmolality.
- The normal osmolar gap is 10–15 mEq/l H_2O.
- *A high osmolar gap with a high anion gap metabolic acidosis may be suggestive of methanol or ethylene glycol poisoning.*

1.5.6 Ammonium Chloride Loading Test

Used for assessment of urinary acidification.

Protocol:

- Ensure that child is not on any bicarbonate supplements.
- Measure blood pH, serum bicarbonates, and urine pH at the beginning of the test (if pH <7.2 and HCO_3 <15 meq/l → no need to perform the test).
- Administer 150 mg/kg of NH_4Cl (can be mixed with fruit juice).
- Check urine pH hourly for 4 h using pH meter.
- Child can be allowed to drink fluids during this time.
- At 4 h check serum bicarbonates and urine pH.

Interpretation:

- Urine pH <5.5 indicates normal urine acidification.
- Failure to achieve urine pH <5.5 indicates distal tubular acidification defect.
- If pH remains above 7 and HCO_3 >15 meq/l at the end of 4 h, then the test is inconclusive and the test may be repeated with higher dose (200 mg/kg) of ammonium chloride.

1.5.7 Furosemide Test

Used for assessment of urinary acidification.

Protocol:

- Ensure that child is not on any bicarbonate supplements.
- Fast from midnight (not required in infants).
- Check urine Na, K, pH, creatinine, plasma Na, K, TCO_2, urea, and creatinine before starting the test.
- Give an oral or intravenous dose of 1 mg/kg furosemide.
- Collect urine every 30 min for 3 h and measure the pH.
- After 3 h, recheck plasma Na, K, TCO_2, urea, and creatinine.
- Prior to discharge, ensure that child is not clinically dehydrated.

Interpretation:

- Urine pH <5.5 indicates normal urine acidification and the test can be stopped.
- Failure to achieve urine pH <5.5 indicates distal tubular acidification defect.

1.5.8 Bicarbonate Loading Test

- The difference in urine and blood CO_2 tension during bicarbonate loading is a useful qualitative index of distal nephron H^+ secretion which helps to differentiate between proximal and distal RTAs.
- The secreted H^+ in the distal tubule reacts with luminal HCO_3^- to form carbonic acid, which forms CO_2 that is trapped in the renal tubule. It is necessary to alkalinize the urine because alkaline urine provides a favorable gradient for H^+ secretion.
- To estimate U-B PCO_2 gradient, alkalinize the urine with 2.75 % $NaHCO_3$ solution infused intravenously at a rate of 4 ml/kg/h. Urine and blood samples are taken at 2-h intervals until the plasma bicarbonate concentration reaches 26 mEq/l.
- The urine is collected under mineral oil. Urine and blood PCO_2 are measured using a blood gas analyzer, and the U-B PCO_2 is calculated when the urine pH is raised to7.5.
- If urine pH is >7.5 and plasma HCO_3- concentration >23–25 mEq/l, the urine PCO_2 should exceed 70 mmHg and the urine to blood PCO_2 gradient should be greater than 20 mmHg.
- Patients with decreased rates of tubular H^+ secretion (classical type 1 RTA) show urine PCO_2 less than 50 mmHg and U-B PCO_2 <10 mmHg.

1.5.9 Fractional Excretion of Bicarbonates $\left(FE_{HCO_3}\right)$

- $FE_{HCO_3} = (Urine_{HCO_3} \times Plasma_{Cr}) \div (Plasma_{HCO_3} \times Urine_{Cr})$.
- Normal FE_{HCO_3} is <5 %.
- >15 % suggests proximal renal tubular acidosis (RTA).
- Usually <5 % in distal RTA.

1.5.10 Tubular (Low Molecular Weight) Proteinuria

Healthy infants excrete about 40–50 μg of protein per day in the urine (109 $\mu g/m^2$/day); urine protein/creatinine ratio is normally <0.49 mg protein/mg creatinine in infants or <0.18 mg protein/mg creatinine in children over 1 year of age. About half of this is albumin and half is constituted by other proteins such as the low molecular weight (LMW) proteins (molecular weight <40 kDa) which are more freely filtered through the glomerular slit pore diaphragm. In renal Fanconi syndrome, urinary excretion of both albumin and LMW proteins increases. Dipsticks (embedded with tetrabromophenol blue) commonly used to detect proteinuria may detect the increased albuminuria, but are relatively insensitive to most LMW proteins. A simple "bedside" test which detects both albumin and LMW protein involves addition of three drops of 20 % sulfosalicylic acid to 5 ml of urine; proteinuria is evident if the urine becomes turbid (due to protein denaturation at low pH). For convincing evidence of proximal tubular dysfunction, however, quantification of a specific LMW is usually required. In normal children, urinary beta-2 microglobulin concentration is less than 0.36 mg/l (less than 0.4 % of the filtered load), whereas it typically ranges from 10 to 30 mg/l in children with renal Fanconi syndrome. Beta-2 microglobulin, normalized for urine creatinine, should be <40 mg/mmol creatinine.

1.5.11 Water Deprivation and Vasopressin (ADH) Test

Protocol:

- Should be done in the morning hours.
- 8 h test is adequate for children.
- Restrict fluid intake, dry food allowed.
- Weigh the child after emptying bladder.
- Insert an indwelling catheter if urine output cannot be measured reliably.
- Measure baseline plasma and urine osmolality.
- Check hourly body weight.
- Measure urine amount and osmolality, serum sodium, and plasma osmolality every 2 h for a maximum of 8 h.
- Stop the test if serum sodium is >150 meq/l, body weight drop >3 %, and serum osmolality >300 mOsm/kg or if specific gravity and osmolality differ <30 mosm/l in two consecutive tests.
- At the end of the test, AVP is given if urinary osmolality remains low (see table). Administer 20 μg (10 IU) DDAVP intranasally (10 μg in infants) or 0.3 units/kg vasopressin intravenous and repeat the parameters after 2 h.

Interpretation (see Table 1.1):

- In normal subjects plasma osmolality remains stable below 300, but the urine output is reduced and urine osmolality rises (800–1,200).

Table 1.1 Water deprivation and vasopressin test interpretation (also see Sect. 2.2.4)

Diagnosis	Thirst at 4 h	Urine volume at 4 h	$Urine_{osm}$ at 4 h mOsmol/l	$Plasma_{osm}$ mOsmol/l	The ratio of $urine_{osm}$ and $plasma_{osm}$ at 4 h	ADH test if urine osmolality low
Normal	±	Decrease	Increase 800–1,400	Stable <300	>2	
Primary polydipsia	Increase	Decrease	Increase	Low normal	>2	
Central DI	Increase	Same	Same or low <300	High	<1.5	$Urine_{osm}$ rises by >50 %
Nephrogenic DI	Increase	Same	Same or low <300	High	<1.5	No increase

- A patient with primary polydipsia, plasma osmolality is low/normal (280) to start with. The urine/plasma osmolality ratio rises to >2 after water deprivation.
- In patients with diabetes insipidus (DI), the plasma osmolality rises but not the urine osmolality and urine to plasma osmolality ratio remains <1.5.
- Concentration of the dilute urine following DDAVP confirms central DI, and no change suggests nephrogenic DI.

1.6 Histopathological Evaluation

The renal histopathology forms an integral part of the clinicopathological correlations that helps to diagnose, to prognosticate, and to plan patient management strategies.

1.6.1 Indications for Kidney Biopsy

Indications for kidney biopsy in some common clinical scenarios are given below:

(a) Nephrotic syndrome
  - Age of onset <1 year
  - Atypical features such as gross hematuria, hypertension, and abnormal renal functions
  - Steroid resistance
  - Prior to use of calcineurin inhibitors (CNI), for monitoring while on CNI therapy
  - Presence of associated systemic features

(b) Acute nephritic syndrome
  - Absence of prior history of sore throat or pyoderma
  - Nephritic–nephrotic presentations

- Progressive deterioration in renal functions
- Failure to normalize renal functions within 2–3 weeks
- Associated systemic features
- Recurrent nephritic features
- Persistence of gross hematuria or hypertension beyond 3–4 weeks
- Persistently low serum C_3 complement levels beyond 8–12 weeks

(c) Hematuria and proteinuria
- Persistent hematuria and proteinuria beyond 3 months
- Recurrent disease
- Associated systemic features
- Positive family history of renal disease or hearing deficit
- Associated with low serum C_3 complement level

(d) Acute kidney injury (AKI)
- Unexplained ARF with normal-sized kidneys
- In patients with suspicion of rapidly progressive glomerulonephritis (histological diagnosis will guide therapy and prognostication)

(e) Chronic kidney disease (CKD)
- CKD of undetermined etiology with normal-sized kidneys

(f) Posttransplant period
- Acute or chronic graft dysfunction
- Glomerulonephritis—recurrent or de novo
- Suspected infections like CMV, polyoma, and parvovirus

The procedural details of kidney biopsy are given in the Appendix. To assure adequate tissue for diagnosis, several cores (for light, immunofluorescent, and electron microscopy) are obtained with an 18-gauge needle, rather than dissection of one or two larger cores obtained with a wider-gauge needle. To assure an adequate number of glomeruli, each core can be examined under a dissecting microscope by an experienced pathologist.

1.6.2 Adequacy of the Renal Biopsy

Light microscopy: >10 glomeruli.
Cortex and medullary regions.
Avoid glomeruli at the biopsy edge where there may be compression artifacts.

1.6.3 Interpretation of Renal Biopsy

Light microscopy, immunofluorescence (IF), and electron microscopic examination of the biopsy specimen are desirable (not mandatory, may not be feasible in every case). IF is especially useful in suspected IgA nephropathy or lupus nephritis. In the diagnosis of hereditary nephritis, thin basement membrane disease is done with electron microscopy.

1.6.3.1 Light Microscopy

Stains used in evaluating renal biopsy specimens by light microscopy are:

1. H&E stain—commonly used
2. PAS—accentuates matrix and basement membrane constituents
3. Trichrome—accentuates matrix and basement membrane constituents and demonstrates immune deposits as fuchsinophilic (red) structures
4. Jones silver stains—accentuates collagenous structures
5. Others—Congo red for amyloidosis

1. Screen H&E-stained biopsy core at low power for number and general appearance of glomeruli and interstitium.
2. Inspect selected H&E-stained glomeruli at high power for:
   - Open capillary loops (suggesting adequate filtration surface)
   - Global or segmental glomerulosclerosis (representing obsolescence or early FSGS, respectively)
   - Increased number of cells (suggesting cellular infiltrate or proliferative glomerulonephritis)
   - Increase in mesangial matrix (common glomerulonephritis)
   - Cellular crescents (a feature of rapidly progressive glomerulonephritis)
   - Patchy red-staining necrosis ± thrombi (as in hemolytic–uremic syndrome)
   - Normal-appearing glomeruli (e.g., minimal change nephrotic syndrome)
3. Inspect H&E-stained renal tubules and interstitium at high power:
   - Widely spaced tubules (suggestive of edema)
   - Thickened tubular basement membrane and dilated tubules (tubular atrophy)
   - Flattened tubular cells, detached cells within tubular lumen (acute tubular necrosis)
   - Cellular infiltrate between tubules (interstitial nephritis)
   - Orange-staining material between tubules (interstitial fibrosis)
   - Pink-staining material within tubular lumen (casts)

1.6.3.2 Immunofluorescent (IF) Microscopy

1. Basic IF microscopy screens for presence of immune reactant deposition in the glomerulus.
   - IgG and C3 in granular pattern along capillary loops and in mesangium (e.g., acute postinfectious nephritis, membranoproliferative glomerulonephritis, or lupus nephritis)
   - IgA in central mesangial areas (e.g., IgA nephropathy and HSP nephritis)
   - Linear deposition of IgG along the capillary loop wall (e.g., Goodpasture syndrome)
2. Special IF staining screens for specific viral pathogens and transplant rejection.
   - Epstein–Barr virus
   - BK virus
   - Peritubular C4d deposition in acute humeral rejection of the renal allograft

1.6.3.3 Electron Microscopy

- Confirm and refine localization of immune deposits to classify glomerulonephritis (e.g., subepithelial “humps” characteristic of acute postinfectious glomerulonephritis or chronic membranous glomerulonephritis).
- Examine integrity of glomerular basement membrane (specific diagnosis of Alport syndrome).

1.6.4 Biopsy findings in various common disease conditions

Biopsy findings in various common disease conditions are given below. Figs. 1.15–1.21 illustrate histological appearances as seen in some of these conditions.

Minimal Change Nephrotic Syndrome

- Essentially normal glomerular appearance on light microscopy. There may be mild mesangial hypercellularity in a few segments.
- Tubular epithelial cells may contain lipid vacuoles and protein reabsorption droplets.
- No immune deposits. Occasionally mesangial IgM and/or C_3 deposits without ultrastructural evidence for electron-dense deposits may be seen.
- There is almost complete effacement of podocyte foot process, often accompanied by microvillous transformation of podocyte cytoplasm.

Focal Segmental Glomerulosclerosis (FSGS)

- One or more glomeruli show segmental sclerosis. They are typically located in deep cortex. A portion of the glomerulus undergoes obliteration of capillary lumens by extracellular matrix.
- Glomerular enlargement, tubular atrophy, and interstitial fibrosis are pointers to underlying FSGS.
- On IF, coarse granular deposits of IgM and C_3 are found in sclerotic glomeruli.
- Electron microscopy of the sclerotic segment shows glomerular capillary collapse, podocyte separation from the underlying basement membrane, and luminal obliteration; other glomeruli disclose foot process effacement.
- Variants of focal segmental glomerulosclerosis include collapsing glomerulopathy, the tip lesion, and the cellular lesion.

IgM Nephropathy

Some consider IgM nephropathy as a discrete entity, in which mesangial hypercellularity is associated with mesangial IgM deposits on IF, while others regard it as part of the spectrum of minimal change disease.

Membranoproliferative or Mesangiocapillary Glomerulonephritis (MPGN)

- Glomeruli have a lobulated appearance. There is mesangial hypercellularity or proliferation, capillary wall thickening, and double contouring of basement membrane.
- In type I MPGN, IF demonstrates peripheral granular or band-like staining of C_3, IgM, and IgG.

- In type II MPGN (dense deposit disease), dense deposits are seen within the basement membrane.
- In type III MPGN, subepithelial deposits are found.

Membranous Glomerulopathy

- Rare in children.
- Thickening of glomerular basement membrane (GBM) is seen.
- Silver staining shows spikes projecting from GBM.
- Tubulo-reticular structures are seen within endothelial cell cytoplasm.
- IF features granular deposits of IgG, C_3 deposits.

Congenital Nephrotic Syndrome (CNS)

- Finnish-type CNS-light microscopy may be normal in early life; tubular dilatation resulting in diffuse micro-cystic change (cysts of 0.1–0.5 mm), progressive glomerular sclerosis, and interstitial fibrosis develops by 6–12 months of age.
- Diffuse mesangial sclerosis-thickened GBM and increase mesangial matrix without hypercellularity, collapsed capillary looks, and dilated Bowman's space.

Postinfectious Glomerulonephritis

- All glomeruli diffusely hypercellular, infiltrated with variable numbers of neutrophils, expansion of mesangial region, increase mesangial and endothelial cell swelling, crescents may be seen.
- IF: C_3 and IgG in glomerular capillary walls and mesangial regions. Typically, a "starry sky" pattern of granular immune deposits are found. Granules can be small or huge and massively distributed in the glomeruli and are immunohistological equivalent of the humps observed on EM. The so-called garland pattern is characterized by huge immune deposits peripherally distributed along glomerular capillary walls.
- EM shows subepithelial hump-shaped deposits.

Crescentic Glomerulonephritis (Proliferative Extra-Capillary)

- A crescent is the presence of at least two layers of cell that fill totally (circumferential) or partially (circumscribed) the Bowman's space, affecting >50 % of the glomeruli.
- Type I—produced by anti-glomerular basement membrane (GBM) antibodies.
- Type II—due to immune complexes deposited in glomeruli.
- Type III—pauci-immune, without deposits of immunoglobulins or complement in glomeruli.
- Crescents can be cellular, fibro-cellular, or fibrous.

IgA Nephropathy

- The histopathological features are very variable, from normal-appearing glomeruli to any type of proliferative or sclerosing lesion, including extra-capillary proliferation.

- IgA mesangial deposits are the characteristic and defining feature of the disease. Other immunoglobulins may be present, but IgA must be dominant or codominant.
- In approximately 25 % of cases, there are variable degrees of IgA deposits in capillary walls.
- EM confirms the presence of large electron-dense deposits in mesangial and para-mesangial regions.

Lupus Nephritis

- Several features that indicate the degree of activity or chronicity of lupus nephritis are important for prognosis and treatment. Abnormalities indicating activity of the disease are cellular proliferation, fibrinoid necrosis, karyorrhexis, cellular crescents, hyaline thrombi, wire loops, leukocyte infiltration, and mononuclear cell infiltration in interstitium. Abnormalities indicating chronicity of the disease are glomerular sclerosis, fibrous crescents, interstitial fibrosis, and tubular fibrosis.
- WHO classification
  - Class I—normal by light microscopy
  - Class II—mesangial involvement
  - Class III—focal proliferative disease involving <50 % of glomeruli
  - Class IV—diffuse proliferative disease where >50 % glomeruli are affected, with segmental (<50 % of glomerular tuft) or global (≥50 % of the glomerular tuft)
  - Class V—membranous changes
  - Class VI—advanced sclerosing lesions
- IF in active renal disease demonstrates a "full house" pattern for IgA, IgG, IgM, C_3, and $C1_q$.
- EM—tubulo-reticular structures are found within endothelial cells and sometimes in monocytes and lymphocytes. A fingerprint pattern of organized deposits is regarded as unique for lupus nephritis.

Thrombotic Microangiopathy

- These lesions are seen in HUS, TTP, malignant hypertension, and scleroderma.
- Glomeruli show swollen endothelial cells with wrinkled capillary walls, mesangiolysis, and luminal thrombi. Arterioles show thrombo-necrotic lesions.
- IF reveals fibrin deposits.
- EM shows glomeruli with subendothelial widening with accumulation of flocculent material.

Alport Syndrome

- Light microscopy variable, ranging from unremarkable histology to presence of interstitial foam cells and segmental sclerosis.
- IF—nonspecific.
- EM changes are diagnostic. Thickening and thinning of GBM with lamellations, basket weaving, interspersed with electron-lucent zones within the basement

membrane and occasional rounded vesicular particles. Scalloping of the subepithelial aspect of the glomerular capillary walls is seen.

Transplant Biopsy

- Acute rejection
  (a) Cell-mediated rejection—tubulointerstitial rejection (lymphocytes within edematous interstitium), tubulitis (lymphocytes within tubular profiles), vascular rejection (arterioles with swollen endothelial cells and subendothelial lymphocytes), glomerular rejection (glomerulitis)
  (b) Antibody-mediated rejection—hyperacute rejections (neutrophils within peritubular capillaries and glomerular, arterial, arteriolar thrombosis), acute rejections (necrotizing arteritis with fibrin within arterial walls), CD4 staining in peritubular capillary walls
- Chronic rejection—double contours of glomerular capillary walls with increased matrix, mesangiolysis, segmental sclerosis, intimal fibrosis as well as foam cells and lymphocytes in vessel wall, tubular atrophy, and interstitial fibrosis
- Acute tubular necrosis—tubular dilatation, flat epithelial, sloughed epithelial cells
- Calcineurin inhibitor nephrotoxicity—vacuoles within tubular epithelial cells, acute tubular necrosis, thrombotic microangiopathy, striped fibrosis, arteriolopathy

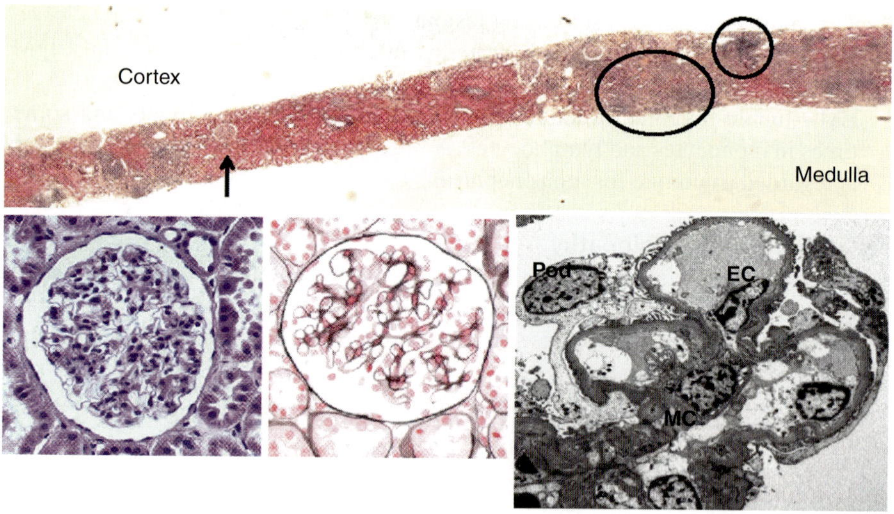

Fig. 1.15 Normal glomeruli (*arrow*): open capillary loops, normal cell number, normal mesangial volume, no cellular crescents, no sclerosis

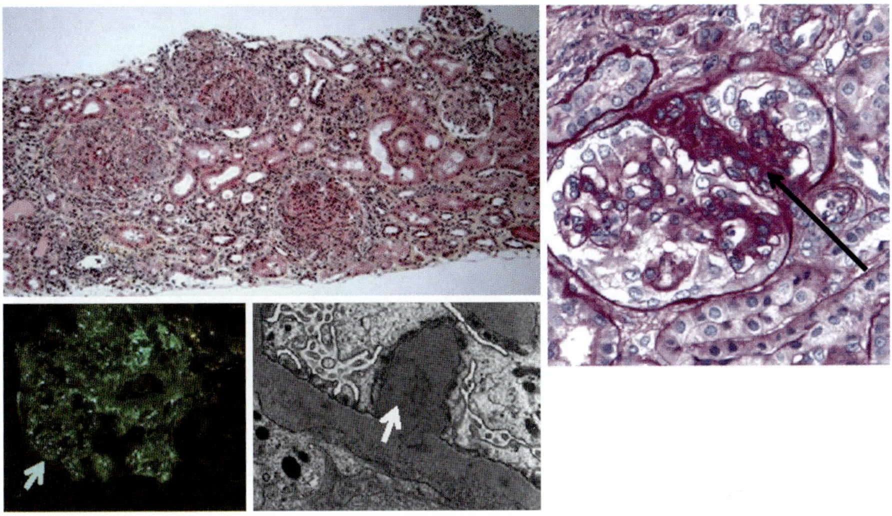

Fig. 1.16 Proliferative glomerulonephritis (*upper left*); focal segmental glomerulosclerosis (*upper right*); immunofluorescent staining for IgG deposition in a glomerulus (*lower left*); subepithelial immune deposit by electron microscopy (*lower right*)

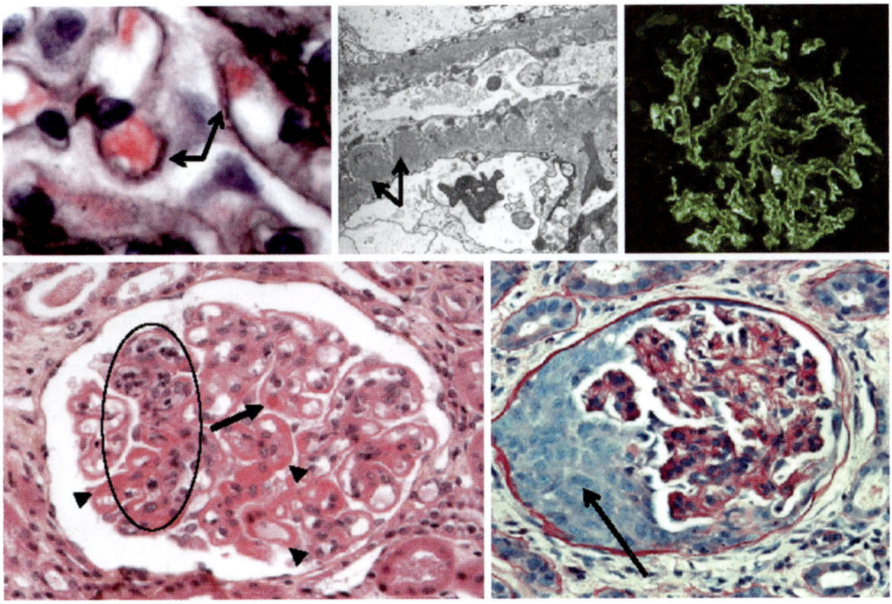

Fig. 1.17 Immune deposits in the capillary membrane by light, electron and immunofluroescent microscopy (*upper panel*); focal proliferative glomerulnephritis (*left lower*); parietal cell crescent in rapidly progressive glomerulonephritis

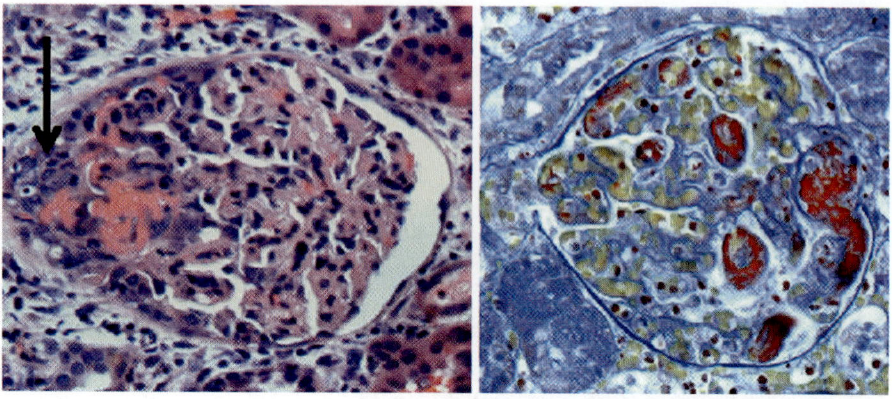

Fig. 1.18 Segmental necrotizing GN: on left fibrinoid necrosis and early cellular crescent (in this case: IGA nephropathy)

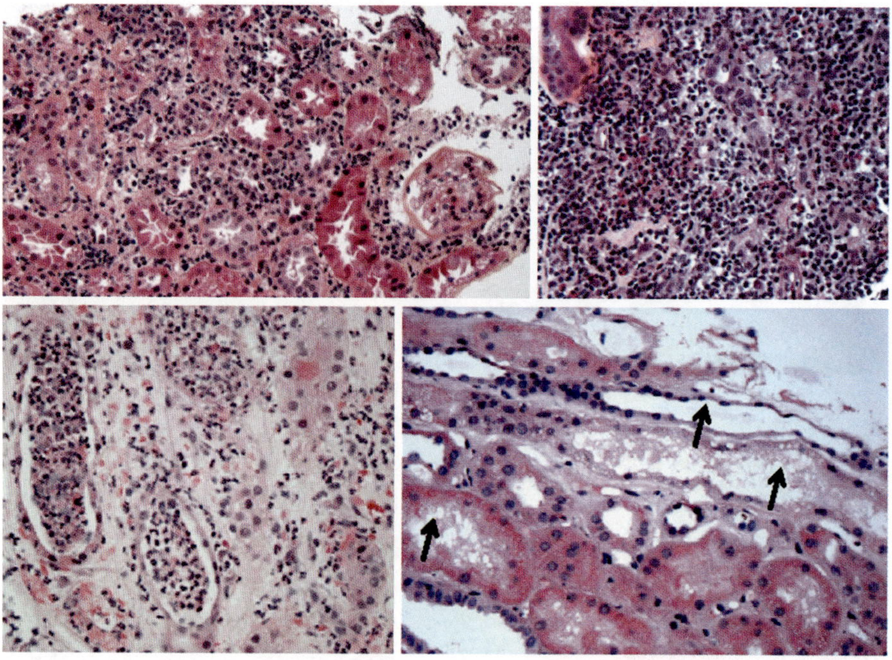

Fig. 1.19 Tubulointerstitial inflammation with tubulitis and predominance of lymphocytes: acute T-cell mediated rejection or tubulointerstitial nephritis (depending on context)

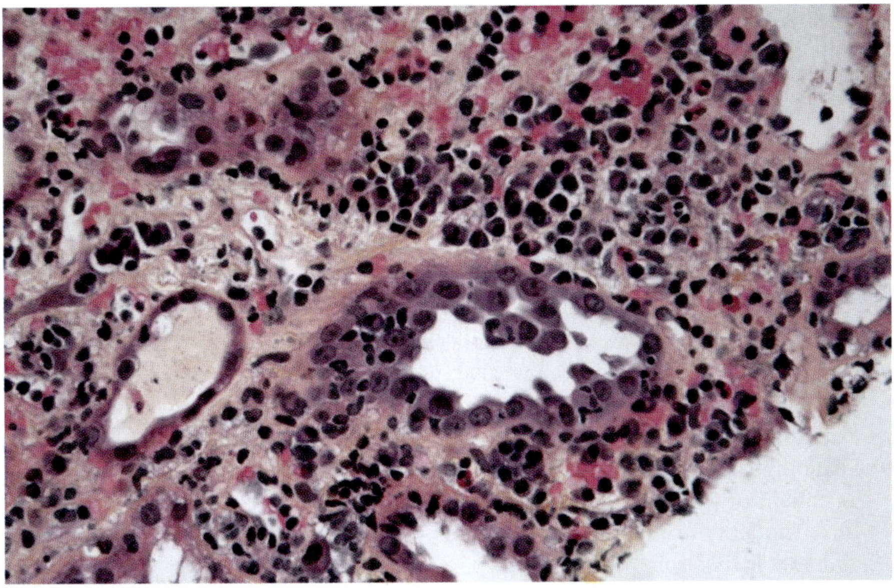

Fig. 1.20 Tubulitis

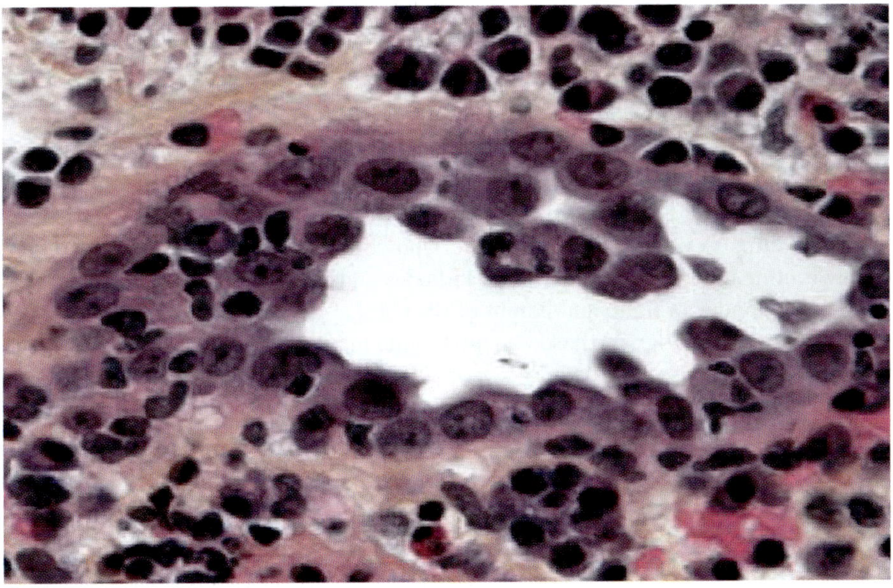

Fig. 1.21 Tubulitis – high power

- Infections—Cytomegalovirus (owl-eye inclusion bodies in tubular epithelial cells), polyoma virus (tubular cell abnormalities, cytopathic changes), parvovirus B-19 virus (collapsing glomerulopathy)
- Glomerulonephritis—recurrent or de novo

1.7 Radiological Evaluation

1.7.1 Ultrasonography

- Ultrasound is the most common initial imaging tool used for evaluation of kidney diseases because it is noninvasive, widely available, and easy to use.
- It does not use ionizing radiation; hence, the safety is ensured even on repeated examinations.
- Scanning is performed with curved array transducers and the obtained image can be enhanced with high-resolution linear transducers.
- It is a modality to evaluate the structure of the kidneys and does not give any clue about their function.
- It is commonly used for aiding the kidney biopsy procedure.

1.7.1.1 Interpreting a Renal Ultrasound Report

Number and Location of Kidneys

- Usually two kidneys should be visualized located in a retroperitoneal position on either side of vertebral column against psoas muscles.
- Absence of kidney in the normal position may indicate an unascended kidney, an ectopic kidney, or renal agenesis/involuted kidney.

Size of Kidneys

- Renal dimensions such as AP diameter and cortical thickness are measured during routine ultrasound evaluation of kidneys, and these measurements depend on the age, gender, weight, and height of the child.
- Renal length nomograms based on ultrasound measurements in pediatric patients may be used to assess kidney size (see Chap. 17).

Renal Parenchymal Architecture

- Echogenicity of the cortex must be compared both to the medulla and to the liver/spleen.
- The medullary pyramids appear prominent and hypoechoic because of a relatively lower cortical volume.
- In healthy children cortex is more echogenic than medulla. This difference is termed as corticomedullary differentiation.
- Increased medullary echogenicity may be because of medullary nephrocalcinosis. In neonates it could be transient, due to the precipitation of Tamm–Horsfall proteins.
- The renal cortex in neonates and infants up to 6 months has echogenicity equal to or greater than that of the liver and spleen, whereas in older children and adults, the cortex is hypoechoic relative to those organs.

Renal Collecting System

Pelvic dilatation is assessed at the level of renal hilum or just beyond it in case of extra renal pelvis. Pelvic diameter should be assessed in anteroposterior diameter after voiding, if the urinary bladder is overdistended.

Ureters

Ureteric diameter can be assessed only if it is dilated. The midportion of ureter is often obscured by bowel gas, whereas the proximal and distal portions are more reliably visualized.

Bladder

Bladder should be filled prior to the examination. It should be assessed for bladder contour, bladder wall thickness, and for pre- and post-void residues.

Figures 1.24, 1.27, 1.28, 1.30 and 1.31 illustrate findings on ultrasound examination of some conditions.

1.7.2 Doppler Studies

Doppler renal ultrasonography can be used to evaluate renal blood flow in native or transplanted kidneys. These include renal vein thrombosis, renal infarction, and renal artery stenosis.

Renal artery stenosis (RAS): There are proximal and distal criteria for diagnosing RAS. Proximal criteria detect changes in the Doppler signal at the site of stenosis, and distal criteria detect changes in the downstream waveform from the stenotic area. The proximal criteria include peak systolic velocity ≥200 cm/s, ratio of peak systolic velocity (PSV) in the aorta to renal artery >3.5, turbulent flow in post-stenotic region, and lack of detectable Doppler signal in the visualized artery. The distal criteria include loss of the early systolic peak, slope of acceleration <300 cm/s, and acceleration time >0.07 s. Based on velocities and intensity of blood flows, resistive index can be calculated in various segments of the vasculature. The normal resistive index is <0.7. A high resistive index may indicate intrarenal vascular disease or obstruction but may also be seen with acute tubular necrosis, obstruction to urine outflow, acute rejection of the transplanted kidney, and in severe renal interstitial edema. Diastolic reversal indicates more severe intrarenal resistance and renal hypoperfusion.

1.7.3 Plain Abdominal X-Ray

- Can identify radiopaque calculi. Small stones, stones overlying bony structures, and radiolucent uric acid stones may be missed.
- Useful for detecting calcifications (including severe nephrocalcinosis).
- Can detect spina bifida occulta and sacral agenesis.
- Can be used to measure renal length.
- Can also be beneficial in determining the correct positioning of various drainage catheters and stents.

1.7.4 Voiding Cystourethrogram (VCUG)

- Active urinary tract infection should be excluded before doing this invasive investigation.
- Gold standard investigation for assessing the lower urinary tract and to detect vesicoureteric reflux.
- Oblique or lateral film without the catheter is necessary to detect posterior urethral valves.
- Films during filling phase are used to document bladder pathology and low-pressure vesicoureteric reflux. Early filling films should be obtained to identify a ureterocele, which may become compressed, on filling of the bladder.
- The film should include the subdiaphragmatic area where the kidneys are situated.
- The details of the procedure are given in Sect. 17.5.7.

Figures 1.25, 1.29 and 1.32 illustrate VCUG appearances in patients with ureterocele, vesicoureteric reflux and posterior urethral valves respectively.

1.7.5 Intravenous Urography (IVU)

- Used relatively infrequently.
- Avoid this procedure in presence of renal failure.
- Avoid IVU in neonates.
- Intravenous low-osmolar contrast medium, e.g., iohexol, should be used in children.
- Useful in malrotation of kidneys, duplex system, helps to visualize the calyces, helps in identification of the site of urinary tract obstructions, e.g., congenital pelviureteric or vesicoureteric obstruction.
- Patient should be well hydrated to reduce nephrotoxicity. The measures that need to be taken to avoid contrast-induced nephrotoxicity are described in Chap. 16.

Figure 1.23 illustrates a non functioning upper pole of left kidney on intravenous urogram.

1.7.6 Nuclear Medicine Investigations

1.7.6.1 Direct Radionuclide Cystography (DRCG)

- Detects vesicoureteric reflux (VUR) with reasonable sensitivity and used as a complementary modality to VCUG.
- VCUG is used to diagnose and grade the VUR. DRCG can be used for follow-up evaluation.
- DRCG provides little anatomical details and is not useful in detecting structural abnormalities (e.g., ureterocele, PUV, duplex collecting systems).
- The radiation dose to the patient would be 1/100 of the dose received during VCUG.
- It involves instillation of ^{99}Tc pertechnetate into the bladder, followed by taking dynamic images while the bladder is filling and while the patient voids on the

table. VUR can be detected either in the bladder filling phase or in the voiding phase.

- A DRCG examination is considered as positive for reflux when radiotracer can be seen in the ureter, renal pelvis, or both.

1.7.6.2 Indirect Radionuclide Cystography

^{99}Tc-MAG 3 is given intravenously and continuous dynamic images of the kidney and bladder are obtained during bladder filling and voiding phase.

1.7.6.3 Radionuclide Scintigraphy

- Three categories of radio tracers are used in radio imaging, which differ in their mode of renal clearance.
- Glomerular filtration agents "cleared by the glomerulus" can be used to measure the GFR (^{99m}Tc DTPA, ^{99m}Tc MAG 3).
- Agents primarily handled by tubular secretion are used to estimate effective renal plasma flow (^{99m}Tc MAG 3).
- Tubular retention agents provide excellent cortical imaging and can be used in suspected renal scarring and infarction (^{99m}TcDMSA). DMSA is taken up though not excreted by renal tubular cells.

1.7.7 Choice of Radionuclides in Renal Imaging

Glomerular filtration rate	^{99m}Tc-DTPA
Glomerular filtration rate with renal impairment	^{99m}Tc-MAG3,^{131}I-OIH
Effective renal plasma flow	^{99m}Tc-MAG3, ^{131}I-OIH
Renal scarring	^{99m}Tc-DMSA,^{99}Tc-GH
Upper renal tract obstruction	^{99m}Tc-DTPA
Upper renal tract obstruction with renal impairment	^{99m}Tc-MAG3

1.7.7.1 DMSA Cortical Scintigraphy

- Highly sensitive to find out the acute lesions (pyelonephritis) and the late sequelae (parenchymal scarring). It can also be used to assess split renal functions.
- Images are acquired 2–3 h after injection of ^{99m}Tc DMSA. Planar images are acquired in the posterior and right and left posterior oblique positions.
- The image produced is that of functional renal cortical mass, and the technique is the gold standard investigation for detection of renal cortical scarring.
- Acute lesions of pyelonephritis can take as long as 3–6 months to resolve scintigraphically.
- Permanent scarring can only be reported when the DMSA is performed at least 3–6 months after acute infection.
- Renal scarring tends to occur at the upper and lower poles of the kidney because of the round-shaped orifices of the compound papillae at these locations.
- Congenital dysplastic kidney may have DMSA appearance similar to that of acquired renal scarring.

- Permanent scarring tends to cause loss of volume, whereas acute infection does not.

  Figure 1.22 illustrates a DMSA scan showing an atrophic left kidney.

1.7.7.2 Dynamic Renography (DTPA or MAG3 Scan)

- Used to detect presence and site of urinary tract obstruction.
- Although 99mTc DTPA is most commonly used for functional renal imaging, 99mTcMAG3 is preferred because of its higher extraction fraction and higher target to background ratio.

Procedure

Immediately after injection of radiotracer, imaging of renal perfusion is performed. Patient should remain well hydrated when the imaging is being done. The patient lies supine with camera positioned posteriorly. Ideally, bladder should be catheterized.

Radioactivity should reach the kidneys in about 1 s after tracer bolus. Maximal parenchymal activity is seen at 3–5 min after injection (T_{max}). Urinary activity in the renal pelvis is typically seen 2–4 min (cortical transit time) after injection. There should be prompt drainage of tracer in to urinary bladder, with less than half of the activity at T_{max} remaining in the renal pelvis 8–10 min after injection ($T_{½}$). Renogram curves are generated by plotting the activity within the regions of interest drawn around the kidney. The renogram is a graphic representation of uptake, excretion, and drainage phases. Renographic curves may show normal uptake and excretion, or they may be pathological (reduced uptake by either or both kidneys indicating poor function or normal uptake but poor excretion indicating obstruction):

$T_{1/2} > 20$ min indicates obstruction.

$T_{1/2}$ 10–20 min indicates equivocal result; test should be repeated.

$T_{1/2} < 10$ min: normal.

1.7.7.3 Diuretic Renogram

- Dynamic urography is combined with administration of furosemide.
- It is useful in determining presence of anatomical obstruction at pelviureteric or vesicoureteric junction.
- The dose of furosemide is 1 mg/kg, with a maximum dose of 40 mg.
- Timing of furosemide administration is variable in different protocols.
- F +20 and F +15 are commonly used protocols. (F +20: furosemide is given 20 min after radiotracer, if normal spontaneous drainage has not occurred.)

1.7.8 CT (Computed Tomography) Scan

CT scanning often provides complementary information to that obtained with ultrasonography. Better image resolution and progressively shorter scanning time have increased the usage of CT scan. Alternatively, MRI scan may be used. Fig 1.26 shows a MRI scan of a patient with Wilm's tumor.

1.7.8.1 Indications

- Used in characterization of renal or perirenal masses and for renal tumor staging.
- Used to differentiate simple cyst from a cyst with suspected malignant changes. Polycystic kidney disease can be diagnosed with a CT scan, with a higher sensitivity than that obtained with renal ultrasonography, particularly in younger patients.
- Used to delineate renal or perirenal collections or abscesses.
- Non-contrast-enhanced helical CT scanning is the gold standard for the radiologic diagnosis of renal stone disease, including for detection of radiolucent stones which are missed on plain films of the abdomen.
- Useful in defining the extent of renal trauma associated with intra-abdominal injuries.
- CT angiography is used for evaluation of renovascular disease.

1.7.9 PET/CT Scan

Positron emission tomography (PET)/computed tomography (CT) is a hybrid medical imaging technique that provides both the metabolic or biochemical activity of the tissue and the anatomic details of the organ scanned. It combines the precision of anatomic localization to functional imaging. The vast majority of PET/CT scans are performed with fluorine-18 fluoro-2-deoxy-D-glucose (FDG), an analogue of glucose. There is significant uptake and excretion of FDG through the kidneys which results in intense activity in the renal collecting system and the bladder. Currently, limited literature exists on the imaging appearances and characterization of renal masses with PET/CT. It has been found to be a useful adjunct tool in the assessment of malignant and inflammatory diseases. Renal involvement by lymphoma, leukemia, or metastatic disease is often intensely avid on FDG PET/CT. Renal cell carcinoma typically shows a low level of FDG uptake comparable to adjacent renal parenchyma. PET/CT is also useful in precise anatomic localization and percutaneous drainage of infected cysts in autosomal dominant polycystic kidney disease (rare in children) because these are difficult to localize with conventional imaging.

1.7.10 Magnetic Resonance Urography (MRU) and Angiography (MRA)

- Can evaluate function, perfusion, excretion, and drainage.
- No exposure to ionizing radiation.
- May substitute formal angiography and venography in some cases.

- Gadolinium contrast should be avoided in patients with GFR <60 ml/min/1.73 m^2 because of the fear of side effects such as nephrogenic systemic fibrosis (described in Chap. 16).
- MR venography is also useful in diagnosing cortical vein or cerebral venous sinus thrombosis.

1.7.11 Arteriography and Venography

- May be used to assist in the diagnosis of renal artery stenosis, Takayasu disease, and systemic vasculitis, e.g., polyarteritis nodosa.
- Renin vein sampling or interventions, e.g., angioplasty, may be possible during the procedure.

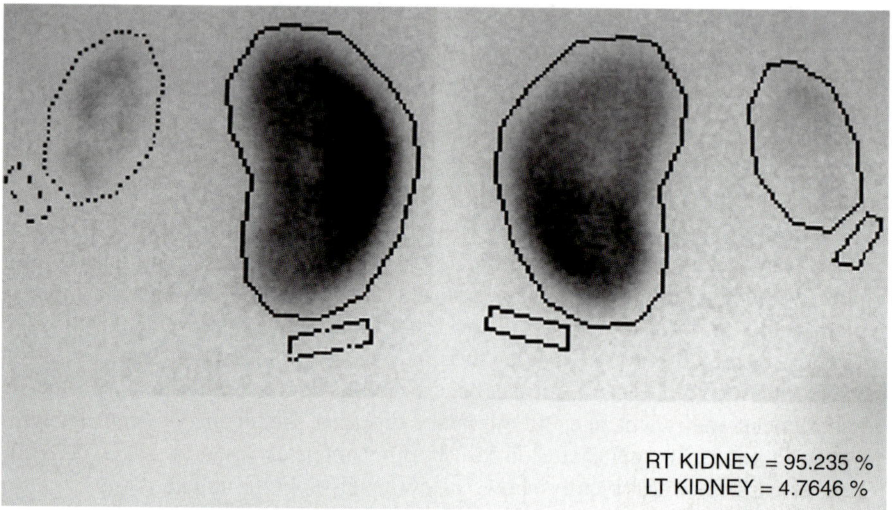

Fig. 1.22 DMSA: atrophic left kidney

Fig. 1.23 Intravenous urogram – left non functioning upper pole

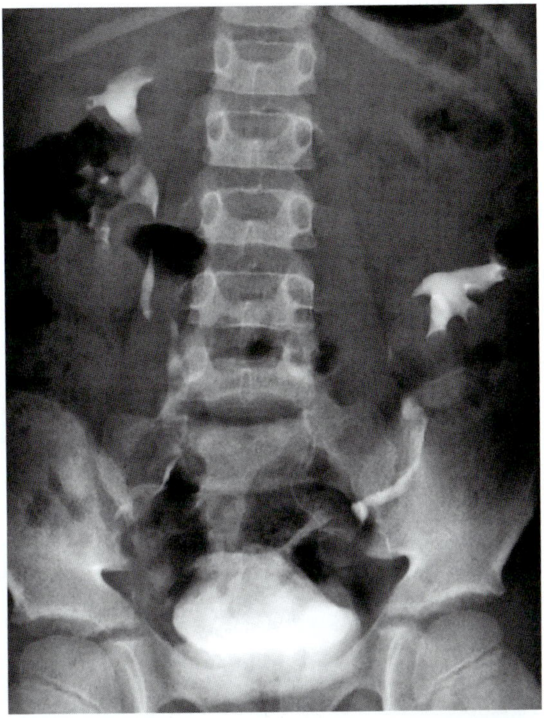

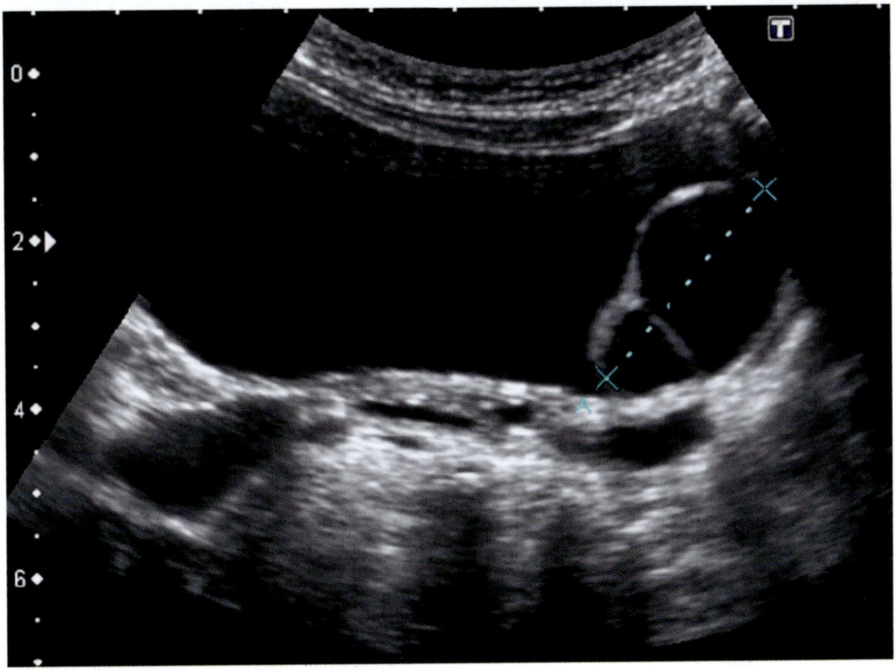

Fig. 1.24 Ultrasound – ureterocele

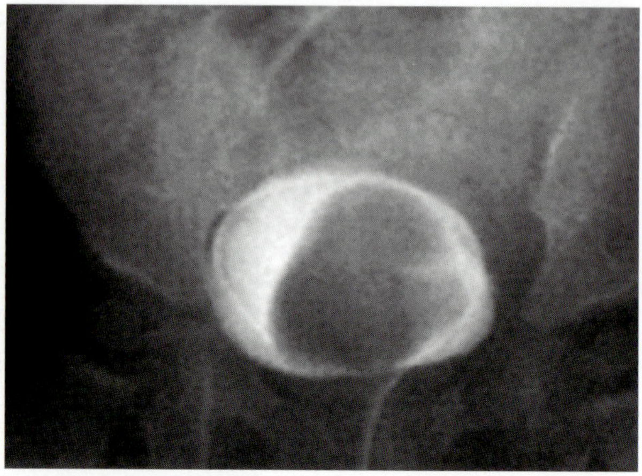

Fig. 1.25 VCUG – ureterocele

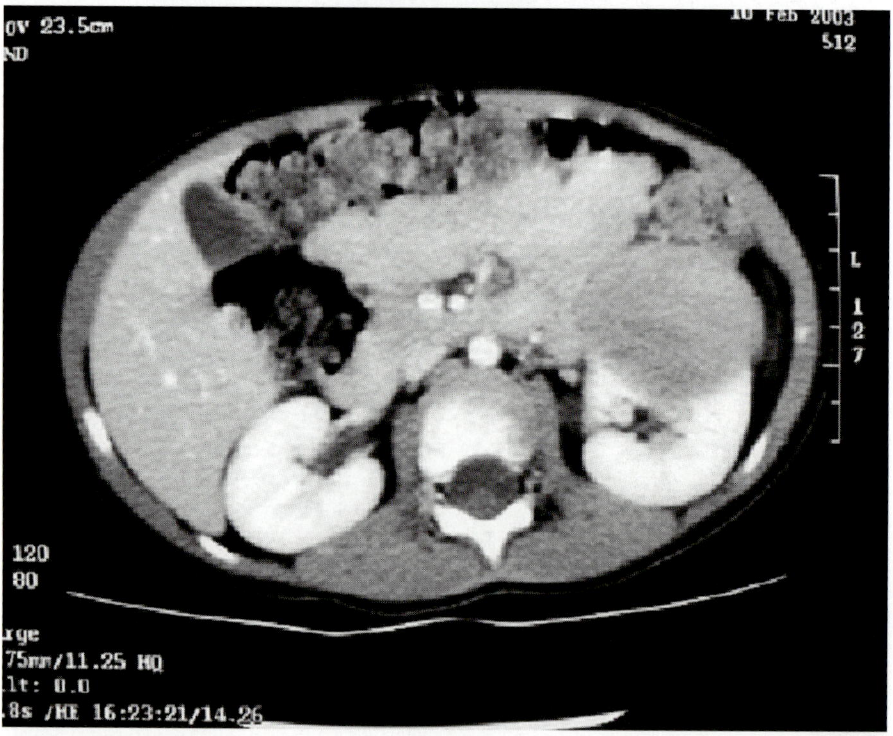

Fig. 1.26 MRI – Wilm's tumour

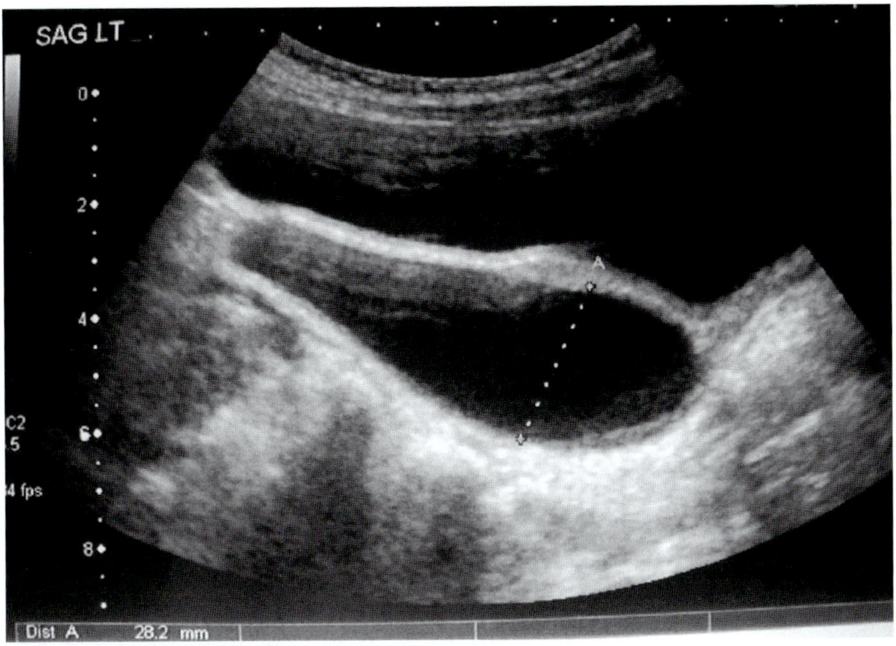

Fig. 1.27 Distal hydroureter (sagittal) – vesico ureteric obstruction

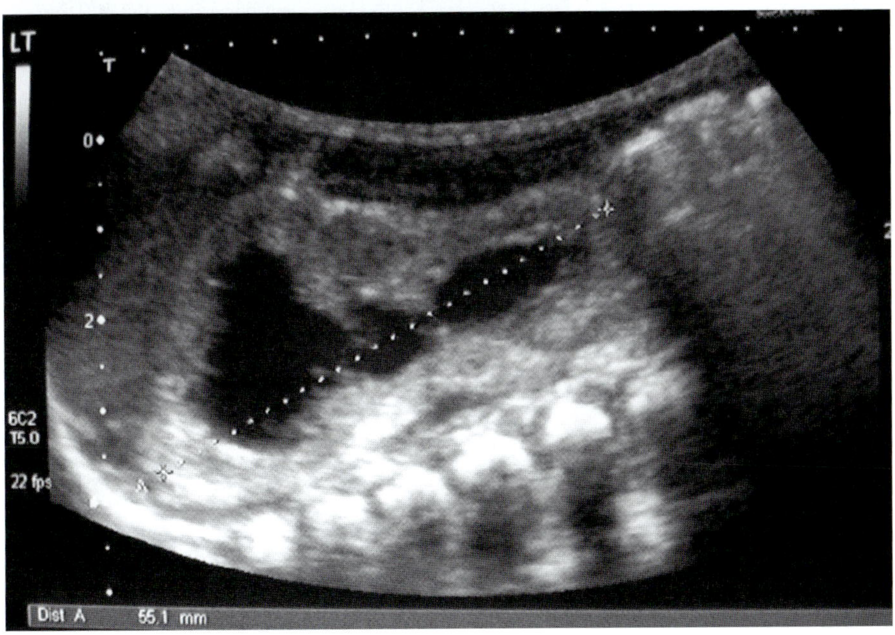

Fig. 1.28 Grade 4 hydronephrosis on renal ultrasound

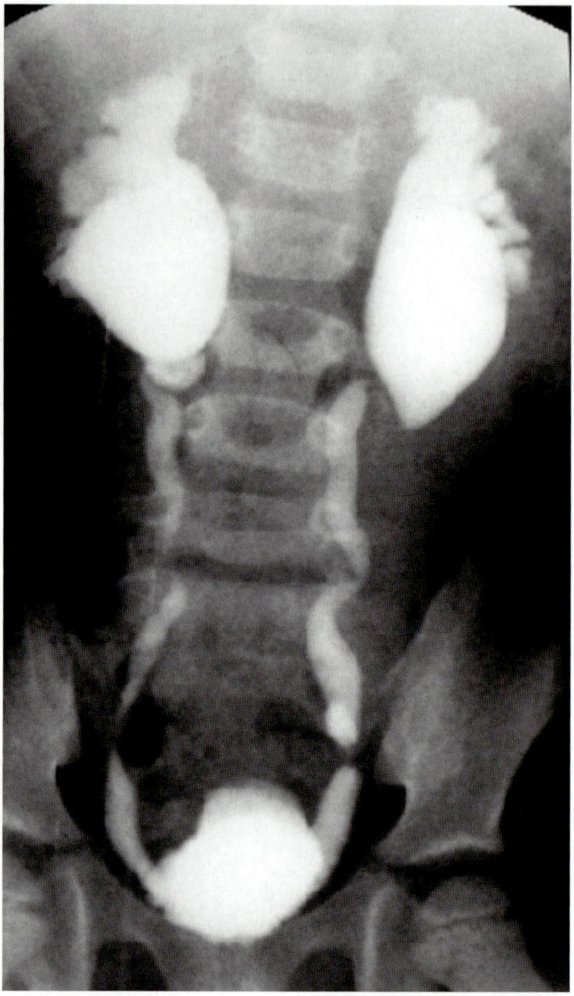

Fig. 1.29 VCUG – bilateral grade 4 VUR

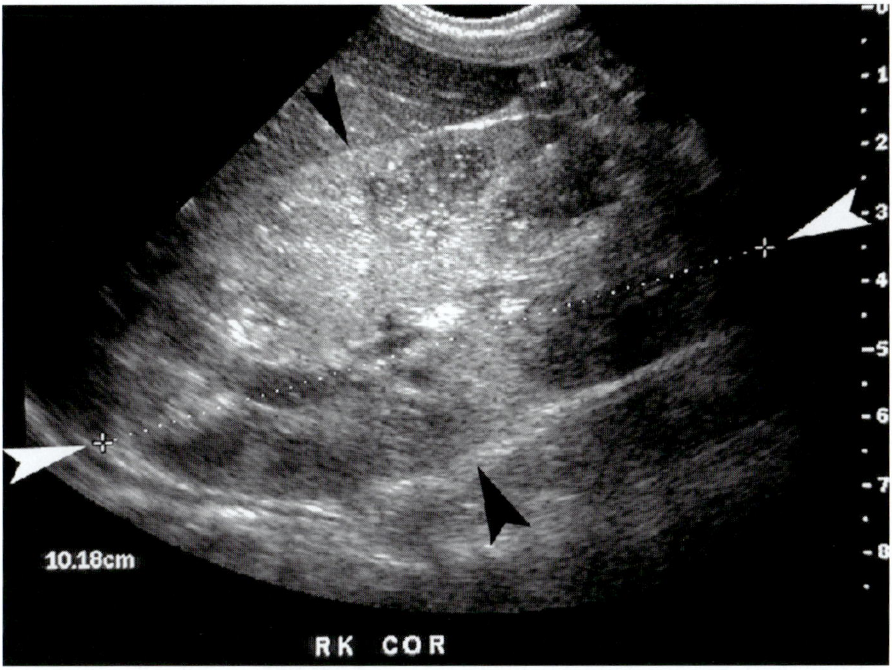

Fig. 1.30 ARPKD on renal ultrasound

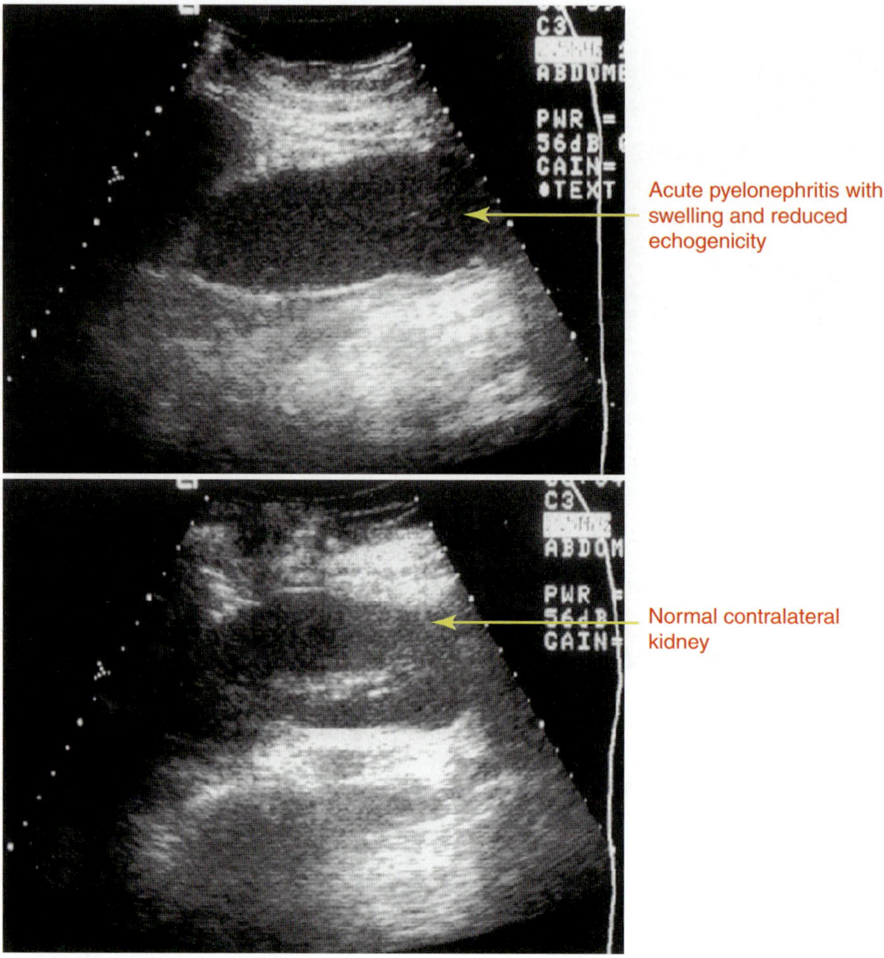

Fig. 1.32 Ultrasound – acute pyelonephritis

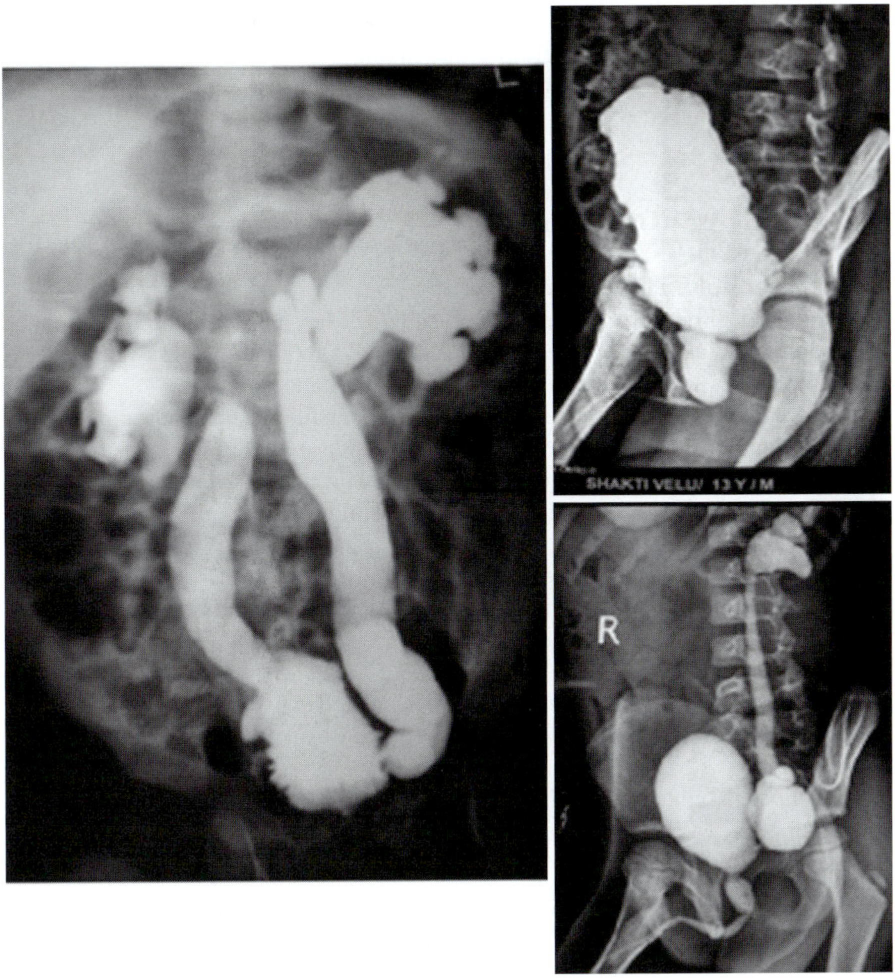

Fig. 1.33 VCUG – posterior urethral valves with VUR

1.8 Molecular Genetics

Gregor Mendel established the principle of classical genetics in the early nineteenth century. Using the classical garden pea experiment, he found that physical characteristics were transmitted by "hereditary units" from one generation to the next in a specific manner. These "hereditary units" are called the genes. Thomas Hunt and his colleagues developed the Mendelian chromosome theory of heredity based on their work on the fruit fly drosophila melanogaster. The discovery of the double helical structure of DNA in early 1950 by Watson and Crick and further experiments on microorganisms like viruses and bacteria marked the beginning of an era of molecular genetics. The regulation of gene expression was the main focus in the 1960s and 1970s. The technique of genetic engineering was developed to control and manipulate gene expression. The current era is focusing on large-scale genetics projects and on sequencing the entire genome.

1.8.1 Patterns of Inheritance

1.8.1.1 Mendelian Inheritance

Single-gene disorders follow inheritance pattern. They may be inherited as autosomal dominant, autosomal recessive, or X-linked dominant or recessive traits.

Examples of various patterns of Mendelian inheritance are:

Autosomal dominant—Denys–Drash syndrome, nail–patella syndrome

Autosomal recessive—congenital nephrotic syndrome, Bartter syndrome

X-linked dominant—X-linked hypophosphatemic rickets, Alport syndrome

X-linked recessive—nephrogenic diabetes insipidus

1.8.1.2 Non-Mendelian Inheritance

Polygenic inheritance: In multifactorial genetic diseases, multiple genes interact with one another to produce a phenotypic trait (e.g., vesicoureteric reflux, type II diabetes).

Genomic imprinting: In these cases there is change in expression of function and a gene due to methylation or other modifications of DNA (e.g., Angelman syndrome).

Mitochondrial inheritance: Mitochondrial genes are inherited only from the mother (e.g., MELAS—myopathy, encephalopathy, lactic acidosis, and stroke-like episodes).

Strategies for Gene Discovery in Renal Diseases

There is a need to identify genes that predispose to renal disease progression or provide renoprotection. Various genetics tools are available to identify potential candidate genes for renal disease and for determining whether these genes actually contribute to disease. Table 1.2 gives an overview of various tools employed for identification of candidate genes.

Genes Involved in Human Renal Diseases

Candidate genes involved in many renal diseases like tubular disorders, inherited glomerular diseases, and nephrotic syndrome have been discovered, but they represent only a small fraction of total spectrum of renal diseases. The most common types of renal disease are the result of a complex interplay between multiple genetic and environmental factors. A meta-analysis of several linkage studies revealed regions on human chromosome 6p21.1–q15 and 20p11–q13.13 associated with systemic lupus erythematosus. Similarly, genome-wide linkage studies of familial IgA nephropathy have identified susceptibility loci on chromosomes 6q22–

Table 1.2 Overview of tools for the identification of candidate genes

Tool	Purpose	Advantages	Limitations
Gene expression array	To profile gene expression	Yields limited number of candidates from genome wide	Complex statistical analysis required
Linkage analysis	To identify a gene or genetic region that has a large effect on phenotype	Can detect causal relationship between genotype and phenotype	Requires rare families
Association analysis	To identify common susceptibility variants of underlying disease	Suitable for study of complex diseases	Large cohorts required, leading to higher costs
Genome-wide analysis study	To identify genetic factors that influence common, complex diseases	High throughput Covers the whole genome	Large number of participants needed

23, 2q36, 4q26–31, 17q12–22, and 3p24–23. Renal injury with a monogenic cause represents only a small fraction of the total spectrum of renal diseases. The Appendix gives a comprehensive overview of genes that have been associated with various renal diseases.

Molecular Genetic Evaluation of Kidney Disease

Hereditary renal diseases comprise an important part of pediatric nephrology. Over 30 different diseases of the kidney have been traced to specific mutant genes, and it is likely that we will continue to identify additional monogenic diseases as well as variants of genes that confer susceptibility to renal disease. Thus, molecular genetics evaluation has become part of the standard of care, in selected situations where the cost of testing may be warranted by the additional information. One example is the identification of hereditary FSGS forms caused by mutant podocyte slit diaphragm genes; in these cases renal transplantation can proceed without high risk of

Example 1. COL4A5 (gene) c.1563A>G p. R554Q (exon 48)

The usual mRNA nucleotide at position A1408 has been substituted by a G. This creates a missense mutation converting an arginine to a glutamine in the glomerular basement membrane collagen protein Col4A5. This missense mutation is pathogenic, since it has been reported in other cases of Alport syndrome.

Example 2. CTNS (gene) c. 198_218del (exon5)

This microdeletion has produced an in-frame deletion of 21 nucleotides from position 198 through 218. This causes a deletion of 7 amino acids in the cystinosis protein. Since the remainder of the protein is intact, it has been reported in association with a milder (juvenile) form of cystinosis.

recurrent disease in the allograft. In severe renal conditions such as recessive polycystic kidney disease or cystinosis, where one affected child has been identified, molecular diagnosis may allow accurate antenatal diagnosis for family planning. Similarly, in conditions such as nephrogenic diabetes insipidus, the risk for future pregnancies may be precise molecular diagnosis to distinguish the X-linked (mutant vasopressin receptor) and autosomal recessive (mutant aquaporin II) forms of the disease. Finally, molecular diagnosis may allow precise early diagnosis of conditions such as Alport syndrome where early medical intervention is thought to improve prognosis. Since few medical centers can support complete laboratory testing for all renal genetic diseases, it is important to gain familiarity with the many commercialized laboratories worldwide that provide these services. An important gateway to these laboratories is provided by the website www.genetests.org, which allows access to about 600 laboratories covering over 2,000 diseases and providing useful clinical and scientific background information on each specific genetic disease.

Samples for DNA Analysis

The most widely used tissue for DNA analysis are the leukocytes in the blood. However, DNA extracted from cultured fibroblasts, oral swabs, hair, and solid tissue samples are increasingly analyzed by many laboratories. A typical procedure for molecular genetic testing is:

1. Discuss implications with family and obtain written informed consent after considering how the information will be used. Many laboratories provide consent forms and assure that the DNA will not be used for other purposes. A plan for counselling the family is recommended.
2. Submit application form to the laboratory, providing synopsis of clinical history and specifying specific test required. A decision should be made as to whether analysis should include (a) sequencing of all exons plus flanking sequences, (b) test for deletions, and (c) screen for only the most common known mutations.
3. Obtain 3–5 ml of whole blood (usually in an EDTA-containing tube) and ship at room temperature to the chosen laboratory within several days.

Molecular Genetics Report

Most laboratories provide a detailed report of the analysis with comparison to background information in their databank of previously identified disease-associated mutations. In most cases, this allows the laboratory to distinguish between benign polymorphisms in the gene sequence and causative mutations. Likely coding sequence mutations are reported in two formats indicating (a) the alteration in the mRNA sequence and (b) the impact on the protein sequence:

When genetic testing does not identify a mutation in the expected gene, the presumptive diagnosis may be incorrect. However, like any laboratory test, there may be other explanations for a negative result:

1. The diagnosis is correct, but the causative mutation does not lie within the coding sequence.

2. If analysis for a deletion has not been performed, the reported "normal" gene sequence comes from the other allele. Thus, the patient carries a heterozygous deletion that cannot be detected by sequence analysis alone.
3. The clinical diagnosis may be correct, but the disease is genetically heterogenous and is caused by an alternative mutant gene in the same pathway or molecular complex.

Genetically Inherited Renal Diseases

See the tables below for various genetically inherited renal diseases.

1.8.2 Nephrotic Syndrome (NS)

1.8.2.1 Isolated NS

Condition	Gene (location)	Protein	Inheritance
Congenital nephrotic syndrome	NPHS1 (19q13.1)	Nephrin	Recessive
Focal segmental glomerulosclerosis	NPHS2 (1q 25-31)	Podocin	Recessive
Focal segmental glomerulosclerosis/ diffuse mesangial sclerosis	NPHS3	Epsilon	Recessive
Focal segmental glomerulosclerosis	ACTN4 (19q13)	α-Actinin 4	Dominant
Steroid-sensitive nephrotic syndrome	Gene located on 2p12-13.2		Recessive

1.8.2.2 Syndromic NS

Denys–Drash syndrome	WT1 (11p13)	WT1 protein	Dominant
Frasier syndrome	WT1 (11p13)	WT1 protein	Dominant
Nail–patella syndrome	LMX1B (9q34)	LIM-homeodomain protein	Dominant

WT1 Wilms' tumor suppressor gene

1.8.2.3 Renal Tubular Acidosis

Primary proximal (type 2) with ocular abnormalities	SLC4A4(4q21)	NBC-1	Recessive
Primary distal (type 1) isolated	SLC4A1(17q21)	AE1	Dominant
With deafness (dRTA1)	ATP6B1	B1 subunit	Recessive
Without deafness(dRTA2)	ATP6N1B(7q33)	116 kd subunit	Recessive
Combined proximal and distal (type3) with osteopetrosis	CA2(8q22)	CA II	Recessive
Hyperkalemic RTA (type 4) pseudohypoaldosteronism type1 renal form	MLR(4q31.1)	Mineralocorticoid receptor	Dominant
Multiorgan form	SNCC1B (16p12) SNCC1A(12p13)	B-ENaC alpha-ENaC	Recessive Recessive

1.8.2.4 Bartter Syndrome

Type 1	SLC12A1 (15q15)	NKCC2	Recessive
Type 2	KCNJ1 (11q21-25)	ROMK	Recessive
Type 3	CLCNKB (1p36)	ClCN-Kb	Recessive
Type 4	BSND (1p31)	Barttin	Recessive
Type 5	CaSR (3q13.3)	CaR	Dominant

SLC12A3 solute carrier family12, member1, *NKCC2* sodium/potassium/chloride transporters, *ROMK* renal outer medullary potassium channel, *CLCN-B* basolateral chloride channel, *CaSR* calcium sensing receptor, *CaR* membrane receptor for Ca

1.8.2.5 Hypomagnesemia

Gitelman syndrome	SLC12A3, CLCNKB(1p3)	NCC ClCN-Kb	Recessive Recessive
Hypomagnesemia with hypercalciuria and nephrocalcinosis	PCLN1 (3q27)	Caludin16/ Paracellin-1	Recessive
Hypomagnesemia with secondary hypocalcemia	TRPM6(9q22)	TRPM6 ion channel	Recessive
Familial hypocalciuric hypercalcemia	CaSR (3q21)	CaSR	Dominant

SLC12A3 solute carrier family12, member3, *NCC* NaCl cotransporter, *CLCN-B* basolateral chloride channel

1.8.2.6 Nephrogenic Diabetes Insipidus

More common	AVPR2(Xq28) AQP2(12Q13)	V2 R AQP2	Recessive Recessive/dominant

V2R vasopressin receptor, *AQP2* aquaporin 2

1.8.2.7 Central Diabetes Insipidus

Idiopathic	AVP(20p13)	AVP	Not known

AVP arginine vasopressin

1.8.2.8 Dent's Disease

Type 1	CLCN5 (Xp11.22)	ClC 5	Recessive
Type 2 X-linked	OCRL (Xp26)		Recessive
Hypophosphatemic rickets	CLCN5 (Xp11.22)	ClC 5	Recessive

ClC 5 chloride channel 5

1.8.2.9 Hemolytic Uremic Syndrome

C3 anomaly	HF1 (1q32)	Complement factor H
I factor	CFI(4q25)	C3b inactivator
CD 46	MCP(1q32)	Membrane cofactor
vWF cleaving protease	ADAMTS(9q34)	vWFcp

vWF von Willebrand factor

1.8.2.10 Monogenic Forms of Hypertension

Condition	Gene (location)	Protein	Inheritance
FH-1	11-βOH+CYP11B2 (8q)	Aldosterone	Dominant
FH-II	(7p22)	Aldosterone	Dominant
CAH (DOC oversecretion)	CYP11B1,CYP17	DOC	Recessive
AME	11β-HSD-2	11β-HSD-2	Recessive
Liddle's syndrome	β- or γ-ENaC(16p)	ENaC	Dominant
Pseudohypoaldosteronism type 2 (Gordon syndrome)	WNK1(12p13.3)	WNK1 kinase	Dominant

FH familial hyperaldosteronism, *DOC* deoxycorticosterone, *CAH* congenital adrenal hyperplasia, *AME* apparent mineralocorticoid excess, *ENaC* epithelial sodium channel

1.8.3 Cystic Kidney Diseases

1.8.3.1 Polycystic Kidney Disease

Recessive	PKHD1(6p21)	Fibrocystin	Recessive
	PKD1(16p13.3)	Polycystin 1	Dominant
Dominant	PKD2 (4q21)	Polycystin 2	Dominant
	PKD3 (8q)		Dominant

1.8.3.2 Nephronophthisis

Infantile	NPHP2 (9q21)	Inversin	Recessive
Juvenile tapetoretinal degeneration	NPHP1(2q13)	Nephrocystin 1	Recessive
	NPHP4(1p36)	Recessive with nephrocystin 4	
Adolescent (late onset)	NPHP3(3q22)	Nephrocystin 3	Recessive
With taporetinal degeneration	NPHP5(3q13)		Recessive
Without hyperuricemia	MCDK1(1q21)		Dominant
With hyperuricemia	MCDK2(16p12)	Uromodulin	Dominant

1.8.3.3 Alport Syndrome

Alport syndrome	COL4A5 (Xp22.3)	Dominant
	COL4A3, COL4A4 (2q36)	Recessive/dominant

1.8.3.4 List of Human Malformation Syndromes with Kidney Hypoplasia/Dysplasia

Gene	Human syndrome	Kidney phenotype
JAG1, NOTCH2	Alagille syndrome	MCDK, kidney dysplasia
BBS1-BBS11	Bardet–Biedl syndrome	Renal dysplasia and calyceal malformations
EYA1, SIX1, SIX2	Branchiootorenal syndrome	Renal agenesis/dysplasia
Del. 22q11	DiGeorge syndrome	Renal agenesis, dysplasia, VUR
GATA3	Hypothyroidism, sensorial deafness anomalies (HDR)	Renal agenesis, VUR, dysplasia
KALL1, FGFR1	Kallmann's syndrome	Renal agenesis, dysplasia
PAX2	Renal coloboma syndrome	Renal hypoplasia, MCDK, VUR
TCF2	Renal cysts and diabetes syndrome	Renal dysplasia, cysts
SALL1	Townes–Brocks syndrome	Renal dysplasia, lower urinary tract malformations
LMX1B	Nail–patella syndrome	Glomerulus malformation, renal agenesis

1.8.3.5 Common Chromosomal Disorders Associated with Renal Agenesis/Hypoplasia

Chromosomal disorders	Other associated anomalies
Patau syndrome (trisomy 13)	Holoprosencephaly, midline anomalies, cleft lip/palate
Miller–Dieker syndrome (17p13 deletion)	MR, lissencephaly, microgyria, agyria, typical facie
Edward syndrome (trisomy 18) 18q deletion	IUGR, CHD, clenched hands, rocker bottom feet SS, MR, microcephaly, narrow external ear canals, long hands
Down syndrome (trisomy 21)	MR, hypotonia, CHD, typical face, clinodactyly
Cat-eye syndrome (tetrasomy 22p)	MR, CHD, colobomas, anal/digital anomalies

Suggested Reading

Dalton RN, Haycock GB (1999) Laboratory investigation. In: Barrat TM, Avner ED, We H (eds) Pediatric nephrology, 4th edn. Williams and Wilkins, Baltimore, pp 343–364

Fogazzi GB Bedside urinary microscopy. Available from URL: http://ndt-educational.org. Accessed 27 Aug 2012

Langlois V (2008) Laboratory evaluation in different ages. In: Geary DF, Schaefer F (eds) Comprehensive pediatric nephrology, 1st edn. Mosby Inc, Philadelphia, pp 39–54

Fluids, Electrolytes, and Acid–Base Disorders

2

Anil Vasudevan and Kishore Phadke

2.1 Acid Base and the Kidney

2.1.1 Interpretation of Blood Gas Abnormalities

2.1.1.1 Overview of Acid–Base Physiology

Under normal condition, 1–3 mmol/kg/day acid is produced in infants and children. Despite the continuous production of acid in the body, the normal pH of the body is maintained over a narrow range (7.35–7.45). As dictated by the Henderson–Hasselbalch equation, $[H^+] = 24 \times PCO_2 / [HCO_3^-]$, disturbances in either the respiratory component (PCO_2) or metabolic component (HCO_3^-) can lead to alterations in pH. Low HCO_3 or high PCO_2 results in acidemia. Likewise an alkalemia can result from either a high HCO_3^- or low PCO_2. Thus, there are four primary disturbances of acid–base balance: metabolic acidosis (too little HCO_3^-), respiratory acidosis (too much PCO_2), metabolic alkalosis (too much HCO_3^-), and respiratory alkalosis (too little PCO_2).

The body's response to a change in acid–base status has two components: The first and immediate defense is buffering. The most important buffer in the body is HCO_3^-. Others include phosphate, hemoglobin, bones, and proteins like albumin. About 60 % of buffering occurs intracellularly (by protein, phosphate, and bicarbonate buffers), and 40 % occurs extracellularly (by bicarbonate & protein buffers). Since buffering has a limited capacity, the extra H^+ ions must be excreted in order to

A. Vasudevan (✉) • K. Phadke
Department of Pediatric Nephrology,
Children's Kidney Care Center, St. John's Medical College Hospital,
Koramangala, Bangalore, KA 560078, India

Department of Pediatrics, Children's Kidney Care Center,
St. John's Medical College Hospital, Koramangala,
Bangalore, KA 560078, India
e-mail: anil.vasudevan@sjri.res.in, anilvasu@hotmail.com; kishorephadke@yahoo.co.in

K. Phadke et al. (eds.), *Manual of Pediatric Nephrology*,
DOI 10.1007/978-3-642-12483-9_2,

Table 2.1 Compensation in various primary acid–base disorders

Primary disturbance	Compensatory disturbance
Metabolic acidosis	Increased ventilation
Metabolic alkalosis	Decreased ventilation
Respiratory acidosis	Increased reabsorption of HCO_3 in the proximal tubule, increased renal excretion of H^+ in the distal tubule
Respiratory alkalosis	Decreased reabsorption of HCO_3 in the proximal tubule, decreased renal excretion of H^+ in the distal tubule

maintain acid–base homeostasis, and both the lungs and kidneys form the second defense. The lungs can remove excess CO_2 formed from H^+ and HCO_3^- in the presence of an acid load. The kidney's role in regulation of acid–base balance involves reabsorption of filtered HCO_3^- and generation of new HCO_3^- following ammonia generation. In addition, the H^+ ions are excreted as titrable acids in the urine.

Thus, in presence of a primary acid–base disorder, the body's defense mechanism triggers a compensatory response that attempts to return the pH towards normal. Primary changes in PCO_2 (respiratory disorder) invoke secondary changes in HCO_3^-, and primary changes in HCO_3^- (metabolic disorder) elicit secondary changes in PCO_2 (see Table 2.1). The metabolic and respiratory compensations can also be predicted using simple equations or nomogram (see Table 2.3, Fig 2.2). It is important to realize that respiratory compensation for metabolic disorders occur rapidly while metabolic compensation for respiratory disorders takes 3–5 days.

2.1.2 Arterial Blood Gas Analysis

2.1.2.1 General Aspects

Arterial blood gas (ABG) analysis is an essential part of diagnosing and managing a patient's oxygenation status and acid–base balance. However, the interpretation of ABG includes a good history and physical examination. Often the presenting symptoms and signs give us a clue regarding the underlying acid–base disorder.

Blood gas machine and CO-oximeter are required to get all the parameters for complete blood gas analysis. Blood gas machine measures pH, PCO_2, and PO_2; the HCO_3 value is derived from the measured parameters. A more direct measurement of bicarbonate is obtained from determining the total venous carbon dioxide (TCO_2). Dissolved carbon dioxide is almost exclusively in the form of bicarbonate, and for practical purposes, the total carbon dioxide content is equivalent (±3 mEq/l) to the bicarbonate concentration. The CO-oximeter can measure the hemoglobin content (in gm/dl) and values related to hemoglobin binding: O_2 saturation (SaO_2), carboxyl hemoglobin (% COHb), methemoglobin (% MethHb). The arterial oxygen content (CaO_2) is calculated from these parameters.

2.1.2.2 Collecting Blood Sample for ABG

Arterial blood gas sampling represents the gold standard method for acquiring patients' acid–base status, and the preferred sites for collection are radial and posterior tibial arteries. Femoral, brachial, and dorsalis pedis arteries should be avoided. Capillary (CBG) and venous (VBG) blood gas samplings may be useful alternatives since these are easier to obtain and are less invasive way of evaluating acid–base status. Various studies have shown significant correlation in pH, PCO_2, PO_2, BE (base excess), and HCO_3 among ABG, VBG, and CBG values. However, PO_2 especially in presence of hypotension may not reflect the actual values in CBG and VBG.

Blood should be collected in a low-friction syringe designed to fill under arterial pressure. Excessive heparin and air bubbles should be expressed from the syringe before collection. Excess heparin may decrease PCO_2 and HCO_3, while air in the sample changes the PO_2 and PCO_2 thereby affecting pH. The sample should be refrigerated if analysis is delayed by more than few minutes.

2.1.2.3 Terminologies

- Acidemia: blood pH <7.35.
- Acidosis: a pathologic process that causes an increase in H^+ ion concentration by increasing PCO_2 or by reducing HCO_3^-.
- Alkalemia: blood pH >7.45.
- Alkalosis: a pathologic process that causes a decrease in H^+ ion concentration by reducing PCO_2 or by increasing HCO_3.
- Simple acid–base disorders: disorders that are either metabolic or respiratory.
- Mixed acid–base disorders: more than one acid–base disturbance present resulting in pH being normal or abnormal. Though acidosis and alkalosis usually lead to acidemia and alkalemia, respectively, a mixed acid–base disorder may lead to a normal pH or a mixed picture.
- Base excess (BE): defined as the number of milliequivalents of acid or base that are needed to titrate 1 l blood to pH 7.40 at 37 °C while the PCO_2 is held constant at 40 mmHg. A typical reference range is –3.0 to +3.0 mEq/l. A negative sign indicates base deficit.

2.1.2.4 Calculations

Various calculations are commonly used in interpreting acid–base disorders and distinguishing between different causes of acid–base disorders. These include anion gap, urinary anion gap, osmolar gap, delta ratio, urine–blood PCO_2 gradient, and fractional excretion of HCO_3. The anion gap and the delta ratio are described below. For others, please refer to Sect. 1.5.

Anion Gap (AG)

AG is defined as the difference between the plasma concentrations of the measured plasma cation (Na^+, K^+) and the measured anions (Cl^-, HCO_3^-). The gap composed of unmeasured anions usually is due to the negatively charged plasma proteins.

- The anion gap is estimated by subtracting the sum of Cl^- and HCO_3^- concentrations from the plasma Na concentration.
- $\text{Anion Gap} = (Na^+) - ([Cl^-] + HCO_3^-)$.
- The normal AG is 8–16 mEq/l (or mmol/l in SI units).

- Because negatively charged plasma proteins account for the normal anion gap, Formatting the normal values should be adjusted for patients with hypoalbuminemia.
- Corrected $AG = (Na^+) - [(Cl^-) + HCO_3^-)] + 2.5 \times [4.0 - \text{measured albumin}\,(g/dl)]$.
- Causes of a low anion gap include a laboratory error, hypoalbuminemia, hypercalcemia, hyperkalemia, hypermagnesemia, lithium toxicity, and multiple myeloma.
- If the anion gap is >20 mEq/l, there is a primary metabolic acidosis regardless of pH or serum bicarbonate concentration. The causes of normal and high anion gap acidosis are discussed in Sect. 2.1.3.

Delta Ratio (Δ/Δ) (see Table 2.3)

Delta ratio = change in anion gap (Δ anion gap)/change in HCO_3 (ΔHCO_3)

$$\frac{\text{Measured anion gap} - \text{normal anion gap}}{\text{Normal}\,[HCO_3] - \text{measured}\,[HCO_3^-]} \text{ OR } \frac{(AG - 12)}{(24 - [HCO_3])}$$

2.1.2.5 Normal Values of ABG

- pH: 7.35–7.45.
- Partial pressure of oxygen (PO_2): 80–100 mmHg
- CO_2 dissolved in arterial blood (PCO_2): 35–40 mmHg
- Calculated value of the amount of HCO_3: 22–24 mEq/l or mmol/l in SI units

Base Excess (BE)	±3 mEq/l
Arterial oxygen saturation (SaO_2)	95–100 %

2.1.2.6 Interpreting a Blood Gas

Step 1: Comprehensive history, clinical examination, and laboratory data

- Clinical information: History and physical examination with emphasis on patient's respiratory rate and vital signs, degree of respiratory effort, mental status, and state of tissue perfusion
- Information about patient's immediate environment: FiO_2 (fraction of oxygen in inspired air)
- Additional laboratory data: Serum electrolytes, blood sugar, BUN, hemoglobin or hematocrit, chest x-ray, and previous ABG reports

Step 2: Look at the pH. Is it acidosis or alkalosis?

- The process that caused pH to shift to whichever side is the primary abnormality because body does not fully compensate for primary acid–base disorders.
- When the pH is below 7.35, the blood is said to be acidic due to elevated PCO_2 (respiratory acidosis) or a lowered bicarbonate (metabolic acidosis).

- When pH is above 7.45, the blood is said to be alkalotic due to lowered PCO_2 (respiratory alkalosis) or a raised bicarbonate (metabolic alkalosis).
- pH may be normal in the presence of a mixed acid–base disorder, particularly if PCO_2 and HCO_3 are abnormal.

Step 3: Look at PCO_2 and HCO_3. Is it primary metabolic or respiratory problem?

Metabolic acidosis: pH <7.35 and HCO_3 <22
Respiratory acidosis: pH <7.35 and PCO_2 >40
Metabolic alkalosis: pH >7.45 and HCO_3 >24
Respiratory alkalosis: pH >7.45 and PCO_2 <35

- Use the direction of pH change to identify the primary change.
- In simple acid–base disorders, both PCO_2 and HCO_3 values are abnormal, and direction of the abnormal change is the same for both parameters (one value will be the initial change and the other will be the compensatory response).
- If pH and PCO_2 are moving in opposite directions, then the problem is primarily respiratory.
- If pH and HCO_3 are moving in the same direction, then the problem is primarily metabolic.

Step 4: Calculate the degree of compensation. Is it a simple uncompensated/-compensated disturbance or a mixed disturbance?

- Use the appropriate formula to determine the degree of compensation (Table 2.2).
- The initial change and the compensatory response move in the same direction.
- If changes occur beyond the predicted values of expected compensation, a mixed disorder should be suspected.

Step 5: Is it acute or chronic respiratory process?

- If the ABG is suggestive of a primary respiratory process, determine the extent of compensation to determine if it is acute or chronic (Table 2.2).
- Acute respiratory acidosis is a medical emergency that may require emergent intubation and mechanical ventilation, whereas chronic respiratory acidosis is often a clinically stable condition.

Step 6: Calculate the anion gap.

- Anion gap > than 16 is suggestive of high anion gap metabolic acidosis.
- If AG is >35, suspect a mixed disorder of metabolic acidosis and metabolic alkalosis.

Step 7: Calculate delta ratio. Determine if other acid–base disorders are present.

- Delta ratio compares the change in the anion gap to the change in bicarbonate (Table 2.3).
- However, always check for other evidences to support the diagnosis, and an unexpected value without any other evidence should always be interpreted with great caution.

Step 8: Generate a differential diagnosis.

Table 2.2 Compensatory responses in simple acid–base disorders

Primary disorder	Initial change	Compensatory response	Expected compensation
Metabolic acidosis[1]	$\downarrow HCO_3$	$\downarrow PCO_2$	$PCO_2 \approx 1.5[HCO_3^-]+8^{@}$ $\downarrow PCO_2 = 1.2 \times \Delta[HCO_3^-]$
Metabolic alkalosis	$- HCO_3^-$	$\uparrow PCO_2$	$PCO_2 \approx 0.9[HCO_3^-]+16$ $- PCO_2 = 0.6 \times \Delta[HCO_3^-]$
Respiratory acidosis[2]	$\uparrow PCO_2$	$\uparrow HCO_3$	For every 10 mmHg Δ in PCO_2, $HCO_3^- \downarrow$ by 1 mEq/l (acute), 4 mEq/l (chronic)
Respiratory alkalosis[3]	$\downarrow PCO_2$	$\downarrow HCO_3$	For every 10 mmHg Δ in PCO_2, HCO_3^- – by 2 mEq/l (acute), 4 mEq/l (chronic)

[1]PCO_2 = last 2 digits of pH
[2]$\downarrow pH = 0.008 \times \Delta PCO_2$ (acute), $\downarrow pH = 0.003 \times \Delta PCO_2$ (chronic)
[3]$\uparrow pH = 0.008 \times \Delta PCO_2$ (acute), $\uparrow pH = 0.003 \times \Delta PCO_2$ (chronic)
[@]Winter's formula

Table 2.3 Interpretation of delta ratio

Delta ratio	Interpretation guideline
<0.4	Hyperchloremic normal anion gap acidosis
0.4–1	High and normal anion gap acidosis Acidosis associated with renal failure
1–2	Uncomplicated high anion gap acidosis Lactic acidosis: average value 1.6 DKA: more likely to have a ratio closer to 1
>2	Suggests a preexisting elevated HCO_3 level so consider a concurrent metabolic alkalosis or a preexisting compensated respiratory acidosis

2.1.2.7 The Summary of Approach to ABG Interpretation

- Check pH.
- Check PCO_2/HCO_3.
- Select the appropriate compensation formula and determine if compensation is appropriate.
- Check the anion gap (correct for hypoalbuminemia).
- If the anion gap is elevated, check the delta ratio.
- Generate a differential diagnosis.

2.1.2.8 Using the Nomogram for the Diagnosis of Acid–Base Disorder

Acid base map may be used as an adjuvant in the diagnosis of acid–base disturbances. A set of confidence bands that represent data for middle 95 % of patients are projected as a graph. The map plots the six zones corresponding to the six primary acid–base (see the Fig. 2.1 below) disturbances and a seventh central zone corresponding to normal.

2.1.2.9 Case Example

A 6-year-old child is hospitalized with severe diarrhea and vomiting. Physical examination revealed severe dehydration and tachypnea. The laboratory investigations are as follows:

ABG: pH 7.12, PCO_2 15 mmHg, HCO_3 4 mmol/l, PO_2 82 mmHg
Serum chemistry: Na 140 mmol/l, K 4 mmol/l, Cl 115 mmol/l, BUN 8.92 mmol/l, Cr 114.4 mmol/l

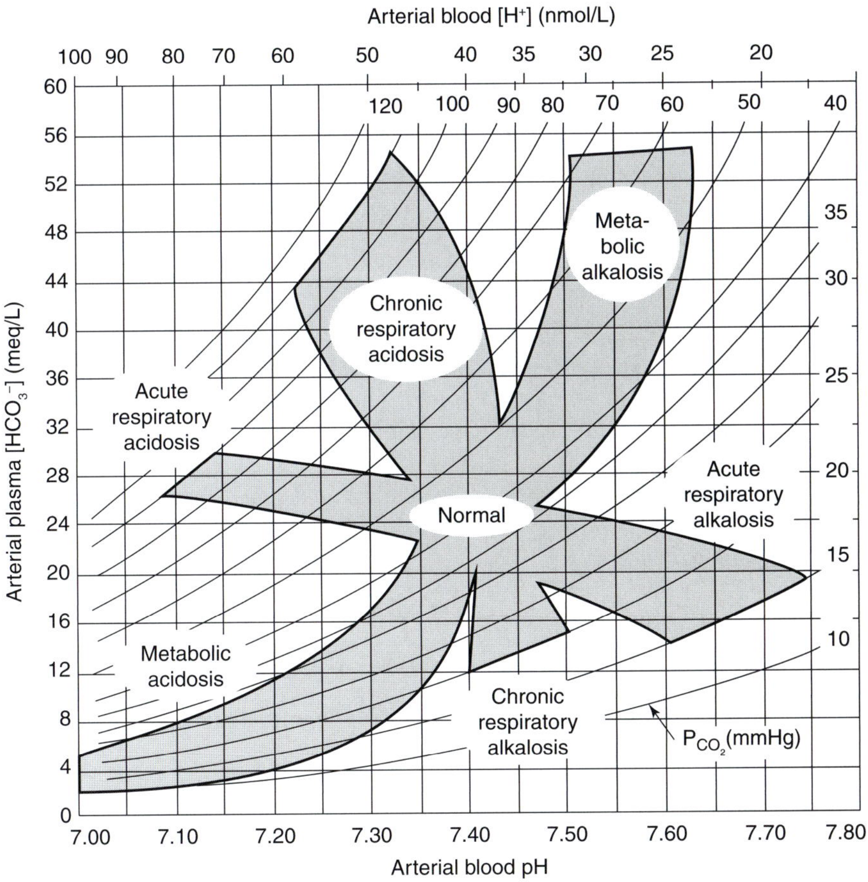

Fig. 2.1 Acid–base nomogram. Shown are the 95 % confidence limits of the normal respiratory and metabolic compensations for primary acid–base disturbances (From Cogan MG (editor): Fluid and Electrolytes: Physiology and Pathophysiology. Appleton & Lange, 1991)

Step 1: *History and clinical examination*

Based on the clinical scenario, the child is severely hypovolemic secondary to diarrhea and has acute kidney injury (AKI) secondary to hypovolemia. The tachypnea may suggest hyperventilation as a compensatory response to metabolic acidosis.

Step 2: *Look at the pH.*

The pH is low (<7.35); hence, the child is *acidemic*.

Step 3: *Look at* PCO_2 *and* HCO_3.

Low PCO_2 suggests alkalosis which is not consistent with pH, whereas a low HCO_3 represents acidosis and is consistent with the pH. Hence low HCO_3^- is the initial change suggesting a primary metabolic acidosis.

Both PCO_2 and HCO_3 values are abnormal, and direction of the abnormal change is the same direction indicating the presence of a simple acid–base disorder.

Step 4: *Calculate the degree of compensation.*

The low PCO_2 is the compensatory response. Apply the formula given in Table 2.2 to calculate the compensation.

Expected PCO_2 (Winter's formula) $= 1.5\,[4] + 8 = 14$

Using the alternative formula, $\Delta PCO_2 = 1.2 \times \Delta HCO_3 = 1.2 \times (24 - 4) = 24$

Expected $PCO_2 = 40 - 24 = 16$

The compensation is appropriate.

Step 5: *Calculate the anion gap.*

The anion gap is $Na - \left(Cl + HCO_3^-\right) = 140 - (115 + 4) = 21$

The anion gap is high, suggestive of high anion gap metabolic acidosis.

In diarrhea we would expect hyperchloremic normal anion gap metabolic acidosis.

To identify the second disorder, proceed to the next step.

Step 6: *Calculate delta ratio.*

$$\frac{(\Delta \text{Anion gap})}{(\Delta HCO_3)} = \frac{(AG - 12)}{(24 - HCO_3)} = \frac{21 - 12}{24 - 4} = \frac{9}{20} = 0.45$$

Since the delta ratio is between 0.4 and 1, we can infer that there is a concurrent normal and high anion gap metabolic acidosis.

Step 7: *Generate a differential diagnosis*

The child has mixed elevated and normal anion gap metabolic acidosis due to diarrhea and acute kidney injury.

2.1.2.10 Physiochemical Approach to Acid–Base Disorders (Stewart's Approach)

Traditional paradigms of acid–base abnormalities rely on the Henderson–Hasselbalch equation to determine the pH and H^+ proton concentration. Steward's approach is not traditional and is too cumbersome for use in day-to-day practice. Stewart et al. described independent determinants of H^+ concentration and pH, enabling the clinician to understand the genesis of each acid–base disturbance. The goal of the Stewart approach is to establish the quantitative relationships that determine $[H^+]$ in any aqueous solution and is based on the principle that **a**n aqueous solution contains the same number of negative and positive charges.

Stewart identified three independent control mechanisms for pH: SID, PCO_2, and ATOT (Table 2.4). All the independent variables are present in concentrations on the order of millimoles or milliequivalents, and their interaction with water dictates the amount of free hydrogen ions, the concentration of which is in the order of nanomoles. Bicarbonate is a dependent variable and as such does not determine the pH which is contrary to the traditional approach of reliance upon bicarbonate as a determinant of the pH.

The physiochemical approach of Stewart depends upon the relationships between ions that completely dissociate at physiologic pH called "strong ions" (cations – Na^+, K^+, Ca^{2+}, and Mg^{2+}; anions – Cl^-, lactate, and sulfate). Normally, strong ion difference, i.e., difference between strong cation and anion (SID), is net strong ion positive (+40). Sodium and chloride are the principal contributors to the strong ion difference.

To maintain the charge balance and normal pH, SID is counterbalanced by an equal and opposing charge termed the effective strong ion difference (SIDe) and is mainly constituted by plasma proteins (~78 % albumin) and phosphate (~20 %). The sum of these weak acids is known as ATOT.

Table 2.4 Variables used in Stewart approach

$\mathrm{SID} = \left[\mathrm{Na^+} + \mathrm{K^+} + \mathrm{Ca^{2+}} + \mathrm{Mg^{2+}}\right] - [\mathrm{Cl^-} + \text{other strong anions}] = 40\ \mathrm{mEq}^{a}$
$\mathrm{SIDe} = \left[\mathrm{HCO_3}^- + \text{charge on albumin} + \text{charge on } \mathrm{PO_4}^- + \text{other weak acids}\right] = 40\ \mathrm{mEq}$
$\mathrm{ATOT} = \text{charge on albumin} + \text{charge on } \mathrm{PO_4^{-2}}$
SIG = SID – SIDe
PCO_2 = carbonic acid content $(H_2CO_3)^c$

SID strong ion difference, *ATOT* total weak acids, *SIG* strong ion gap, PCO_2 partial pressure of carbon dioxide

[a]↑SID will ↓H^+ liberation and cause metabolic alkalosis, ↓SID will ↑H^+ causing acidosis

[b]↓ albumin or PO_4 leads to metabolic alkalosis, ↑PO_4^- leads to metabolic acidosis

[c]Respiratory acidosis and alkalosis are caused by changes in PCO_2

The strong ion gap (SIG), the difference between [SID] and [SIDe], may be taken as an estimate of unmeasured ions and may be a better indicator of unmeasured anions than the anion gap. When SIG (SID–SIDe) = 0, the plasma pH is exactly 7.4 at a PCO_2 of 40 mmHg.

Change in SID+ is equal to base excess (BE) when nonvolatile buffers are held constant; BE is not equal to ΔSID+ when nonvolatile acids vary.

Six simultaneous equations (Fencl–Stewart equation) were constructed and solved for H^+.

Work by Figge's group has further modified the Fencl–Stewart equation for the base excess effect of albumin.

An alternative approach was developed by Story et al. They used two equations to calculate the effect of change in the sodium chloride component of the strong ion difference on the base excess and the effect of albumin on the base excess.

- *Sodium chloride effect (mEq/liter)* $= [Na^+] - [Cl^-] - 38$
- *Albumin effect (mEq liter* $\pm 1) = 0.25 \times [42 - \text{albumin (g/liter)}]$

The classification of acid–base disturbance according to Stewart's approach is given in Table 2.5.

2.1.2.11 Case Example Using Stewart's Approach

A 10-year-old male is hospitalized following a crush injury to right leg and septic shock. Four days on mechanical ventilation, the following laboratory reports are obtained:

ABG: pH 7.47, PO_2 106 mmHg, PCO_2 39 mmHg, HCO_3 28, BE +3.3
Na^+ 146 mmol/l, Cl^- 114 mmol/l, K^+ 4.4 mmol/l
Serum albumin 6 g/l, creatinine 105.6 μmmol/l

Based on traditional analysis, the child has metabolic alkalosis and may be the result of volume contraction.

Table 2.5 Classification of acid–base disturbances according to Stewart's approach

Acid–base disturbance	Disease state	Examples
Metabolic alkalosis	Low serum albumin	Nephrotic syndrome, hepatic cirrhosis
	High SID^+	Chloride loss: vomiting, gastric drainage, diuretics, post-hypercapnea, Cl^- wasting diarrhea due to villous adenoma, mineralocorticoid excess, Cushing's syndrome, Liddle's syndrome, Bartter's syndrome, exogenous corticosteroids, licorice Na^{2+} load (such as acetate, citrate, lactate): Ringer's solution, TPN, blood transfusion
Metabolic acidosis	Low SID^+ and high SIG	Ketoacids, lactic acid, salicylate, formate, methanol
	Low SID^+ and low SIG	RTA, TPN, saline, anion exchange resins, diarrhea, pancreatic losses

RTA renal tubular acidosis, *SIG* strong ion gap, *SID^+* strong ion difference, *TPN* total parenteral nutrition (©Cowdery HE, Critical Care 2005)

Using the Fencl–Stewart approach modified by Story et al.:

- *Sodium chloride effect on base excess* $= [Na^+] - [Cl^-] - 38 = -6$
- *Albumin effect on base excess* $= 0.25 \times [42 - albumin\ (g/l)] = +9$

The child in addition to contraction metabolic alkalosis also has significant hypoalbuminemic alkalosis and hyperchloremic acidosis.

2.1.3 Metabolic Acidosis

Metabolic acidosis is characterized by a decrease in plasma bicarbonate concentration due to loss of bicarbonate from the body or an impaired ability to excrete acid by the kidney or an addition of acid (exogenous/endogenous) to the body that exceeds normal excretory capacity of the kidneys. The compensatory mechanism for the reduction in blood pH causes a secondary decrease in partial pressure of carbon dioxide (PCO_2).

2.1.3.1 Etiology

For discussion on anion gap, please refer to Sect. 2.1.1. Metabolic acidosis can be divided into normal anion gap and high anion gap types.

Normal anion gap acidosis (hyperchloremic)

A. Loss of bicarbonate
- Diarrhea
- Intestinal, pancreatic, and biliary drains
- Proximal renal tubular acidosis
- Ureterosigmoidostomy
- Carbonic anhydrase inhibitors

B. Failure to replenish bicarbonate stores
- Distal renal tubular acidosis
- Renal tubular acidosis type 4
- Decreased mineralocorticoid activity (Addison's disease)
- Potassium-sparing diuretics

C. Exogenous infusions
- Ammonium chloride
- L arginine and L lysine during parenteral nutrition
- Rapid infusion of sodium chloride

High anion gap metabolic acidosis (normochloremic)

A. Excessive acid load – endogenous source
- Ketoacidosis – diabetes, starvation
- Organic acidemias
- Lactic acidosis – tissue hypoxia, liver failure, inborn errors of metabolism, thiamine deficiency, drugs (some antiretroviral agents)

B. Defective renal excretion of fixed acids – renal failure

C. Poisonings – salicylate, methanol, ethylene glycol

- Hyperchloremic normal anion gap metabolic acidosis can be divided into disorders associated with high/normal K^+ (e.g., parenteral nutrition, hypoaldosteronism, type IV RTA) and those associated with low K^+ (e.g., diarrhea, proximal and distal RTAs).
- In cases of diarrhea with severe hypovolemia, hyperchloremic metabolic acidosis with hypokalemia and alkaline urine may be observed, mimicking RTA. The acidemia and coexisting hypokalemia stimulate renal $NH4^+$ generation and result in very high urine $NH4^+$ levels and high urine pH. Urine anion gap can be used to differentiate between MA caused by acute gastroenteritis and renal tubular acidosis (refer Sect. 1.5).

2.1.3.2 Consequences of Metabolic Acidosis

Acute Metabolic Acidosis

- Reduces cardiac contractility and cardiac output
- Arterial vasodilatation and hypotension
- Resistance to effect of catecholamine (at pH <7.2)
- Decreased affinity of hemoglobin for oxygen tissue hypoxia
- Impaired leukocyte, lymphocyte function
- Stimulates interleukins and increases inflammation
- Hyperkalemia, decrease in ionized calcium levels

Chronic Metabolic Acidosis

- Growth retardation
- Demineralization of bones
- May contribute to progression of renal disease

2.1.3.3 Clinical Features

Acute metabolic acidosis
Tachypnea, Kussmaul's breathing
Fruity odor of breath (in diabetic ketoacidosis)
Increased risk of cardiac arrhythmias (when pH <7.2)
Exacerbation of hypotension
Lethargy, stupor, coma
Vomiting, anorexia, drowsiness (in infants)
Chronic metabolic acidosis
Osteopenia, muscle wasting, growth failure

2.1.3.4 Evaluation

ABG
Serum electrolytes, ionized calcium
Serum creatinine
Serum and urine ketones
Random blood sugar
Serum osmolality

Serum lactate
Urine pH, osmolality
Urine glucose, electrolytes
Urine–blood PCO_2 gradient
Urine organic acids
Fractional excretion of HCO_3

2.1.3.5 Approach to Metabolic Acidosis

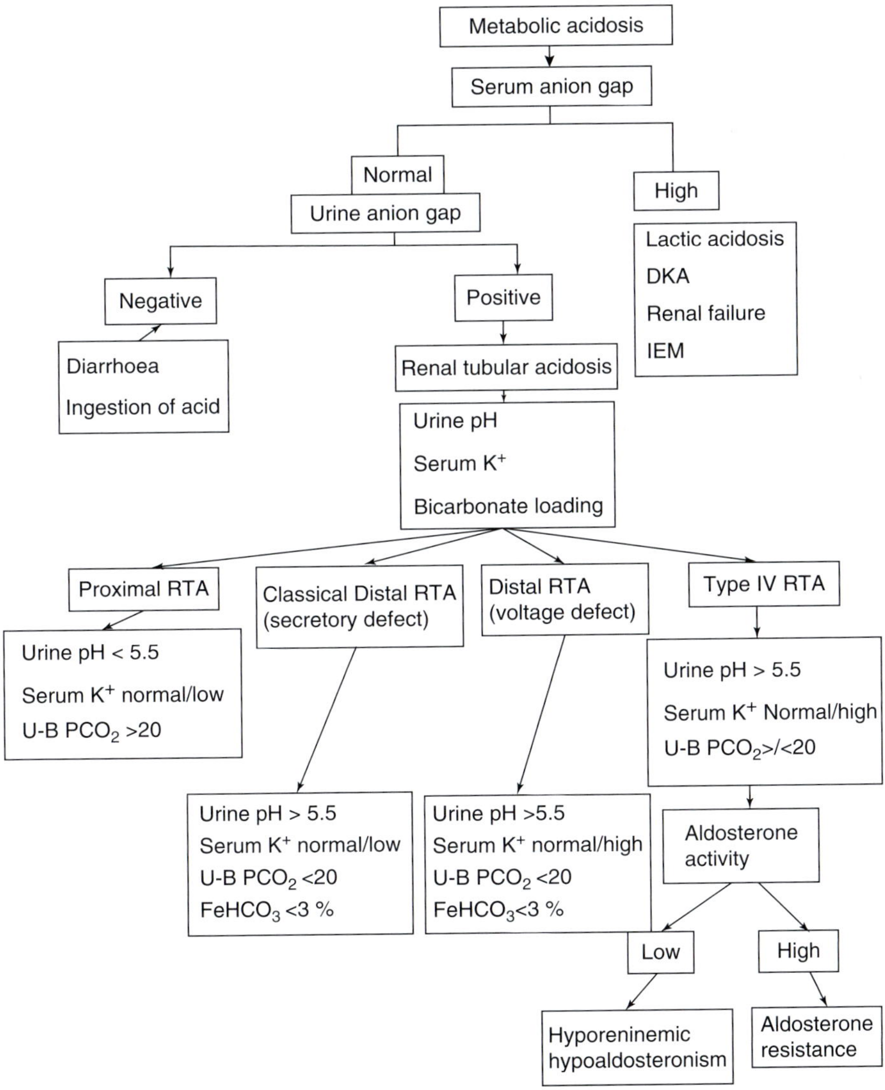

U-B PCO$_2$ urine–blood PCO_2 gradient, *FeHCO$_3$* fractional excretion of HCO_3, *K^+* potassium

2.1.3.6 Management

In addition to correcting the underlying cause of metabolic acidosis, the following measures may be taken in some cases:

Bicarbonate Therapy

- Intravenous bicarbonate should be used very judiciously if the pH is <7.1 with cardiovascular compromise, with the aim to raise pH to 7.2 (serum $HCO_3^- < 10$ mEq/1).
- Adequate ventilation should be established since PCO_2 is expected to rise after $NaHCO_3$ administration; avoid severe hypokalemia when $NaHCO_3$ is given.
- Intravenous 7.5 % $NaHCO_3$ (1:1 dilution) is administered as a slow infusion.
  Amount of bicarbonate to be given = 0.5 × body weight (kg) × base deficit.
  Half of the calculated dose is given over 1–2 h, and the remaining is given over next 4–6 h.
- Complications of sodium bicarbonate therapy: hyperosmolality, hypernatremia, hypokalemia, decrease in ionized calcium, intracerebral acidosis, and shift of oxygen dissociation curve resulting in worsening of tissue hypoxia and worsening of intracellular acidosis.
- Sodium bicarbonate administration does not reduce morbidity or mortality in children with lactic acidosis or ketoacidosis.
- Oral bicarbonate therapy is given to children with chronic acidosis in the form of sodium bicarbonate, sodium citrate, or potassium citrate. This can be started as 1–2 mEq/kg/day of base. Some conditions like proximal RTA may require up to 20 mEq/kg/day of base for correction of acidosis.

Tris-Hydroxymethyl Aminomethane (THAM)

- THAM is a weak alkali that reduces arterial $[H^+]$ without producing CO_2.
- It is an alternative to bicarbonate therapy especially if acidosis is associated with severe hypernatremia and high PCO_2. However, there are few studies regarding its efficacy.

Hemodialysis (HD) or Peritoneal Dialysis (PD)

- Renal replacement therapy (HD or PD) is indicated in refractory acidosis. Bicarbonate-based peritoneal dialysate solutions (instead of acetate or lactate based) may be used in cases of lactic acidosis (for details of these dialysate solutions, please refer to Sect. 17.6.4).

2.1.4 Metabolic Alkalosis

Metabolic alkalosis is the result of an increase in plasma HCO_3 due to either gain of HCO_3 or extracellular volume contraction. This can be either saline responsive or saline non-responsive.

2.1.4.1 Etiology

A. *Chloride responsive*: *loss of acid* (spot urine chloride <20 mmol/l)

Extra renal losses:

- Gastric losses – vomiting, nasogastric drain, pyloric stenosis
- Diarrhea – villous adenoma, congenital chloride diarrhea
- Post-hypercapnia
- Cystic fibrosis (chloride loss in sweat)
- Dietary chloride depletion

Renal losses: diuretic use (remote)

B. *Chloride resistant*: *gain of base* (spot urine chloride >20 mmol/l)

Normotensive: Bartter syndrome, Gitelman's syndrome, diuretics (recent)

Hypertensive

- Mineralocorticoid excess: associated with hypokalemia, hypertension
- Primary aldosteronism: adenoma, hyperplasia
- Apparent mineralocorticoid excess: 11β and 17α hydroxylase deficiency
- Glucocorticoid remediable hypertension, Liddle's syndrome, drugs: licorice, carbenoxolone
- Secondary hyperaldosteronism: reninoma, renovascular hypertension, malignant hypertension

Others: laxative abuse, milk alkali syndrome, bicarbonate use

- Hypercalcemia, hypokalemia
- Hypoalbuminemia
- Blood transfusion (citrate)

2.1.4.2 Phases of Metabolic Alkalosis

Initiation and maintenance are the two phases of metabolic alkalosis. The alkalosis can persist after the initiating process has resolved only if there are additional factors maintaining it.

Initiation

- Renal or extra renal losses of H^+ (vomiting, nasogastric suction, use of diuretics)
- Gain of HCO_3 ($NaHCO_3$ administration, citrate in transfused blood)

Maintenance

- Chloride depletion: There is increased reabsorption of HCO_3 in order to maintain electroneutrality. Decrease in luminal chloride decreases the activity of the β intercalated cells and decreases bicarbonate excretion.
- Potassium depletion: Bicarbonate reabsorption in both the proximal and distal tubules is increased in the presence of potassium depletion.
- Volume contraction augments fluid reabsorption in the proximal tubule increasing bicarbonate reabsorption and maintains alkalosis.
- Reduced glomerular filtration rate (GFR) due to volume contraction limits the filtration of HCO_3.

2.1.4.3 Clinical Features

Mild metabolic alkalosis (HCO_3 <36 mEq/l): asymptomatic
Moderate metabolic alkalosis (HCO_3 36–42 mEq/l): paresthesias, weakness, orthostatic hypotension, fatigue, muscle cramps, lethargy, hyporeflexia, muscular irritability
Severe metabolic alkalosis: (HCO_3 >45–50 mEq/l): arrhythmias, tetany, seizures, delirium, stupor
Complications: hypoventilation, hypoxemia, difficulty in weaning from ventilator, increased digoxin toxicity, worsening of hepatic encephalopathy
Features of hypokalemia: muscle weakness, paralytic ileus, arrhythmias
Features of decrease in ionized calcium: neuromuscular irritability, tetany

2.1.4.4 Evaluation

- ABG
- Blood urea, serum creatinine
- Serum electrolytes, serum magnesium
- Serum ionized calcium, serum albumin
- Urine electrolytes
- Plasma renin activity
- Serum aldosterone levels

2.1.4.5 Approach to Metabolic Alkalosis

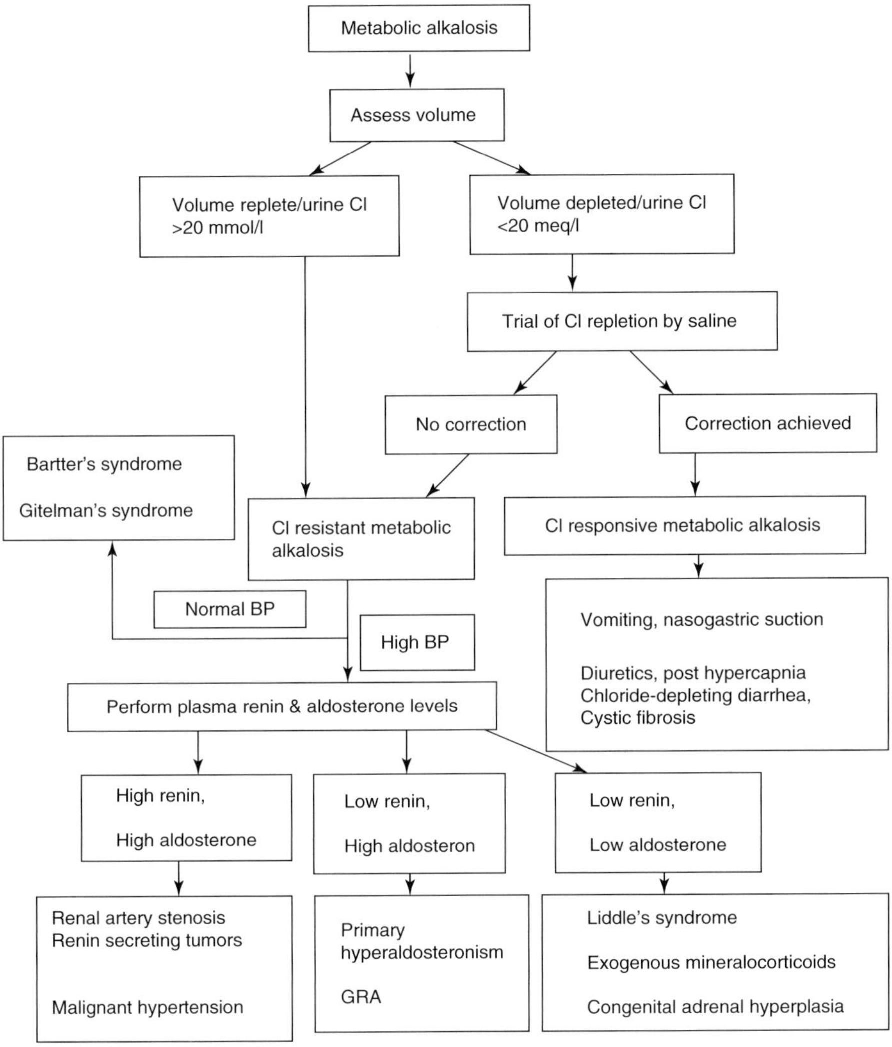

2.1.4.6 Management

Chloride-Responsive Metabolic Alkalosis

- Correct the hydration status with normal saline infusion @ 10 ml/kg over 10–30 min. May repeat the bolus, if indicated. Do not use Ringer's lactate.
- Associated hypokalemia should be corrected.
- For GI losses: decrease frequency of nasogastric drainage, use antiemetics and drugs that inhibit gastric acid secretion.
- In diuretic-induced metabolic alkalosis: stop or decrease the dose of diuretics, use of K^+ -sparing diuretics and KCl supplementation.

Chloride-Resistant Metabolic Alkalosis

- Treat the underlying cause.
  - Adrenal adenoma – surgical removal
  - Primary hyperaldosteronism – NaCl restriction, KCl supplementation, spironolactone
  - Glucocorticoid remediable aldosteronism – low-dose dexamethasone
  - Apparent mineralocorticoid excess – K^+ supplements, K^+-sparing diuretics
  - Bartter syndrome – K^+ supplementation, K^+-sparing diuretic, indomethacin
  - Gitelman's syndrome – K^+ supplementation, K^+-sparing diuretics, magnesium replacement
  - Liddle's syndrome – salt restriction, K^+ supplementation, K^+-sparing diuretics (triamterene, amiloride)

Treatment of Refractory Metabolic Alkalosis

- Acetazolamide orally @ 5 mg/kg OD or up to 8–30 mg/kg/day in 2–3 divided doses or intravenously @ 8–30 mg/kg/day in 2–3 divided doses; monitor serum K^+.
- Life-threatening metabolic alkalosis (HCO_3 >50 mmol/l) with problems in mechanical ventilation warrants the following options:
  - Renal replacement therapy (hemodialysis or peritoneal dialysis) dialysate fluid may be modified with reduced/absent base. Continuous form of renal replacement therapy (e.g., CVVH) may be preferred.
  - Direct titration with HCl infusion.

    The goal of HCl therapy is to decrease HCO_3 by 50 % aiming at reducing the pH <7.55 and HCO_3 <40 mEq/l. Intravenous 0.1 M HCl (100 mEq H^+ per liter) via central vein is infused or added to dextrose/amino acids/electrotype solution. Pediatric dose not firmly established. Rate of infusion should not exceed >0.2 mEq/kg/h.

    Limitations: volume of fluid required, hemolysis, venous thrombosis.

    For example, 30-kg child, HCO_3=50, pH=7.60

$$\begin{aligned}\text{HCl required} &= 0.5 \times \text{body weight} \times (\text{observed} - \text{desired bicarbonate}) \\ &= 0.5 \times 30 \times (50 - 40) \\ &= 150\ \text{mEq} @ 10\ \text{mEq/h}\ (0.1\ \text{M HCl} @ 100\ \text{ml/h})\end{aligned}$$

  - Ammonium chloride

    It is given orally in a dose of 75 mg/kg in 4 divided doses. It is contraindicated in liver failure.

    - Peritoneal dialysis using chloride-based peritoneal dialysis solution may be done. (For details on chloride-based PD solutions, please refer to Sect. 17.6.4.)

2.2 Sodium and Water Balance

2.2.1 Sodium Handling and Dysnatremias

Dysnatremias are one of the common electrolyte abnormalities seen in children. They usually result from disorders of water metabolism. It is the brain that suffers from all the consequences of alteration in water metabolism. In hyponatremia, there is an inability of the kidney to generate dilute urine and excrete free water. It may also be due to excessive salt losses. Hyponatremia is an independent predictor of mortality in a critically ill child. It is also a significant risk factor for sensorineural hearing loss and cerebral palsy. Hospital-acquired hyponatremia may be iatrogenic and in large part are due to the administration of hypotonic fluids to sick children who may have elevated arginine vasopressin levels. In hypernatremia, there is a net deficit of water in relation to sodium. It may be caused by water loss, sodium gain, or a combination of both.

2.2.1.1 Renal Handling of Sodium

- Sodium, the major extracellular cation in the body is freely filtered and then reabsorbed, but not secreted. More than 99 % of the filtered sodium is reabsorbed.
- Most sodium reabsorption occurs in the proximal tubule. Nearly 60 % is reabsorbed at the proximal tubule, 30–40 % at thick ascending limb of loop of Henle and 5–10 % actively at the distal tubule.
- Sodium reabsorption is driven by the $3Na^+/2K^+$ ATPase enzyme in the three tubular segments mentioned above.
- The main factors that regulate sodium reabsorption and excretion are extracellular volume status, delivery of sodium to the distal tubule, and aldosterone levels.

2.2.2 Hyponatremia

Hyponatremia is defined as serum Na^+ <135 mEq/l. Mild hyponatremia (serum Na^+ <135 mEq/l) occurs in 25 % of hospitalized children, while moderate hyponatremia (Serum Na^+ <130 mEq/l) is seen in 1 % of hospitalized children.

2.2.2.1 Applied Physiology

Development of hyponatremia typically requires a relative excess of free water in conjunction with an underlying condition that impairs the ability to excrete free water. Rarely, excess ingestion of free water or excess loss of urinary sodium causes hyponatremia. Excretion of free water will be impaired when there is either:

- A marked reduction in glomerular filtration rate (acute or chronic renal failure)
- Renal hypoperfusion (diarrhea, vomiting, cardiac failure, nephrotic syndrome)
- Arginine vasopressin (AVP) excess (SIAD, mutations in AQP2 receptors) Hyponatremia may result from increased non-osmotic AVP production.

2.2.2.2 Etiology

1. Hypovolemic hyponatremia
   - Extrarenal losses:
     - Gastrointestinal – vomiting, diarrhea
     - Transcutaneous – excessive sweating, cystic fibrosis
     - Third-space losses – burns, trauma, septic shock
   - Renal losses:
     - Diuretics
     - Tubulointerstitial diseases – medullary cystic disease, polycystic kidney disease
     - Tubular: proximal RTA, Bartter syndrome
     - Polyuric phase of AKI, post-obstructive diuresis
     - Prematurity
   - Mineralocorticoid deficiency
   - Pseudohypoaldosteronism
   - Cerebral salt wasting
2. Euvolemic hyponatremia
   - SIAD
   - Glucocorticoid deficiency
   - Hypothyroidism
   - Psychogenic polydipsia
   - Drugs (increased ADH release) – desmopressin, carbamazepine, chlorpropamide, vincristine, haloperidol, cyclophosphamide
3. Hypervolemic hyponatremia (increase in effective circulating volume or increased salt and water retention)
   - Nephrotic syndrome
   - Renal failure (acute/chronic)
   - Congestive cardiac failure
   - Cirrhosis of liver

2.2.2.3 Clinical Features

- The symptoms depend not only on the level of sodium but also on the rapidity of development (acute versus chronic).
- Sometimes, children present with symptoms of primary disease and recognition of hyponatremia may be incidental.
- The primary symptoms of hyponatremia are mostly due to cerebral edema, and the severity of neurologic symptoms correlates well with the rapidity and severity of the drop in serum sodium:
  - Early or mild hyponatremia – headache, nausea and vomiting, lethargy, confusion, agitation, and gait disturbances
  - Advanced or severe hyponatremia – seizures, coma, non-cardiogenic pulmonary edema, papilledema, and rarely cardiac arrhythmias
- Signs of dehydration may be exaggerated in presence of hypovolemic hyponatremia.
- Asymptomatic chronic hyponatremia in preterm neonates is associated with poor growth and development and sensorineural hearing loss.

2.2.2.4 Evaluation

Serum electrolytes
Spot urinary sodium and potassium
Serum osmolality
Urine osmolality
Renal function tests
Serum uric acid and urea[a]
Arterial blood gas
TSH and cortisol levels

[a]Important supportive information in differentiating between syndrome of inappropriate antidiuresis (SIAD) and cerebral salt wasting (CSW)

2.2.2.5 Approach to Hyponatremia

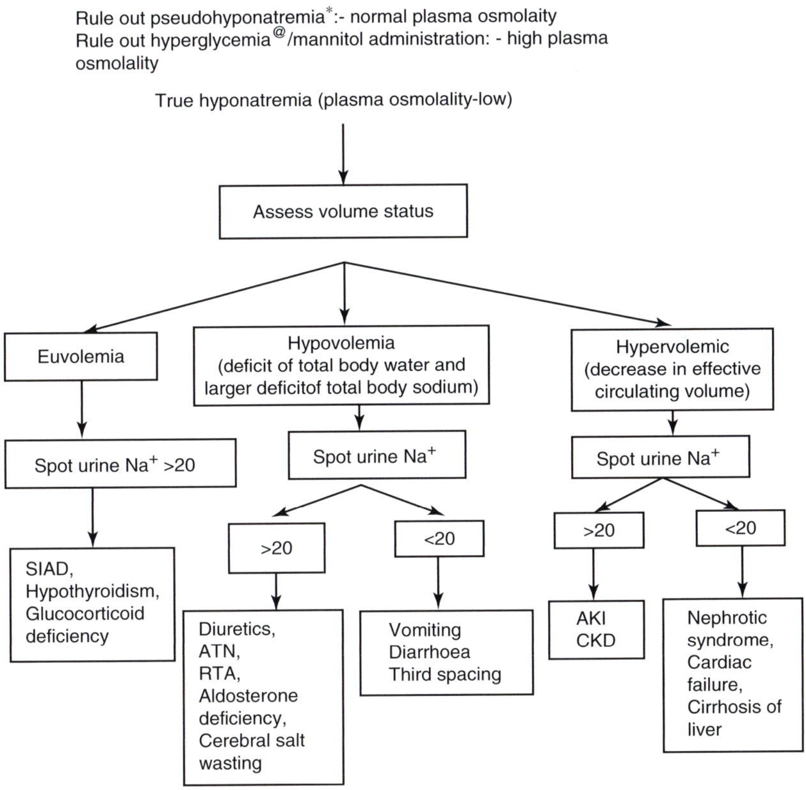

*Hyperproteinemia and hyperlipidemia can produce spuriously low serum sodium values (pseudo-hyponatremia) if it is measured by flame emission spectrophotometer. Readings obtained by ion-selective electrode method may not have an effect on lipid or protein levels in the serum. @A rise in serum glucose by 100 mg/dl (5.55 mmol/l) more than baseline of 100 mg/dl will decrease serum Na^+ by 1.6 mEq/l (1.6 mmol/l). *SIAD* syndrome of inappropriate antidiuresis, *ATN* acute tubular necrosis, *RTA*, renal tubular acidosis, *AKI* acute kidney injury, *CKD* chronic kidney disease; spot urine values are in mEq/l (mmol/l in SI units)

2.2.2.6 Treatment

- It is important to ensure that the patient has associated hypoosmolality. The treatment of hypertonic and pseudohyponatremia is directed at the underlying disorder.
- While treating hyponatremia, three factors should be taken into consideration: severity and duration of hyponatremia, neurological symptoms, and volume status of the child.
- Asymptomatic hyponatremia is usually chronic (>48 h duration), while symptomatic hyponatremia is acute (<48 h duration).
- If the child is in shock or volume depleted, treat with isotonic saline in sufficient amounts to restore the intravascular volume before correcting serum sodium.
- Acute hyponatremia, especially those with hyponatremic encephalopathy, requires early recognition and treatment (see box).
- Children with chronic hyponatremia are at significant risk for developing cerebral pontine demyelination, if hyponatremia is treated aggressively.
- Asymptomatic hyponatremia (chronic hyponatremia) should be corrected gradually, and recommended safe limits for the correction of hyponatremia is <10 mmol/l in 24 h or <20 mmol/l in 48 h (see box).

Management of Symptomatic Hyponatremia
Goal: 5–6 mmol/l increase in serum sodium (SNa) in first 1–2 h.
End point: Resolution of neurological symptoms or acute rise in SNa of 5 mmol/l in first 4–6 h.
Dosage: 2 ml/kg of 3 % NaCl over 10 min (maximum 100 ml). Repeat bolus 1–2 times as needed until symptoms improve.
Monitoring: SNa q 2–4 h, signs of fluid overload, urine output, acid base status, correction in first 48 h should not exceed 15–20 mmol/l.

Management of Asymptomatic Hyponatremia (Chronichyponatremia)
Treat the underlying cause
Fluid restriction (½ to 2/3 maintenance fluids/day)
Oral salt supplementation
Furosemide (to increase free water loss) + 0.45 % normal saline (to replace sodium loss in the urine)
Demeclocycline
V2-receptor antagonists (vaptans) could be used to treat euvolemic or hypervolemic hyponatremia that do not respond to fluid restriction.

Formulae to Calculate no of Mmol of Na Necessary to Achieve the Desired Change in Serum Sodium (SNa) Concentration

1. (0.6) × body weight in kg × (desired Na – present Na) – commonly used method

2. $$\text{Change in serum Na} = \frac{\text{infusate Na} - \text{current serum Na}}{\text{TBW} + 1}$$

   (Nicholas–Madias formula which estimates change in S Na with 1 l of infusate)

2.2.2.7 Case Example for Correction of Hyponatremia

An infant weighing 10 kg with symptomatic hyponatremia (SNa: 120 mmol/l), the goal is to increase SNa to 125 mmol/l over a period of 1–2 h.

Step 1: Assess the volume status: if the child is hypovolemic, treat with isotonic saline in sufficient amounts to restore the intravascular volume.

Step 2: Calculate the rise in sodium required using the formulae and the optimal rate.

<u>*Formula 1*</u>

Number of mmol of Na^+ required increasing serum Na to 125 mmol/l

$= 0.6 \times 10 \times (125 - 120) = 6 \times 5 = 30$ mmol.

1 ml of 3 % NaCl = 0.5 mmol of Na^+, so to give 30 mmol of Na, 60 ml of 3 % NaCl should be given over a period of 1–2 h (i.e., 30–60 ml/h).

<u>*Formula 2*</u>

By applying the Nicholas–Madias formula, if we use 3 % NaCl (513 mmol/l) for correction,

$$\text{Change in SNa} = \frac{513\ (\text{infusate Na}^+) - 120}{(0.6 \times 10) + 1}$$

$$= \frac{513 - 120}{6 + 1} = 56\ \text{mmol}$$

That means 1 l of 3 % NaCl will increase the serum Na concentration by 56 mmol/l. Thus, in order to increase the SNa^+ concentration by 5 mmol/l, dividing the target. Na (5 mmol/l) by the change in SNa^+ obtained by this formula (56 mmol/l), 0.089 l, i.e., 89 ml (5/56) over a period of 2 h or 40 ml/h of 3 % NaCl is required.

Step 3: Once symptom-free, hyponatremia can be corrected more slowly over a period of 48 h with a goal of not to increase the serum Na^+ concentration by more than 10–20 mmol/l over 24–48 h by using the same formulae.

2.2.3 Syndrome of Inappropriate Antidiuresis

- Syndrome of inappropriate antidiuresis (SIAD) is characterized by clinical euvolemia, low plasma osmolality, and inappropriately concentrated urine, with normal renal, adrenal, and thyroid function.
- The term SIAD has replaced syndrome of inappropriate antidiuretic hormone secretion (SIADH) because not all patients with the syndrome have inappropriately elevated circulating levels of arginine vasopressin (ADH).
- The degree of water retention that leads to hyponatremia is determined by both the fluid intake and the severity of the impairment in water excretion.
- ADH regulation is impaired in SIAD, and four different patterns have been described.
  - Type A – unregulated release of ADH that varies widely with no relation to the plasma osmolality.
  - Type B – constant release of ADH with little or no variation in ADH levels.
  - Type C – resetting of the osmostat, plasma sodium concentration is normally regulated at a lower level (between 125 and 135 mmol/l).
  - Type D – ADH level is undetectable and is secondary to activating mutations in V2 vasopressin receptor.
- In SIAD, there is an initial phase of water retention and hyponatremia followed by partial escape from antidiuresis.

2.2.3.1 Diagnostic Criteria (Bartter and Schwartz 1967)

Essential criteria
Hyponatremia(serum Na <135 mmol/l)
Decrease extracellular fluid effective osmolality (<270 mOsm/kg H_2O)
Inappropriate urinary concentration (>100 mOsm/kg H_2O)
Clinical euvolemia
Elevated urinary Na (>20 mmol/l) concentration under conditions of normal salt and water intake
Absence of adrenal, thyroid, pituitary, or renal insufficiency or diuretic use
Supplemental criteria
Plasma vasopressin level inappropriately elevated relative to plasma osmolality
(Any detectable AVP level when serum osmolality is <270 mOsm/kg H_2O itself denotes inappropriate elevation.)
Abnormal water load test – inability to excrete at least 90 % of a 20 ml/kg water load in 4 h and/or failure to dilute urine osmolality to <100 mOsm/kg H_2O
No significant correction of serum sodium with volume expansion but improvement after fluid restriction

2.2.3.2 Etiology

CNS disorders – infection, trauma, hypoxic ischemic encephalopathy, Guillain–Barre syndrome, cerebral malformations, intracranial hemorrhage, and malignancy (primary or secondary)
Pulmonary disorders – infections, malignancy, cystic fibrosis, and positive pressure ventilation
Postsurgery – anesthetic or premedication induced, abdominal, cardiothoracic and neurosurgery procedures, pain
Drugs – desmopressin, carbamazepine, chlorpropamide, vincristine, haloperidol, cyclophosphamide
Miscellaneous – acute intermittent porphyria, leukemia, lymphoma

2.2.3.3 Evaluation and Differential Diagnosis

SIAD may be difficult to distinguish from cerebral salt wasting (CSW), a syndrome characterized by hyponatremia and extracellular fluid depletion due to inappropriate urinary sodium wasting in patients with intracranial bleeding or following neurosurgical procedures. It is postulated that unregulated release of brain natriuretic peptide (BNP) results in impaired renal tubular sodium reabsorption. CSW tends to be transient and usually resolves within 3–4 weeks.

The primary feature that differentiates cerebral salt wasting from SIAD is extracellular fluid volume depletion, but clinical assessment of volume status is imprecise (Table 2.6).

It is important to distinguish SIAD from CSW because fluid restriction is the mainstay of treatment in SIAD while volume repletion with isotonic saline is the definitive treatment in CSW.

Table 2.6 Differentiating between SIAD and CSW (cerebral salt wasting)

	SIAD	CSW
Sodium	Low	Low
Body water	Increased	Decreased
Serum urea	Decreased	Increased
Serum uric acid	Decreased	Increased
Serum osmolality	<280 mOsm/l	Decreased
Urine osmolality	>500 mOsm/l	Increased
Urine to serum osmolality ratio	>1	>1
Urine output	Low	High
Urine Na concentration	Increased	Increased

2.2.3.4 Treatment

- Correct the underlying cause.
- Fluid restriction with appropriate sodium-containing fluids to avoid worsening of hyponatremia is the mainstay of therapy. Fluid restriction to less than 2/3 of maintenance and decreased to ½ maintenance or lower if no improvement in 4–6 h.
- Use 0.45 sodium chloride solution with 5 % dextrose, if intravenous fluids are indicated.
- Severe symptomatic patients with SIAD often initially require administration of 3 % NaCl.
- The use of furosemide with 0.45 or 0.9 N sodium chloride solution to replace urinary losses of sodium can be successful in some children.
- Demeclocycline may be used in those who do not respond to fluid restriction. The dose in children >8 years is 6–12 mg/kg/day divided into 2–3 doses orally. However, it has unpredictable renal clearance, and onset of the response varies and ranges between 5 and 8 days.
- Osmotic diuretics like urea have been used in adults with refractory SIAD, but safety and efficacy in children has not been established.
- The efficacy and safety of vasopressin receptor antagonists (tolvaptan, conivaptan) in children has not been established.

2.2.4 Hypernatremia

Hypernatremia, defined as serum Na^+ >145 mmol/l, always represents a hypertonic state.

The ability to release ADH (AVP) and intact thirst mechanism are two mechanisms by which hypernatremia or increased effective blood osmolality is prevented in a normal child. In hypernatremia, there is a net deficit of water in relation to sodium, and it may be caused by water loss or sodium gain or a combination of both.

2.2.4.1 Etiology

1. *Water deficit in excess of sodium (clinically dehydrated)*
Diarrhea, emesis/nasogastric tube suction, burns
2. *Free water deficit (clinically dehydrated/normal hydration)*
Central diabetes insipidus (CDI) – may be partial or complete; Hereditary: autosomal dominant
Acquired: trauma, craniopharyngioma, postsurgical, radiation
Nephrogenic diabetes insipidus (NDI) – hereditary: X-linked dominant, autosomal recessive; acquired: hypercalcemia, hypokalemia, tubulointerstitial nephritis, obstructive uropathy, amphotericin B, demeclocycline
Inadequate intake – ineffective breast feeding, lack of thirst (adipsia)
Increased insensible water loss – preterm newborns on radiant warmer/phototherapy, excessive sweating

3. *Sodium excess (clinically normal hydration/mild hypervolemia)*
   Improperly mixed formula or rehydration solutions
   Excessive sodium bicarbonate administration
   Hypertonic saline enema
   Primary hyperaldosteronism

2.2.4.2 Clinical Features

- Hypernatremic dehydration – increased thirst, poor skin turgor, dry mucus membranes, and doughy feel of abdomen are observed in a child with hypernatremic dehydration. Signs and symptoms of dehydration may be masked because of better preservation of intravascular volume.
- CNS symptoms – high-pitched cry, irritability, hyperpnea, and increase in muscle tone; eventually progress to seizures, coma, and death.

2.2.4.3 Evaluation

The kidneys' normal response to hypernatremia is excretion of a minimal amount of maximally concentrated urine. If urine osmolality is >600 mOsm/kg in a child with hypernatremia, suspect extrarenal hypotonic fluid losses (e.g., vomiting, diarrhea, burns). Isotonic urine osmolality may be observed with diuretics.

CT scan or MRI of brain is suggested in all patients with severe hypernatremia.

Serum osmolality
Urine osmolality
Serum electrolytes
Renal function tests
Arterial blood gas
Spot urinary sodium and potassium
CT/MRI imaging of brain

2.2.4.4 Treatment

- Identify and treat the underlying cause.
- Stabilize hypovolemic children who have unstable vital signs with isotonic saline before correcting free water deficits.
- Correct free water deficit/sodium excess by calculating the free water deficit and replacing water or by calculating the required rate of sodium reduction for the chosen infusate (see box).
- Free water deficits can be replaced either orally or intravenously depending on the child's status.
- Do not decrease serum sodium level by more than 0.5 mmol/l/h or 12 mmol/l/day.
- Hyperglycemia may also accompany hypernatremia. Insulin treatment is not recommended because it may increase brain "idiogenic osmoles" content.

- Hypocalcemia is common; addition of calcium gluconate to rehydration fluid is often indicated.
- Dialysis if conservative measures fail.
- If child develop seizures during correction (suggestive of rapidly falling S. Na), give 3 % NaCl (4–6 ml/kg over 30 min).

2.2.4.5 Approach to Hypernatremia

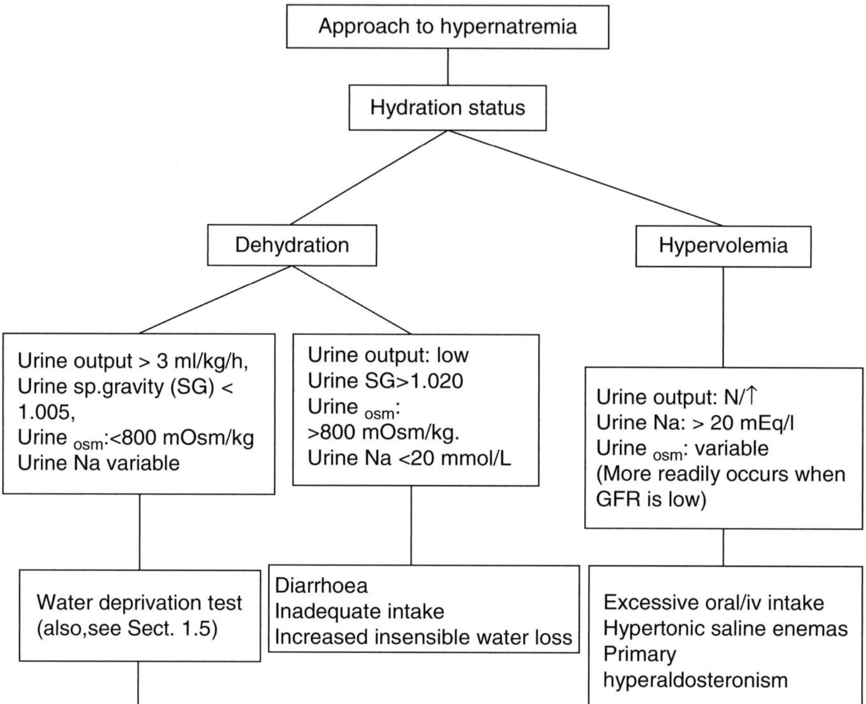

Disease	Urine osmolality with water deprivation	Plasma AVP after dehydration	Increase in urine osmolality after exogenous AVP administration at one hour
Complete CDI	Low (<300)	Undetectable	>10 % increase in Uosm
Partial CDI	Same or low (300–800)	<1.5 pg/ml	>50 % increase in Uosm
NDI	Same or low	>5 pg/ml	No increase
Primary polydypsia	Increase (800–1400)	<5 pg/ml	Little or no increase

Formulae to Calculate Desired Rate of Drop in Sodium

1. 1.5 times the maintenance intravenous (IV) fluid is given at a constant rate over the time for correction. 0.45 % DNS is the preferred fluid for children.
2. Volume of fluid to be administered over 48 h = 2 × maintenance fluid + calculated total body free water deficit.

   Free water deficit: total body water – total body water at the time of hypernatremia

   TBWD × weight (kg)–normal serum Na × TBWD × weight (kg)

   $$\text{TBWD} \times \text{weight}(\text{kg}) - \frac{\text{normal serum Na} \times \text{TBWD} \times \text{weight}(\text{kg})}{\text{Current serum Na}}$$

   TBWD = total body water distribution =>0.6 for children and 0.7 in case of infants

   The free water deficit calculated by this formula is equivalent to 4 ml/kg for each mmol > the expected Na^+.
3. $$\text{Change in serum Na} = \frac{\text{infusate Na} - \text{current serum Na}}{\text{TBW} + 1}$$

(Nicholas – Madias formula which estimates change in S Na with 1 l of infusate)

2.2.4.6 Case Example for Correction of Hypernatremia

An infant weighing 10 kg presents with symptomatic hypernatremia (serum Na – 170 mmol/l).

Sodium correction based on the various methods is shown below:

Step 1: Restoration of intravascular volume if there is evidence of shock

Step 2: Calculation of desired rate of SNa drop and fluid requirements

Formula 1:

$$\begin{aligned}\text{Amount of fluid to be given}&\\ \text{over next 24 h} &= 1.5 \times \text{maintenance IV fluid}\\ &= 1.5 \times 1{,}000 = 1{,}500/24\\ &= 62.5\,\text{ml/h } 0.45\% \text{ DNS to be given.}\end{aligned}$$

Formula 2:

According to the formula, the free water deficit will be

$$0.6 \times 10 - \frac{150 \times 0.6 \times 10}{170} = 6 - \frac{900}{170} = 6 - 5.3 = 0.7\,\text{l} = 700\,\text{ml}$$

The volume of fluid required to be given over 48 h will be 2 × 1,000 ml (maintenance fluid) + 700 ml (calculated deficit) = 2,800 ml over 48 h, i.e., 1,400 ml/24 h, i.e., 58 ml/h. So, the child needs to be given 0.45 % DNS at 58 ml/h for correction of hypernatremia.

Formula 3:

By applying Nicolas–Madias formula, if we use 0.45 % DNS for correction,

$$\text{change in } S_{Na} = \frac{77\left(\text{infusate Na}^{+}\right) - 170\left(\text{SNa}\right)}{\left(0.6\times 10\right)+1} = \frac{-93}{7} = -13$$

That means 1 l of 0.45 % NS will lower the SNa^+ concentration by 13 mmol/l.

So, to reduce the SNa^+ concentration by 10 mmol/l over next 24 h, 770 ml of 0.45 % DNS 1,000 × 10/13 to be given in addition to the maintenance iv fluids.

Maintenance iv fluid = 1,000 ml (100 ml/kg, i.e., 1,000 ml), total 1,770 ml of 0.45 % DNS at 73 ml/h

Step 3: Replacement of ongoing losses as they occur

Diarrhea => replace with D5 1/4 NS + 15 mmol/l $NaHCO_3$ +20 mmol/l of KCl; replace stool ml/ml every 1–6 h.

Vomiting/Nasogastric tube losses => D51/2 NS + 10 mmol/l of KCL, replace output ml/ml

Step 4: Frequent monitoring and management of complications

If child develop seizures during correction (suggestive of rapidly falling S. Na), give 3 % NaCl (4–6 ml/kg)

2.3 Disorders of Potassium Homeostasis

2.3.1 Potassium Balance

Potassium is the major intracellular cation. Ninety-eight percent of the potassium in the body is within cells, primarily in skeletal muscles and to a lesser extent in liver. The maintenance of distribution of potassium across cells is largely dependent on the activity of the sodium pump (Na^+ K^+ ATPase). The ratio of intracellular and extracellular potassium is the primary determinant of the resting membrane potential. All of the excitable cells (muscle cells, nerve cells) rely upon this resting membrane potential or K^+ gradient to set their basal voltage for their function. Hence, there are profound clinical effects whenever this K^+ gradient gets disturbed.

The three components for defense against abnormalities in potassium balance are:

- Shift K^+ in and out of cells
- Excretion by the kidney
- Excretion into the GI tract

2.3.1.1 Renal Handling of Potassium

Cortical Collecting Duct

There are two main regulators of potassium secretion in the cortical collecting duct:

- Mineralocorticoid activity
  A combination of high mineralocorticoid and high distal delivery of sodium results in high K^+ secretion and hypokalemia, seen in aldosterone-secreting tumor. A combination of low mineralocorticoid and low distal delivery of sodium leads to low K^+ secretion and hyperkalemia, classically seen in Addison's disease.
- Distal delivery of sodium
  A diuretic that works proximal to the cortical collecting duct causes an increase in distal delivery of sodium; a lot of that sodium goes out in the urine and causes volume depletion. The volume depletion then leads to an increase in mineralocorticoids leading to increased K^+ secretion, resulting in hypokalemia. In acute glomerulonephritis, there is volume expansion and decreased distal delivery of sodium due to decreased GFR. This suppresses mineralocorticoids secretion causing hyperkalemia.

Medullary Collecting Duct

- The potassium absorption occurs via H^+ K^+ ATPase.
- It may contribute to hypokalemia in the condition of hypokalemic distal RTA, where defect in hydrogen secretion causes defective K^+ reabsorption.

2.3.1.2 Urinary Indices Used in Evaluation of Disorders of Potassium Homeostasis

- Assessing renal K^+ excretion is an important step in evaluation of hypokalemia or hyperkalemia.
- The 24-h urine and/or spot urine have been used to assess renal K^+ excretion rate. However, 24-h urine collection is often difficult in children and is prone to errors because of inaccuracies in timing and collection.
- Four spot urine indices of renal potassium excretion are commonly used:
  - Spot urine K^+ concentration: Value <15 mmol/l in presence of hypokalemia suggests appropriate renal conservation, while >15 mmol/l suggests renal wasting of potassium.
  - Urine potassium/creatinine (K^+/Cr) ratio: Values less than 1.5 suggest renal conservation of potassium during hypokalemia. However, the ratio can vary with age, renal failure, and muscle mass and hence should be interpreted with caution.
  - Fractional excretion of K^+ (FeK^+): It measures the amount of filtered potassium that is excreted in urine. Normally, it is less than 3 %.
    FeK^+ = urinary potassium/serum potassium × serum creatinine/urinary creatinine ×e100

Potassium excretion in normal infants is slightly higher than in older children and adults. Among normal infants, mean FEK = 12.2 % (range 5–27 %); values above 27 % indicate potassium wasting (Rodrigues-Soriano Ped Nephrol 1990).

– Transtubular potassium gradient (TTKG): The transtubular potassium gradient (TTKG) is used to assess renal potassium secretion by the cortical collecting duct, indirectly assessing aldosterone activity in patients who have hypo- or hyperkalemia. For details, refer to Sect. 1.5.

2.3.2 Hypokalemia

Serum potassium concentration <3.5 mmol/l is defined as hypokalemia.

2.3.2.1 Applied Physiology

Hypokalemia is typically due to increased aldosterone activity or increased delivery of sodium to distal tubules of loop of Henle. Hypokalemia seen with vomiting and prolonged nasogastric suction is not due to increased losses from GI but is due to increased urinary potassium loss secondary to intravascular volume depletion and metabolic alkalosis which result in secondary hyperaldosteronism.

2.3.2.2 Etiology

Spurious hypokalemia: (Abnormal white blood cells take up potassium from extracellular compartment when stored at room temperature)

Leukemia

Redistribution: (Movement of potassium from extracellular to intracellular compartment)

Aldosterone, beta-adrenergic agonists, hypokalemic periodic paralysis, alkalosis, exogenous insulin, hyperthyroidism

Extrarenal losses:

Excessive sweating, diarrhea, burns, fistula and ostomies, short bowel syndrome, malabsorption syndromes

Renal loss:

Drugs: thiazide and loop diuretics, carbenicillin, Amphotericin B

Hormones: aldosterone, cortisol

Magnesium depletion: aminoglycosides, cisplatin

Intrinsic renal defect: Bartter syndrome, Gitelman's syndrome, Liddle's syndrome

Bicarbonaturia: metabolic alkalosis, proximal renal tubular acidosis

2.3.2.3 Clinical Features

- Mild hypokalemia is often asymptomatic.
- Patients with more severe hypokalemia (serum K^+ <3 mmol/l) present with generalized weakness, fatigue, and constipation.
- Severe hypokalemia can precipitate rhabdomyolysis and impair urinary concentrating mechanism. It can also cause life-threatening cardiac arrhythmias and respiratory paralysis due to weakness of respiratory muscles.
- Moderate and severe hypokalemia can induce electrocardiographic changes, including a prominent U wave, a flattened T wave, low ST segment, and a widened QRS complex.

Acute
Skeletal muscle weakness involving limbs, trunk, and respiratory muscles
Smooth muscle weakness: paralytic ileus and gastric dilatation
Cardiac arrhythmia: premature ventricular contractions, sinus bradycardia
Ventricular tachycardia or fibrillation
Atrioventricular block
Rhabdomyolysis
Chronic
Growth failure
Tubulointerstitial and cystic changes
Polyuria
Metabolic alkalosis
Impaired glucose tolerance

2.3.2.4 Evaluation

Serum potassium, sodium and chloride
EKG (see Fig. 2.4)
Serum magnesium, calcium, phosphorous, alkaline phosphatase
Blood urea/serum creatinine
Urine potassium, urine creatinine
Arterial blood gas
Plasma and urine osmolality to estimate transtubular potassium gradient

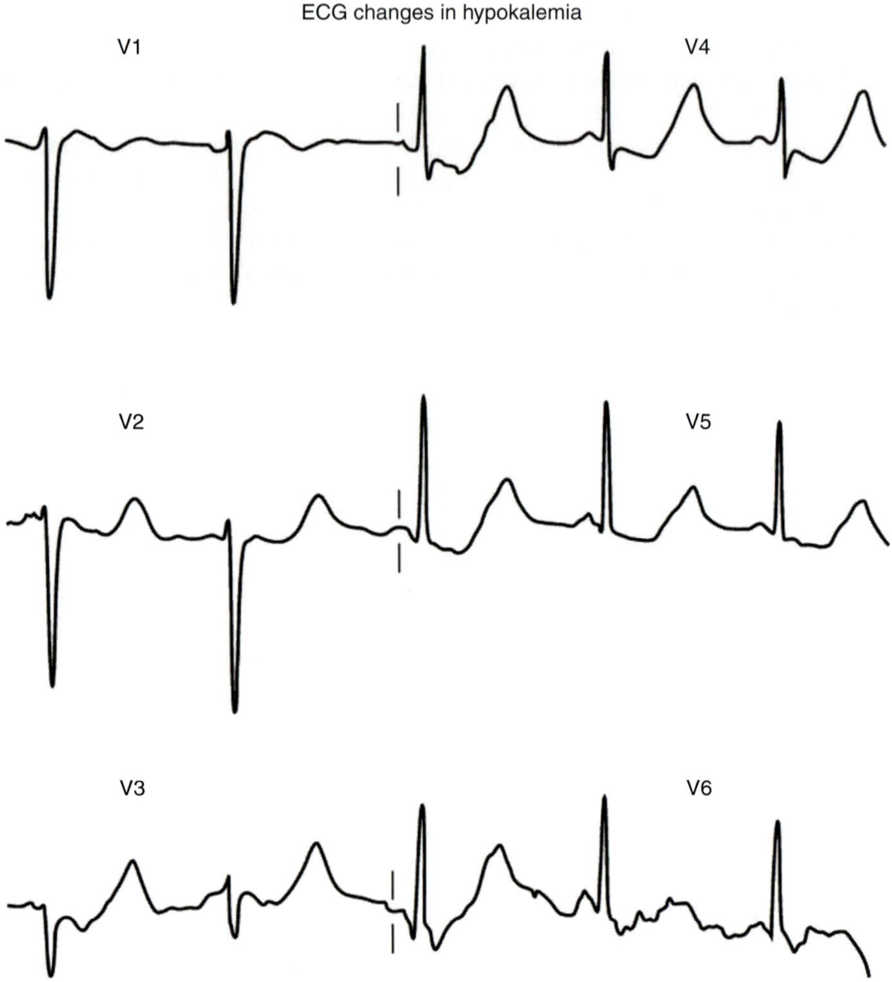

Fig. 2.3 EKG changes of hypokalemia: Sinus rhythm. Normal axis. Narrow QRS complex. ST depression V3–V5. "Apparent" prolonged QT interval. T-waves unseparable from giant U-waves seen V2–6 (Webster A et al. Emerg Med J 2002; 19:74–77)

2.3.2.5 Approach to Hypokalemia

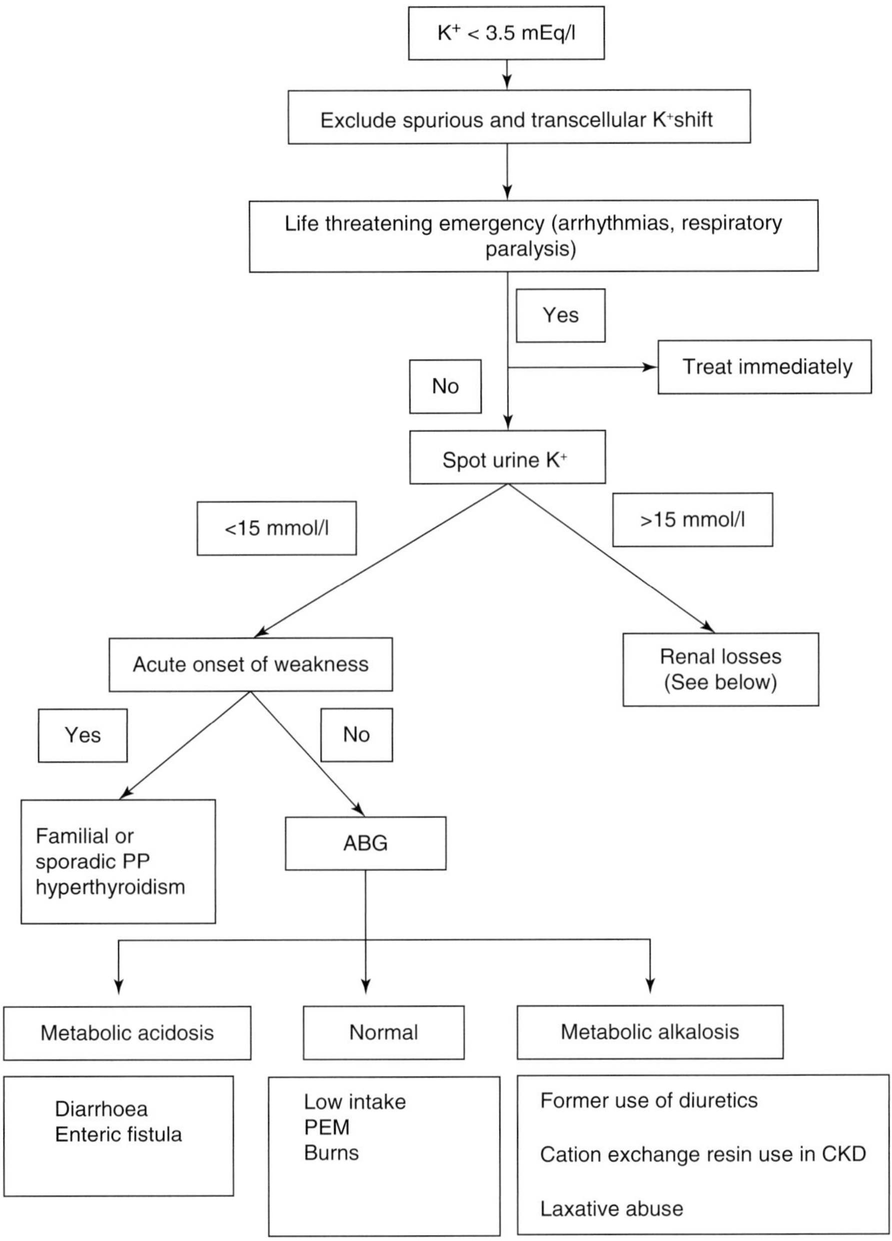

PP periodic paralysis, *PEM* protein energy malnutrition, *ABG* arterial blood gas, *CKD* chronic kidney disease

2.3.2.6 Approach to Hypokalemia Due to Increased Renal Losses

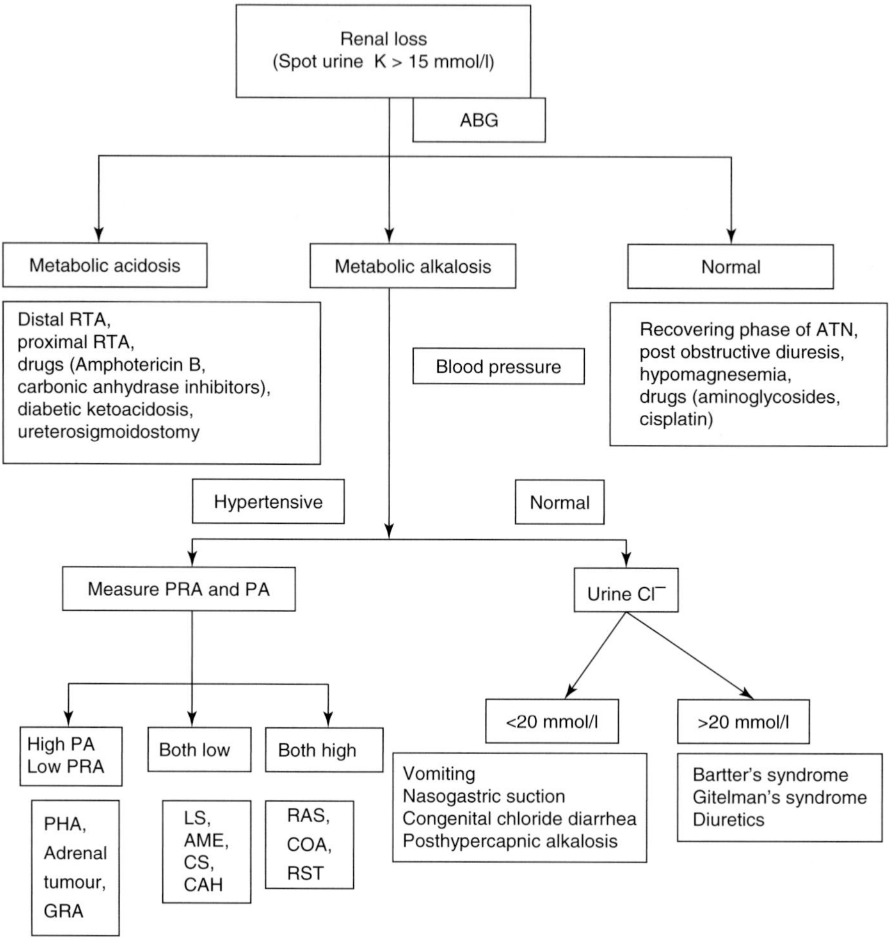

RTA renal tubular acidosis, *ATN* acute tubular necrosis, *PRA* plasma renin activity, *PA* plasma aldosterone, *PHA* primary hyperaldosteronism, *LS* Liddle's syndrome, *AME* apparent mineralocorticoid excess, *CS* Cushing's syndrome, *CAH* congenital adrenal hyperplasia, *RAS* renal artery stenosis, *COA* coarctation of aorta, *RST* renin-secreting tumor, *GRA* glucocorticoid remediable aldosteronism

2.3.2.7 Treatment of Hypokalemia

Symptomatic Hypokalemia

Management in emergencies (EKG changes, respiratory paralysis)

The initial aim of therapy is to raise serum potassium to a safe range (>3 mEq/l).

- Potassium chloride (KCl) as intravenous bolus dose (given in 1–2 min) at a dose calculated as: [3 − measured K^+ × body weight × 0.04] followed by an infusion at rate of 0.015 mEq/kg/min.
- Concentration of K^+ in IV fluid should not exceed 60 mmol/l while giving through peripheral line, 80 mmol/l via central line, and should not be mixed with dextrose solution.
- The infusion should also not contain HCO_3 because this might aggravate the degree of hypokalemia by increasing redistribution of K^+ from extracellular fluid space into intracellular space.
- Caution should be exercised in children with hypokalemia due to increased shift K^+ into cells as aggressive KCl therapy may be associated with a potential risk of rebound hyperkalemia, due to K^+ rapidly released from cells when the K^+ shift resolves.
- Hypokalemia needs to be corrected prior to correcting metabolic acidosis.
- Concomitant magnesium deficiency may exacerbate hypokalemia and render it refractory to treatment with K^+ supplementation.
- Cardiac monitoring and a central venous catheter are essential for aggressive treatment.

Management in Nonemergent Situations

The infusion rate of potassium chloride should not exceed 0.5–1 mEq/kg/h and should be replaced by oral or nasogastric supplementation of potassium chloride (1–3 mmol/kg in divided doses) as soon as the child starts taking orally, titrating with serum K levels.

Asymptomatic Hypokalemia

- The mainstay of therapy is oral potassium supplementation (3–4 mmol/Kg/day).
- Dietary supplementation with foods having high potassium content like coconut water, banana, citrus fruits, and potatoes should be encouraged.
- Potassium-sparing diuretics (spironolactone, amiloride) may be used in children on loop diuretics to counteract diuretic-induced hypokalemia.
- Treatment of underlying cause.

Formulations of Potassium Salts Available in the Market

- Potassium chloride (20 % KCl 1 ml = 2 mmol) – It is most commonly preferred.
- Potassium citrate (1 ml = 2 mmol) – Useful in children with renal tubular acidosis.
- Potassium phosphate (94 mg PO_4 and 4.4 mmol K^+/ml) – Useful in children who also have hypophosphatemia (diabetic ketoacidosis, children on continuous renal replacement therapy).

2.3.3 Hyperkalemia

Hyperkalemia is defined as serum concentration of K^+ >6 mmol/l in newborn and >5.5 mmol/l in older children.

2.3.3.1 Etiology

Pseudohyperkalemia: Hemolysis
Severe leukocytosis/thrombocytosis
Redistribution: Hyperglycemia
Acidosis due to nonorganic acids
Excess intake: Potassium supplements
Impaired renal secretion:
Chronic kidney disease
Primary decrease/resistance in mineralocorticoid activity
    Tubulointerstitial disease, Addison's disease, Type IV RTA
Primary decrease in sodium delivery
  Oliguric acute kidney injury
  Acute glomerulonephritis
  Gordon's syndrome
Abnormal cortical collecting duct
  Pseudohypoaldosteronism type 1
  Tubulointerstitial nephritis
  Obstruction
Drugs: Spironolactone, amiloride, triamterene
Trimethoprim, pentamidine
NSAIDs, COX2 inhibitors
Cyclosporine, tacrolimus
ACEI, ARBs, heparin

RTA renal tubular acidosis, *ACEI* angiotensin-converting enzyme inhibitor, *ARB* angiotensin receptor blockers, *NSAIDs* nonsteroidal anti-inflammatory drugs, *COX2*: cyclooxygenase

2.3.3.2 Clinical Features

Acute: Cardiac standstill
Neuromuscular weakness
Chronic: Asymptomatic
ECG Findings: Diminished to absent p waves
Tall peaked t waves
Widened QRS complex
Sine wave pattern of QRS widening

2.3.3.3 Evaluation

EKG (see Fig. 2.5)
Serum bicarbonate
Serum sodium, potassium, chloride
Serum creatinine
Urine spot potassium
Transtubular potassium gradient: TTKG

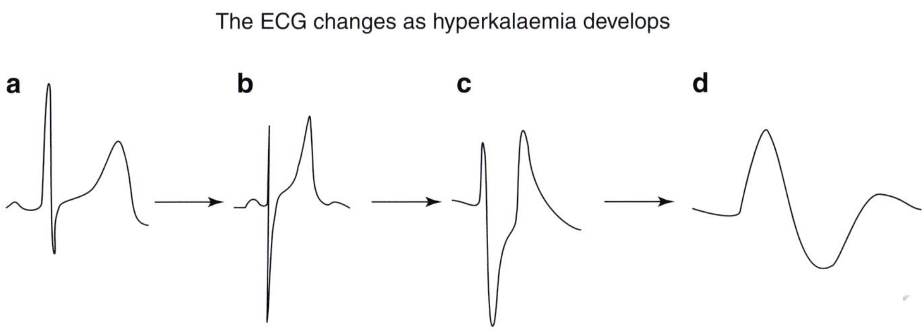

Fig. 2.4 The EKG changes as hyperkalaemia develops. (**a**) A normal complex. (**b**) Loss of P-waves, tenting of the T-waves. (**c**) Broadening of the QRS complex. (**d**) Sine wave appearance (Webster A et al. Emerg Med J 2002; 19:74–77)

2.3.3.4 Approach to Hyperkalemia

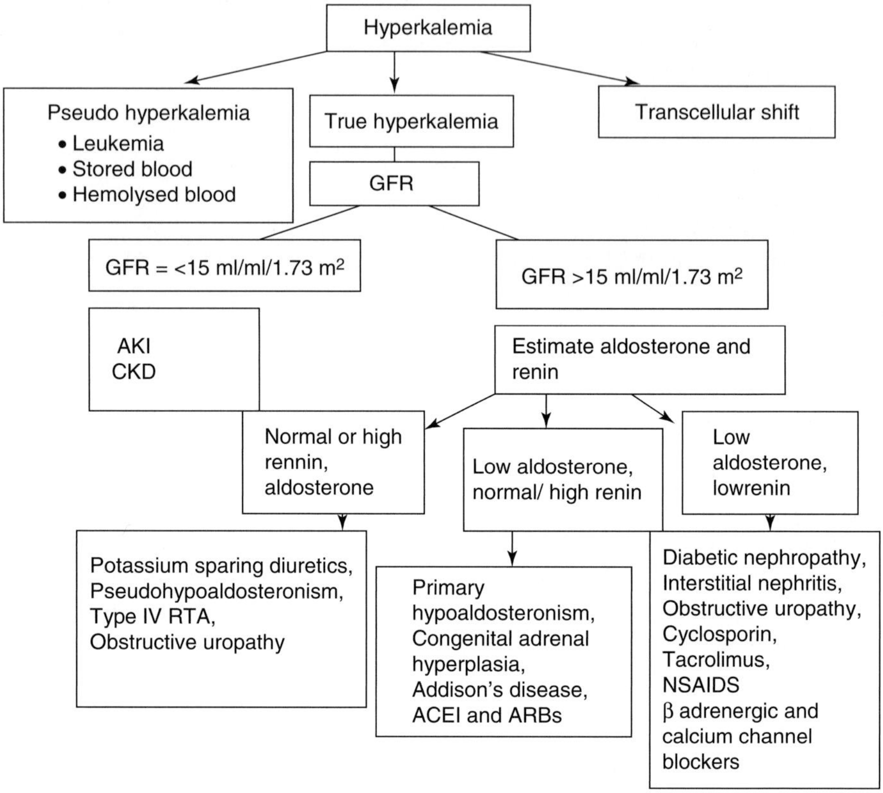

GFR glomerular filtration rate, *AKI* acute kidney injury, *CKD* chronic kidney disease, *RTA* renal tubular acidosis, *ACEI* angiotensin-converting enzyme inhibitor, *ARB* angiotensin receptor blockers, *NSAIDs* nonsteroidal anti-inflammatory drugs

2.3.3.5 Treatment

Immediate Treatment (Also See Chap. 8)

- Eliminate potassium from diet and fluids and discontinue drugs causing hyperkalemia.
- Calcium gluconate (10 % solution) – 1 ml/kg/dose diluted in saline over 10 min under cardiac monitoring. (The onset of action is within 2–3 min and the effect lasts for 1 h.)
- Sodium bicarbonate – 1–2 mmol/kg IV over 10 min.
- Insulin bolus dose at 0.1 unit/kg with 5 % dextrose at 2 ml/kg over 30 min
  or
- Insulin infusion of 5 % dextrose 1–2 ml/kg/h with regular insulin 0.1 U/kg/h. The insulin glucose infusion causes cellular shifts of potassium which occur by 30 min and lasts for 2–4 h.

- Potassium binders – sodium or calcium polystyrene sulfonate 1 g/kg/dose every 4–6 h, with 20 % sorbitol orally or mixed with 250 ml of water as retention enema.
- Peritoneal dialysis or hemodialysis – potassium content of dialysate could be zero or 1–2 mmol/l against a normal content of 3–4 mmol/l.

Long-Term Treatment

- Measure aldosterone levels, and if they are low treat with fludrocortisone. If the levels are normal, treat with a diuretic.
- Assess the volume status. If the volume is low, treat with fludrocortisone, and if the patient is volume expanded, treat with a diuretic.

2.4 Calcium, Phosphate and Magnesium

2.4.1 Calcium Disturbances

2.4.1.1 Calcium Metabolism

Introduction

Calcium (Ca) exists in three forms in plasma: calcium bound to protein, predominantly albumin (40 %); ionized calcium (48 %); and calcium that is complexed with anions like phosphate, citrate, and bicarbonate (12 %). A change in serum albumin of 10 g/l causes a change in serum calcium in the same direction by 0.8 mg/dl (0.2 mmol/l). Calcium stores depend on dietary Ca intake, absorption of Ca from the GI tract, and renal Ca excretion.

Renal Handling of Calcium

- Bone, intestine, and kidney are key organs involved in Ca homeostasis and is regulated principally by parathyroid hormone (PTH) and 1, 25 dihydroxyvitamin D (1, $25(OH)_2D$), and to a lesser extent by calcitonin.
- Sixty percent of plasma calcium is freely filtered at the glomerulus. Seventy percent of this is passively reabsorbed at the proximal tubule, 20 % at thick ascending limb of loop of Henle by the transepithelial electrochemical gradient created by sodium reabsorption, 5–10 % actively at the distal tubule by calcium channels TRPV5, and 5 % in the collecting tubules via TRPV6.

2.4.1.2 Hypocalcemia

Definition

- Preterm newborn – serum calcium <7 mg/dl (1.75 mmol/l) or ionized calcium <1 mmol/l
- Term newborn – serum calcium <8 mg/dl (2 mmol/l) or ionized calcium <1.1 mmol/l
- Children – serum calcium <8.5 mg/dl (2.12 mmol/l) or ionized calcium <50 % of serum calcium

Etiology

Vitamin D deficiency or impaired metabolism
Nutritional vitamin D deficiency, vitamin D-dependent rickets, bone mineral disease of CKD
Hypoparathyroidism
DiGeorge syndrome (22q11 deletion), CHARGE association, HDR association, HRD syndrome, KCS syndrome,
X-linked, autosomal or recessive hypoparathyroidism
PTH gene mutations
Calcium sensing receptor (CASR) abnormality – gain of function mutations or antibodies to the receptors
Hypomagnesemia
Neck surgery/post-parathyroidectomy
Mitochondrial diseases (MELAS, Kearns–Sayre syndrome)
Others – thalassemia, Wilson's disease, iodine 131 therapy
Resistance to PTH
Pseudohypoparathyroidism type IA, IB, II
Redistribution of plasma calcium
Tumor lysis syndrome
Hyperphosphatemia
Hungry bone syndrome
Acute pancreatitis
Poor calcium intake
Parenteral nutrition
Presence of dietary calcium chelators
Malabsorption
Others
Septic shock
Drugs – furosemide, steroids, phenytoin, phenobarbitone, rifampicin
Massive blood transfusions

CHARGE coloboma, heart anomaly, choanal atresia, mental retardation, genital hypoplasia, and ear anomalies, *HDR* hypoparathyroidism, deafness, and renal dysplasia, *HRD* hypoparathyroidism, mental and growth retardation, and dysmorphic features, *KCS* Kenny–Caffey syndrome, *MELAS* mitochondrial encephalopathy, lactic acidosis, and stroke-like episodes, *CKD* chronic kidney disease

Clinical Features (See Table 2.10)

- Hypocalcemia may often be asymptomatic. In children with symptoms, the signs and symptoms are related to the severity and duration of hypocalcemia. Acute hypocalcemia often results in symptoms due to neuromuscular irritability or cardiac arrhythmias.
- Tetany and seizures are more common in children with acute hypocalcemia.
- Rickets, candidiasis, cataracts, skin and dental changes, and extrapyramidal abnormalities are usually seen with chronic hypocalcemia and hypoparathyroidism.

Table 2.10 Clinical features of hypocalcemia

Acute

Neuromuscular irritability
  Paresthesias of lips, extremities (fingers and toes)
  Tetany
  Laryngeal stridor, apnea in neonates
  Seizures

Cardiac
  Congestive cardiac failure
  Arrhythmias
  ECG: prolonged QT interval, heart block

Chronic   Candidiasis, subcapsular cataracts, basal ganglia calcifications, extrapyramidal symptoms, enamel hypoplasia, papilledema
Features of rickets
Latent signs   Signs of Chvostek and Trousseau

Eliciting Signs of Chvostek and Trousseau

Chvostek's Sign

A sphygmomanometer cuff is inflated above systolic pressure and maintained for 3 min. A positive sign is flexion of the wrist and metacarpophalangeal joints and extension of the interphalangeal joints and adduction of the fingers due to carpopedal spasms.

Trousseau's Sign

Tap gently and repeatedly with a forefinger on the lateral cheek over the course of the facial nerve 0.5–1.0 cm below the zygomatic process and 2 cm anterior to the earlobe. A positive sign is twitching of the corner of the mouth on the ipsilateral side due to contractions of the circumoral muscles.

Evaluation of Hypocalcemia

Serum ionized calcium, phosphate, and magnesium
Serum albumin
Serum alkaline phosphatase
Serum electrolytes, creatinine
Arterial blood gases
Plasma 25-hydroxyvitamin D (25 OH D)

Serum intact parathyroid hormone
Urine analysis
pH, glucose, protein
Calcium/creatinine ratio
Fractional excretion of phosphate
ECG for prolonged QT interval
X-ray of wrist or knee
Renal ultrasound for nephrocalcinosis
Maternal vit D3 levels
1, 25 dihydroxy D3 level
Auto antibody screen for autoimmune polyendocrinopathy
Genetic studies (22q11 deletion, CASR mutations)

Approach to Hypocalcemia

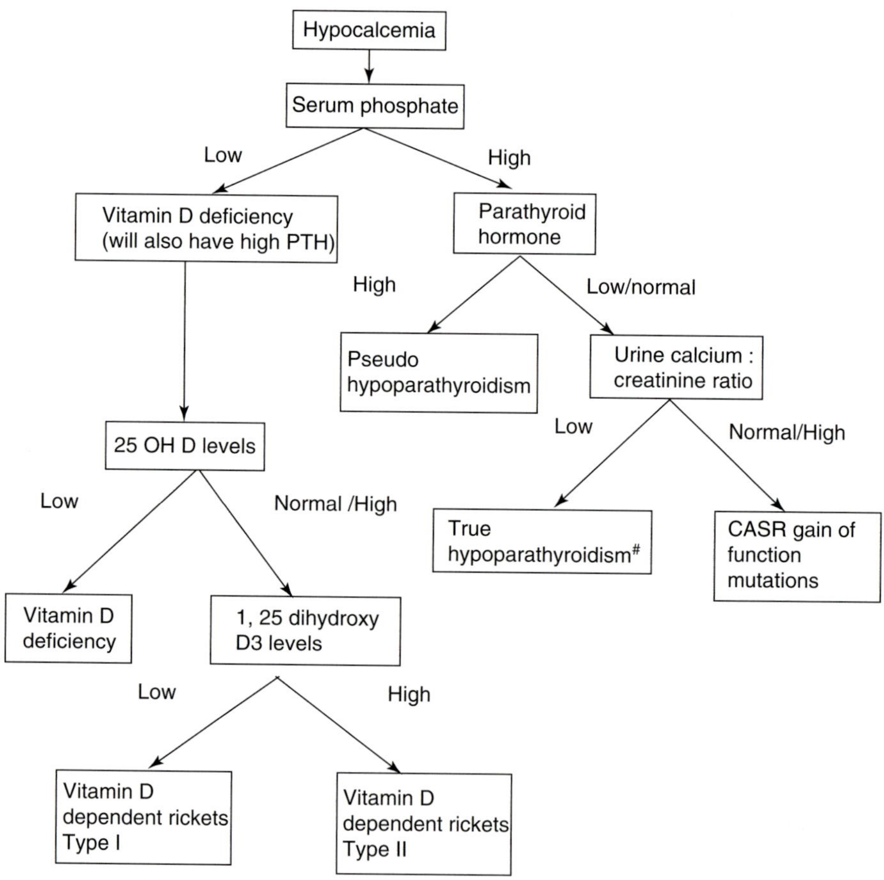

Treatment

- Symptomatic hypocalcemia
  Elemental calcium at 100–200 mg per kg (1–2 ml/kg/dose of 10 % calcium gluconate diluted to twice the volume in dextrose; maximum dose 10 ml/dose) is given intravenously under cardiac monitoring at a rate of not more than 100 mg/min. Do not mix IV calcium with $NaHCO_3$.The same dose is then repeated every 6–8 h. Once the symptoms have resolved, oral supplements can be initiated at 50–100 mg/kg/day of elemental calcium in 3–4 divided doses.
  While administering the intravenous dose, ensure patency of the venous access as calcium extravasations can cause tissue necrosis. The intravenous infusion should be immediately discontinued if there is a gradual decrease or sudden slowing of heart rate.
- Asymptomatic hypocalcemia
  Oral supplements can be initiated at 50–100 mg/kg/day of elemental calcium in 3–4 divided doses.
- Treatment of underlying cause of hypocalcemia
  For example, vitamin D deficiency should be treated with ergocalciferol (D2) or cholecalciferol (D3) (see Sect. 2.4.3). Hypomagnesemia if present should be treated (see Sect. 2.4.4). Vitamin D analogue (1α-hydroxyvitamin D (alphacalcidol) or 1, $25(OH)_2D_3$ (calcitriol)) in a dose of 25–50 ng/kg/day helps in increasing intestinal calcium absorption in hypoparathyroidism or pseudohypoparathyroidism. Management of vitamin D-dependent rickets type I and II has been described in Sect. 2.4.3

2.4.1.3 Hypercalcemia

Definition

Hypercalcemia is defined as serum calcium >12 mg/dl (>3 mmol/l). Severe hypercalcemia is defined as serum calcium >15 mg/dl (3.75 mmol/l).

Etiology

Hyperparathyroidism
Primary – adenoma, multiple endocrine neoplasia, calcium-sensing receptor mutation (loss of function)
Secondary and tertiary hyperparathyroidism (e.g., chronic kidney disease)
Excess vitamin D
Hypervitaminosis D
Sarcoidosis
Granulomatous diseases (Wegener's, Crohn's disease)
Cat scratch disease
Tuberculosis
Factors releasing calcium from bone
Thyrotoxicosis
Immobilization

Low turnover renal osteodystrophy on vitamin D
Malignancy-associated ectopic PTH/PTH-related products
Systemic lupus erythematosus
Drugs
Thiazides, lithium, calcium and vitamin D supplements, vitamin A
Others
Idiopathic infantile hypercalcemia
William's syndrome
Jansen's metaphyseal dysplasia
Milk alkali syndrome
Addison's/Cushing's disease
Phosphate depletion in preterm newborns

Clinical Features

- The clinical features are often due to the underlying disease causing hypercalcemia.
- The symptoms and signs depend on the severity and duration of hypercalcemia.

Clinical Features of Hypercalcemia

Gastrointestinal: nausea, vomiting, constipation, poor feeding
Cardiac: hypertension, arrhythmias, shortened QT interval
Neurological: hypotonia, poor activity, psychiatric disturbances, coma
Renal: polyuria, polydipsia, nephrocalcinosis, nephrolithiasis, distal renal tubular acidosis, acute renal injury
Ocular: Band keratopathy, conjunctival and palpebral calcification
Others: Weakness, anorexia

Evaluation

Serum total and ionized calcium, phosphate
Calcium × phosphate product
Serum alkaline phosphatase
Serum parathyroid hormone
Plasma 25 hydroxy vitamin D_3
Urine calcium creatinine ratio
Serum creatinine
Thyroid function test
Ultrasound neck for parathyroids

Approach to Hypercalcemia

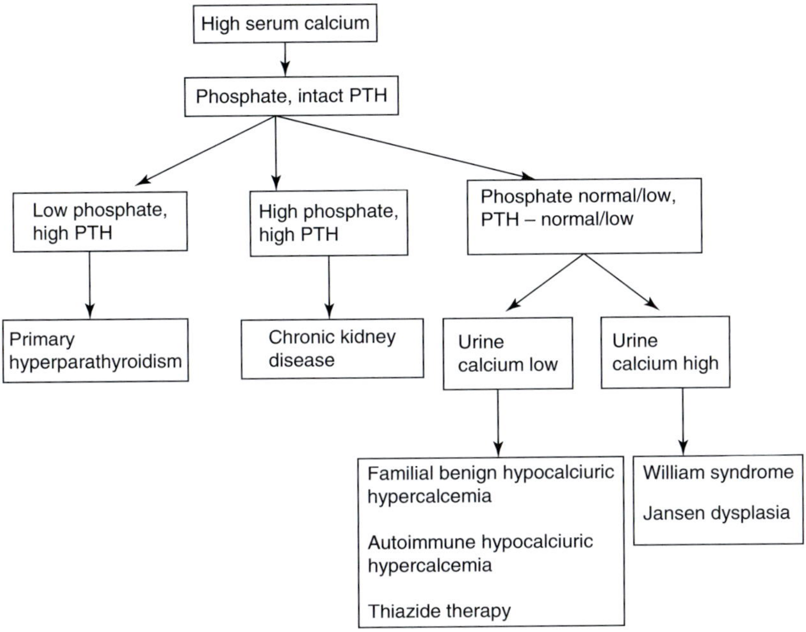

Treatment

- The four main strategies in management of hypercalcemia are to decrease intestinal calcium (Ca) absorption, increase urinary Ca excretion, decrease bone resorption, and remove excess Ca with the help of dialysis.
- Hydration with 3,000 ml/m^2/day of isotonic saline if renal functions are normal.
- Loop diuretics – furosemide 1 mg/kg/dose q 6 h.
- Hydrocortisone 1 mg/kg/dose every 6 h or equivalent dose of glucocorticoids in case of vitamin D intoxication, granulomatous disease, or paraneoplastic syndrome.
- Bisphosphonates:

  Pamidronate: Mild hypercalcemia: 0.5–1 mg/kg/dose IV

  Severe hypercalcemia: 1.5–2 mg/kg/dose IV

  Dilute pamidronate initially in water but infuse in saline or 5 % dextrose. The final concentration should not exceed 12 mg/100 ml of diluent. It is given as an infusion over 4 h initially and later over 2–4 h for three consecutive days. Repeat infusion every 2–3 weeks or every 2–3 months according to the degree and severity of hypercalcemia.
- Calcitonin: Start at 4 IU/kg 12–24 hourly intramuscular or subcutaneous and may increase up to 8 IU/kg q 6–12 h. The effect, although rapid, is short lasting, and prolonged use may lead to tachyphylaxis.
- Dialysis (hemodialysis or peritoneal dialysis using low dialysate calcium concentrations) for hypercalcemia associated with renal failure or if above measures fail.
- Surgical subtotal parathyroidectomy in cases of primary/tertiary hyperparathyroidism.

2.4.1.4 Hypercalciuria

Measurement of urinary calcium is a part of evaluation of patients with hematuria, nephrocalcinosis, and nephrolithiasis. Frequency urgency syndrome, recurrent urinary tract infections, and decreased bone density have been loosely associated with idiopathic hypercalciuria.

Hypercalciuria is defined as calcium excretion >4 mg/kg/24 h or >0.1–0.125 mmol/kg/24 h. Calcium creatinine ratio with a value of >0.2 mg/mg (>0.6 mmol/mmol) is suggestive of hypercalciuria. The ratio is higher in newborns and infants (refer Chap. 17).

Approach to hypercalciuria is given below. Some genetic conditions associated with hypercalciuria are given at the end of this chapter.

Evaluation of Hypercalciuria

An evaluation for secondary disorders should be considered in the presence of positive family history, failure to thrive, growth retardation, rickets, acid–base disturbances, renal dysfunction, proteinuria, electrolyte imbalance, dysmorphic features, or poor response to therapy.

Approach to Hypercalciuria

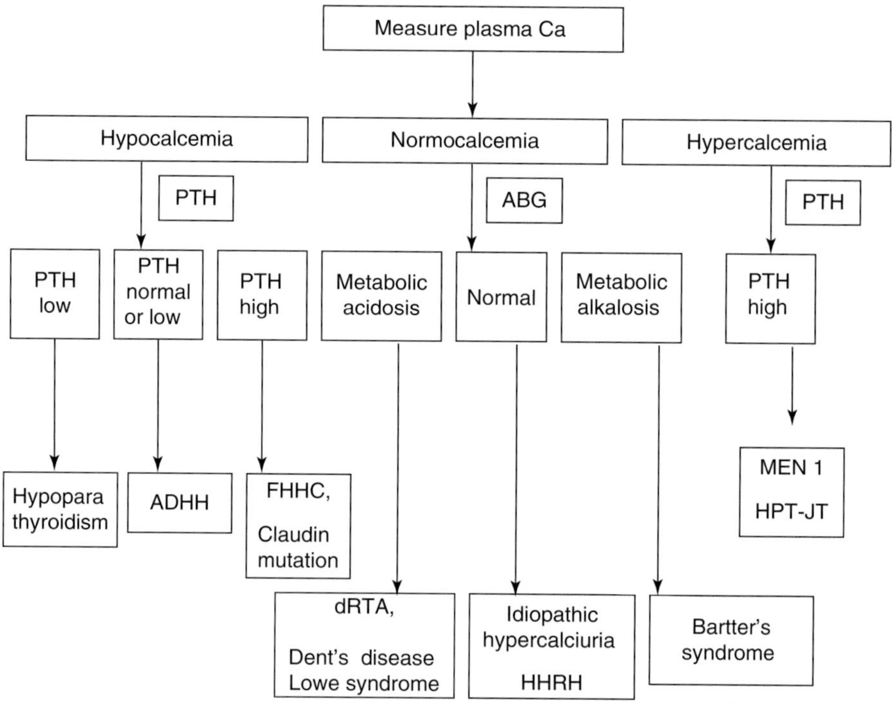

ABG arterial blood gas, *PTH* parathyroid hormone, *ADHH* autosomal dominant hypocalcemic hypercalciuria, *FHHC* familial hypomagnesemia with hypercalciuria, *dRTA* distal RTA, *HHRH* hereditary hypophosphatemic rickets with hypercalciuria, *MEN* multiple endocrine neoplasia, *HPT-JT* parathyroid tumors with ossifying fibromas of the jaw, *FIH* familial isolated hyperparathyroidism (Modified from Michael J. Stechman & Nellie Y. Loh & Rajesh V. Thakker **Genetic** causes of hypercalciuric nephrolithiasis: *Pediatr Nephrol* (2009) 24:2321–2332)

Idiopathic Hypercalciuria

Idiopathic hypercalciuria (IH): Elevated urinary calcium excretion without concomitant hypercalcemia when secondary causes have been ruled out. It is a common disorder seen in 3–6 % of children.

Clinical Features

In children, hypercalciuria can cause manifestations such as recurrent hematuria, voiding dysfunction (frequency–dysuria syndrome), flank pain, abdominal pain, nephrolithiasis, urinary tract infection, and decreased bone mineral density. Many of these symptom complexes have been only loosely associated with IH with no definite established causal relationship.

Twenty-six to 36 % of children have no identifiable basis for hematuria other than hypercalciuria. The type of hematuria (gross or microscopic) is not related to the severity of hypercalciuria.

Hypercalciuria is found in 28–79 % of children with urolithiasis and nephrocalcinosis. The risk of urolithiasis in children with idiopathic hypercalciuria varies from 0 to 16 % and increases with increasing duration of follow-up. The presence of gross hematuria, a family history of urolithiasis, and severity of hypercalciuria increase the risk for progression to urolithiasis.

Children with idiopathic hypercalciuria have decreased bone mineral content which is more marked in children with stones.

Treatment

- Dietary modifications form the mainstay of therapy in children with IH because urinary calcium excretion is significantly affected by sodium, protein, potassium, phosphorus, and calcium in the diet. Limiting excessive sodium and supplementing potassium in diet are important in management of hypercalciuria.
- Protein restriction is not suggested in children as it could impair growth. Similarly, a dietary restriction of calcium is not advised in these children because of risk of negative calcium balance and poor bone mineralization.
- Thiazide diuretics may be used in children who fail to normalize urinary calcium excretion with dietary modifications and/or have persistent symptoms attributable to hypercalciuria. Chlorothiazide 15–25 mg/kg/day or hydrochlorothiazide 1.5–2.5 mg/kg/day can be used. Children on long-term therapy with thiazides should be regularly monitored for dyselectrolytemia, hyperuricemia, hypomagnesemia, hyperlipidemia, and hyperglycemia.
- Potassium citrate can be used in children with persistent hypercalciuria who are at risk of stone formation and in children with secondary causes like renal tubular acidosis.
- Neutral phosphate salts should be used in children in whom hypercalciuria is secondary to severe tubular phosphate wasting (hypophosphatemic rickets with hypercalciuria and Lowe syndrome).
- Bisphosphonates may be considered in children with severe osteopenia and persistent hypercalciuria to improve bone density, but the data is limited.

Genetic Conditions Associated with Hypercalciuria

Disease	Gene	Key features
Autosomal dominant hypocalcemia	CASR	Hypocalcemia with hypercalciuria
Familial isolated hypoparathyroidism	CASR	Hypocalcemia with hypercalciuria, low PTH
Bartter syndrome – type I	SLC12A1/NKCC2	Hypercalciuria, nephrocalcinosis, metabolic alkalosis
Bartter syndrome – type II	KCNJ1/ROMK	Hypercalciuria, nephrocalcinosis, metabolic alkalosis
Bartter syndrome – type III	CLCNKB	Hypercalciuria with no nephrocalcinosis
Bartter syndrome – type IV	BSND	Also has congenital deafness
Bartter syndrome – type IV	CASR	Type similar to autosomal dominant, hypocalcemia
dRTA (distal RTA)	SLC4A1	Autosomal dominant, nephrocalcinosis, renal stones
dRTA with sensorineural deafness	ATP6B1/ATP6V1B1	Nephrocalcinosis, hypercalciuria
Dent's disease	CLCN5	Hypercalciuria, phosphaturia tubular proteinuria, Fanconi syndrome
Lowe syndrome	OCRL1	Hypercalciuria, aminoaciduria, phosphaturia, Fanconi syndrome, cataracts, CNS manifestations
Hereditary hypophosphatemic rickets with hypercalciuria	NPT2c/SLC34A3	Hypercalciuria, phosphaturia
Familial hypomagnesemia, hypercalciuria, nephrocalcinosis	PCLN1/CLDN16	Hypomagnesemia, hypercalciuria, magnesuria
Familial hypomagnesemia, hypercalciuria, nephrocalcinosis with ocular abnormalities	CLDN19	Myopia, fundal changes, hypomagnesemia, hypercalciuria, magnesuria

2.4.2 Disorders of Phosphate Metabolism

Phosphates exist as organic and inorganic forms. Inorganic phosphate (Pi) accounts for about 30 % of total plasma phosphorous; 10–15 % of this is protein bound and the remainder is freely filtered at the glomeruli. The intestine and kidney play important roles in the absorption of phosphates from the diet and in the excretion of phosphate in the urine, respectively.

Parathyroid hormone, vitamin D, and phosphatonins – fibroblast growth factor 23 (FGF 23), frizzled-related protein (FRP-4), matrix extracellular phosphoglycoprotein (MEPE) – are important regulators of phosphate homeostasis. The phosphatonins inhibit the activity of 1 α hydroxylase enzyme resulting in decreased formation of calcitriol [1, 25 $(OH)_2D_3$]. Fibroblast growth factor FGF23 acts via FGF receptor and a transmembrane protein Klotho and causes phosphaturia. The activity of FGF 23 is controlled by PHEX gene, located on the X chromosome.

Dietary phosphate absorption occurs in duodenum and jejunum and is regulated by dietary phosphate content and 1, 25 dihydroxy D3 levels which act via Na-Pi co-transporter.

Seventy percent of filtered phosphate is reabsorbed in the proximal tubule, and about 10 % is reabsorbed in the distal tubule. This occurs via sodium phosphate co-transporter and is regulated by PTH. PTH and PTH-related proteins inhibit this co-transporter and cause phosphate loss.

Phosphates play an important role in cellular functions, providing energy to cells with ATP (adenosine triphosphate).

Hyperphosphatemia occurs commonly in chronic kidney disease and is described in the chapter on chronic kidney disease. Hypophosphatemia is described in this chapter.

2.4.2.1 Hypophosphatemia

The serum phosphate level depends on age. Hence, there is no single cutoff value for hypophosphatemia. Serum phosphate levels according to age are given in the Chap. 17.

Hypophosphatemia can occur in the setting of low, normal, or high total body phosphate since more than 99 % of total body phosphorus stores are located intracellularly and serum phosphorus concentration does not adequately reflect total body phosphate stores.

2.4.2.2 Etiology

Transcellular shift
Re-feeding syndrome in malnutrition
Hungry bone syndrome
Respiratory alkalosis
Decreased intake
Nutritional deficiency
Premature infants
Phosphate binders
Renal losses
Hyperparathyroidism
X-linked hypophosphatemic rickets
Autosomal dominant and recessive hypophosphatemic rickets
Hereditary hypophosphatemia with hypercalciuria
Fanconi syndrome, Dent's disease
Steroids, diuretics, metabolic acidosis
Post-renal transplant
Fibrous dysplasia – McCune–Albright syndrome
Miscellaneous
Vitamin D deficiency
Tumor-induced osteomalacia
During CRRT (continuous renal replacement therapy)

2.4.2.3 Clinical Features

- Weakness of skeletal or smooth muscle is the most common clinical manifestation of phosphate deficiency. Hypophosphatemia also causes rhabdomyolysis via ATP depletion.
- Respiratory failure or failed weaning from the ventilator may occur in patients with severe hypophosphatemia.
- Hypophosphatemia can present with growth retardation and skeletal deformities with rickets. Lower extremities are involved more than upper extremities (genu varum or genu valgum). Dental (enamel/dentin) abnormalities are characteristically seen.

2.4.2.4 Clinical Features of Hypophosphatemia

Acute
Proximal myopathy, impaired myocardial contractility
Paresthesias, tremors, peripheral neuropathy, and features similar to Guillain–Barre syndrome
Chronic
Symptoms and signs of rickets
Rhabdomyolysis
Cardiac failure, respiratory failure
Hemolysis

2.4.2.5 Evaluation

Serum calcium, phosphorous, alkaline phosphatase
Serum 25 (OH) D3
PTH
Urine phosphate excretion: $FePO_4$, $TmPO_4/GFR$
Urine calcium creatinine ratio

FePO4 fractional excretion of phosphate, *TmPO4/GFR* maximal tubular reabsorption of phosphate; these have been described in Sect. 1.5

Various types of hereditary hypophosphatemic rickets, their clinical presentations, genetic aspects, and management are described in detail in chapter on tubular disorders – Chap. 4.

2.4.3 Rickets

2.4.3.1 Overview

- Rickets is a condition in which there is defective mineralization of growing bone and accumulation of non-mineralized osteoid tissue.
- Defective mineralization of bone matrix after the growth plates have fused is known as osteomalacia.
- Osteopenia refers to subnormal bone mineral density (BMD). Severe form of osteopenia is known as osteoporosis.
- Defective mineralization is generally caused by a lack of mineral supply which can be as a result either of deficiency of calcium (calcipenic rickets) or of phosphate (phosphopenic rickets). The commonest cause of rickets in developing countries is vitamin D deficiency.
- Disorders of vitamin D metabolism or responsiveness may also cause rickets. It is referred to as "non-nutritional rickets." Lack of response to two doses of 6×10^5 units of vitamin D given 2 weeks apart is termed as "resistant or refractory rickets."

2.4.3.2 Sources of Vitamin D and Its Metabolism

- Vitamin D is primarily made in the skin, and <10 % is derived from dietary sources.
- Vitamin D2 – ergocalciferol is plant derived.
- Vitamin D3 – cholecalciferol is synthesized by animals. The sources include fish like salmon and sardines, cod liver oil, and egg yolk. Cow's milk, yogurt, and butter are also good sources of vitamin D.
- Vitamin D content in breast milk ranges from 15 to 50 IU/l in a vitamin D-sufficient mother.
- In the skin, 7-dehydrocholesterol is activated to vitamin D3 on exposure to ultraviolet rays (UVR). It is transported to liver bound to vitamin D-binding protein. It is hydroxylated to 25-OH cholecalciferol (25 hydroxylase) and subsequently undergoes a second hydroxylation in renal cortex to 1, 25-dihydroxycholecalciferol or calcitriol (1 hydroxylase), the active form of vitamin D.

2.4.3.3 Etiology

Calcium deficiency with secondary hyperparathyroidism
Decreased vitamin D synthesis – lack of exposure to sunlight, dietary deficiency of vitamin D, altitude, air pollution, shade, skin pigmentation, clothing habits, sunscreen application
Malabsorption – celiac disease, cystic fibrosis
Low maternal stores of vit D and delayed weaning during infancy
Chronic liver disease
Drugs – anticonvulsant drug therapy, rifampicin, isoniazid, steroids
Vitamin D-dependent rickets type I

Primary phosphate deficiency with no secondary hyperparathyroidism
Primary hypophosphatemia (X-linked, autosomal dominant, Associated with hypercalciuria)
Fanconi syndrome
Renal tubular acidosis type II
Phosphate deficiency or malabsorption
Oncogenic hypophosphatemia
Renal osteodystrophy – bone mineral disease of chronic kidney disease
End organ resistance to 1, 25 $(OH)_2$ D_3
Vitamin D-dependent rickets type II

2.4.3.4 Diagnosis and Evaluation of Rickets

Symptoms and Clinical Signs

Nutritional Rickets

- Nutritional rickets usually appear during late infancy and second year of life. However, it may be seen as early as 2 months of age in breast-fed infants of vitamin D-deficient mothers.
- Infants who are at risk of vitamin D deficiency rickets are those who are born preterm, low birth weight, have delayed weaning, and are on supplemental feeds, low in vitamin D.
- Adolescence, dark-skinned population, and children residing at high altitude are also risk factors for rickets.
- Children and infants usually present with symptoms and signs related to bony deformities, may be associated with hypocalcemia and associated clinical features like seizures, tetany, stridor, muscular weakness, and hypotonia.
- The symptoms of rickets can range from being asymptomatic to varying degrees of irritability, delay in gross motor development, bone pain, poor growth, and recurrent respiratory infections.

Skeletal and Extra Skeletal Signs of Rickets
Craniotabes – earliest manifestation, indentable softening of skull bones
Anterior fontanel large and closure is delayed
Bossing of frontal and parietal bones – hot cross bun appearance
Rachitic rosary – prominent costochondral junctions
Pigeon-shaped chest
Harrison's sulcus
Widening of wrists
Double malleoli
Genu varum/genu valgum/coxa vara
Kyphoscoliosis, lordosis
Pathological fractures

Delayed eruption of primary tooth
Pot belly – visceroptosis, hypotonia of abdominal muscles
Bilateral lamellar cataract – rare
Increase sweating over forehead in infants

Non-nutritional Rickets

Rickets seen in chronic kidney disease (chronic kidney disease) is described in detail in Chap. 9. Some pointers to non-nutritional or refractory rickets are given below:

Pointers to Non-nutritional Rickets or Refractory Rickets

- Age <6 months or >3 years
- Associated failure to thrive with marked motor delay and short stature
- Positive family history
- History of polyuria, polydipsia, nocturia, salt craving, vomiting, seizures, pallor, hypertension
- Marked lower limb deformities in infancy
- Alopecia and enamel deformities
- H/O bone pains and weight loss
- Ultrasonography suggestive of nephrocalcinosis
- Elevated serum creatinine
- Very low or very high levels of $1,25(OH)D_3$
- Failure of response to vitamin D therapy

Biochemical Parameters

Investigations	Calcium-deficient rickets	Phosphate-deficient rickets (hereditary)	End organ resistance to $1,25\ (OH)_2\ D_3$
Serum calcium	Normal/low	Normal	Low
Serum phosphorus	Usually low	Low	Normal
Alkaline phosphatase (ALP)	Elevated	Elevated	Elevated
PTH	Elevated	Normal	Elevated

Note: Serum alkaline phosphatase may be normal in children who are malnourished and have zinc deficiency

In non-nutritional rickets, additional investigations such as PTH, 25-hydroxyvitamin D levels, and TMP/GFR (depending on suspected etiology) may be required. These have been given in other relevant chapters.

Biochemical Profile at Different Stages of Nutritional Rickets

	Serum Ca^{++}	Serum PO_4	ALP	PTH
Phase I	N/↓	N/↓	↑	↑
Phase II	↓	↓	↑↑	↑↑
Phase III	↓↓	↓↓	↑↑↑	↑↑↑

N Normal; ↑ increase; ↓ decrease

Radiological Findings

The radiological changes follow biochemical changes but precede clinical changes. They are best seen at end of long bones especially radius and ulna (ulna is affected prior to radius), knee joint, and costochondral junctions since they are the sites of rapid growth.

Osteopenia is the earliest sign followed by widening of growth plate (increased distance between epiphysis and the visible end of shaft due to uncalcified metaphysis) and metaphyseal changes:

- Changes at metaphysis: widening/cupping/fraying/flaring
- Changes in epiphysis: rarefaction, delayed bone age
- Changes in diaphysis: thinning of cortex resulting in green stick fractures and looser zones
- Changes during healing of rickets: appearance of a dense line of provisional calcification, normal density of bone is restored, starting from subperiosteal layer

Note: In non-nutritional rickets, especially in renal osteodystrophy secondary to chronic kidney disease (CKD stages 2–5), effects of secondary hyperparathyroidism may be seen and specific radiological findings such as cystic lesions and slipped epiphyses may be noted. These are described in detail in Chap. 9.

2.4.3.5 Treatment

Nutritional Rickets

- Vitamin D (cholecalciferol) is given in daily doses of 1,000–10,000 IU (depending on the age of the child) for a 2- to 3-month period (8–12 weeks).
- It is recommended to give 1,000 IU/day for infants <1 month old, 1,000–5,000 IU/day for infants 1–12 months old, and 5,000–10,000 IU/day for children >12 months old.
- 600,000 IU orally over 1–5 days or as single intramuscular (equally divided to each of the buttocks) dose may be used if noncompliance is suspected.
- Calcium supplements (30–75 mg/kg/day in 2–3 divided doses) should always be given with vitamin D therapy.
- Symptomatic hypocalcemia requires parenteral calcium replacement (1–2 ml/kg of 10 % calcium gluconate intravenously slowly over 5–10 min, repeat doses based on calcium levels). In addition, calcitriol may be necessary (20–100 ng/kg/day in divided doses) until calcium levels normalize.
- The vitamin D dose is reduced to 400–1,000 IU/day after the acute phase of management. Calcium supplementation is usually not necessary during the maintenance therapy.

- A satisfactory response to vitamin D therapy is indicated by a line of healing on a radiograph performed 2–3 weeks later. If no radiological healing is observed after a second course of therapy, the patient should be investigated for the cause of refractory rickets (see Fig. 2.5 – algorithm).
- Preparations of vitamin D and calcium are given in the Chap. 17.
- Monitoring of therapy: serum calcium, phosphorus, and ALP levels 1 and 3 months after initiating therapy. Increase in serum phosphate, the first sign of biochemical response is seen as early as 1–2 weeks. 25(OH) D_3 and PTH levels at end of therapy (3 months), x-ray wrist at 2 weeks and 3 months to confirm healing, 25(OH) D_3 levels should be monitored yearly.
- Be aware of "hypervitaminosis D" – Excess of vitamin D therapy may lead to intoxication (25(OH) D_3 levels >150 ng/l). Symptoms include anorexia, irritability, constipation, polydipsia, and polyuria. The child may be hypertensive secondary to hypercalcemia. Laboratory investigations reveal hypercalcemia and hypercalciuria. Nephrocalcinosis may be observed on renal ultrasonography. Treatment includes discontinuation of vitamin D and management of hypercalcemia (Sect. 2.4.1.3).

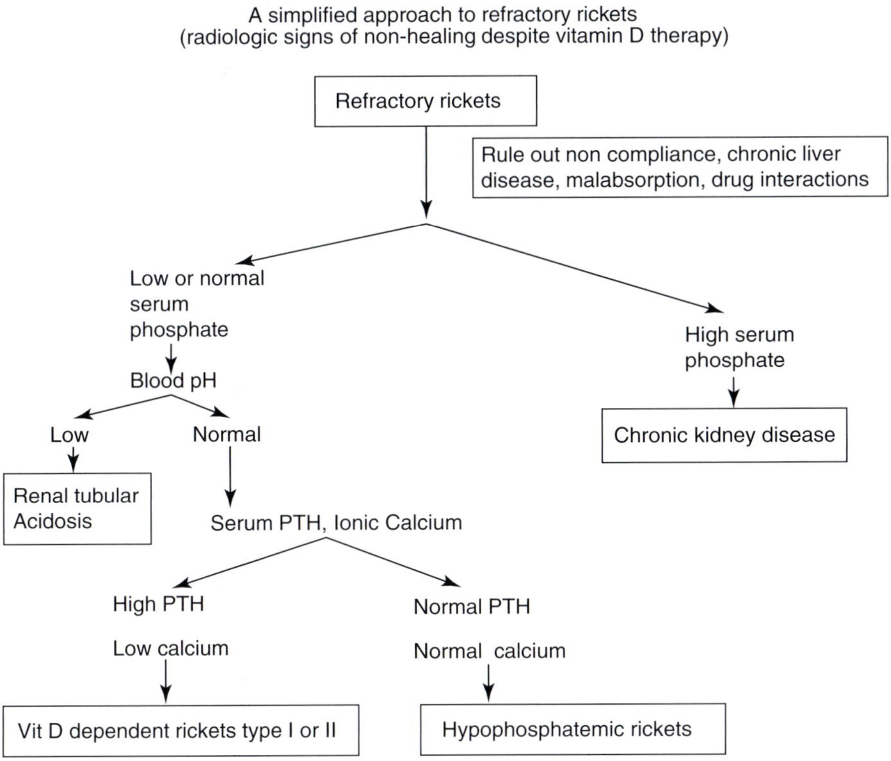

Fig. 2.5 A simplified approach to refractory rickets. *Note*: (1) Vitamin D deficiency may coexist in a child with refractory rickets. Blood levels of 25 hydroxyvitamin D_3 levels will help to identify coexistent vitamin D deficiency. (2) 1, 25-dihydroxyvitamin D_3 blood levels will help to differentiate between VDDR type I and type II

Prevention of Nutritional Rickets

1. Sunlight exposure – Exposure to sunlight is the principal source of vitamin D. Thirty minutes of sun exposure per week for infants in diapers and 2 h of sun exposure per week for fully clothed infants without a hat have been reported to maintain adequate vitamin D levels. Safe sun exposure between 11:00 and 15:00 h is important to ensure production of vitamin D in the skin.
2. Supplementation – All breast-fed infants and non-breast-fed infants and children who do not ingest at least 1 l of vitamin D-fortified milk per day receive 400 IU vitamin D per day as a supplement. Premature infants, dark-skinned infants and children, and children who reside at higher latitudes or live in countries with severe winter may given supplementation with up to 800 IU of vitamin D per day. Pregnant and lactating mothers should also be supplemented with vitamin D.
3. Vitamin D-fortified foods – Food-fortification practices vary around the world. Infant formulas contain 40–100 IU of vitamin D per 100 kcal of formula. However, food-fortification strategies in current practice may not be sufficient to prevent vitamin D deficiency in high-risk infants and children.

Non-nutritional Rickets

The therapy depends on the underlying disease. Management of renal osteodystrophy secondary to chronic kidney disease is described in Chap. 9. Features of vitamin D-dependent rickets have been described below, whereas hereditary hypophosphatemic rickets is discussed in Chap. 4.

2.4.3.6 Vitamin D-Dependent Rickets (VDDR)

These rare disorders present usually at 3–6 months of age with refractory rickets and features of hypocalcemia. They are autosomal recessively inherited. Two forms are seen:

VDDR Type I Rickets

- Deficient 1 alpha-hydroxylase activity due to loss of function mutations in the human CYP27B1 gene, localized to chromosome 12q13.3.
- Normal blood levels of 25(OH) D_3 but 1, 25(OH)$_2$ levels are markedly decreased.
- May present with seizures due to hypocalcemia. Dentition is delayed and enamel is hypoplastic.
- Associated with aminoaciduria, glycosuria, and proximal renal tubular acidosis.
- Also known as hereditary pseudovitamin D deficiency rickets.
- It is treated with physiological doses of alphacalcidol or calcitriol (1–2 μg/day). Most patients will require calcium supplements as well.

VDDR Type II Rickets

- End organ resistance to 1, 25(OH)$_2$D$_3$ due to point mutations in the vitamin D receptor gene, located on chromosome 12q.
- Raised blood levels of 1,25(OH)$_2$D$_3$

- High prevalence of alopecia and ectodermal defects such as epidermal cysts, milia, oligodontia.
- Poor and variable response to large doses of calcitriol and calcium supplements. Long-term nocturnal calcium transfusions may be required.

2.4.4 Magnesium

Magnesium is the second most abundant cation, next to calcium in the body. The normal serum values range from 1.5 to 2.3 mg/dl (0.62–0.95 mmol/l). Magnesium homeostasis depends on dietary intake, intestinal absorption, and renal excretion.

2.4.4.1 Renal Handling of Magnesium

- Eighty percent of magnesium is filtered and 95 % of filtered magnesium is reabsorbed, 15–20 % reabsorbed in the proximal tubule, 70 % by thick ascending limb of loop of Henle, and 5–10 % in the distal tubule. The distal tubule reabsorption rate determines the final concentration of magnesium excreted in urine.
- Magnesium reabsorption in the loop of Henle occurs by passive paracellular reabsorption due to a lumen-positive transcellular gradient created by absorption of sodium chloride. In the distal tubule, magnesium reabsorption is active via TRPM6 channel at the luminal surface.
- Calcium-/magnesium-sensing receptors are responsible for PTH secretion as well as for regulation of magnesium reabsorption in the kidney.

2.4.4.2 Hypomagnesemia

- Hypomagnesemia is defined as a serum magnesium concentration of less than 0.74 mmol/l (<1.8 mg/dl).
- Hypomagnesemia may be due to renal or extrarenal losses of magnesium. Rarely, it is due to decreased intake.
- The magnesium content of intestinal fluid is high. Hence, Mg depletion may be observed in children with acute or chronic diarrhea.
- Hypomagnesemia can cause hypocalcemia by impaired release of parathyroid hormone (PTH) and impaired response of tissues to PTH.

2.4.4.3 Etiology

Reduced intake: malnutrition, parenteral nutrition
Gastrointestinal losses
Acute/chronic diarrhea
Malabsorption syndrome

Prolonged vomiting, nasogastric tube suction
Bowel resection/fistula
Acute pancreatitis
Renal losses
Diuretic phase of acute tubular necrosis
Post-obstructive diuresis
Renal tubular acidosis
Gitelman's syndrome
Bartter syndrome
Familial hypomagnesemia with hypercalciuria and nephrocalcinosis with or without ocular involvement
Autosomal dominant hypocalcemia
Isolated dominant and recessive hypomagnesemia
Hypomagnesemia with secondary hypocalcemia
Drugs: diuretics, calcineurin inhibitors, aminoglycosides, cisplatin, amphotericin B, post-renal transplantation
Metabolic acidosis, hypercalcemia
Tubular diseases: chronic pyelonephritis, interstitial nephritis
Endocrine disorders
DKA
Hyperparathyroidism
Hyperthyroidism
Syndrome of inappropriate antidiuresis (SIAD)

2.4.4.4 Clinical Features

- Early symptoms of hypomagnesemia are nonspecific and include lethargy and weakness. Hypomagnesemia may also remain asymptomatic.
- The clinical features of magnesium depletion are usually due to associated hypocalcemia and hypokalemia.
- Hypocalcemia is common in patients with severe hypomagnesemia <1.2 mg/dl (<0.5 mmol/l) because of blunting of PTH secretion.

Symptoms and Signs of Hypomagnesemia

Neuromuscular
Tetany, seizures, muscle cramps, tremors, weakness, positive Chvostek sign, Trousseau sign, ataxia, nystagmus
Cardiovascular
Tachycardia, premature beats, arrhythmias – atrial fibrillation, ECG: prolonged PR and QT interval, U wave
Psychiatric
Depression, psychosis

Nonspecific
Nausea, vomiting, anorexia

2.4.4.5 Evaluation

Serum magnesium, calcium, phosphate
Serum electrolytes
Serum creatinine
Intact PTH
Fractional excretion of urinary magnesium
24-h urinary calcium
Renal ultrasound for nephrocalcinosis
EKG
Ophthalmic evaluation – severe myopia, macular coloboma

Fractional Excretion of Magnesium (FeMg)

The urinary Mg^{2+} is an important investigation during evaluation of hypomagnesemia. It helps to differentiate renal losses from extrarenal losses. Measurement of serum magnesium and creatinine and spot urinary magnesium and creatinine should be done simultaneously. The normal value is 3–5 %.

$$\text{FeMg}\left(\%\right) = \text{urine Mg} / \text{plasma Mg} \times \text{plasma Cr} / \text{urine Cr} \times 100$$

During magnesium depletion, the FeMg is <1 % and value >1 % suggests renal losses of magnesium as the cause of hypomagnesemia.

2.4.4.6 Clinical and Biochemical Features of Genetic Disorders of Magnesium Handling

Disorder	Gene	Age at onset	Key features
Gitelman's syndrome	SLC12A3	Adolescence	Hypomagnesemia, normocalcemia, hypomagnesuria, hypocalciuria, metabolic alkalosis, hypokalemia
Isolated dominant hypomagnesemia	FXYD2	Childhood	Hypermagnesuria, hypocalciuria, normal potassium, calcium, and blood pH
Autosomal dominant hypocalcemia	CASR	Infancy	Hypocalcemia, hypermagnesuria, hypercalciuria, normal K^+, may have metabolic acidosis, nephrocalcinosis, and renal stones during calcium and vitamin D therapy

Disorder	Gene	Age at onset	Key features
Familial hypomagnesemia with hypercalciuria, nephrocalcinosis	CLDN 16 CLDN 19	Childhood	Severe hypermagnesuria and hypercalciuria; normocalcemia; may have incomplete RTA, nephrocalcinosis, and renal stones; ocular involvement
Hypomagnesemia with secondary hypocalcemia	TRPM6	Infancy	Most severe hypomagnesemia of all listed disorders, hypocalcemia, magnesuria, normal urinary calcium excretion

2.4.4.7 Treatment

- Symptomatic hypomagnesemia
  Intravenous magnesium sulfate (50 % $MgSO_4$) @35–50 mg/kg (maximum dose 2 g) slowly, over 20–30 min. The dose is repeated every 6–8 h, monitoring magnesium levels. Alternatively, continuous infusion of 100–200 mg of $MgSO_4$/kg over 24 h may be used. The maximum infusion rate is 1 mEq/kg/h or 125 mg of $MgSO_4$/kg/h. This regimen can be used for 3–5 days if hypocalcemia is present. The aim of treatment is to achieve relief from symptoms though Mg levels may not reach normal values.
  Special caution is required during renal insufficiency. Intravenous calcium gluconate should be available as an antidote. Blood pressure, heart rate, and respiratory rate should be monitored during the intravenous therapy. Close monitoring of serum Mg is advised to avoid toxicity.
  Associated hypokalemia and hypocalcemia is refractory to potassium and calcium replacements, respectively, until magnesium level normalizes.
- Asymptomatic hypomagnesemia
  Oral replacement is usually the preferred route of therapy. The various salts available are magnesium gluconate, magnesium oxide, and magnesium sulfate. The oral dose for magnesium sulfate is 100–200 mg/kg/dose q 4–6 h. Alternatively, 0.2 ml/kg of 50 % magnesium sulfate may be given intramuscularly. The maintenance dose is 30–60 mg/kg/day or 0.25–0.5 mEq/kg/day. The dose should be increased gradually as diarrhea is commonly seen at higher dosages. Therapy should be titrated based on symptoms as it would be difficult to achieve normal magnesium level in disorders associated with renal wasting of magnesium.

Available Preparations

Magnesium sulfate ($MgSO_4$): parenteral – 500 mg/ml (4 mEq/ml), 250 mg/ml (2 mEq/ml), and 125 mg/ml (1 mEq/ml); oral – 50 % solution (500 mg/ml)

Magnesium oxide: tablets – 400 mg, 500 mg (400 mg = 241.3 mg of elemental Mg or 20 mEq Mg)

2.4.4.8 Hypermagnesemia

- A relatively rare condition and most commonly due to excessive intake of magnesium.

- May be seen in neonates born to mothers who have received magnesium sulfate for preeclampsia, abuse of laxatives and antacids, and children on parenteral nutrition.
- Can also be seen in children with chronic renal insufficiency, neonatal severe hyperparathyroidism, familial hypocalciuric hypercalcemia, milk alkali syndrome, tumor lysis syndrome, and lithium toxicity.
- Clinical features: The child may present with hypotonia, hyporeflexia, paralysis, drowsiness, and hypotension. ECG may show prolonged PR and QRS and QT interval. Rarely, heart block can occur.
- Treatment:
  In acute situations with cardiac abnormalities, intravenous calcium gluconate, 100 mg/kg, is to be administered. Hydration along with loop diuretics helps in magnesium excretion. Hemodialysis may be required in those with renal insufficiency. Peritoneal dialysate using chloride-based peritoneal dialysis solution may be done in patients with hypermagnesemia and metabolic alkalosis. For preparation of chloride-based solution, please see the Sect. 17.6.

2.5 Fluid Therapy in Select Situations

2.5.1 Maintenance Intravenous Fluids

- The term "maintenance fluids" is used when prescribing intravenous fluids for children with normal hydration who have no oral intake.
- Volume of maintenance fluid per day – insensible losses (sweat, stools, and losses with breathing) + volume required to excrete solutes (urea, creatinine) in volume of urine osmotically similar to plasma.
- Insensible losses are approximately 400 ml/m^2 in normal children. It increases by 12 % for each degree rise of body temperature >37.8 °C. The amount of fluid decreases by 25 % if child is lying inactive in bed or is on ventilator with humidified gases.
- The Holliday–Segar formula based on caloric expenditure is used to calculate the maintenance fluids in children (>4 weeks old) as given in Table 2.7.
- Alternatively, the maintenance fluid can also be calculated using the body surface area (BSA). Based on BSA, the fluid requirements per day are 1,500 ml/m^2.
- The maintenance electrolytes to be added to the IV fluids are as follows: sodium, 3 mmol/100 ml (50 mmol/m^{2+}); potassium, 2 mmol/100 ml (30 mmol/m^2); and chloride, 2 mmol/100 ml (30 mmol/m^2).

Table 2.7 Maintenance fluids according to the weight of the child

Weight (kg)	ml/kg/day	ml/h[a]
0–10	100/kg/day	4 ml/kg/h
11–20	1,000 + 50/kg/day (For each kg >10 kg)	(40) + 2 ml/kg/h (For each kg >10 kg)
>20	1,500 + 20/kg/day (For each kg >20 kg)	(60) + 1 ml/kg/h (For each kg >20 kg)

hr hour
[a]100 ml/h or 2,500 ml/day is the normal maximum amount

- Maintenance fluid must contain glucose (usually as 5 % dextrose) to prevent hypoglycemia and to prevent catabolism by providing calories.
- The maintenance requirements for well children with normal hydration are usually met using 0.2 % NaCl in 5 % dextrose with 20 mmol of potassium per liter as KCl (isolyte P).
- It is increasingly being recognized that very sick children which are prescribed 0.2 % NaCl in 5 % dextrose (which is hypotonic) may be at risk of developing hyponatremia. The recommendation is to use 0.45 % NaCl in 5 % glucose with 20 mmol KCl per liter in these critically ill children because they excrete less free water due to non-osmotic activation of antidiuretic hormone (ADH), predisposing them to hyponatremia.
- Maintenance fluid volume will need to be adjusted in the following situations:
  Unwell children with no activity – ↓ 25 %
  Mechanically ventilated children (with humidified gases) – ↓ 25 %
  Children with SIAD – ↓ 30–60 %

2.5.2 Fluid Therapy in Diabetic Ketoacidosis (DKA)

Fluids and electrolyte management in DKA is described below. For discussion on insulin therapy and other aspects of management of DKA, please refer to the relevant literature on the subject.

Fluid Resuscitation

- Initial hydrating fluid is isotonic saline. Dehydration is usually approximately 10 % of body weight, and the initial fluid prescription is based on this rough estimate, with subsequent adjustments, to be related to clinical and laboratory data.
- The fluid deficit correction is done evenly over 48 h.
- If hypoperfusion is present, replace approximately 10–20 % (10–20 ml/kg) of the fluid deficit over the first 1–2 h. Patients with DKA rarely require >20 ml/kg as boluses.
- After initial stabilization with isotonic saline, change to half-normal saline (0.45 % NS matches losses due to osmotic diuresis).
- Severity of dehydration may be difficult to assess; hence, infuse fluid each day at a rate rarely in excess of 1.5–2 times the usual daily maintenance requirements, based on age, weight, or body surface area.
- Change to 5 % dextrose containing IV fluid once blood sugar is <250 mg/dl.
- Urinary losses should not routinely be added to the calculation of replacement fluids except in severe polyuric states.

Electrolyte Replacement

Potassium

- If the patient is hypokalemic, start potassium replacement (KCl) at the time of initial volume expansion and before starting insulin therapy; otherwise, add potassium to fluids concurrent with insulin therapy. Defer potassium replacement if the serum level is >5.5 mmol/l or if the patient is anuric.

- Start KCl at a concentration of 40 mmol/l if body weight is <30 kg or 60 mmol/l if >30 kg.
- Anticipate rapid fall in serum potassium during therapy due to dilution and intracellular shifting.
- EKG may be done to help determine whether the child has hyper- or hypokalemia if the lab results are delayed.
- The maximum recommended rate of intravenous potassium replacement is usually 0.5 mmol/kg/h.
- If hypokalemia persists despite a maximum rate of potassium replacement, then the rate of insulin infusion can be reduced.

Sodium

- Spuriously low serum sodium may be estimated because of lipemia and hyperglycemia which reduce the aqueous phase of blood in which sodium predominantly resides.
- If the (corrected) serum sodium rises dramatically during therapy, then it is advisable to change to hypotonic fluids to avoid hypernatremia.

Phosphate

- Profound hypophosphatemia caused by renal losses from osmotic diuresis is common at presentation and during early treatment of DKA.
- As the acidosis gets corrected, the effects of hypophosphatemia may become more pronounced.
- Severe hypophosphatemia in conjunction with unexplained weakness should be treated with phosphate supplements.
- Potassium phosphate salts may be safely used as an alternative to or combined with potassium chloride or acetate provided that careful monitoring of serum calcium is performed to avoid hypocalcemia.

Magnesium

- DKA may be associated with significant hypomagnesemia, and it may contribute to refractory hypokalemia.

Correction of Acidosis

- Bicarbonate administration is not recommended unless the acidosis is profound (pH <7.1).
- If bicarbonate is considered necessary, cautiously give 1–2 mmol/kg over 60 min.

Identification of Early Features of Cerebral Edema and Treatment

In children younger than 10 years of age (especially less than 5 years), anticipate possibility of cerebral edema after 4–6 h of treatment. Look for the clinical features of heralding cerebral edema such as headache, change in level of consciousness, unequal dilated pupils, delirium, incontinence, vomiting, and bradycardia. Key features in management of cerebral edema are:

- Reduce IV fluid flow rate (decrease to ½ maintenance and correct deficit over 72 h instead of 48 h)
- Give mannitol 0.25–1 g/kg (1.25–5 ml/kg 20 % mannitol) IV or 5–10 ml/kg of 3 % saline slow IV over 30 min, and it can be repeated in 2–4 h if indicated
- Assess vital signs and neurologic status hourly or more frequently as indicated
- Assess accurately hourly fluid input and output
- Reassess serum electrolytes, glucose, calcium, magnesium, phosphorus, blood gases, anion gap, and urine ketones every 2–4 h (or more frequently if indicated) and BUN, creatinine, and hemoglobin every 6–8 h until they are normal

2.5.3 Fluid Therapy in Shock

Shock is an acute syndrome that occurs because of cardiovascular dysfunction and inability of circulatory system to provide adequate oxygen and nutrients to meet the metabolic needs of the vital organs.

Types of Shock

Hypovolemic – diarrhea, blood loss.
Cardiogenic – with preexisting myocardial disease or injury, shock with myocardial dysfunction.
Distributive shock – distributive shock occurs when blood is redistributed among organs such as secondary to sepsis, anaphylaxis, or neurogenic shock.
Septic shock is the prototype combination of hypovolemia, cardiogenic, and distributive shock.

Management of a Child with Shock

Initial evaluation and management in emergency room: "*The Golden Hour*"

Recognition of shock state by rapid cardiopulmonary assessment	0–5 min
Early fluid resuscitation	5–15 min
Recognition of fluid refractory shock and initiation of inotropes	15–60 min
Recognition of catecholamine-resistant shock and consideration of steroids	60 min

- Fluid resuscitation is given a lot of importance in the golden hour of shock management to achieve cardiopulmonary stability.
- Rapid intravascular volume expansion should be guided by frequent clinical examinations and urine output measurements.
- Crystalloids (0.9 % NS or Ringer lactate) are recommended as the routine initial resuscitation fluid. In children with nephrotic syndrome and shock, if the response to initial resuscitation is not adequate, early use of albumin infusion is recommended in view of hypoalbuminemia.

- The role of colloids (albumin, hydroxyethyl starch) in resuscitation of shock is not clear.
- A 60-ml syringe filled with fluid drawn via the fluid bag with a three-way connection can be conveniently used to push fluid boluses in the absence of a volumetric pump.
- For details on the "golden hour of shock management," please refer to standard textbooks of Pediatric Critical Care.

Management of Shock in PICU

A few practical points regarding "shock management in PICU" are given below:

- Electrolyte abnormalities (such as hypocalcemia) that might impair cardiac performances and hypoglycemia should be corrected to ensure appropriate response to inotropes.
- Goals at the end of 6 h in PICU management are normalized MAP (mean arterial pressure) for age, normalized CVP (central venous pressure) for age, $S_{SVC}O_2$ >70 % (mixed venous blood saturations), and resolving lactic acidemia.
- Inotropes/vasopressors

Infusion pumps should be used, and all infusions with their rates should be carefully labeled.

Dopamine

It is the first drug of choice in children with septic shock. Young infants (<6 months) may be insensitive to dopamine possibly due to lack of complete development of synaptic vesicles. The infusion dose varies from 2 to 20 μg/kg/min. The effects of dopamine are dose dependent. Infusion may be increased by 1–4 μg/kg/min at 10- to 30-min intervals until optimal response is obtained. *At low rates of infusion (0.5–2 mcg/kg/min)*, dopamine causes vasodilatation due to agonist action on dopamine receptors in the renal, mesenteric, coronary, and intracerebral vascular beds. *At intermediate rates of infusion (2–10 mcg/kg/min)*, dopamine acts to stimulate the beta-1 adrenoceptors, resulting in improved myocardial contractility. *At higher rates of infusion (10–20 mcg/kg/min)*, there is some effect on alpha-adrenoreceptors, with consequent vasoconstrictor effects.

Preparation: 40 mg per 5 ml (6 mg/kg in 100 ml 5 % dextrose, 1 ml/kg/h = 1 μg/kg/min)

Dobutamine

The infusion dose varies from 2.5 to 20 μg/kg/min. It increases contractility and, to a lesser extent, heart rate by its action on β-1 receptors with direct effect on blood pressure.

Preparation: 250 mg per vial (6 mg/kg in 100 ml 5 % dextrose: –1 ml/kg/h = 1 μg/kg/min)

Epinephrine

The dosing varies from 0.05 to 2 μg/kg/min.

Epinephrine is a potent α- and β-adrenergic agent. It is the drug of choice for dopamine-resistant septic shock.

Preparation: 1 mg/ml 1:1,000 (0.6 mg/kg in 100 ml 5 % dextrose –1 ml/kg/h=0.1 μg/kg/min)

Norepinephrine

The dosing varies from 0.05 to 2 μg/kg/min.

It acts on both α- and β-1 receptors and is the most potent vasoconstrictor, effective in vasodilatory shock.

Preparation: 1 mg/ml (0.6 mg/kg in 100 ml 5 % dextrose:–1 ml/kg/h=0.1 μg/kg/min)

Milrinone

The dosing varies from 0.375 to 0.75 μg/kg/min.

It is a phosphodiesterase inhibitor with positive inotropic and vasodilator activity.

It is useful in children who have high vascular resistance shock and low cardiac output but remain normotensive.

Preparation: 10 mg/ml

Vasopressin

Recommended dosing is 0.3 to 2 milliunits/kg/min (equivalent to 0.00053–0.002 units/kg/min or 0.01 to 0.12 units/kg/h).

Vasopressin acts on V1, V2, and V3 receptor sites. The vasoconstrictive effects of vasopressin are mediated through vascular V1 receptors. Vasodilation within the coronaries, as well as the cerebral, pulmonary, and renal vascular beds, is likely the result of a complex interplay of vasopressin activity at V1 and endothelial V3 and oxytocin receptor sites.

Vasopressin may also enhance or restore catecholamine sensitivity.

Preparation: 20 U/ml (0.2 U/kg in 100 ml isotonic saline, 1 ml/h=0.002 U/kg/h)

- Steroids: Stress-dose steroids should be reserved for use in children with catecholamine-resistant septic shock who have suspected or proven adrenal suppression.

  Dose recommendation varies from 1 to 2 mg/kg (based on clinical suspicion of adrenal insufficiency). A cosyntropin stimulation test may be performed to identify patients with relative adrenal insufficiency.
- Recombinant human activated protein C: Administration of recombinant activated protein C inhibits thrombosis and inflammation, promotes fibrinolysis, and modulates coagulation and inflammation. The therapy is expensive, limiting its use.
- Extracorporeal therapies:

  Continuous renal replacement therapy (CRRT) has been used in managing children with septic shock who have either volume overload or acute kidney injury. CRRT may also have the additional advantage of removing inflammatory mediators from children with sepsis.

  Other forms of extracorporeal therapies that have been used in children with catecholamine refractory septic shock are plasmapheresis and extracorporeal membrane oxygenation (ECMO) (Fig. 2.6).

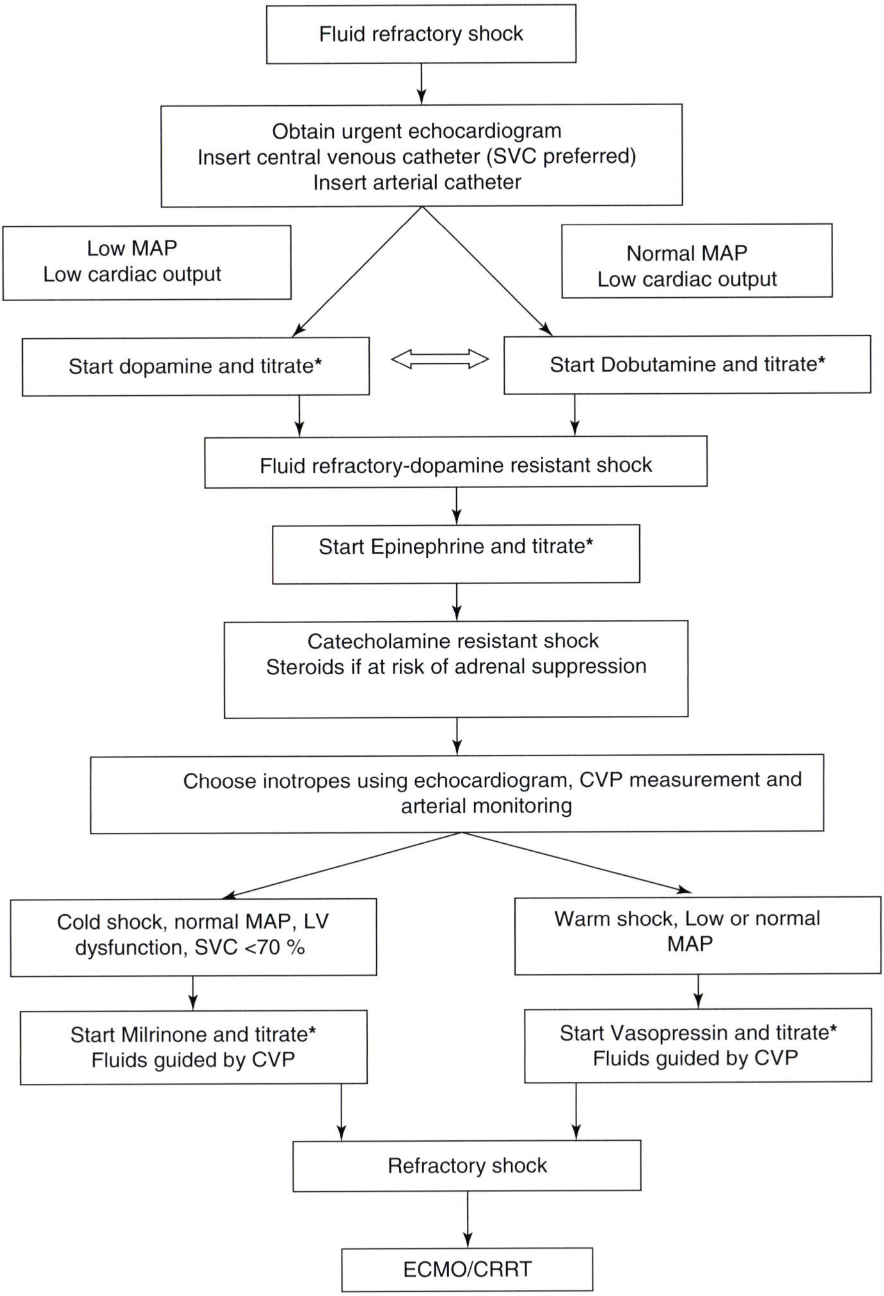

Fig. 2.6 Algorithm for management of shock in PICU. *Titration of inotropes aimed at normalized MAP for age, normalized CVP for age, $S_{svc}O_2$ >70 %, and resolving lactic acidemia. *MAP* mean arterial pressure, *CVP* central venous pressure, *LV* left ventricle, *ECMO* extracorporeal membrane oxygenation, *CRRT* continuous renal replacement therapy

2.5.4 Fluid Therapy in Acute Diarrhea

History

- Character of the stool – watery/blood stained
- History of fever/vomiting, acceptability of oral rehydration therapy (ORT)
- Urine output in last 6 h
- Whether received ORT (oral rehydration solution) before reaching hospital
- Whether receiving breast feeding/normal diet after the onset of diarrhea

Rehydration Therapy

Oral Rehydration Solutions (ORS) see Table 2.9

- Oral rehydration therapy (ORT) uses a simple, inexpensive, glucose and electrolyte solution promoted by the World Health Organization (WHO).
- The gastrointestinal reabsorption of ORS depends on three factors: the concentration of sodium, the concentration of glucose, and the osmolality of the solution.
- The types of oral rehydration solutions (ORS) that may be used are:
  Glucose-based ORS – low-osmolality ORS, standard ORS, rehydration solution for malnourished (ReSoMal)
  Rice-based ORS
  Home-available ORS (rice gruel, lemon water)
  ORS with other nutrients like amino acids
- The advantages of ORS are that it is physiological, easy to administer, cost-effective, and is readily available. It can also be prepared easily at home using salt, sugar, and water.
- ORS is ineffective in children who have high stool purge rate (>5 ml/kg/h), persistent vomiting, paralytic ileus, or underlying malabsorption states.
- The low-osmolality ORS allows for quicker absorption of fluids, reducing the need for intravenous fluids, and also decreases the stool volume due to lesser tonicity as compared to standard ORS. It has replaced standard ORS in the management children with acute non-cholera diarrhea.

Treatment According to Severity of Dehydration (Also See Table 2.8)

Plan A

- Oral rehydration therapy should be initiated.
- ORT includes:
  1. Complete oral rehydration salt solution with composition as per the WHO recommendation (WHO ORS)
  2. Solutions made from sugar and salt (40 g sugar + 4 g salt + 1 l of drinking water)
  3. Food-based solutions (rice approximately 50 g + salt 4 g + 1 l of drinking water)
  4. Variety of commonly available and culturally acceptable fluids (lemon water, coconut water, soups, thin rice gruel)
- Report if diarrhea persists for more than 3 days or any of the danger signs (many watery stools, repeated vomiting, marked thirst, eating or drinking poorly, fever and blood in stool) develop.

Table 2.8 Dehydration severity based on clinical signs and symptoms

Look at	Condition	Well alert	"Restless, irritable"	"Lethargic or unconscious"
	Eyes	Normal	Sunken	Very sunken and dry
	Tears	Present	Absent	Absent
	Mouth and tongue	Moist	Dry	Very dry
	Thirst	Drinks normally/ not thirsty	"Thirsty, drinks eagerly"	"Drinks poorly or not able to drink"
Feel	Skin pinch	Goes back quickly	"Goes back slowly"	"Goes back very slowly"
Decide		No signs of dehydration	Patient has two or more signs with at least one "*sign*," there is some dehydration	Patient has two or more signs with at least one "*sign*," there is some dehydration
Treat		Plan A	Plan B	Plan C

- Commercially available ORS preparations and its ingredients:
  1. WHO low-osmolality ORS
  2. WHO standard ORS
  3. Rehydration solution for severely malnourished children – ReSoMal
  4. Cereal-based ORS – rice water electrolyte solution

     Put 2 finger scoops of rice powder in 1 l water and boil it. Add a pinch of salt and 1/4 medium-sized lemon juice to make rice–water electrolyte solution.
  5. Amount of ORS or other culturally acceptable ORS fluids to be given after each loose stool:

     <24 months – 50–100 ml

     2–10 years – 100–200 ml

     >10 years – as much as child wants

Plan B

- All patients with evidence of dehydration to be treated at a health center or hospital.
- Fluid therapy includes (a) deficit correction, (b) replacement of ongoing losses, and (c) maintenance fluid therapy.
- Deficit correction – Give 75 ml/kg of oral rehydration solution (ORS) in first 4 h. Use the child's weight for calculating fluids. Encourage breast-feeding during this period.
- Maintenance fluid therapy (breast feeding/semisolid foods/milk mixed with cereals) is started when the signs of dehydration disappear, usually at the end of 4 h. If the child continues to have evidence of some dehydration at the end of 4 h, repeat rehydration with ORS solution.
- Replacement of ongoing losses – 10–20 ml/kg for each liquid stool as ORS.

Plan C

- Start intravenous (IV) fluids immediately. While the drip is being set up, give ORS solution if the child can drink.
- Deficit replacement – Ringer's lactate or 0.9 % saline solution:
  <12 months age – 30 ml/kg[1] in 1 h and 70 ml/kg in next 5 h
  12 months up to 5 years – 30 ml/kg[2] in 30 min and 70 ml/kg in 2 ½ h
- If one is unable to give IV fluids (for reasons of access, logistic availability, or during transport), immediately start rehydration with ORS using nasogastric tube at 20 ml/kg/h (total of 120 ml/kg) and try to start IV fluids as early as possible.
- Reassess the child every 15–30 min. Blood sample to be sent for BUN, creatinine, serum electrolytes (Na, K, Cl, and HCO_3), arterial gas, and serum lactate.
- If there is evidence of shock, the fluid therapy guidelines of septic shock should be followed.
- Continue maintenance therapy and replacement of ongoing losses.

2.5.5 Management of Dehydration and Shock in a Malnourished Child

Challenges in Managing Malnourished Children with Dehydration and Shock

- It is often difficult to estimate dehydration status in a severely malnourished child using clinical signs alone.
- Hypovolemia can coexist with edema.
- Shock from dehydration and sepsis are likely to coexist in severely malnourished children. Those with septic shock and no dehydration will not respond to fluids.
- The amount of fluid given is determined by the child's response, and overhydration must be avoided.
- *Re*hydration *So*lution for *Mal*nutrition (ReSoMal) is preferred. The ReSoMal contains less sodium and higher amounts of potassium (see Table 2.9).

Management of Dehydration

- *Re*hydration *So*lution for *Mal*nutrition (ReSoMal) 5 ml/kg is initially given every 30 min for 2 h, orally or by nasogastric tube, then 5–10 ml/kg/h for the next 4–10 h: the exact amount to be given should be determined by how much the child accepts, stool losses, and vomiting.
- Replace the ReSoMal doses at 4, 6, 8, and 10 h with F-75 (please find below the composition of F-75 and F-100 WHO solutions).
- F-75 is the "starter" formula used during initial management of malnutrition, beginning as soon as possible and continuing for 2–7 days until the child is stabilized. F-100 is used as a "catch-up" formula to rebuild wasted tissues.

[1] Repeat the same volume again if the radial pulse is weak/not detectable.

[2] See footnote 1.

Table 2.9 Composition of ORS

	WHO low-osmolality ORS (mEq/l)	WHO standard ORS (mEq/l)	ReSoMal (mEq/l)
Na	75	90	45
K	20	20	40
Cl	65	80	70
Citrate	10	10	7
Glucose	75	111	
Mg	–	–	3
Zn	–	–	0.3
Copper	–	–	0.045
Osmolality (mOsm/l)	245	311	300

- During treatment, rapid respiration and pulse rates should slow down, and the child should begin to pass urine. Return of tears, moist mouth, eyes and fontanel appearing less sunken, and improved skin turgor are also signs that rehydration is proceeding well.
- Monitor progress of rehydration: Observe half hourly for 2 h, then hourly for the next 6–12 h, recording pulse rate, respiratory rate, urine frequency, and stool/vomit frequency.
- Continuing rapid breathing and pulse during rehydration suggest coexisting infection or overhydration. Signs of excess fluid (overhydration) are increasing respiratory rate and pulse rate, increasing edema, and puffy eyelids.

Management of Shock

- Administer sterile 10 % glucose (5 ml/kg) by IV.
- IV fluid at 15 ml/kg over 1 h. Use Ringer's lactate with 5 % dextrose, or half-normal saline with 5 % dextrose, or half-strength Darrow's solution with 5 % dextrose, or if these are unavailable, use Ringer's lactate.
- Measure and record pulse and respiration rates every 10 min.
- Empirical IV antibiotics.

  If there are signs of improvement (pulse and respiratory rates fall):
- Repeat IV 15 ml/kg over 1 h.
- Switch to oral or nasogastric rehydration with ReSoMal, 10 ml/kg/h for up to 10 h. Give ReSoMal every 2 h with starter F-75 solution.
- Continue feeding with starter F-75 solution.

  If the child fails to improve after the first hour of treatment (15 ml/kg):
- Assume that the child has septic shock.
- Give maintenance IV fluids (4 ml/kg/h) and whole blood if indicated at 10 ml/kg slowly over 3 h.
- Begin feeding with starter F-75 solution while waiting for blood.

F-75 and F-100 Diet

F-75 contains 75 kcal and 0.9 g protein per 100 ml.

F-100 contains 100 kcal and 2.9 g protein per 100 ml.

Ingredient	Amount F-75[a–d]	F-100[e–f]
Dried skimmed milk	25 g	80 g
Sugar	70 g	50 g
Cereal flour	35 g	–
Vegetable oil	27 g	60 g
Mineral mix[g]	20 ml	20 ml
Vitamin mix[g]	140 mg	140 mg
Water to make	1,000 ml	1,000 ml

Reference: Management of severe malnutrition: a manual for physicians and other senior health workers. World Health Organization Geneva 1999

[a]Prepare the F-75 diet; add the dried skimmed milk, sugar, cereal flour, and oil to some water; and mix. Boil for 5–7 min. Allow to cool, then add the mineral mix and vitamin mix, and mix again. Make up the volume to 1,000 ml with water

[b]A comparable formula can be made from 35 g of whole dried milk, 70 g of sugar, 35 g of cereal flour, 17 g of oil, 20 ml of mineral mix, 140 mg of vitamin mix, and water to make 1,000 ml. Alternatively, use 300 ml of fresh cows' milk, 70 g of sugar, 35 g of cereal flour, 17 g of oil, 20 ml of mineral mix, 140 mg of vitamin mix, and water to make 1,000 ml

[c]Isotonic versions of F-75 (280 mOsm/l), which contain maltodextrins instead of cereal flour and some of the sugar and which include all the necessary micronutrients, are available commercially

[d]If cereal flour is not available or there are no cooking facilities, a comparable formula can be made from 25 g of dried skimmed milk, 100 g of sugar, 27 g of oil, 20 ml of mineral mix, 140 mg of vitamin mix, and water to make 1,000 ml. However, this formula has a high osmolality (415 mOsm/l) and may not be well tolerated by all children, especially those with diarrhea

[e]To prepare the F-100 diet, add the dried skimmed milk, sugar, and oil to some warm boiled water and mix. Add the mineral mix and vitamin mix and mix again. Make up the volume to 1,000 ml with water

[f]A comparable formula can be made from 110 g of whole dried milk, 50 g of sugar, 30 g of oil, 20 ml of mineral mix, 140 mg of vitamin mix, and water to make 1,000 ml. Alternatively, use 880 ml of fresh cows' milk, 75 g of sugar, 20 g of oil, 20 ml of mineral mix, 140 mg of vitamin mix, and water to make 1,000 ml

[g]The mineral mix contains potassium, magnesium, and other essential minerals. Combined Mineral Vitamin Mix (CMV) is available commercially

Suggested Reading

Bhatnagar S, Lodha R, Choudhury P, Sachdev HP, Shah N, Narayan S, Wadhwa N, Makhija P, Kunnekel K, Ugra D, Indian Academy of Pediatrics (2007) IAP guidelines 2006 on management of acute diarrhea. Indian Pediatr 44(5):380–389

Bianchetti MG, Bettinelli A (2008) Differential diagnosis and management of fluid, electrolyte and acid base disorders. In: Geary D, Schafer F (eds) Comprehensive pediatric nephrology. Elsevier/Mosby Inc, Philadelphia, p 461

Brodehl J (1994) Assessment and interpretation of the tubular threshold for phosphate in infants and children. Pediatr Nephrol 8:645

Devuyst O, Konrad M, Jeunemaitre X, Zennaro MC (2009) Tubular disorders of electrolyte regulation. In: Avner D, Harmon WE, Niaudet P, Yoshikawa N (eds) Pediatric nephrology. Springer, Berlin, p 929

Ellison DH, Berl T (2007) Clinical practice. The syndrome of inappropriate antidiuresis. N Engl J Med 356:2064

Ewout J, Zietse HR (2008) Hyponatremia revisited: translating physiology to practice. Nephron Physiol 108:46–59
Halperin and Goldstein: Fluid, electrolyte and acid base physiology: a problem based approach
http://motherchildnutrition.org/malnutrition-management/info/feeding-formulas-f75-f100.html
http://rehydrate.org
Mishra M et al (2008) Vitamin D deficiency in children and its management: review of current knowledge and recommendations. Pediatrics 122:398–417
Williams AJ (1998) ABC of oxygen assessing and interpreting arterial blood gases and acid base balance. BMJ 317:1213–1216
World Health Organization (2009) Management of severe malnutrition: a manual for physicians and other senior health workers. World Health Organization, Geneva

Glomerular Diseases

3

Martin Bitzan

3.1 Approach to Hematuria

3.1.1 Abstract

The goal of the initial assessment is to decide if the hematuria is due a medically important cause while avoiding unnecessary investigations.

Important differential laboratory and clinical criteria are the presence or absence of glomerular (deformed) red blood cells or casts, concomitant, persistent proteinuria, systemic features, hypercalciuria, urine crystals, pain, and the patient's age.

This section provides several diagnostic approaches based on the clinical presentation and simple laboratory observations.

3.1.2 Definitions

- Presence of red blood cells (RBC) in urine (>10 RBC per mm^3 of freshly voided, unspun urine or >5 RBC per high power field (HPF) of 10 ml of fresh urine, centrifuged at 2,000 rpm and resuspended in 0.5 ml).
- Macroscopic (gross) hematuria refers to urine that is visibly bloody (bright red to brown or tea (cola) colored). The color depends on the amount of blood, the source of bleeding, and urine acidity. One ml of blood per 1 l of urine is sufficient to render urine visibly "bloody."
- Microscopic hematuria (microhematuria) refers to the presence of RBC without urine discoloration, detected by microscopy or chemical (dipstick) analysis. Threshold for a positive readout is a hemoglobin concentration of approximately 0.6 mg/l.

M. Bitzan
Division of Pediatric Nephrology, Montreal Children's Hospital, McGill University, 2300, rue Tupper, Montreal, QC H3H 1P3, Canada
e-mail: martin.bitzan@mcgill.ca

K. Phadke et al. (eds.), *Manual of Pediatric Nephrology*,
DOI 10.1007/978-3-642-12483-9_3,

- A positive dipstick reaction in the absence of RBC in urine by microscopy suggests hemolysis or myoglobinuria.
- Glomerular diseases, if associated with gross hematuria, usually present with dark-brown (tea or cola) colored urine. Acute, non-glomerular hematuria is generally bright red, often with clots and painful voiding.
- Active glomerulonephritis and acute interstitial nephritis present with increased numbers of dysmorphic RBCs or RBC casts compared with hematuria originating from the lower urinary tract.
- Not all red urine is due to hematuria. Blood may be of menstrual origin or be due to hematospermia. Red urine in the absence of RBC or hemoglobin/myoglobin suggests excretion of other agents that color the urine (see Box 3.1 and Sect. 1.3).

3.1.3 Introduction

- Microscopic hematuria is much more frequent than gross hematuria. It may be transient or chronic. It is often discovered incidentally, e.g., at a routine check during the workup for dysuria, abdominal/flank pain, or extrarenal disease.
- The prevalence of significant disease in children with isolated microhematuria found at random screening is low (<1 to 7.2 %).
- While malignancies of the urogenital tract are an important differential diagnosis in adults, they are rare in children (e.g., Wilms tumor).
- Macroscopic hematuria can be the presenting sign of parenchymal kidney disease (e.g., membranoproliferative glomerulonephritis, Alport syndrome, IgA nephropathy, polycystic kidney disease), yet >40 % of children presenting gross hematuria have no identifiable cause.
- Fifteen to 20 % of patients with painless micro- or macrohematuria have hypercalciuria.
- The prognosis of microhematuria depends on the underlying etiology; it is favorable in most instances.
- The differential diagnosis is wide (Box 3.1). Careful history and complete physical examination are a prerequisite for a focused diagnostic approach.
- Extensive and invasive random laboratory investigations in a child with isolated hematuria are unnecessary and discouraged.
- In contrast, the presence of concomitant proteinuria can indicate clinically important kidney disease and may warrant diagnostic workup and treatment that should be coordinated with a pediatric renal specialist.

3.1.4 Baseline Investigations for Hematuria

- Urine microscopy
- Confirm that urine discoloration is due to blood (dipstick analysis and microscopy)
- Rule out extra-urinary sources of the blood
- Differentiate between glomerular and non-glomerular hematuria (Table 3.1; Figs. 3.1 and 3.2)

Box 3.1 Etiology of Hematuria

1. Glomerular causes
   - Acute postinfectious glomerulonephritis (APIGN)
   - IgA nephropathy (IgAN)
   - Membranoproliferative GN (MPGN)
   - Focal-segmental glomerulosclerosis (FSGS)
   - Thin basement membrane nephropathy (TBMN) and benign familial hematuria
   - Alport syndrome (hereditary nephritis)
   - Systemic diseases, immunological causes
     - SLE, HUS, Schönlein-Henoch purpura (SHP), anti-glomerular basement membrane (anti-GBM) disease and Goodpasture's disease, infective endocarditis, shunt nephritis
2. Non-glomerular causes
   - Nephrolithiasis, hypercalciuria
   - Infections
     - Bacterial urinary tract infection (UTI), leptospirosis, tuberculosis
     - Viral (polyomavirus [BKV] hemorrhagic cystitis; HIV nephropathy)
     - Parasitic (malaria, bilharziosis [*S. haematobium*])
   - Tumor/malignancy
     - Wilms tumor/nephroblastoma
     - Renal carcinoma (extremely rare in childhood)
   - Polycystic kidney disease (PKD) and other cystic renal diseases
   - Hematologic causes (sickle cell anemia with renal papillary necrosis, hemophilia, disseminated intravascular coagulation)
   - Vascular anomalies
   - Medications (NSAIDs, warfarin, heparin, cyclophosphamide, ifosphamide, hydralazine, propyl thiouracil, allopurinol, penicillamine, etc.)
   - Physiological (exercise, fever)
   - Trauma, bladder catheterization, surgery
3. Rare or debated causes
   - Young girls with recurrent hematuria: suspect abuse, foreign body insertion
   - Loin pain-hematuria syndrome is a diagnosis of exclusion
   - Nutcracker syndrome: hematuria due to trapping of the left renal vein between the superior mesenteric artery and the abdominal aorta
4. Newborns
   - Renal venous thrombosis
   - Renal artery thrombosis
   - Autosomal recessive polycystic kidney disease (ARPKD)
   - UTI
   - Obstructive uropathy
   - Bleeding and clotting disorders
5. Common causes of "dark urine" mimicking hematuria
   - Drugs: rifampin, nitrofurantoin, metronidazole; methyldopa, levodopa
   - Pigments: hemoglobin, myoglobin, bilirubin; urate
   - Nutrients: beets, blackberries

Table 3.1 Glomerular versus non-glomerular hematuria

Features	Glomerular hematuria	Non-glomerular hematuria
History		
Dysuria	Absent	Present in urethritis, cystitis
Systemic signs	Edema, fever, pharyngitis, rash, arthralgia	Fever with UTI, pain with calculi
Family history	Possible diagnoses: Isolated hematuria in TBMN Hematuria plus deafness, ESRD in Alport syndrome IgAN, SHP, HUS, SLE	Renal stones, hypercalciuria
Physical examination		
Hypertension, edema	Usually present	Less common
Abdominal mass	Absent	Present in Wilms tumor, obstructive uropathy
Rash, petechiae or purpura, arthritis	SLE, SHP	Absent unless part of drug-induced interstitial nephritis
Urinalysis		
Color	Brown, tea, cola	Bright red; clots may be seen
Proteinuria	2+ or more (≥1 g/l)	<2+ (<1 g/l)
Dysmorphic RBCs	>20 %	<15 %
RBC casts	Common	Absent
Crystals	Absent	May be present

Abbreviations: *TBMN* thin basement membrane nephropathy, *SHP* Schönlein–Henoch purpura, *HUS* hemolytic uremic syndrome

- Check for protein (dipstick analysis, chemistry)
- Look for WBC (dipstick, microscopy); rule out urinary tract infection
- Imaging (ultrasonography; CT scan)

3.1.5 Management

Hematuria is a clinical (or laboratory) sign, not a diagnosis. The most common cause of glomerular gross hematuria in children is APIGN, frequently due to streptococcal infection of the throat or skin (Fig. 3.1). The most common causes of non-glomerular gross hematuria are UTI and hypercalciuria or stones (Fig. 3.2). Management of the underlying disorders will be discussed in the following chapters.

3.2 Approach to Proteinuria

3.2.1 Abstract

Proteinuria heralds glomerular and occasionally tubular renal injury. The aim of the initial workup is to discern between transient or functional proteinuria and clinically significant, acute and chronic (progressive) proteinuria. This section provides a

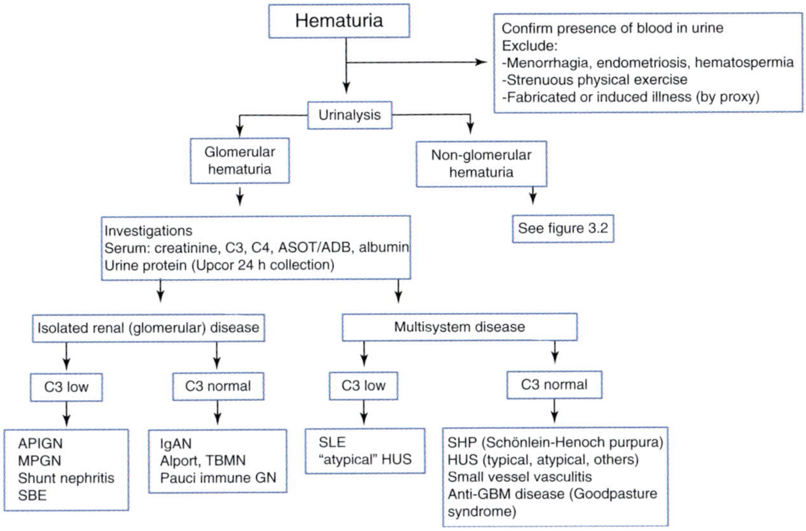

Fig. 3.1 Approach to hematuria. *Abbreviations*: *APIGN* acute postinfectious GN, *ASOT* antistreptolysin O titer, *GBM* glomerular basement membrane, *GN* glomerulonephritis, *HUS* hemolytic uremic syndrome, *IgAN* IgA nephropathy, *MPGN* membranoproliferative GN, *SBE* subacute bacterial endocarditis, *SLE* systemic lupus erythematosus, *TBMN* thin basement membrane nephropathy, *Upc* urine spot protein to creatinine ratio

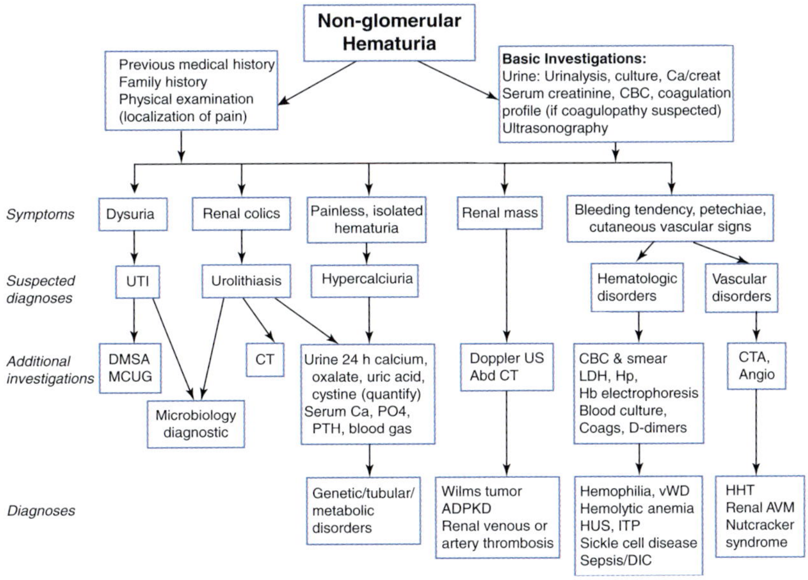

Fig. 3.2 Approach to non-glomerular hematuria. *Abbreviations*: *Abd* abdominal, *ADPKD* autosomal dominant polycystic kidney disease, *AVM* arteriovenous malformation, *Ca* calcium, *CBC* complete blood count, *creat* creatinine, *CT* computer tomogram, *DIC* disseminated intravascular coagulation, *DMSA* dimercaptosuccinic acid renal scan, *Hb* hemoglobin, *HHT* autosomal dominant hereditary hemorrhagic telangiectasia, *Hp* haptoglobin, *ITP* idiopathic thrombocytopenia, *LDH* lactate dehydrogenase, *MCUG* micturition cystourethrogram, *US* ultrasonography, *UTI* urinary tract infection, *vWD* von Willebrand disease

framework for the differentiation of proteinuria and their association with renal parenchymal disease. Specific glomerular diseases are discussed in the remaining sections of this chapter.

3.2.2 Introduction

- Proteinuria is a hallmark of glomerular and/or tubular injury. Both can be associated with hematuria.
- Most acute inflammatory glomerular diseases present with macro- or microhematuria (glomerulonephritis; nephritic–nephrotic syndromes).
- Proteinuria can signal acute disease or be the result of chronic kidney disease secondary to parenchymal fibrosis or scarring with nephron loss and hyperfiltration of the remaining nephrons.
- The aim of evaluating a patient with proteinuria is to differentiate clinically significant, generally persistent (or recurrent) proteinuria from transient or physiological proteinuria.
- Proteinuria can be isolated or present with peripheral edema, hypertension, and (other) extrarenal manifestations.
- For differential etiologies of proteinuria refer to Box 3.2.

3.2.3 Definitions

- Estimation of protein excretion from spot urine samples is best accomplished by the "urine protein to creatinine ratio" (U prot/creat or Upc). It is expressed as g protein/mmol creatinine (normal <0.02) or g protein/g creatinine (normal <0.2). The ratio normalizes urine protein excretion to urine density (concentration of urine creatinine). The units should be added to avoid confusion between conventional and SI unit definitions.
- The use of the ratio circumvents problems of timed urine specimens, such as inaccurate sampling periods, missed samples, or enuresis.
- If practical, obtain first morning urine samples to avoid collection errors and pitfalls due to orthostatic proteinuria.
- The numerator of the Upc (g/g) correlates with the daily protein excretion (per 1.73 m^2 body surface area; multiply by 8.84 (or by 10 for a quick estimate), if the urine creatinine is expressed in mmol/l).
- Physiologic proteinuria: normal urinary protein excretion <50 $mg/m^2/day$ with an upper limit of 100 $mg/m^2/day$ or 4 $mg/m^2/h$ (adults 150 mg/day) (Table 3.2).
- Physiological proteinuria originates from plasma (60 %), consisting of albumin (30–40 %), IgG (5–10 %), light chains (5 %), and IgA (3 %), and the tubule (predominantly Tamm–Horsfall protein).
- Transient or functional proteinuria: associated with fever, exercise, stress, seizures, or congestive heart failure. It does not reflect renal disease.
- Orthostatic proteinuria can be assumed when proteinuria is limited to periods of upright position (absent in the recumbent position). It rarely exceeds 600 $mg/m^2/day$

Box 3.2 Etiology of Proteinuria

1. Glomerular proteinuria
   - Resulting from lesions of the glomerular filtration barrier
   - Disorders with prominence of glomerular basement membrane (GBM) changes
     - Hereditary: Alport syndrome, laminin β2 mutation
     - Acquired/immunological: Goodpasture's syndrome, membranous nephropathy
   - Disorders with prominence of podocyte lesions
     - Hereditary (genetic mutation): congenital nephrotic syndromes (Finnish-type [NPHS1], podocin [NPHS2], etc.)
     - Idiopathic/acquired: minimal change disease, some forms of focal segmental glomerulosclerosis
   - Complex inflammatory causes
     - C3 nephropathies (membranoproliferative glomerulonephritis (MPGN), dense deposit disease (DDD)), a HUS, APIGN
   - Systemic vasculitides: lupus nephritis (LN), Schönlein–Henoch nephritis (SHN), ANCA-associated vasculitis (AAV)
   - Disorders with prominent mesangial involvement: IgAN, SHN, C1q nephropathy (C1qN), LN
   - Infection-associated: hepatitis B and C, endocarditis, shunt infection
   - Other immunological and secondary forms
   - Miscellaneous
     - Hematological disorders: sickle cell disease
     - Reflux nephropathy
2. Tubular proteinuria
   - Inflammatory tubular injury: ATN, interstitial nephritis, reflux nephropathy, acute cellular kidney transplant rejection, polyomavirus nephropathy
   - Toxic tubular injury: aminoglycosides, chemotherapeutics, antiviral (HIV) medications, heavy metals
   - Proximal tubular injury: Fanconi syndrome, proximal tubular acidosis, Dent's disease, nephropathic cystinosis
   - Developmental and chronic changes: renal dysplasia, reflux nephropathy, chronic kidney disease
3. Microalbuminuria
   - Important parameter of glomerular injury due to diabetes mellitus, possible marker in reflux nephropathy and CKD (associated with glomerular hyperfiltration)

(1 g/day in adults) or Upc 0.1 g/mmol creatinine (1 g/g creatinine). The prevalence of orthostatic proteinuria is highest in adolescents. The prognosis is benign. In the absence of other findings, no additional investigations and follow-up are needed (Fig. 3.3).

Table 3.2 Proteinuria (threshold values)

Proteinuria measurements	Timed sample	Protein to creatinine ratio (Upc) Conventional units	Protein to creatinine ratio (Upc) Alternative units
Normal urinary protein excretion	<4 mg/m²/h (<100 mg/m²/day)	<0.2 g protein/g	<0.02 g/mmol
Proteinuria	>4 mg/m²/h (>100 mg/m²/day)	> 0.2 g/g	>0.02 g/mmol
Nephrotic-range proteinuria	>40 mg/m²/h (>1,000 mg/m²/day)	>2 g/g	>0.2 g/mmol
Microalbuminuria	30–300 mg/day or 20–200 μg/min (adults) 20–200 mg/m²/day	30–300 mg/g (0.03–0.3 g/g)	3–30 mg/mmol (0.003–0.03 g/mmol)

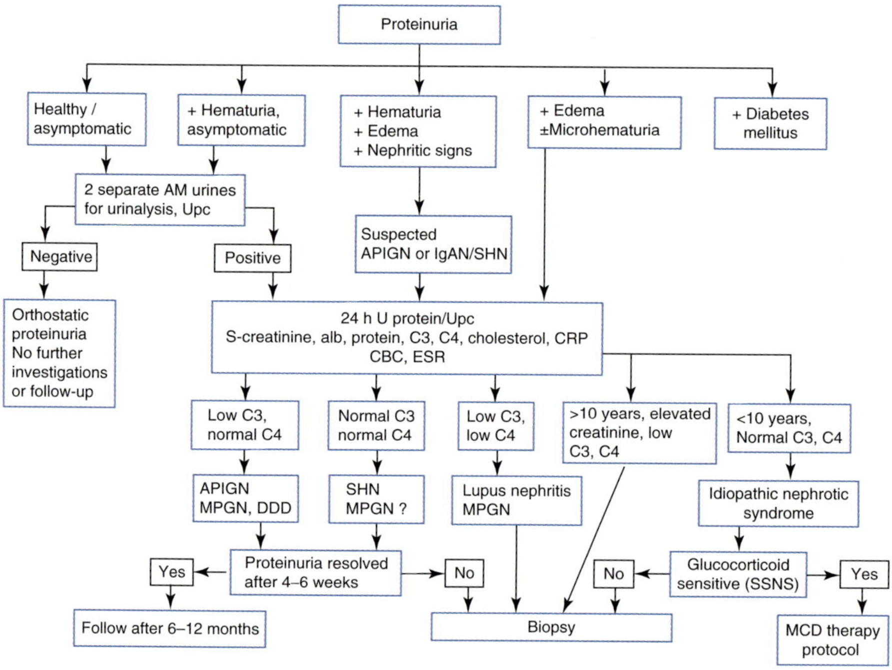

Fig. 3.3 Approach to proteinuria. *Abbreviations*: *APIGN* acute postinfectious GN, *creat* creatinine concentration, *CRP* C-reactive protein, *DDD* dense deposit disease or MPGN type II, *GN* glomerulonephritis, *IgAN* IgA nephropathy, *MPGN* membranoproliferative GN, *SHN* Schönlein–Henoch nephritis, *SSNS* steroid [glucocorticoid]-sensitive nephrotic syndrome, *Upc* urine protein to creatinine ratio

- Glomerular proteinuria results from altered permeability selectivity ("permselectivity") of the glomerular filtration barrier due to various mechanisms often due to genetic or acquired changes of components of the glomerular filtration barrier, such as nephrin in the interpodocyte slit diaphragm or type IV collagen or laminin β2 in the glomerular basement membrane.

- Toxic effects of drugs and environmental agents, such as aminoglycosides, chemotherapeutics, or herbal ingredients may affect tubular cells or glomerular endothelial and epithelial cells (podocytes).
- Glomerular proteinuria can be selective or nonselective. Albumin, IgG, and transferrin are used to characterize the selectivity of glomerular proteinuria.
- In selective proteinuria, the clearance ratio of IgG/albumin is <0.10 (nonselective proteinuria >0.5).
- Microalbuminuria denotes an albumin excretion above the normal range but below a level quantifiable by conventional dipstick analysis (0.06 g/l or 6 mg/dl). It is defined as urine albumin (U alb) excretion of 20–200 μg/min (30–300 mg/day) in a timed sample (in adults) or 3–30 mg/mmol creatinine (30–300 mg/g of creatinine) in a spot urine sample (see Table 3.2).
- Microalbuminuria is a risk factor for progressive renal insufficiency in patients with diabetes and (possibly) reflux nephropathy or chronic kidney disease.
- *Tubular proteinuria* refers to impaired proximal tubular reabsorption of low molecular weight proteins.
- Markers of tubular proteinuria are $ß_2$ microglobulin, α_1 microglobulin, retinol-binding protein and lysozymes.
- Tubular proteinuria is generally <1 g/1.73 m^2/day.
- It is seen in acute tubular necrosis, interstitial nephritis, aminoglycoside and other drug toxicity, heavy metal intoxication, Fanconi syndrome and proximal renal tubular acidosis, Dent's disease, and renal hypoplasia/dysplasia.
- It can also be observed as overflow proteinuria when excessive amounts of low molecular weight (LMW) protein overwhelm the (proximal) tubular reabsorption capacity, e.g., Bence Jones proteins.

3.2.4 Proteinuria Methods

- Current mehodology uses colorimetric assays (e.g., pyrogallol red for total protein) or immunological assays (e.g., immunotubidimetry for albumin) and automated equipment. Urine creatinine is measured by the Jaffé method or by precipitation reaction (e.g., pricric acid).
- Selective U alb assays are substantially more expensive than measuring total protein, but add little information for most indications.
- U protein dye binding assays can be established where expensive commercial equipment and reagents are lacking.
- U protein can be estimated using sulfosalycilic acid (SSA), even by families after proper instruction; its accuracy is similar to that of (expensive) dipsticks.

3.2.5 Clinical Signs and Symptoms

Proteinuria is often asymptomatic. High protein content lets urine appear frothy, bubbly, and dark yellow. Large (nephrotic-range) proteinuria can result in peripheral edema and other signs and symptoms associated with the underlying glomerular disease.

3.2.6 Basic Investigations

For methods of urine protein determination, see above Sect. 3.2.4 and Chap. 1. The evaluation of children with proteinuria is shown in Fig. 3.3.

3.3 Primary Nephrotic Syndrome

Nephrotic syndrome results from inherited or acquired disturbances of the podocyte and/or glomerular basement membrane (GBM). It is an important reason for nephrology consultations. Primary nephrotic syndrome (nephrotic syndrome without an identifiable systemic or extrarenal disorder) has a cumulative prevalence of about 16/100,000 population <16 years. Reported annual incidence figures range from 1–3 to 8 per 100,000 children.

Sect. 3.3.1 describes diagnostic approaches and management of children presenting with (primary) nephrotic syndrome, followed by brief summaries of the histological diagnoses of minimal change nephrotic syndrome (MCNS) or minimal change disease (MCD) and focal-segmental glomerulosclerosis (FSGS) in Sects. 3.3.2 and 3.3.3. Examples of inherited and genetically defined nephrotic syndromes, including congenital and syndromic forms, are highlighted in Sect. 3.3.4. Current standard (first-line) treatment regimens for idiopathic nephrotic syndrome are based on pioneering cooperative studies in North America and Europe between 1970 and 1990. An important source for diagnostic and treatment recommendations in this and the following sections is the 2012 Kidney Disease Improving Global Outcomes (KDIGO) Clinical Practice Guideline for Glomerulonephritis.

3.3.1 Idiopathic Nephrotic Syndrome (INS)

3.3.1.1 Introduction

- INS is more prevalent in boys than in girls, with onset between 2 and 8 years of age.
- Up to 80 % of children with INS respond to daily glucocorticoid therapy.
- Differentiation between glucocorticoid (steroid)-sensitive (responsive) syndrome (SSNS) and glucocorticoid (steroid)-resistant nephrotic syndrome (SRNS) has important therapeutic and prognostic implications.
- The long-term prognosis (renal function) of children with primary glucocorticoid-sensitive nephrotic syndrome is good.
- The underlying histopathological lesion is minimal changes (MCNS) in the large majority, but some have FSGS or different glomerular diseases, such as membranous nephropathy (MN; Sect. 3.5.3), membranoproliferative glomerulonephritis (MPGN; Sect. 3.5.1).
- In contrast, a large proportion of patients with glucocorticoid-resistant nephrotic syndrome has FSGS and is at risk of developing chronic kidney disease (CKD).

- Etiology and histopathologic lesions of nephrotic syndromes change with age of onset (inherited forms and diffuse mesangial sclerosis during the first 3 to 12) months, MCNS 1–10 years, other forms of primary NS and of secondary forms during adolescence and young adulthood).

3.3.1.2 Definitions

- Nephrotic syndrome (NS) is defined clinically by the combination of large (nephrotic-range) proteinuria, hypoalbuminemia (<25 g/l), and generalized, pitting edema. The accompanying hypercholesterolemia is likely secondary.
- The degree of edema may not be proportional to the proteinuria or hypoalbuminemia. 24-h urine collection is not necessary to establish the diagnosis.
- Nephrotic-range proteinuria may be present in other glomerular diseases or cystinosis, usually not associated with edema or (significant) hypoalbuminemia.
- "Primary" nephrotic syndrome is used synonymously with "idiopathic" nephrotic syndrome (INS). The designation requires exclusion of primary infectious, systemic or malignant diseases (Box 3.3).

Box 3.3 Nephrotic Syndrome: Definitions

Nephrotic syndrome	Clinical syndrome defined by (1) large proteinuria of 3 to 4+ by dipstick or Upc >2 g/g creatinine (>0.2 g/mmol) or >4 mg/m^2/h in a timed urine specimen, (2) hypoalbuminemia <25 g/l, and (3) generalized edema
Primary nephrotic syndrome	Requires exclusion of systemic diseases and other forms of glomerulonephritis (see below)
Secondary nephrotic syndrome	Nephrotic syndrome secondary to systemic disease (e.g., SLE, lymphoma) or infection
Idiopathic nephrotic syndrome (INS)	Primary nephrotic syndrome, where etiology and disease mechanism are not well defined or known
Urinary remission	Urine albumin nil or trace (or proteinuria <4 mg/m^2/h) for three consecutive days
Relapse	Urine albumin 3+ or 4+ (or proteinuria >40 mg/m^2/h) for three consecutive days, having been in remission previously
Frequent relapses (FRNS)	Two or more relapses during 6 months, or more than three relapses during any 12-month period
Glucocorticoid (steroid) dependence (SDNS)	Two consecutive relapses during alternate-day prednisone therapy or within 14 days of its discontinuation
Glucocorticoid resistance (SRNS)	Persistent proteinuria (>2 g/g creatinine) despite high-dose prednisone therapy with 60 mg/m^2 (2 mg/kg) daily for 4 weeks, in the absence of infection or nonadherence to medication
Secondary glucocorticoid resistance	Refers to patient who was previously responsive to glucocorticoid therapy

- The term "idiopathic" implies that etiology and disease mechanism are not known in a large percentage of children with primary nephrotic syndrome.

3.3.1.3 Pathology of Idiopathic Nephrotic Syndrome (INS)

- The common histopathological variety seen in children with idiopathic nephrotic syndrome is "minimal change disease" (MCD) or minimal change (or minimal lesion) nephrotic syndrome (MCNS; both terms are used interchangeably). Less commonly seen are focal segmental glomerulosclerosis (FSGS), membranoproliferative (or mesangiocapillary) glomerulonephritis (MPGN or MCGN), or (rarely) membranous nephropathy (MN) as causes of nephrotic syndrome.
- MCNS is characterized by the lack of histological changes by bright-field and immunofluorescence microscopy. Electron microscopy reveals generalized effacement of podocyte foot processes.
- The term FSGS refers to sclerotic lesions that initially affect some glomeruli while sparing others ("focal"). Glomeruli are partially affected ("segmental" sclerosis), but the lesions may progress to global sclerosis with progressive nephron loss. Immunofluorescence is negative. In contrast to MCNS, foot process effacement is not generalized. Up to 25 % of patients with FSGS may not present with nephrotic syndrome.
- The biopsies of some patients with nephrotic syndrome demonstrate mesangial proliferation and/or mesangial deposition of IgM or (dominant) C1q, or collapsing glomeruli with abnormal podocyte morphology. Some pathologists consider them variants of MCNS and FSGS, while others regard them as separate diseases, i.e., mesangial proliferative glomerulonephritis, IgM nephropathy, C1q nephropathy, and collapsing glomerulopathy.

3.3.1.4 Clinical Features

Typical Presentation

- Patients with nephrotic syndrome typically present with periorbital swelling (puffiness), more noticeable in the morning, which progresses to generalized edema or anasarca over days or weeks. Abdominal wall edema and ascites with a "smiling" umbilicus or pleural effusions and scrotal or vulval edema may be seen.
- Microscopic hematuria is found in up to 30 %, but gross hematuria is unusual in INS and suggests an alternative primary diagnosis.
- Nephrotic patients are at risk of intravascular volume depletion despite a fluid gain of up to 20 % of body weight. The presence of edema makes assessment of the intravascular volume status difficult.
- Patients occasionally present with hypertension due to intravascular volume depletion and activation of the renin–angiotensin system.

Atypical Features of Nephrotic Syndrome Suggesting Alternative Diagnoses

- Age <3–12 months and >12 years
- Sustained serum creatinine elevation
- Hypertension
- Gross hematuria

- Low serum C3 or C4
- Evidence of specific infection (HBV, HCV, HIV)

3.3.1.5 Investigations at First Presentation of Nephrotic Syndrome

- Urinalysis and microscopy. Microhematuria is noted in up to 30 % of patients with INS and does not predict poorer outcome. Mild "sterile" pyuria can be present.
- Urine protein to creatinine ratio (Upc) or 24-h (timed) urine protein estimation.
- Serum albumin, total protein, cholesterol, and creatinine.
- Infectious disease workup including PPD (Mantoux) skin test and chest X-ray in Tb endemic areas, and HIV, HBV, or HCV serology or PCR for patient at risk.
- Kidney biopsy is reserved for infants and older children, those with "atypical" presentation and those unresponsive to 4 weeks of daily high-dose glucocorticoid therapy (Box 3.4).

3.3.1.6 Treatment of Idiopathic Nephrotic Syndrome

First Episode

- Prednisone (or prednisolone, used interchangeably): 60 mg/m^2 once daily or in 2–3 divided doses (~2 mg/kg/day, max. 60 mg/day) for 4–6 weeks followed by 40 mg/m^2 (~1.5 mg/kg, max. 40 mg) on alternate days as a single morning dose for the next 4–6 weeks with or without taper. Some authors recommend prolonged glucocorticoid therapy for 6 months after the initial, intense therapy (Fig. 3.4).
- A focus of infection must always be searched and treated. Control of underlying infection can achieve remission in some cases.

Relapse Treatment

- About 70 % of patients with INS will have one or more relapses. Treatment is directed to suppress proteinuria and restore normal serum protein concentrations and to reduce the frequency of future relapses, both with minimal short- and long-term adverse effects.

Box 3.4 Indications for Renal Biopsy in Patients with Nephrotic Syndrome

- Age <12 months or >12 years at presentation
- Glucocorticoid resistance (defined in Box 3.3)
- Proteinuria associated with malformations or "syndromes" (e.g., nail patella syndrome, Lowe syndrome)
- Persistently low plasma C3 and/or C4 (see Fig. 3.3)
- Sustained hypertension not related to glucocorticoid or calcineurin inhibitor therapy
- Serum creatinine elevation (renal failure) for >1 week, not attributable to intravascular volume depletion
- Secondary nephrotic syndrome with features of systemic disease (e.g., SLE, SHP, HIV infection, hepatitis B or C)

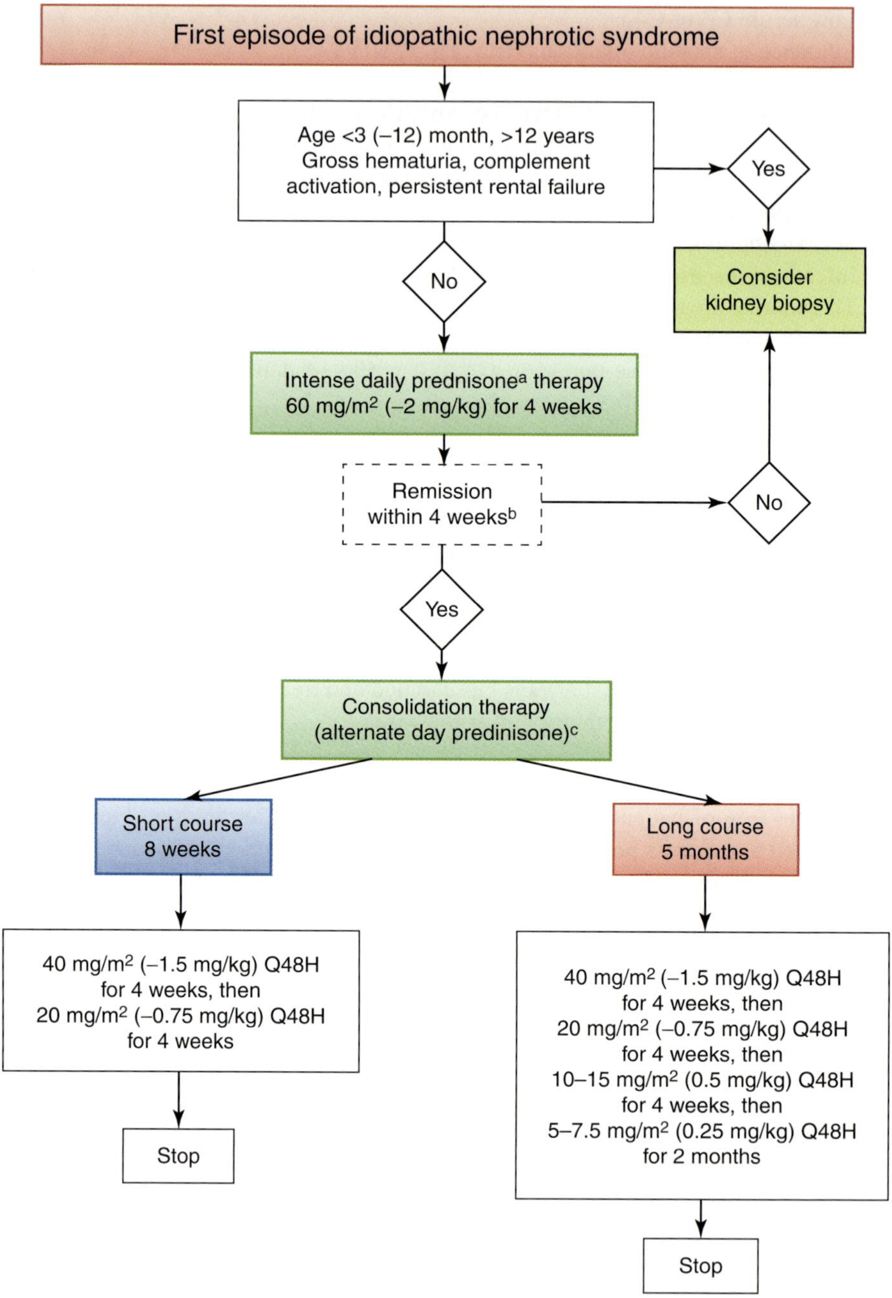

Fig. 3.4 Algorithm for the treatment of a first episode of nephrotic syndrome. [a]Prednisone or prednisolone used interchangeably; max. 60 mg/day, [b]Remission defined as three consecutive days of "negative" or "trace" urine protein (by dipstick). [c]The 2012 KDIGO Clinical Practice Guideline recommends glucocorticoid therapy for the first episode of glucocorticoid-sensitive INS over a total period of 3–6 months

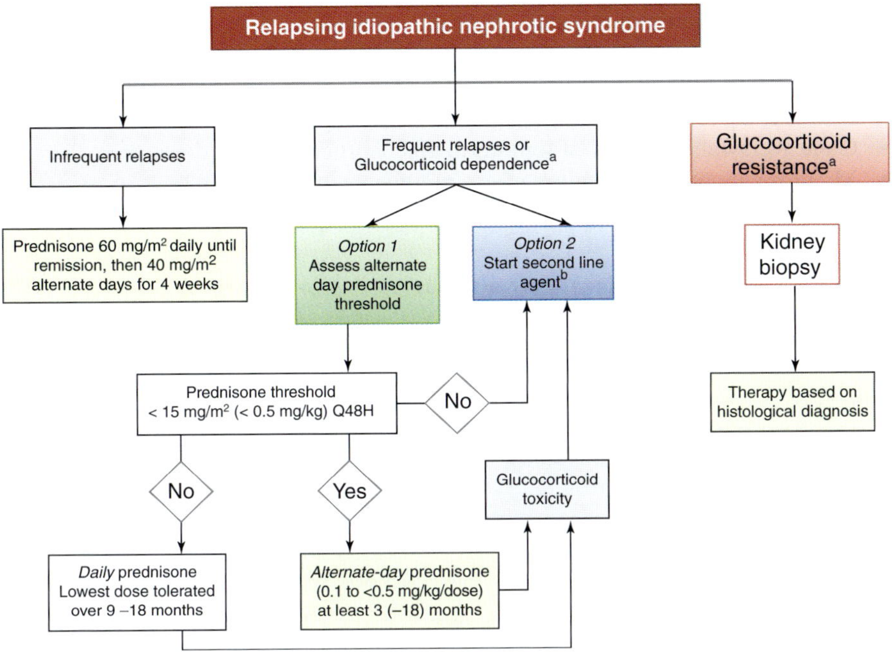

Fig. 3.5 Treatment choices in patients with relapsing idiopathic nephrotic syndrome[a]. [a]As defined in Box 3.3. [b]See Fig. 3.6 and Table 3.4

- Prednisone remains the only medication to effect remission quickly in patients with glucocorticoid-sensitive, relapsing INS. Prednisone 60 mg/m^2 per day (see above) usually achieves urinary remission within 7–10 days. Once urine is protein-free for three consecutive days, daily prednisone is switched to a single morning dose of 40 mg/m^2 (~1.5 mg/kg) on alternate days for 4 weeks and then stopped (Fig. 3.5).

Frequent Relapses and Glucocorticoid (Steroid) Dependence

- Upon achieving remission with daily high-dose prednisone, patient is switched to alternate-day prednisone as above. However, there is no clear consensus about the best long-term approach.
- Option 1: identification of a "threshold" dose of prednisone. Alternate-day prednisone is tapered to 0.5 mg/kg every 48 h. If stable, taper is continued until a dose is reached that still prevents relapses. When a relapse occurs, aim at a maintenance dose just above the last dose where the patient relapsed and continue this dose for 6 months.
- Option 2: introduction of second-line agent, usually in conjunction with prednisone tapering, intended to minimize long-term glucocorticoid adverse effects (Fig. 3.5).

Glucocorticoid Adverse Effects

- Prednisone and prednisolone have similar potency (1:1 conversion) and toxicity profiles.
- "Threshold" for glucocorticoid toxicities varies among individuals.
- Controversy about safety of long-term glucocorticoid at low dose.
- Monitor patients receiving long-term prednisone (see Table 3.3).

Table 3.3 Major adverse effects of glucocorticoids

Organ system	Adverse effect	Remarks
Skin, soft tissue	Skin thinning, striae, purpura, acne, alopecia, hypertrichosis	
	Cushingoid, weight gain (increased appetite)	Dose and duration dependent, within first 2 months of treatment. May occur with 7.5 mg/1.73 m²/day
Eye	Posterior subcapsular cataract	Noted in 10–38 % of children treated chronically
		Generally bilateral, develops slowly, may stabilize with lowering of prednisone dose
		Dose and duration dependent (no minimal safe dose)
		Annual ophthalmological exam
Cardiovascular	Fluid retention, blood pressure rise	Mineralocorticoid effect
	Ischemia, heart failure	Accelerated atherosclerosis (elevated lipoprotein levels)
Bone	Osteoporosis, avascular necrosis of bone (AVN), vertebral fractures	May occur with "normal" bone mineral density (accumulation of microfractures)
		Supply vitamin D, calcium supplements
Muscle	Myopathy	Proximal motor weakness upper and lower extremities
Growth	Impaired growth	
GI tract	Gastric ulcer, GI bleeding	Elevated in combination with NSAIDs. Patients may benefit from addition of ranitidine or proton pump inhibitor (e.g., lansoprazole)
CNS	Mood swings, insomnia, pseudotumor cerebri	Mood changes (euphoria, depression) occur within days of treatment
Endocrine	Hyperglycemia, diabetes	Dose dependent; may need insulin injections; reversible with glucocorticoid discontinuation
	Growth retardation	More with daily than alternate-day dosing
		Some loss of height can be permanent
		Monitor height Q 3 months
Immune system	Suppresses proinflammatory cytokines and phagocyte function	Avoid live virus vaccines if prednisone dose >20 mg/1.73 m²/day for ≥14 days
		Risk of severe varicella, tuberculosis exacerbation

- *Methylprednisolone* is derived from hydrocortisone. The biological $T_{1/2}$ is 12–36 h, relative potency 1.25× versus prednisolone, suitable for IV use.
- *Dexamethasone* is a fluoridated glucocorticoid with a biological half-life of 36–72 h, anti-inflammatory potency ratio 6.7 versus prednisolone, and minor mineralocorticoid effects (less sodium retention).
- *Deflazacort* is an oxazoline derivative and prodrug of prednisolone that has been claimed to cause less adverse effects during long-term use than prednisone/prednisolone. Based on the potency ratio of deflazacort versus prednisolone of 1.28, the initial dose is 1.5 mg/kg/day followed by down titration according to clinical need. It is not widely prescribed due to cost and limited availability and experience.

Second-Line Agents and Strategies (Fig. 3.6)

- Second-line agents are introduced to avoid long-term glucocorticoid related adverse effects or as alternative for glucocorticoid resistance. A summary of second-line drugs is given in Table 3.4.

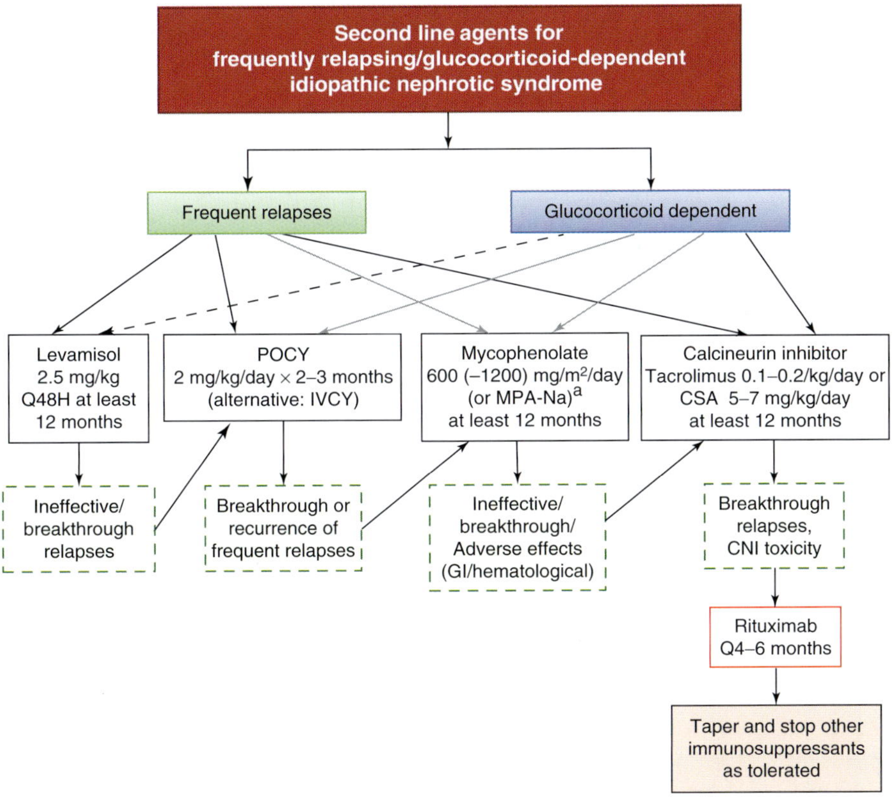

Fig. 3.6 Algorithm for second-line agents for frequently relapsing/glucocorticoid-dependent idiopathic nephrotic syndrome. [a]Switch from the prodrug MMF to MPA-sodium may alleviate MMF-induced diarrhea and oral ulcers. *CNI* calcineurin inhibitor, *CSA* cyclosporin A, *IVCY* intravenous cyclophosphamide, *MPA-Na* mycophenolate-sodium, *POCY* oral cyclophosphamide

Table 3.4 Second-line drugs for idiopathic nephrotic syndrome (MCNS, FSGS)

Drug	Dose [trough level]	Important adverse effects	Remarks
Levamisole	2–2.5 mg/kg on alternate days	Neutropenia, flu-like symptoms, skin rash, gastrointestinal symptoms	Limited availability, not recommended for glucocorticoid-resistant nephrotic syndrome Monitor CBC and differential Q 6–8 weeks
Cyclophosphamide[a]	2–3 mg/kg/day for 8–12 weeks (POCY)	Neutropenia, anemia, gonadal toxicity (more in males than in females)	Start POCY after induction of remission. Cumulative dose over lifetime ≤168 mg/kg to reduce risk of gonadal toxicity (equals 12 weeks of 2 mg/kg)
		Less frequent: thrombocytopenia, transient alopecia. Hemorrhagic cystitis (with higher doses and insufficient fluid)	Monitor CBC Q2wks and stop or reduce dose when absolute neutrophils $<1.5\times10^9$/l
	500 mg/m² IV pulses every 4 weeks (6 doses) (IVCY)	Hemorrhagic cystitis (rare with this dose and good hydration)	Ensure pre- and post-hydration (IV or PO 2,500 ml/m²/24 h) Possibly better tolerated than POCY Indicated where oral therapy is not reliable
Cyclosporine A (CSA)	5–7 mg/kg/day÷q12h [100–150 ng/ml]	Nephrotoxicity, hypertension, hepatotoxicity, hyperkalemia, hypomagnesemia, gingival hyperplasia, hirsutism, tremor	Once stabilized, reduce to lowest effective dose Monitor creatinine, electrolytes
Tacrolimus	0.1–0.25 mg/kg/day ÷q12h [5–8 ng/ml]	Nephrotoxicity, hypertension, hepatotoxicity, impaired glucose tolerance, hyperkalemia, hypomagnesemia, tremor	Once stabilized, reduce to lowest effective dose. Monitor creatinine, electrolytes
Mycophenolate mofetil (MMF)	600–1,200 mg/m²/day ÷ BID	Gastrointestinal (colitis, oral aphthous ulcers), anemia, neutropenia	Dose decrease or discontinuation if ANC $<1.3\times10^9$/l. Teratogenicity (pregnancy risk)
Rituximab (RTX)	375 mg/m² per infusion	Allergic-type (cytokine release) reaction with first infusion. Suppression of de novo antibody responses. Suspected risk of JC virus progressive multifocal leukoencephalopathy	1–2 doses 1 week apart. If possible, induce remission before initiating RTX. Relapse may occur with recovery of peripheral B cells

[a]A alternative alkylating agent (chlorambucil, 0.1–0.2 mg/kg/day PO × 8 weeks) has similar efficacy, but a lower safety margin than cyclophosphamide (malignancy risk, azoospermia)

- Treatment with second-line drugs depends on availability and affordability, adverse effect profile, physician comfort and family preference.
- Literature and common practice suggest efficacy of (oral) alkylating agents in patients with frequently relapsing or glucocorticoid-dependent nephrotic syndrome (oral cyclophosphamide [POCY], chlorambucil). The reported duration of remission after POCY varies. Early relapses after an alkylating agent are more common in SDNS and FSGS than in FRNS. Although affordable and widely available, there are concerns of drug safety, specifically gonadotoxicity, bone marrow suppression, and severe infection.
- The efficacy of *calcineurin inhibitors* (CNI) is firmly established. Tacrolimus lacks the adverse cosmetic effects of cyclosporin A (CSA), but the latter is more affordable. Both are similarly effective. Many centers perform a renal biopsy after 24 months of CNI treatment.
- *Mycophenolic acid*: diarrhea and colitis due to mycophenolate mofetil (MMF) may be alleviated by switching to mycophenolate sodium (MPA-Na). Note that 1,000 mg MMF is equivalent to 720 mg MPA-Na.
- Experience with *rituximab* (RTX), a monoclonal antibody targeting $CD20^{+}$ B lymphocytes, is still evolving. Costs and uncertainties about long-term infection risks need be considered. RTX appears to have a long-lasting effect in patients with frequently relapsing and glucocorticoid-dependent nephrotic syndrome. Patients who relapse immediately after the recovery of B cells may receive additional (preemptive) RTX infusions after 5–6 months. Patients may discontinue or substantially reduce current second-line agents. Adverse effects include infusion-related allergic-type reactions and delayed onset neutropenia and lung injury. JC virus progressive multifocal leukoencephalopathy has been associated with rituximab treatment in a few patients.

Management of Glucocorticoid (Steroid)-Resistant Idiopathic Nephrotic Syndrome (SRNS)

- Chances of remission diminish drastically after 3 weeks of high-dose daily prednisone treatment. Preparations should be made for a kidney biopsy and genetic testing to avoid excess glucocorticoid toxicity.
- Kidney biopsy is mandatory in patients who do not achieve remission after 4 weeks of prednisone treatment with or without a short course (3 pulses) of 10 mg methylprednisolone (Fig. 3.5).
- The majority of patients with SRNS will have FSGS, diffuse mesangial proliferation, or MCNS by biopsy. The differential diagnoses include membranoproliferative (mesangiocapillary) glomerulonephritis (MPGN) and membranous nephropathy (MN).
- Children (or adolescents) with pathogenic mutations of genes encoding structural podocyte proteins do not benefit from immunosuppressive therapies but require supportive treatment and frequent monitoring. Examples are podocin (*NPHS2*) (in children), α-actinin 4 (*ACTN4*), and transient receptor potential cation channel type 6 (*TRPC6*) mutation (in adolescents and young adults).

- *Methylprednisolone or dexamethasone pulses* with cyclophosphamide have been used in patients where induction of remission has been difficult to achieve (so-called Mendoza protocol). The 2012 KDIGO guideline advises against the use of cytotoxic agents for SRNS.
- In an attempt to minimize overall toxicity, the following modified protocol is proposed for patients with SRNS (Fig. 3.7):
  - Glucocorticoid pulse therapy with IV methylprednisolone (3 pulses of 10 mg/kg Q 48 h) or PO/IV dexamethasone (three doses of 1.5–3 mg/kg or 50–100 mg/m^2 Q 3 days).
  - Alternate-day PO prednisone.
  - Calcineurin inhibitor (tacrolimus or CSA), to be started in the upper dose range with target (trough) plasma concentrations (C0) of 5–10 or 150–250 ng/ml, respectively.
  - If patient enters remission, taper prednisone. Adjust CNI dosage according to therapeutic effect.
  - In case of CNI toxicity, consider reducing CNI dose or switch to alternative CNI. Addition of MMF may spare glucocorticoid or CNI.
  - Rituximab does not appear to be effective in the majority of patients resistant to glucocorticoids and other second-line agents.

Adjunctive Therapies

- Patients with glucocorticoid-dependent and glucocorticoid-resistant nephrotic syndrome may develop hypertension as a treatment complication or with progressive chronic kidney disease. Treatment consists of sodium restriction, diuretics, and blockade of the renin–angiotensin system with ACE inhibitor (ACEi) and/or angiotensin receptor blocker (ARB).
- ACEi, such as enalapril, and ARB, such as losartan, decrease proteinuria and are a useful adjunct for patients with SRNS. The antiproteinuric effect is dose dependent. ACEi and ARB can lead to a reversible rise of serum creatinine and potassium and to anemia.
- Lipid-lowering drugs such as the HMG-CoA reductase inhibitors (statins, e.g., atorvastatin) are used in glucocorticoid-resistant patients.
- Consider thrombosis prophylaxis.
- Vitamin D, specifically for patients receiving long-term glucocorticoid therapy or prophylaxis.

Management of Edema, Fluid Balance, and Hypertension

- *Sodium salt restriction.* "No added salt" and avoidance of foods rich in sodium (papads, pickles, baked products, dried and salted fish or meat) to control edema formation and blood pressure.
- *Fluid management.* Do not miss hypovolemia (may be difficult to diagnose in edematous patient). It can lead to acute kidney injury and thrombosis. In children with vomiting, diarrhea, fever, or sepsis, 10–20 ml/kg of 5 % albumin or other colloids are effective.

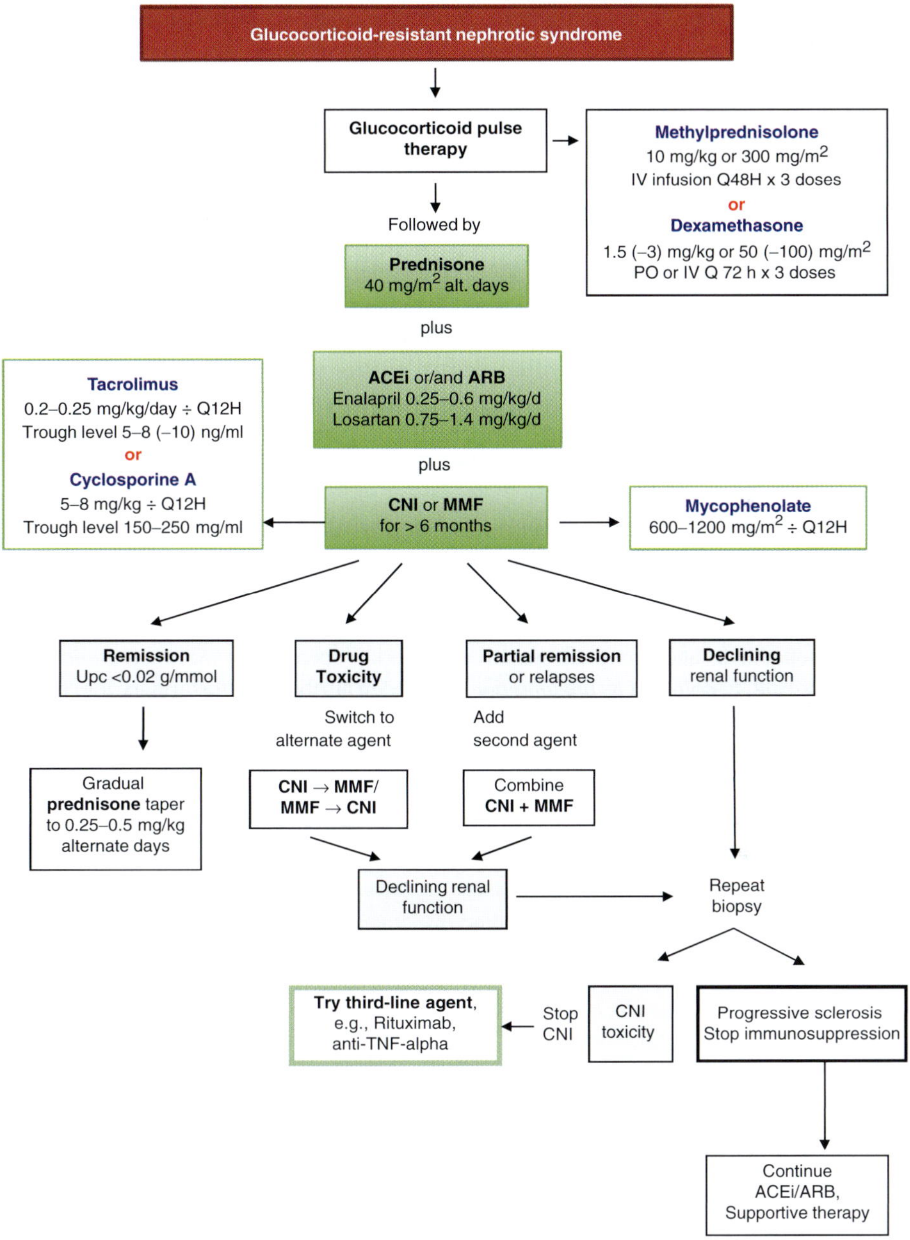

Fig. 3.7 Algorithm for treatment of glucocorticoid-resistant nephrotic syndrome

- *Albumin infusion*. Temporarily increases intravascular oncotic pressure and improves renal perfusion. 0.5–1 g/kg of salt-poor 20 or 25 % albumin over 4 h in patients who are volume depleted and have severe edema. Albumin is often combined with IV furosemide 0.5–1 mg/kg once or twice during and at the end of the albumin infusion. Note that albumin is rapidly lost in the urine, and additional doses may be needed.
- *Diuretics*. If albumin is unavailable, diuretics alone can be given when edema, pleural effusion, or severe ascites cause respiratory distress and scrotal swelling/skin breaks. *Exercise caution* and ensure that child is not intravascularly depleted. Regimens include intermittent IV furosemide at doses up to 1–2 mg/kg every 8–12 h with careful monitoring of vital signs in hospital or as a continuous infusion of 0.05 mg/kg/h (titrate to effect). Monitor renal function and electrolytes.
- *Outpatients* may receive oral furosemide, with or without a *thiazide* (hydrochlorothiazide 1–2 mg/kg/day).
- *Metolazone* (0.2–0.4 mg/kg/d ÷ QD or BID) is a thiazide-like diuretic with action at both the proximal and distal tubules.

Complications in Children with Primary Nephrotic Syndrome

Infections

- In the pre-antibiotic and pre-steroid era, many children with nephrotic syndrome died of infection and/or malnutrition. Bacterial infections, commonly due to encapsulated gram-positive and or gram-negative bacteria, specifically *S. pneumoniae*, *H. influenzae*, *E. coli*, and *K. pneumoniae*, have been attributed to the urinary loss of IgG and complement components. They present as spontaneous bacterial peritonitis, septicemia, cellulitis, diarrhea, upper and lower respiratory, or urinary tract infection.
- If a serious bacterial infection is suspected, cultures must be taken and broad-spectrum antibiotics initiated until bacterial culture results become available (see Table 3.5).

Table 3.5 Infections in children with nephrotic syndrome and antibiotic therapies

Presentation	Organism	Choice of antibiotics
Peritonitis	*S. pneumoniae*, group A hemolytic streptococci (*S. pyogenes*), *E. coli*	Cefotaxime or ceftriaxone for 7–10 days[a] Ampicillin + aminoglycoside for 7–10 days
Pneumonia	S. *pneumoniae*, *H. influenzae*, *S. aureus*	PO amoxicillin, amoxicillin/clavulanate (co-amoxiclav) IV ampicillin and aminoglycoside, or cefotaxime/ceftriaxone for 7–10 days
Cellulitis	Staphylococci, *S. pyogenes*, *H. influenzae*	PO cloxacillin, cephalexin, or amoxicillin/clavulanate (co-amoxiclav) Severe/complicated cellulitis IV/IM ceftriaxone for 7–10 days[a]
Fungal infections	*Candida*, *Aspergillus* spp.	Skin, mucosa: PO fluconazole for 10 days Systemic: IV fluconazole or amphotericin for 14–21 days

[a]Initial therapy may be parenteral for 5 days; once patient is nontoxic and accepting orally, the medication may be administered orally

- Antibiotic prophylaxis for all children with nephrotic syndrome is not recommended but may be indicated in individual patients and under specific circumstances.
- Common viral infections, mostly of the upper respiratory tract, may trigger relapses. Exposed children should be monitored for proteinuria.
- Glucocorticoids and other immunosuppressants increase the susceptibility to life-threatening varicella-zoster virus (VZV) infection. Nonimmune children should receive immunoglobulin (VZIG) within 96 hours of exposure and/or acyclovir (intravenously, if poor absorption or compliance is suspected).
- Immunosuppressed patients may develop fungal infections, such as oral thrush and Candida esophagitis, tinea versicolor, and tinea corporis.
- Note that immunosuppressive therapy can mask clinical signs of infection.

Hypercoagulopathy

- Nephrotic syndrome increases the risk of thrombosis and thrombosis-related complications, such as deep venous thrombosis, renal venous thrombosis, pulmonary emboli, and cerebral infarction.

Acute Kidney Injury

- May be due to intravascular volume depletion (prerenal failure) or renal hypoperfusion, use of nephrotoxic drugs, renal venous thrombosis, or sepsis.

Electrolyte Disturbances

- Spurious hyponatremia may be seen due to hyperlipidemia or where the laboratory measures electrolytes by flame photometry. True hyponatremia may develop due to diuretics.

3.3.1.7 Prognosis

- Seventy percent of patients with glucocorticoid-responsive nephrotic syndrome relapse at least once. Around 50 % of the latter will have frequent relapses or become glucocorticoid dependent.
- Outcome is often poor in glucocorticoid-resistant patients (SRNS). They are at risk of chronic or end-stage kidney disease and recurrence of nephrotic syndrome after renal transplantation (see Sect. 3.3.3).

3.3.1.8 Long-Term Management of Children with Nephrotic Syndrome

Nutrition

- No change of diet other than sodium salt restriction is needed in children with initial presentation or relapse of nephrotic syndrome and normal kidney function.
- Prednisone stimulates appetite and weight gain. Encourage physical activity and avoidance of calorie-rich snacks and soft drinks.
- Patients with persistent proteinuria receive normal protein intake in a balanced diet.

Immunization of the Child with Nephrotic Syndrome

- Live vaccines are contraindicated in children receiving immunosuppressive or cytotoxic medication (e.g., varicella, measles, mumps, rubella, rotavirus, oral polio).
- Live vaccines should be deferred until
  - Prednisone dose is <1 mg/kg/day (<20 mg/day) or <2 mg/kg/dose on alternate days (<40 mg/dose)
  - More than 3 months after the last cyclophosphamide or chlorambucil dose
  - More than 4 weeks after the last calcineurin inhibitor or mycophenolate dose
- Immunosuppression is not a contraindication for inactive (killed) vaccines, but the vaccine response is likely to be reduced.
- *Hepatitis B* vaccine should be given to all unvaccinated or non-immune children
  - Higher glucocorticoid doses at the time of immunization appear to diminish the short-term, but not the long-term vaccine response
- Immunization, particulalry against encapsulated bacteria including *H. influenzae*, *S. pneumoniae* and *N. meningitidis* should be initiated, if they have not been obtained previously.
- *Pneumococcal* vaccine: Unimmunized children up to 2 years of age should receive 2–4 doses of the 13-valent (or at least the 7-valent) conjugate pneumococcal vaccine. For previously unimmunized children between 2 and 5 years old, give two doses of the available conjugate vaccine 4–8 weeks apart, followed 8 weeks later by administration of one dose of the 23-valent polysaccharide vaccine. Children older than 5 years receive a single dose of the 23-valent polysaccharide vaccine. Revaccination every 5 years should be considered for children who continue to have active nephrotic syndrome.
- Not all pneumococcal serotypes are included in the vaccines, and antibody levels may fall during a relapse; hence, previously vaccinated children may develop pneumococcal peritonitis and sepsis, as well as infections by other pathogens, despite having been vaccinated.
- *Seasonal Influenza vaccines* are given to patient and family to reduce preventable relapses and morbidity.
- *Varicella* vaccine is given as 2 doses, 1–3 months apart.
- Defer *oral polio vaccine* (OPV) to patients and to siblings unless patient is in stable remission off immunosuppressants or can be isolated from vaccinated family members.

Adrenal Suppression and Dosing of Glucocorticoids During Stress

- Patients who have received high-dose glucocorticoids daily for more than 2 weeks in the past 1 year or those with a morning cortisol level <10 nmol/l require supplementation of cortisol during surgery, including dentistry, anesthesia, or serious infections or burns (Box 3.5).
- A physiological hydrocortisone dose is 10 mg/m^2/day corresponding to 2.5 mg/m^2/day of prednisolone and 0.25 mg/m^2/day of dexamethasone.

Box 3.5 Recommendations for Patients with Adrenal Insufficiency

Name of patient ____________________

Record # __________ Date of birth __________

Weight ______ kg Height ______ cm Surface area ________ m^2

IN CASE OF STRESS (temperature >38.5 C, infection, diarrhea, surgery)

- Double each dose of prednisone/prednisolone or hydrocortisone for the duration of the episode or give 2.5 mg/m^2 BID (AM, afternoon)
- Triple each dose for a more important stress (e.g. temperature >39 C) or give 3.75 mg/m^2 BID (AM, afternoon)

IN CASE OF VOMITING: give dose parenterally in HOSPITAL

- Hydrocortisone 50 mg/m^2/dose (maximum 50 mg/dose)
- =______mg hydrocortisone IV or IM with volume expansion (saline bolus) Q 4–6 h until vomiting has stopped

IN CASE OF ADRENAL CRISIS (fatigue, weakness, hypotension, tachycardia, abdominal pain, nausea, vomiting):

- Patient has to go to HOSPITAL immediately.
- Administer hydrocortisone IV or IM with volume expansion (saline bolus). Repeat Q 4–6 h until patient has recovered and is able to take PO medication

For questions, contact ____________________

At the ______________________________ (hospital/office) Tel ________

________	________	________	________
Date	Name of physician	Signature	License #

3.3.1.9 Support and Information for Patients and Families

- Provide written information about nephrotic syndrome (e.g., website)
- Examples:
  - Teach Albustix testing of (morning) urine and early detection of relapses.
  - Provide diary (calendar) with medication dosing schedules, appointments, and space to enter urine dipstick results and record clinical events.
  - Patients may create their own manual or electronic spreadsheets.

  - Provide form sheet for "Recommendations for patients with adrenal insufficiency" to be carried in wallet (Box 3.5).
- Avoid self-medication. Encourage patient/family to speak to designated contacts (MD, nurse).

3.3.2 Minimal Change Nephrotic Syndrome (MCNS)

- The majority of children with INS have MCNS (MCD).
- MCNS incidence peaks between 2 and 6 years of age.
- Tell-tale signs are periorbital and dependent edema. Ascites, pleural effusion, and scrotal or labial edema may also occur. Patients are usually not hypertensive. Upto 30 % have microhematuria.
- Probability of MCNS (and glucocorticoid responsiveness) is greater than 90 % for a young child with typical features of nephrotic syndrome. Hence, kidney biopsy is reserved to children with unsatifactory glucocorticoid response and/or "atypical" presentation.
- On light microscopy, the glomeruli are normal with normal capillary walls and normal cellularity. A mild mesangial hypercellularity may be noted. Immunofluorescence microscopy is negative, although some cases show deposits of IgM, IgG, and C3. The significance of IgM deposits (and whether they represent a separate entity) is not known. Ultrastructural changes are always present in MCNS, involving podocytes and mesangial cells. Podocyte foot process fusion is constant and generalized.
- MCNS, diffuse mesangial proliferation, and focal segmental glomerulosclerosis (FSGS) are considered separate diseases because of differences in response to glucocorticoids and subsequent clinical course. However, some think of MCNS and FSGS as a spectrum of the same disease. Transition of MCNS to FSGS has been reported.
- More than 90 % patients with MCNS will respond to glucocorticoid therapy. Proteinuria will resolve within 10 days of initiation of glucocorticoid therapy in the majority of children. In late responders, it may take up to 4 weeks.
- Relapses are common and are often triggered by viral respiratory tract infections. Seventy percent of glucocorticoid-responsive nephrotic syndrome will have at least one relapse. Half of these will have frequent relapses or become glucocorticoid-dependent. Relapses of proteinuria continue till onset of puberty or even into adulthood.
- Glucocorticoid sensitivity is the most important prognostic indicator. Renal function remains normal in children with (frequent) relapses who do not exhibit secondary glucocorticoid resistance.

3.3.3 Focal Segmental Glomerulosclerosis (FSGS)

- FSGS is a histological description without etiological specificity.
- It is characterized by proteinuria with or without full-blown nephrotic syndrome; patient may demonstrate "atypical" features, such as hypertension and hematuria, poor response to glucorticoids and progression to CKD. Progression

to end-stage renal disease. Depending on the populations studied, up to 70 % of patients with FSGS fail to respond to glucocorticoid therapy.

- Risk factors for progression to CKD include black ethnicity, poor response to glucocorticoids and other immunosuppressive agents, persistance of proteinuria, elevated serum creatinine at presentation, and important of interstitial fibrosis by kidney biopsy.
- FSGS may be primary or secondary. Causes of secondary FSGS include hyperfiltration injury (decreased nephron mass), reflux nephropathy, morbid obesity, sickle cell nephropathy, HIV or parvovirus infection, and heroin abuse.
- There is a concern that the incidence of FSGS is increasing worldwide.
- Genetic forms of FSGS have been described. They are generally glucocorticoid resistant (see Sect. 3.3.4). FSGS lesions due to known mutations do not recur in the transplanted kidney unlike other forms of primary FSGS.
- Renal biopsy shows segmental scarring involving some but not all of the sampled glomeruli. Affected glomeruli are initially localized in deep cortex and may be missed. The glomerular scars are composed of collapsed glomerular capillaries, adhesions between the tuft and Bowman's capsule, and hyaline deposits. Podocyte dysregulation is accompanied by podocyte detachment from the glomerular basement membrane. Uninvolved areas of the glomerulus appear normal.
- A pathological classification of FSGS has been proposed – the "Columbia" classification – with five histological variants: "FSGS not otherwise specified," perihilar variant, cellular variant, tip variant, and collapsing variant. Glomerular tip variants have been associated with better outcomes and the collapsing variant with the worst outcome.
- Collapsing glomerulopathy is a distinct form of FSGS. These lesions are also seen in HIV associated nephropathy, recurrent nephrotic syndrome after renal transplantation, and parvovirus B19 or CMV infection. The prognosis is poor.
- The management of FSGS can be challenging. Specific treatment options include high-dose methylprednisolone, intravenous cyclophosphamide, calcineurin inhibitors, mycophenolate mofetil, rituximab, anti-TNF-alpha antibody, plasmapheresis, and ACE inhibitors/ARB to reduce proteinuria (see Fig. 3.7).
- Recurrence risk of FSGS after renal transplantation is highest in patients with disease onset between 6 and 12 years of age and progression to ESRD within 18 to 36 months in the absence of an identifiable genetic mutation (see also Chap. 11).

3.3.4 Inherited Forms of Nephrotic Syndrome

3.3.4.1 Introduction

- Defects in various genes have been associated with the development of nephrotic syndromes that are generally glucocorticoid-resistant (Table 3.6)
- Affected individuals may present postnatally ("congenital nephrotic syndrome") or during childhood or adolescence ("late-onset FSGS")
- The percentage of children with primary nephrotic syndrome and FSGS due to currently identifiable genetic mutations beyond the first year of life is <10 %

Table 3.6 Genetic forms of nephrotic syndrome

Gene locus	Inheritance	Encoded protein	Protein localization	Clinical manifestation
NPHS1	AR	Nephrin	Podocyte and slit diaphragm	Congenital (Finnish-type) nephrotic syndrome
NPHS2	AR	Podocin	Podocyte and slit diaphragm	Childhood-onset FSGS
PLCE1 / NPHS3	AR	Phospholipase C ε-1	Podocyte	Non-syndromic DMS (28 % all DMS), FSGS
WT1 / NPHS4	AD	Wilms' tumor 1 protein	Podocyte (transcription factor)	Denys–Drash (DMS), Frasier (FSGS)
LAMB2 / NPHS5	AR	Laminin β2	GBM	Pierson syndrome (DMS), isolated FSGS
ACTN4 / FSGS1	AD	α-actinin 4	Podocyte	Adult-onset FSGS (incomplete penetrance, slow progression to ESRD)
TRPC6 / FSGS2	AD	Transient receptor potential cation channel 6	Podocyte	Adult-onset FSGS
CD2AP / FSGS3	AR or AD	CD2-associated protein	Podocyte and slit diaphragm	Early and adult-onset FSGS
INF2 / FSGS5	AD	Actin polymerization regulatory protein inverted formin 2	Podocyte	Familial FSGS (variable penetrance, onset from child- to adulthood)
LMX1B	AD	LIM homeobox transcription factor 1-beta	Podocyte	Nail patella syndrome: dystrophic nails, absent or hypoplastic patella, iliac horns, FSGS, moth-eaten appearance of mesangium and GBM
MYH9	AR	Non-muscle myosin heavy chain IIA	Podocyte	FSGS (May–Hegglin, Sebastian, Fechtner, and Epstein syndromes)
SCARB2	AR	Lysosome membrane protein 2	Lysosome	Syndromic FSGS
SMARCAL1	AR	SWI/SNF-related matrix-associated actin-dependent regulator of chromatin subfamily A-like protein 1	Podocyte	Schimke immuno-osseous dysplasia

Abbreviations: *AD* autosomal dominant, *AR* autosomal recessive, *DMS* diffuse mesangial sclerosis, *FSGS* focal segmental glomerulosclerosis, *GBM* glomerular basement membrane

- Affected genes encode for proteins involved in the development, structure and function of podocytes
- All hereditary proteinuric syndromes show typical flattening (effacement) of podocyte foot processes and loss of a normal slit diaphragm
- They usually do not respond to glucocorticoids or other immunosuppressants and do not recur in the transplanted kidney

3.3.4.2 Congenital Nephrotic Syndrome (CNS)

- Congenital nephrotic syndrome (CNS) is defined as the presence of nephrotic syndrome within the first 3 months of life
- CNS can be inherited or caused by spontaneous mutation, or acquired due to maternal (transplacentally transmitted) antibodies or cytokines, or congenital infections (Box 3.6)

3.3.4.3 Finnish-Type Congenital Nephrotic Syndrome (FCNS)

- Autosomal recessive disorder with highest incidence in Finland
- It is caused by a defect in the *NPHS1* gene, which codes for the protein nephrin, a podocyte transmembrane protein and structural component of the slit diaphragm between podocyte foot processes
- FCNS is resistant to immunosuppressive therapy
- Infants with FCNS are born prematurely; placental weight >25 % of their birth weight; edema is present at birth or shortly afterward
- Massive proteinuria leads to malnutrition and poor somatic growth
- Patients are highly susceptible to bacterial infections including peritonitis, pneumonia and cellulitis
- Very low serum albumin levels and net loss of immunoglobulin G (IgG), vitamin D, thyroglobulin-binding protein (leading to hypothyroidism), antithrombin III and transferrin

Box 3.6 Etiologies of Congenital Nephrotic Syndromes

Primary (genetic)	Identifiable or suspected genetic mutation	Finnish-type (FCNS) Denys-Drash syndrome (DDS) Frasier syndrome (FS) WAGR syndrome Galloway-Mowat syndrome Secondary Primary FSGS
Secondary (acquired)	Transplacental transmission (very rare)	Fetal nephrotic syndrome due to maternal antibodies or cytokines to (e.g. FSGS, SLE)
	Congenital infection	Cytomegalovirus (CMV) Hepatitis B virus (HBV) Rubella virus *T. gondii* (toxoplasmosis) *T. pallidum* (syphilis)

- Thromboembolic complications are common
- Renal function is normal at birth, but declines after the first year of life
- Histological lesions are characterized by irregular dilatation of the proximal convoluted tubules and increased mesangial matrix and hypercellularity, leading to glomerular sclerosis and interstitial fibrosis
- Genetic analysis obviates need for kidney biopsy
- High amniotic fluid alpha-fetoprotein levels aid in prenatal diagnostic
- Management is challenging: Daily infusions of albumin may be needed, diuretics, gamma globulin infusions, tube feeding for adequate nutrition, thyroxin supplementation, and ACE inhibitor and indomethacin therapy to reduce proteinuria
- Many infants require uni- or bilateral nephrectomy to stop massive protein losses and malnutrition
- No disease recurrence in the graft, parents can be organ donors

3.3.4.4 Denys–Drash Syndrome (DDS)

- DDS presents in infancy with proteinuria or nephrotic syndrome and ambiguous genitalia in a chromosomally male (46, XY) child
- DDS is caused by a heterozygous, generally spontaneous, point mutation of the Wilms tumor suppressor gene (*WT1*) resulting in loss or altered structure of the functionally important zinc finger domain (encoded by exons 8 and 9). WT1 is also a critical regulator of kidney and gonadal development
- The typical histological lesion is diffuse glomerular mesangial sclerosis, identified by kidney biopsy
- The glomerular lesion progresses to end-stage renal failure by 4 years of age
- The Wilms tumor risk is 90 %
- Frequent, proactive echographic monitoring (e.g. every 3 months) and nephrectomy with the first appearance of suspected tumor lesions are recommended. Preemptive (pretransplant) bilateral nephrectomy if hemodialysis or peritoneal and back-up hemodialysis are feasible
- Most centers wait 1 year to kidney transplantation following Wilms tumor removal (and chemotherapy)

3.3.4.5 Frasier Syndrome (FS)

- FS should be suspected in any child with glucocorticoid-resistant nephrotic syndrome and ambiguous genitalia, and in phenotypically females with nephrotic syndrome and amenorrhea (male pseudohermaphroditism: normal-appearing female external genitalia, streak gonads 46, XY caryotype)
- FS is caused by an intronic mutation of *WT1* (intron 9)
- The histopathological lesion is focal segmental glomerulosclerosis
- Proteinuria begins between age 2 and 6 years, progression to ESRD during or after adolescence
- FS is not associated with Wilms tumor, but with an increased risk of gonadoblastoma

3.3.4.6 WAGR Syndrome

- Acronym of Wilms tumor, aniridia, genitourinary malformations, and mental retardation
- WAGR syndrome is caused by a microdeletion in chromosome 11p13 affecting *WT1* and *PAX6* that encode proteins involved in eye development
- Many patients with WAGR syndrome eventually develop ESRD
- Wilms tumor risk is ~50 %

3.3.4.7 Pierson Syndrome (PS)

- PS is characterized by congenital nephrotic syndrome with microcoria and buphthalmos
- It is due to a mutation in *LAMB2* coding for the GBM protein laminin β2
- The histopathological lesion is diffuse glomerular mesangial sclerosis
- Patients progress rapidly to ESRD

3.4 Acute Glomerulonephritis

Acute GN, defined by hematuria (characteristically macroscopic), proteinuria, acute renal dysfunction, hypertension and fluid retention, requires an etiological diagnosis. It may follow an acute or sustained focal infection and often involves activation of complement. The course can be self-limited or require immunosuppressive, at times aggressive treatment.

The approach to a child with acute GN is depicted in Fig. 3.8.

3.4.1 Acute Post-Infectious (Poststreptococcal) Glomerulonephritis (APIGN/APSGN)

3.4.1.1 Abstract

- APIGN/APSGN is the most common form of acute glomerulonephritis in childhood.
- *Pathogenesis*: Immunologically mediated, inflammatory disorder of the renal parenchyma that is characterized by alternative complement pathway activation and exudative, proliferative glomerulonephritis. Manifestation after a latent period of 1–3 weeks after upper respiratory tract infection/pharyngitis or 3–5 weeks after pyoderma, caused by group A hemolytic streptococci (*S. pyogenes*) and other infectious organisms.
- *Clinical Features*: Triad of (gross) hematuria, arterial hypertension, and generalized edema (acute nephritic syndrome). Spectrum ranges from microhematuria to nephrotic syndrome, severe renal failure, and encephalopathy or seizures due to hypertension (posterior reversible encephalopathy syndrome, PRES).
- *Investigations*: Basal tests include urinalysis and microscopy (red blood cell casts), serum creatinine, electrolytes, and C3. Plasma C3 is almost always

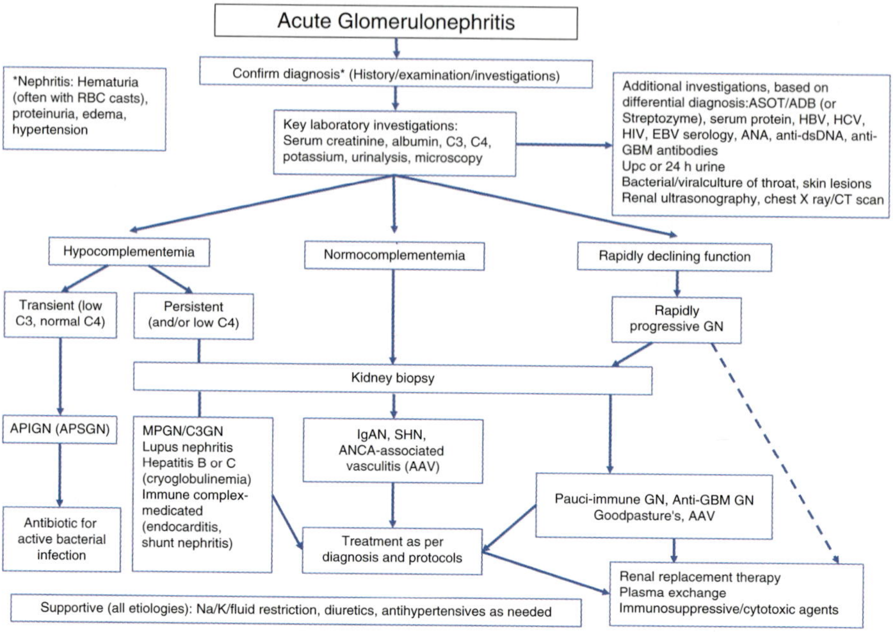

Fig. 3.8 Suggested approach to children with acute nephritis. *Abbreviations*: *ASOT* anti-etreptolysin O titer, *ADB* anti-DNAse B, *GBM* glomerular basement membrane, *APIGN* acute post-infectious glomerulonephritis (GN), *APSGN* acute post-streptococcal GN, *MPGN* membranoproliferative GN, *LN* lupus nephritis, *SHN* Schönlein–Henoch nephritis

decreased during acute illness. Elevated antistreptolysin (ASOT) or anti-DNAse B (ADB) antibody titers (or streptozyme test) indicate preceding streptococcal infection.

- *Histological Findings*: Kidney biopsy shows endocapillary proliferation by light microscopy, granular deposits of C3 and IgG in capillary loops by immunofluorescence, and typical, large subepithelial "humps" by electron microscopy. Renal biopsy is indicated if C3 remains low after 6–8 weeks and with persisting proteinuria or declining kidney function.
- *Treatment*: Symptomatic therapy, including control of blood pressure and edema. Dialysis, although rarely indicated, is needed for severe AKI with oligoanuria, uncontrolled hyperkalemia, or fluid overload unresponsive to loop diuretics.
- *Antibiotics*: Antibiotic treatment does not change course of (or prevent) disease but may limit spread of nephritogenic strains of β-hemolytic *streptococci*.
- *Prognosis*: Excellent outcome in >95 % of cases. Progression to end-stage renal disease or recurrence of APSGN is extremely rare.

Vignette

A 5-year-old boy presents with acute onset of bloody urine which frightens the family. Parents also report that their child lost energy and appetite over the last 2 days, that he complains of headache and one-time vomiting without diarrhea, and that he looks swollen. He was previously healthy, except that some mosquito bites on his leg became infected about 3 weeks ago.

You quickly determine that the child has moderate facial and limb edema. There is no rash but cellulitis on his left shin. He is afebrile. Blood pressure is 135/95 mmHg, and he appears irritable. You ask for urine and blood samples. While awaiting the results, the child has a seizure.

3.4.1.2 Introduction

Postinfectious glomerulonephritis is one of the earliest described renal diseases. While group A β-hemolytic streptococci (GAS) are responsible for the vast majority of APIGN, other organisms can lead to a similar presentation. APIGN (APSGN) is one of the commonest causes of community-acquired, acute kidney injury in children. The prognosis is excellent in most cases. The exact disease mechanism is still debated.

3.4.1.3 Definition

APSGN is the prototype of an acute nephritic syndrome. It is an immune-mediated, glomerular inflammatory disorder leading to acute kidney injury (AKI), often with gross hematuria, hypertension, and generalized edema. About 85 % of cases follow an infection by beta-hemolytic streptococci. Hence, the terms APIGN and "post-streptococcal GN" (APSGN) are often used synonymously. The hallmark of all forms of APIGN is the transient activation of the alternative complement pathway with subepithelial glomerular deposition of C3 (and IgG/IgM) and depletion of plasma C3.

3.4.1.4 Epidemiology

- APIGN affects school children with a peak from 4–10 years of age.
- The disease burden is highest in resource-poor countries and disadvantaged populations.
- More than 80 % of cases are linked to infections by Lancefield group A (GAS) and occasionally C or G beta-hemolytic streptococci.
- Incidence 9.5–28.5 new cases per 100,000 person-years.
- Glomerulonephritis risk approaches 5 % of pharyngitis and 25 % of pyoderma cases in epidemics of nephritogenic *S. pyogenes* infections.
- The serotype most frequently associated with pyoderma-associated APSGN is M49; others are M2, M42, M56, M57, and M60. Common pharyngitis APSGN-associated M types are 1, 4, (12) and 25. Newer studies use molecular-based

typing of the *emm* gene encoding the hypervariable M protein and multilocus sequence typing.

- APIGN due to streptococcal pharyngitis peaks during winter and early spring; APIGN due to pyoderma peaks in late summer and early fall. The latter is more common in tropical and subtropical regions.
- APIGN occurs at any age but peaks in children ages 6–10 (2–12) years.
- Male to female ratio 2:1.1.
- APIGN is associated with conditions that favor spread of the causative organism.
- Siblings are at risk of developing subclinical nephritis.

3.4.1.5 Etiology and Pathogenesis

- Exact mechanism of glomerular injury is debated.
- Pattern of hypocomplementemia in APIGN reflects activation of the alternative complement pathway (AP): plasma C3, C5, and properdin levels are transiently decreased in the presence of preserved concentrations of C4.
- Current hypotheses:
  - Antibodies bind to streptococcal antigen(s) planted in the glomerular basement membrane leading to alternative complement pathway activation.
  - Two streptococcal proteins, glyceraldehyde phosphate dehydrogenase (also known as nephritis-associated plasmin receptor) and cationic proteinase exotoxin B (SPEB) with its zymogen precursor, have been identified in the GBM of APSGN patients and proposed as pathogenic antigens.
  - M-like and non-M proteins including fibronectin-binding (Fba) and streptococcal collagen-like proteins (Scl) bind complement factor H (CFH) and/or CFH-related protein 1 (CFHR-1), regulators of the C3 and C5 convertases of complement activation pathways. While some of theses proteins have been associated with bacterial immune evasion, their role for the pathogenesis of APIGN remains speculative.

3.4.1.6 Clinical Features

- AKI with classical triad of gross hematuria, hypertension, and edema (classical nephritic syndrome).
- The clinical spectrum ranges from asymptomatic microhematuria to severe disease. Complications due to hypertension, renal failure, and cardiac insufficiency (Table 3.7).
- Hypertension (60 %) can be associated with headache, vomiting and altered mental status, hypertensive encephalopathy with risk of seizure, and hypertensive congestive cardiac failure.
- Abnormal urinalysis, transitory hypocomplementemia, and increased ASOT indicate subclinical nephritis (e.g., in siblings).

3.4.1.7 Laboratory Investigations

- Useful investigations are detailed in (Table 3.8)

Table 3.7 Clinical manifestations of APIGN

Condition	Remarks
Hypertension	Headache, vomiting, seizures, somnolence/altered mental status Risk of posterior reversible encephalopathy syndrome (PRES) with visual changes and focal neurological signs
Edema	Facial/periorbital, dependent, or generalized edema (more frequently in young children) Ascites, pleural effusion Cardiac insufficiency (orthopnea, dyspnea, cough, pulmonary crackles/edema, and gallop rhythm)
Hematuria	Dark-brown urine (cola- or tea-colored) in one-third of patients; remainder microscopic hematuria
Proteinuria	Mild to moderate, rarely nephrotic range (>1 g/m²/day)
Oliguria	Transient oliguria in 50 %, complete anuria rare
Acute kidney injury	Nausea, vomiting fatigue, weakness, pallor
Others	Back pain and abdominal discomfort, fever, weight gain (edema)

Table 3.8 Investigations in APIGN

Investigation	Comments

Urine	Dipstick analysis
	  Hematuria, proteinuria
	Urine microscopy
	  Red blood cell (RBC) and mixed cellular casts
	  Dysmorphic RBCs
	  Leukocytes (sterile pyuria)
	Proteinuria
	  <2 g/l in 85 % of cases (U protein/creatinine <2 g/g)
	  Nephrotic presentation may herald poor renal outcome

Complement	Reduced plasma C3 and CH50 in >90 % of cases Normalize within 6–12 weeks after presentation Plasma C4 generally normal

Bacterial/viral identification	Pharyngeal swab
	  Index patient and siblings (opportunity of preventing spread of nephritogenic strain)
	  Culture of beta-hemolytic steptococci
	  Rapid streptococcal antigen test
	Skin swab
	  Suspected pyoderma
	Alternative etiologies
	  S. pneumoniae (rare), *S. aureus* and other non-streptococcal bacteria
	  Viral infections (e.g., EBV, parvovirus B19)

(continued)

Table 3.8 (continued)

Investigation	Comments
Serology	Antistreptolysin O titer (ASOT) Elevated in 70–80 % of APIGN cases 1–5 weeks after infection, decrease to preinfection levels after several months Unreliable for streptococcal pyoderma or infection by other organisms Streptozyme test Simple, sensitive hemagglutination assay detecting antibodies against several streptococcal antigens (streptolysin O, DNaseB, hyaluronidase, streptokinase, anti-nicotinamide adenine dinucleotidase (NADase)) Anti-Dnase B (ADB) Elevated in 80–90 % of cases of pyoderma-associated APSGN
Kidney biopsy	Indications (rare): Alternative diagnosis (e.g., MPGN, IgAN) Normal serum C3/CH50 Persistently low serum C3 or CH50 (>12 weeks after onset) Persistent GN/deteriorating renal function

Table 3.9 Spectrum of histological finding in APIGN

Modality	Findings
Bright-field microscopy	Endocapillary proliferative glomerulonephritis with diffusely increased cellularity, occasionally with abundant polymorphonuclear neutrophils (exudative GN) Enlarged, bloodless glomeruli secondary to capillary occlusion, normal-appearing glomerular basement membrane Infiltration of macrophages and lymphocyte in glomeruli and tubulointerstitial compartment
Immunofluorescence	Discrete deposits of C3, IgG, and IgM in the mesangium and in the glomerular basement membrane ("starry sky") Heavy, "garland"-like GBM deposits (associated with nephrotic-range proteinuria and poorer outcome)
Electron microscopy	Subepithelial electron-dense deposits ("humps," a hallmark lesion of APSGN) containing mainly C3 and IgG/IgM (and streptococcal antigens, e.g., SPEB) Note that "humps" may also be found in other nephritides, e.g., lupus nephritis

3.4.1.8 Kidney Biopsy

- Kidney biopsy is indicated (1) when kidney function fails to recover or (2) declines rapidly, and (3) when C3 levels fail to normalize or (4) proteinuria persist beyond 2–3 months
- Expected biopsy results are shown in Table 3.9

3.4.1.9 Treatment of APIGN

Treatment is based on the clinical severity of the illness focusing on control of blood pressure, edema, and consequences of acute renal failure (Table 3.10). Patients with

Table 3.10 Treatment of APIGN

Indications and treatment modalities	Remarks
Hypertension and fluid overload	Restriction of sodium and fluid intake Loop diuretics (furosemide) Antihypertensive drugs If blood pressure is not controlled with diuretics Preferably calcium channel blocker or angiotensin-converting enzyme inhibitor (ACEi)
Pulmonary edema (rare) Hypertensive urgency or emergency (with or without CSN symptoms)	Loop diuretics, O_2 therapy Oral agents (nifedipine, hydralazine, minoxidil) Intravenous agents (nitroprusside, nicardipine labetalol – dosing see Chap. 7)
Hyperkalemia	Loop diuretic K restriction, sodium polystyrene sulfonate Inhaled bronchodilator, IV calcium or bicarbonate, or insulin drip If refractory, dialysis
Dialysis or continuous venovenous hemofiltration	Life-threatening hyperkalemia Severe fluid overload unresponsive to diuretics Rapidly progressive GN with persistent oligoanuria
Antibiotics	Obtain throat cultures from patient, family members, and close contacts Treat those infected to minimize spread of nephritogenic strain Oral penicillin V for 10 days (<25 kg = 250 mg twice daily, >25 kg 500 mg twice daily) Erythromycin (40 mg/kg for 10 days) or derivative for patients allergic to penicillin
Glucocorticoids, other immunosuppressants	Rarely indicated

milder disease, i.e., normal BP and mild renal failure, may not be hospitalized but require BP monitoring. Patients with elevated BP, oliganuria, hyperkalemia, or severe edema should be treated as inpatients.

3.4.1.10 Prognosis and Outcome

- Short- and long-term prognosis of APIGN in children is excellent.
- >95 % of the patients recover renal function within 3–4 weeks.
- Chronic or progressive kidney disease <1 % of children (higher percentage in adults).
- The superimposition of APSGN in patients with diabetes mellitus or metabolic syndrome may increase risk of CKD.
- Recurrence of APSGN extremely rare due to streptococcal type-specific, long-lasting immunity and limited number of nephritogenic GAS strains.

3.4.2 Infection-Induced Immune Complex Glomerulonephritis (ICGN)

3.4.2.1 Abstract

Sustained, focal infections can result in glomerulonephritis. Classical examples are subacute bacterial endocarditis (SBE) and ventriculo-atrial (and rarely ventriculo-peritoneal) shunt nephritis.

Infectious organisms release soluble antigens that are deposited in glomerular structures, either directly or after complexing with specific antibodies.

ICGN has also been described after acute infective carditis and chronic otitis media, tonsillitis and abscesses, and associated with portal fibrosis or portocaval shunts, or congenital and acquired syphilis.

The diagnosis involves bacterial culture, serological or molecular antigen detection, urinalysis, and biochemical testing and evidence of complement activation.

Treatment targets the primary infection and occasionally the inflammatory processes directly.

The risk of recurrence in the absence of persistent or new infections is negligible.

Vignette (1)

A 17-year-old adolescent presents to the emergency room because of gross hematuria following several weeks of intermittent fever, night sweat, decreasing energy, non-defined weight loss, and myalgia. Medical history is significant for a small, muscular ventricular septum defect (VSD). She has been well at the time of her last cardiology checkup 3 months earlier. A week prior to her current illness, she had pireced her navel. On physical examination, she appears acutely ill, dyspneic, and moderately edematous. The temperature is 38.5 °C, pulse 120/min. A pansystolic murmur of Levine III/IV is noted at the fourth left sternal border. She has mild splenomegaly and dark red, painful papules on her finger tips. The umbilical area is indolent. Urine is positive for blood (+++) and protein (1 g/l). Laboratory exam reveals serum creatinine 180 μmol/l (2.0 mg/dl), neutrophilia and anemia (hemoglobin 90 g/l [9 g/dl]), elevated sedimentation rate and C-reactive protein. No antinuclear (ANA), anti-glomerular basement membrane (GBM), and anti-neutrophil cytoplasmic antibodies (ANCA) are detected. Repeat blood cultures grow *Propionibacterium acnes*.

Vignette (2)

A 7-year-old boy presents with malaise, headache, vomiting, fever, and gross hematuria. He has a ventriculoatrial shunt for hydrocephalus that had been changed 3 years prior to the current presentation. Physical examination reveals lethargy, pallor, skin rash and hepatosplenomegaly. BP is 130/90 mmHg. Laboratory findings include normocytic anemia (hemoglobin 83 g/l [8.3 g/dl]), elevated serum creatinine 185 μM [2.1 mg/dl], estimated GFR 0.39 ml/s/1.73 m^2 [23 ml/min/m^2]), and abnormal urinalysis with large hematuria and proteinuria (>3 g/l by dipstick). Serum C3 and C4 are profoundly decreased. Repeat blood cultures grow coagulase-negative Staphylococcus.

3.4.2.2 Definition

ICGN is caused by immunologically mediated inflammatory processes linked to the deposition of a microbial antigen, immunoglobulin and C3 in glomerular basement membranes and mesangium, induced by focal intra- or extravascular infection. It is commonly associated with classical (CP) or alternative pathway (AP) complement activation and depletion of serum C3, C4 and total hemolytic complement (CH_{50}). Best-known examples are subacute/infective endocarditis (SBE/IE) and "shunt nephritis" due to an infected ventriculoatrial (VA) shunt.

3.4.2.3 Etiology and Pathogenesis

- Subacute or chronic infection by bacterial or other microbial agents that release soluble antigens into the circulation.
- The most common organisms are low-virulence bacterial pathogens, such as *Streptococcus viridians* and coagulase-negative staphylococci (*S. epidermidis*).
- Other organisms associated with ICGN are *S. aureus*, *S. pyogenes*, *S. pneumoniae*, anaerobic streptococci, *Salmonella spp.* (S. typhi) and *Brucella spp.* and *Treponema pallidum*.
- Primary infections include abscesses of the brain or other organs, ventriculo- and portosystemic shunt infections, osteomyelitis, pyelonephritis, pneumonia/pleuroempyema, otitis media, and enterocolitis.
- Congenital syphilis causes GN along with rash, rhinitis, and osteochondritis and full-blown nephrotic syndrome with anasarca 2–3 months postnatally.
- Chronically released antigen(s) elicit a humoral immune response and formation of antigen–antibody (immune) complexes (IC). Circulating ICs become trapped in the glomerulus or form in situ after antigen deposition in the glomerular basement membrane and mesangium.
- CP and AP complement activation lead to local inflammation due to chemokine production, such as C3a and C5a, and expression of adhesion molecules.
- Sustained inflammation results in focal necrotizing or diffuse proliferative glomerulonephritis with progressive renal injury.
- Some forms of infective carditis cause localized infarcts and glomerular vasculitis without apparent immune deposits.

3.4.2.4 Clinical Features

- Systemic signs: picture of chronic infection, primary organ impairment, generalized inflammation, and renal injury.
- Intermittent or persistent fever, weight loss, lethargy, arthralgia, lymphadenopathy, and hepatosplenomegaly.

- VA shunt infections may present with lethargy and seizures.
- Renal and urinary findings: gross or microscopic hematuria, large proteinuria, arterial hypertension, and acute kidney injury.
- Classic picture of SBE: peripheral stigmata such as (conjunctival) petechiae, splinter hemorrhages (linear hemorrhagic lines in the nail beds, images see http://199.231.142.148/dermnet/Splinter-Hemorrhage), Roth spots (retinal hemorrhages with pale or yellow center image see http://www.aao.org/theeyeshaveit/optic-fundus/roth-spot.cfm), Osler's nodes (painful, palpable, erythematous lesions most often involving the pads of the fingers and toes, image), and Janeway lesions (nontender, macular lesions most commonly involving the palms and soles; images, see: http://www.childrenshospital.org/cfapps/mml/index.cfm?CAT=media&MEDIA_ID=1887).

3.4.2.5 Investigations

- Basic Laboratory Investigations
  Blood culture (preferably repeat cultures)
  CBC and differential with blood smear (peripheral leukocytosis/neutrophilia)
  Serum creatinine
  C-reactive protein or sedimentation rate (elevated), C3, C4 and CH50 (decreased)
  Urinalysis with quantitative assessment of proteinuria and microscopy
  Cerebrospinal fluid (CSF) in case of suspected cranial pathology or shunt infection
- Extended Laboratory Investigations:
  Serological (specific antibody or antigen detection) and nucleic acid-based tests (e.g., bacterial DNA and RNA).
- Kidney Biopsy:
  In cases of persistent renal disease or worsening renal function, see Table 3.11.
- Imaging Studies:
  Cardiac echography (to detect vegetations on valves and/or tips of VA shunt), CT scan (VP shunt integrity), enhanced head CT or MRI for brain abscess, targeted ultrasound, gallium scan (osteomyelitis, occult abscess)

Table 3.11 Histological findings of shunt nephritis in kidney biopsy

Bright-field microscopy	Endocapillary proliferation, double-countered capillary walls, lobular accentuation in MPGN-type lesions
	Focal necrotizing or diffuse mesangial or membranoproliferative GN. Crescent formation in up to 50 % of proliferative GN following SBE
	Congenital and acquired syphilis can present as proliferative or membranous GN
	Interstitial nephritis or cortical necrosis in 10 % of renal biopsies or autopsies
Immunofluorescence/ immunohistochemistry	Granular IgM, IgG, (IgA), and C3
Electron microscopy	Subendothelial, mesangial, and subepithelial electron-dense (immune) deposits

3.4.2.6 Treatment

- Subacute Bacterial Endocarditis/Infectious Carditis:
  Intravenous (IV) antibiotics directed by bacterial culture and sensitivity
  Empiric therapy with vancomycin due to ubiquitous penicillin (methicillin)-resistant staphylococci and streptococci
  Total duration of antibiotics (IV and PO) 4–6 weeks
- Shunt Nephritis
  IV antibiotics until surgical removal of infected VA or VP shunt.
  Antibiotics alone are rarely able to eliminate the biofilm on implanted devices.
- Other Infections
  Effective treatment of brain abscesses, pleural empyema, and other focal or systemic infections will resolve associated GN.
- Crescentic or progressive GN
  Anecdotal use of glucocorticoids or cytotoxic agents.

3.4.2.7 Prognosis and Outcome

- Renal outcome of GN associated with SBE, shunt nephritis, or other focal or chronic infections is favorable with early diagnosis and treatment.
- Delayed removal of infected VA shunt may result in chronic renal injury and progression to ESRD.
- Urinary findings persist during weeks to months following the eradication of the bacterial organism in cases of SBE.
- Complement levels normalize after eradication of the infection and healing of the renal lesions.

3.4.3 Rapidly Progressive Glomerulonephritis (RPGN)

RPGN must be considered a medical emergency that requires a rapid (etiological) diagnosis and aggressive treatment in an attempt to divert irreversible loss of kidney function.

3.4.3.1 Definition

RPGN is a clinical entity characterized by acute GN with progressive loss of renal function over days to weeks. The histopathological hallmark is the presence of crescents; hence, it is also called crescentic glomerulonephritis. The diagnosis of crescentic GN rests on the detection of crescents in >50 % of glomeruli.

3.4.3.2 Etiology and Pathogenesis

- RPGN can be classified in 3 groups based on the pathophysiology and histopathological presentation: anti-GBM disease, immune-complex GN and pauci-immune GN (see Box 3.7).
- The spectrum of diseases underlying RPN and crescentic GN include
  - SHP (Sect. 3.6.2) and IgAN (Sect. 3.5.2)
  - Anti-GBM GN and Goodpasture's disease (very rare in children)
  - ANCA associated vasculitis (AAV) and pauci-immune vasculitis (Sect. 3.6.3)

Vignette
A 12-year-old boy is brought with worsening generalized edema, oliguria, and gross hematuria since 4 days. There is no history of sore throat, skin rash, joint pain or fever in the recent past. Blood pressure is 150/100 mmHg. Urine analysis shows protein +++, plenty of RBCs, RBC casts and occasional WBC. His serum creatinine is 185 mcmol/l (2.1 mg/dl). Family history is non-contributory. Two days later, his creatinine has risen to 334 mcmol/l (3.4 mg/dl).

Box 3.7 Classification of RPGN

Anti-glomerular basement membrane disease

Anti-GBM GN, Goodpasture's syndrome, post kidney transplantation in Alport syndrome

Pauci-immune RPGN

- ANCA-associated vasculitis and renal limited vasculitis (see Box 3.10 and Sect. 3.6.3)
- Idiopathic crescentic GN
- Medications: penicillamine, hydralazine, propylthiouracil

Immune complex RPGN

- IgA nephropathy, SHN, membranoproliferative GN, membranous nephropathy
- Infection associated GN: acute poststreptococcal/postinfectious GN, subacute bacterial and infective endocarditis, shunt nephritis, visceral abscesses, human immunodeficiency virus, hepatitis B and C, syphilis
- Systemic disease: SLE, Schönlein–Henoch purpura, cryoglobulinemia, mixed connective tissue disorder, juvenile chronic arthritis

3.4.3.3 Pathogenesis of Crescent Formation

- Crescent formation starts with a break in the glomerular capillary basement membrane leading to influx of macrophages, T cells into the Bowman's space.
- The influx of cells causes release of inflammatory mediators such as interleukin-1 and tumor necrosis factor-alpha.
- Proinflammatory cytokines contribute to epithelial cell proliferation and crescent formation.
- Fibroblast growth factor and transforming growth factor-beta (TGF-beta) induce deposition of collagen resulting in fibro-cellular and fibrous crescents.

3.4.3.4 Clinical Features

- Renal:
  - Most patients (80–90 %) present with signs of acute GN, including gross hematuria, oliguria, hypertension, and edema and, occasionally, with hypertensive emergency with encephalopathy or congestive heart failure.

- Extrarenal:
  - Upper (nasal discharge, polyps, sinusitis) and lower respiratory tract involvement (pneumonitis, pulmonary nodules, asthma, pulmonary hemorrhage) with or without vasculitic rash: ANCA-associated vasculitis (AAV), pauci-immune vasculitis (see Sect. 3.6.3)
  - Hemoptysis, pulmonary hemorrhage: Goodpasture's disease, AAV
  - Arthralgia, skin rash/purpura, anemia: systemic lupus erythematosus, SHP
  - History of sore throat, pyoderma: acute poststreptococcal nephritis

3.4.3.5 Investigations

- Urine analysis: moderate to large proteinuria (2+ to 4+), RBC, WBC, RBC or granular casts
- Serial, frequent monitoring of serum creatinine, electrolytes
- Serology:
  - Antistreptolysin O: poststreptococcal RPGN
  - Complement: C3 consumption in APIGN/APIGN, SLE and MPGN/C3 GN
  - ANA, anti-dsDNA: positive in SLE
  - Antineutrophil cytoplasmic antibodies (ANCA): perinuclear (pANCA/MPO) and cytoplasmic (cANCA/PR3): pauci-immune vasculitis (see Sect. 3.6.3, Box 3.10)
  - Circulating anti-glomerular basement membrane (GBM) antibody: anti-GBM nephritis, Goodpasture's syndrome (with pulmonary involvement)
  - Hepatitis serology
- X-ray, CT chest: ANCA-associated vasculitis (AAV), Goodpasture's disease
- Renal biopsy

3.4.3.6 Renal Histopathology

- Crescents are the pathognomonic feature of RPGN (see Table 3.12 and Sect. 3.4.3.3).

Table 3.12 Renal biopsy findings in RPGN

	Anti-GBM GN	Immune complex RPGN	Pauci-immune RPGN
Light microscopy	Focal glomerular capillary vasculitis to diffuse, exudative (crescentic) and necrotizing GN (CNGN)	Diffuse exudative glomerular proliferation (APIGN/LN) Duplication/splitting of glomerular basement membrane (MPGN/C3 GN) Mesangial proliferation (IgAN/SHN)	Segmental fibrinoid necrosis, karyorrhexis and crescents
Immunofluorescence (IF)	Linear deposits of IgG along the capillary walls	C3/IgG (APIGN) C3 deposits (MPGN/CE GN) Full-house IF (SLE) IgA deposits (IgAN/SHN)	No or scanty immune deposits

Abbreviations: *RPGN* rapidly progressive glomerulonephritis (GN), *APIGN* acute post-infections GN, *LN* lupus nephritis, *MPGN* membranoproliferative GN, *SHN* Schönlein–Henoch nephritis

- They may be circumferential or segmental, with compression of the glomerular tuft.
- Crescents may be cellular, fibro-cellular or fibrous, based on the duration of the disease.

3.4.3.7 Treatment

- RPGN must be diagnosed promptly and treatment initiated urgently to preserve renal function.
- An etiological diagnosis, usually by means of kidney biopsy and serology, is important as specific treatments evolve.
- For the treatment of specific underlying diseases presenting as RPGN, refer to Sect. 3.6.
- Aggressive immunosuppressive therapy is inappropriate in patients with mainly chronic versus active lesions by kidney biopsy.
- Extrarenal manifestations should prompt adequate immunosuppressive therapy regardless of the degree of kidney disease.

Induction phase:

  - Three to five doses of IV methylprednisolone (10–20 mg/kg/day) followed by 1.5–2 mg/kg/day of oral prednis(ol)one for 4–6 weeks with gradual tapering to 0.5 mg/kg/day by 3 months
  - Cyclophosphamide IV (500–750 mg/m^2/dose every 4 weeks for 3–6 doses) or PO (2 mg/kg for 8 weeks).

Maintenance phase:

  - Prednisone 0.5–1 mg/kg alternate days, with slow tapering
  - Azathioprine 2 mg/kg/day or mycophenolate mofetil at 800–1,200 mg/m^2/day for 12–24 months

Antibody mediated or refractory disease:

  - Plasmapheresis: e.g., in patients with anti-GBM disease or pauci-immune vasculitis presenting with RPGN and/or diffuse pulmonary hemorrhage
  - The therapeutic role for B-cell depleting (rituximab), anti-cytokine and anti-complement antibodies is evolving

3.4.3.8 Prognosis

- The prognosis depends on the underlying etiology, severity of disease, and time to initiation of treatment.
- With adequate treatment, >50 % of patients show partial or complete recovery of renal function

3.5 Chronic Glomerulonephritis and Immune Nephropathies

This section combines an etiologically diverse group of (chronic) nephropathies that display varying degrees of glomerular inflammation.

3.5.1 Membranoproliferative Glomerulonephritis

Membranoproliferative glomerulonephritis (GN), also known as mesangiocapillary GN, is a chronic disease characterized by thickening and splitting of the glomerular basement membrane (GBM) with mesangial proliferation and mesangial interposition into the GBM. Median age at onset is 10 years, but ranges from 5 years to young adulthood.

Based on light and electron microscopic features, such as location of the immune deposits and GBM appearance, MPGN is classified as MPGN type I, MPGN type II and MPGN type III. Subsequently, type II MPGN has been recognized as a distinct disorder and termed dense deposit disease (DDD; Box 3.8).

An evolving, immunofluorescence (IF) microscopy-based nomenclature refers to the demonstration of isolated or dominant C3 deposits (C3 GN) versus the mixed presence of IgG and complement. The new diagnostic term C3 GN encompasses DDD and MPGN type III, as well as a proportion of MPGN type I cases. Excluded are secondary forms of MPGN that are more frequently seen in adult patients.

3.5.1.1 Etiology and Pathogenesis

- Persistent consumption of complement and low circulating concentrations of C3 in plasma are found in 80–95 % of (primary) type I and type III MPGN and essentially all DDD patients
- Complement activation via the classical pathway (CP) is present in > 40 % of type I MPGN, often associated with hepatitis C virus (HCV) infection and cryoglobulinemia. Conversely, in one large series > 80 % of patients with HCV infection and cryoglobulinemia had MPGN type I lesions
- C4 is not depleted in plasma nor deposited in the kidney in patients with DDD or type III MPGN (see Table 3.13)
- Activation of the terminal complement components C5-C9 is common in type III, but rare in type I MPGN or DDD

Box 3.8 Traditional Classification of Membranoproliferative Glomerulonephritis (MPGN)

MPGN type I

- Primary/idiopathic
- Secondary
  - Infections: hepatitis B, hepatitis C, HIV, schistosomiasis, malaria
  - Auto-immune: cryoglobulinemia, SLE, Sjogren's syndrome
  - Malignancy: B cell lymphoma, non-Hodgkin's lymphoma, chronic lymphocytic leukemia

MPGN type II (dense deposit disease, DDD)

- Primary/idiopathic
- Partial lipodystrophy

MPGN type III

Table 3.13 MPGN renal histology

Modality	MPGN type 1	MPGN type 2 (DDD)	MPGN type 3
Light microscopy	Endocapillary and mesangial proliferation (proliferative GN) Lobular accentuation of glomerulus, mesangial matrix expansion Silver stain: double contour of GBM, "tram track" appearance, mesangial interposition	Enlarged glomeruli due to increased cellularity (proliferation) Silver stain: thickened GBM	Complex laminal lesions caused by iterative subepithelial and subendothelial deposits
Immunofluorescence	IgG and/or C3 (and often C4) present in the periphery of glomerular lobules ("fringe" pattern)	Abundance of C3 deposits in GBM and mesangium, rarely IgG/A/M or C4	C3 deposits in capillary loops and mesangium. C4 is rarely present, IgG only in small amounts in 50 %
Electron microscopy	Intact GBM with subendothelial and mesangial deposits, mesangial proliferation, and matrix expansion/ interposition	Intramembranous dense deposits (DD) in GBM; DD also in Bowman's capsule and tubular basement membrane	Thickened GBM with patchy dense deposits

- MPGN has been linked to the detection of autoantibodies to complement components
- The autoantibodies C3 nephritic factor (C3Nef or NF), stabilize physiological C3 and C5 convertases, presumably by interfering with the control of classical (NFc), alternative (NFa) or terminal (C5 convertase) pathway regulation (NFt)
- This may lead to the deposition of C3 fragments in the glomerulus and generation of complement-derived proinflammatory chymokines
- Genetic mutations or functional inactivation of critical AP regulators have been found to underly the occurrence of all types of MPGN/C3 GN (see Sect. 3.7.6 for a schematic diagram of the complement cascade and its regulators)
- The term C3 GN hence separates "primary" or "idiopathic" MPGN of all types from secondary forms of type I MPGN (see Box 3.8)

3.5.1.2 Clinical Presentation

- MPGN types cannot be differentiated clinically due to widely overlapping features.
- They may present as asymptomatic microhematuria and proteinuria, nephrotic syndrome or acute GN (nephritic syndrome) with gross hematuria and hypertension
- Acute nephritic syndrome with gross hematuria, hypertension, mild hypoalbuminemia and initially normal renal function can be found in all forms of MPGN (20–30 %)

- Nephrotic syndrome is present in 1/3 of type I and type III MPN and 50 % of DDD. It has been associated with a poor prognosis
- In contrast, clinically mild or asymptomatic presentation has been reported in about 60 % of type III, 20 % of type I and rarely in type II/DDD

3.5.1.3 Laboratory Evaluation

- Urinalysis, microscopy, 24-hour collection for protein and creatinine or spot urine protein/creatinine
- Renal function and related biochemical markers
- Kidney biopsy (see Table 3.13)
- Search for infectious or malignant causes (see Box 3.8)
- Serology: ANA, other antibodies and markers of primary autoimmune disorders (see Box 3.8)
- Serum complement studies: C3, C4, CH50 and, where available, C3Nef (C3 nephritic factors), CFH (factor H), SC5b-9 (soluble terminal complement complex or MAC)
- Alternative complement pathway regulator gene mutation screen

3.5.1.4 Therapy

- Treatment options are limited
- Mainstay is initially daily, then alternate-day prolonged oral prednisone over several years
- Mycophenolate or calcineurin inhibitor can be tried as second-line agents
- The 2012 KDIGO guideline suggests PO cyclophosphamide or MMF plus low-dose alternate-day or daily prednisone for up to 6 months in patients with idiopathic MPGN with nephrotic presentation and renal function decline
- Indications for the use of rituximab (MPGN type I) and of eculizumab are evolving
- Angiotensin-converting enzyme inhibitors (ACEi) and/or receptor blockers (ARB) should be used to control hypertension and reduce proteinuria
- Statins are recommended to control hyperlipidemia
- Consider thrombosis prophylaxis for recalcitrant nephrotic syndrome with profound hypoalbuminemia

3.5.1.5 MPGN Type 1

- MPGN can present as asymptomatic hematuria or proteinuria (40–50 %), acute nephritic syndrome (25 %), nephrotic syndrome (25–30 %), rapidly progressive glomerulonephritis, or CKD.
- MPGN may manifest in the context of an acute (upper respiratory tract) infection ("syninfectious GN") may also present as syninfectious glomerulonephritis.
- Secondary type I MPGN is associated with hepatitis C, SLE, or neoplasia.
- Serum C3 is reduced in 70–80 % of patients with type I MPGN, and 40 % will have low C4 levels
- Renal histopathology: see Table 3.13

Prognosis

- More than 50 % of patients progress to end-stage renal disease in 10 years; risk factors are nephrotic range proteinuria and hypertension.
- Recurrence risk following renal transplantation is 20–30 %.

3.5.1.6 Type II MPGN (Dense Deposit Disease)

- Type II MPGN/DDD accounts for <20 % of pediatric MPGN.
- DDD has been linked to the presence of an autoantibody, C3NeF (C3 nephritic factor), that binds to and stabilizes the alternative C3 convertase C3bBb, thus preventing degradation of this complex and resulting in continuous consumption of C3. The complement abnormality precedes development of GN.
- C3 nephritic factor may also be associated with partial lipodystrophy, an occasional precursor to type II MPGN.
- The presence of C3 nephritic factor suggests a role for complement dysregulation in the pathogenesis of MPGN type II. The presence of C3NeF or mutated comlement factor H (CFH) or other alternative pathway regulators may lead to excess C3 activation and glomerular deposition of C3 metabolits, the "dense deposits".

Clinical Features

- Age of onset is the second decade of life. Males and females are equally affected.
- Patients may present with mild proteinuria and microscopic hematuria. 50 % of patients are nephrotic, and about 1/3 have hypertension. AKI and rapid progression to ESRD are unusual.
- Dense deposits of C3 are known as "Drusen"; found as yellow and white dots between Bruch's membrane and the retinal epithelial cell layer, the deposits lead age related macular degeneration.
- DDD can be associated acquired partial lipodystrophy due to complement-mediated destruction of adipocytes.

Prognosis

- Progression to ESRD is seen within 1 year of onset with proteinuria and hypertension.
- Recurrence risk after renal transplantation is high (about 50–100 %).

3.5.1.7 MPGN Type III

- Rare variant of MPGN associated with unregulated alternative complement pathway activation
- Typically less (often focal) mesangial proliferation compared with type I MPGN, but clinical and histological differentiation from the latter is not reliable.
- Presentation with nephrotic proteinuria and/or crescents have portends an increased risk of CKD progression.
- Subendothelial, intramembranous, and subepithelial deposits and a frayed and disrupted GBM.
- In comparison to other types of MPGN, patients with type III MPGN are more likely to have asymptomatic proteinuria with hematuria.

3.5.2 IgA Nephropathy

3.5.2.1 Abstract

IgA nephropathy (IgAN) represents worldwide the most common primary glomerulopathy.

Secondary IgAN is rare.

IgAN is typically diagnosed during teenage years and young adulthood. Natural disease progression leads to end-stage renal disease within 20 years of diagnosis in 30–35 % of patients (range 20–50 %).

The rate of disease progression is modifiable.

Pathogenesis has been related to the mesangial deposition of hypoglycosylated IgA1 resulting in glomerular and related tubulointerstitial inflammation and fibrosis.

Familial occurrence has been reported and genetic factors postulated, but no causal gene mutation has been identified.

Kidney biopsy is important to estimate the degree of acute and chronic tissue injury.

Treatment focuses on antiproteinuric and antihypertensive medications through the blockade of the renin–angiotensin–aldosterone system (ACE inhibitors, ARB) and glucocorticoids. The role of (other) immunosuppressants, cytotoxic agents, polyunsaturated fatty acids (fish oil), coagulation or platelet modifying agents, and tonsillectomy remain controversial.

IgAN may recur after kidney transplantation.

Vignette

An 11-year-old boy presents to the emergency room with gross hematuria 2 days after the beginning of a sore throat with a 1-day fever. He has mild flank pain. Parents report that their child experienced 2 similar episodes over the preceding year. Family history is significant for an uncle who started chronic dialysis at the age of 35 years. Physical examination reveals a healthy appearing, normally grown boy with no edema, rash, purpura or petechiae, and no pallor. He is presently afebrile. The manual blood pressure is 105/75 mmHg. Urinalysis reveals >100 RBC/μl, occasional WBC, and no cellular casts; protein is 1 g/l per dipstick analysis. Repeat urinalysis 2 weeks later shows <5 RBC/μl and no protein.

3.5.2.2 Introduction

IgA nephropathy, first described by Berger and Hinglais in 1968, is worldwide the most common primary glomerulopathy. It represents between 20 and 40 % of glomerular diseases in Asia and Europe. Biopsy practices and genetic factors may contribute to the reported geographic variation. Most children with progressive IgAN do not reach ESRD until adulthood.

3.5.2.3 Definition

Primary IgAN is a primary immune-complex glomerulopathy characterized immunohistologically by the presence of dominant glomerular (mesangial) IgA deposits, often associated with C3 and IgG deposits and inconsistently with morphological evidence of local inflammation.

3.5.2.4 Etiology and Pathogenesis

- Exacerbation of symptoms (macroscopic hematuria with or without proteinuria and, occasionally, flank pain), is triggered by non-specific mucosal viral or bacterial infections.
- Mesangial IgA deposits are composed of polymeric IgA1. The frequent detection of C3 (and, if searched for, properdin and the terminal membrane attack complex C5b-9), but not C1q and C4, suggest alternative complement pathway activation in IgAN.
- Abnormal galactosylation and sialylation at the hinge region of IgA1 molecules changes their mesangial cell binding. However, it remains unclear, whether hypoglycosylated IgA1 is sufficient to induce IgAN. Diagnostic testing for abnormally glycosylated IgA is not routinely available.
- Genetic factors have been implicated in disease susceptibility and progression. Familial clustering is known. Aberrant IgA1 galactosylation appears to be inherited in some families. A causal genetic mutation remains to be identified.

3.5.2.5 Clinical Features

- Recurrent macroscopic hematuria with or without proteinuria is the hallmark of childhood IgA nephropathy and is the most common presenting symptom.
- For other disease manifestations, see Table 3.14.

3.5.2.6 Laboratory Investigations

- Investigations focus on differential causes of hematuria and (occasional) loin pain (see Figs. 3.1 and 3.2 in Sect. 3.1 and Table 3.15).
- Decreasing kidney function and nephrotic-range proteinuria are of prognostic importance.
- Serial follow-up is recommended to identify progression to CKD.
- IgAN is largely a diagnosis of exclusion. A positive diagnosis requires a kidney biopsy.
- Extended laboratory evaluation if secondary IgAN is suspected or to be ruled out.

3.5.2.7 Pathological Diagnosis

- Diagnosis of IgA nephropathy requires a kidney biopsy (see Table 3.16).
- Biopsies can be graded according to the amount of mesangial cell proliferation on the basis of WHO criteria as (1) minimal glomerular lesions, (2) focal mesangial proliferation, (3) diffuse mesangial proliferation.
- The International IgA Nephropathy Network has identified four histopathological lesions of independent prognostic importance, abbreviated as "MEST": mesangial (M) and endocapillary hypercellularity (E), segmental glomerulosclerosis (S) and tubular atrophy and interstitial fibrosis (T) (Table 3.16)

Table 3.14 Clinical features of IgA nephropathy

Features	Comments
Age of presentation and gender preference	Diagnosis during second and third decade of life. Male predominance (2:1–6:1) Uncommon in persons of African descent Familial predisposition (up to 20 %)
Microscopic hematuria	Associated with (mild) proteinuria in 20–60 %
Macroscopic hematuria	Up to 60 % of patients have at least one, usually more episodes of macrohematuria Manifests 1–2 days after mucosal (upper respiratory tract) infection Generally painless, occasionally with loin pain Duration (24–48 h), occasionally up to a week
Acute nephritic syndrome	In 23 %, associated with (severe) acute glomerular injury with or without AKI, usually reversible
AKI with macroscopic hematuria	Uncommon, may represent first manifestation of IgAN Kidney function to baseline after normalization of urine color Incomplete recovery of renal function in 25 % Duration of macroscopic hematuria >10 days is a risk factor of persistent kidney impairment
Nephrotic syndrome	Uncommon presentation (<10 %), with unfavorable prognosis Differentiate from minimal change NS wih incidental IgA staining
Flank or abdominal pain	Occasionally with macroscopic hematuria
Rapid progressive GN	Characterized by extensive crescents and rapidly progressive course 40 % of patients with IgA RPGN are ≤16 years old
Hypertension	Infrequent in pediatric IgAN, unless patient has CKD
End-stage renal disease (CKD 5)	25 % of patients 10 years after diagnosis, 40–50 % after 20 years

Table 3.15 Diseases associated with diffuse mesangial deposits of IgA ("secondary IgAN")

Primary diagnosis	Comments
Schönlein–Henoch purpura nephritis	Renal histological findings indiscernable from IgAN
Systemic lupus erythematosus (lupus nephritis)	
Chronic liver disease/cirrhosis	
Celiac disease	
Inflammatory bowed disease	Crohn's disease, ulcerative colitis
Infections	Disseminated tuberculosis, leprosy, mycoplasma infection and toxoplasmosis
Dermatitis herpetiformis	
Ankylosing spondylitis	
Cystic fibrosis	
Bronchiolitis obliterans	
Mixed cryoglobulinemia	
Monoclonal IgA gammopathy	
Neoplasms	Hodgkin and T cell lymphoma, mycosis fungoides, solid cancers of lungs and colon

Table 3.16 Spectrum of histological finding in IgA nephropathy

Modality	Morphological findings[a]
Light microscopy	Characteristic finding is mesangial enlargement due to hypercellularity and increased matrix *Glomerular* findings *Mesangial* proliferation (>4 cells/peripheral mesangial area) with varying degrees (defined as diffuse >50 %) glomeruli, focal (<50 % of glomeruli), global (involving more than half of the glomerular tuft), or segmental (involving less than half of the glomerular tuft) *Endocapillary* hypercellularity (hypercellularity due to increased number of cells within glomerular capillary lumina) Cellular and fibrocellular crescents (*extracapillary lesions*). Crescents (see Sect. 3.4.3.3) if present, usually affect <50 % of glomeruli. Crescentic IgAN requires that >50 % glomeruli are affected) *Tubulo-interstitial changes* (interstitial fibrosis and tubular atrophy; acute tubular injury) *Vascular* (arterial) lesion *Other changes* include segmental and global *glomerulosclerosis* and interstitial lymphocytic infiltration
Immunofluorescence	*Mesangial IgA deposits* (predominant) May extend to mesangio-capillary junctions and into capillary wall Can be associated with C3 (about 2/3 of biopsies), IgG (1/3), IgM (10 %) or IgG/IgM (10 %)
Electron microscopy	*Electron-dense deposits* in mesangium (granular masses beneath lamina densa in perimesangium and expanded mesangium [matrix]) Deposits in glomerular capillary wall (mainly subendothelial and subepithelial, adjacent to mesangium) Lysis of glomerular basement membrane (GBM) Diffuse foot process effacement limited to patients with (large) proteinuria

[a]The International IgA Nephropathy Network has identified four histopathological lesions of independent prognostic importance: *mesangial* (M) and endocapillary hypercellularity (E), segmental glomerulosclerosis (S) and tubular atrophy and interstitial fibrosis (T), which have been validated for children and adults (Oxford MEST score). Endocapillary hypercellularity appears to be responsive to immunosuppressive therapy

3.5.2.8 Therapeutic Management

- There is presently no curative treatment for IgAN.
- Pathological risk factors identified in the Oxford Classification have not been validated to guide treatment choices.
- *Graded treatment recommendations* include antiproteinuric and antihypertensive therapies, glucocorticoids, and immunosuppressive/cytotoxic agents.
- Antiproteinuric and antihypertensive therapy
  - Normalize BP to <90th (ideally 50th percentile) percentile for age and height (<120/80 mmHg) using ACE inhibitors or ARBs as first-line agents.
  - Start ACE-I or ARB, if proteinuria is >0.5 g/1.73 m^2/day.
  - Titrate ACE-I or ARB as tolerated to keep proteinuria <1 g/1.73 m^2/day.

- Glucocorticoid therapy
  - Add glucocorticoids if proteinuria of ≥1 g/1.73 m²/day persists despite 3–6 months of optimized RAS targeting therapy (ACEi or ARB).
  - A suggested regimen consists of methylprednisolone pulses on 3 subsequent days at months 1, 3, and 5, and oral prednisone (or equivalent) at a dose of 0.5 mg/kg on alternate days for 6 months.
  - An alternative regimen starts with oral prednisone at 0.8–1 mg/kg/day for 2 months, followed by a reduction every month by 0.2 mg/kg/day over the next 4 months.
  - There are no published recommendations on how to proceed after 6 months. Options include (1) to continue antiproteinuric and antihypertensive therapy, if proteinuria remains between 0.5 and 1 g/1.73 m²/day, with or without continued alternate-day prednisone (e.g., 0.25 to 0.5 mg/kg QOD) or with fish oil (see below).
- Immunosuppressive and cytotoxic agents
  - There is insufficient evidence that immunosuppressive agents other than glucocorticoids are beneficial in the majority of patients.
  - According to the 2012 KDIGO practice guideline, combining prednisone and azathioprine (or cyclophosphamide), with or without antiplatelet agents, does not add benefit, but may increase occurrence of adverse effects. Japanese experience suggests improved outcome with the combination treatment (prednisolone, azathioprine, warfarin, and dipyridamole) in cases of *severe* IgA nephropathy.
  - Clinical trials employing MMF in (adult) patients with IgAN are heterogeneous and inconclusive. MMF was reported to be beneficial in a Chinese trial, but ineffective in placebo-controlled studies involving Caucasian patients. The KDIGO Guideline does not suggest the use of MMF in IgAN.
- Fish-oil supplements/Omega-3 (polyunsaturated) fatty acids
  - Beneficial cardiovascular effects in part by lowering BP and triglyceride levels
  - Typically supplied as 460 mg EPA and 380 mg DHA (1 g, for children <50 kg) and 920/760 mg (2 g, for children >50 kg)
  - Randomized controlled trials with omega-3 fatty acid supplements for IgAN showed no clinically significant improvement of kidney survival
  - The KDIGO guideline suggests trying fish oil in patients with persistent proteinuria ≥1 g/day (per 1.73 m²) despite 3–6 months of optimized renin/angiotensin blockade. Despite higher-quality evidence for treatment with glucocorticoids as step-up therapy than with fish oil, the latter may be used in patients with glucocorticoid toxicity.
- Antiplatelet/anticoagulation agents
  - KDIGO advises against use these agents for IgAN.
- Tonsillectomy
  - Tonsillectomy has no proven benefit in IgAN.
- Atypical forms of IgAN
  - *MCNS with mesangial IgA deposits*

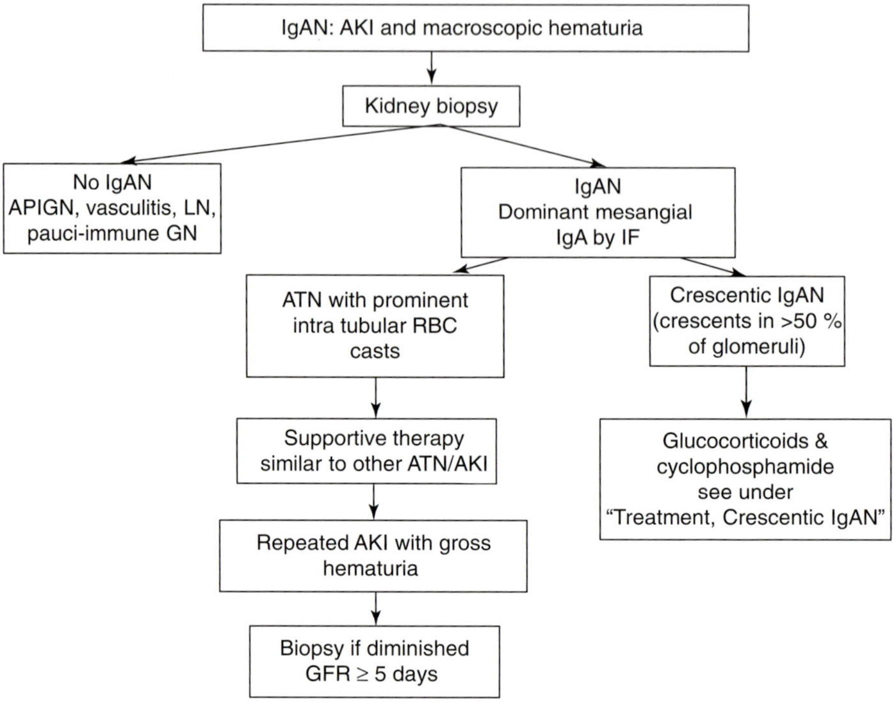

Fig. 3.9 Management of IgA with AKI and macroscopic hematuria. *AKI* acute kidney injury, *ATN* acute tubular necrosis, *APIGN* acute postinfectious GN, *GN* glomerulonephritis, *IF* immunofluorescence/immunohistology, *LN* lupus nephritis

Patients with nephrotic syndrome and coincidental histological findings of minimal lesions and IgAN should be treated like MCNS (see Sects. 3.3.1.6 and 3.3.2).

– *Macroscopic hematuria and AKI* (see Fig. 3.9)

IgAN patients presenting with macroscopic hematuria and AKI should undergo kidney biopsy if renal function fails to improve within 5 days. If histological changes are limited to ATN and intratubular RBC casts, provide supportive treatment only.

Macroscopic hematuria longer than 10 days heralds persistent renal impairment and requires supportive care as other forms of ATN/AKI.

– *Crescentic IgAN*

Defined as IgAN with crescents in >50 % of glomeruli.

Long-term prognosis is poor if associated with rapidly progressive deterioration of kidney function.

Treatment with high-dose glucocorticoids and cyclophosphamide is potentially useful and recommended (see Sect. 3.4.3.7).

A published regimen (Tumlin et al. 2003) consists of 15 mg/kg methylprednisolone pulses for 3 days, followed by daily oral prednisone for a total of 6 months, combined with six monthly IV cyclophosphamide infusions of 0.5 (–0.75) g/m^2. Oral prednisone dose 1 mg/kg/day for 2 months is tapered every second month to 0.6, 0.3, and 0.15 mg/kg/day, followed by 10 mg/1.73 m^2 daily.

3.5.2.9 Prognosis

- Proteinuria is the strongest prognostic indicator for ESRD or accelerated decline of kidney function. In adults, proteinuria above a threshold of 1 g/1.73 m^2/day (24 mg/m^2/h) has a "dose-dependent" effect, independent of other risk factors.
- Reduction of proteinuria below this threshold (or 50 % reduction of baseline proteinuria) improves long-term outcome.
- Proteinuria cutoffs for partial and complete remission in children are 0.5 g/1.73 m^2/day (12 mg/m^2/h) and <0.16 g/1.73 m^2/day (<4 mg/m^2/h), respectively.
- Decline of GFR is faster in patients with poorly controlled hypertension.
- The Oxford Classification of IgAN identified (1) mesangial hypercellularity, (2) segmental glomerulosclerosis, (3) endocapillary hypercellularity, and (4) interstitial fibrosis/tubular atrophy (IF/TA) as independent pathological variables predicting kidney outcome in patients with an estimated GFR of >30 ml/min/1.73 m^2.

3.5.3 Membranous Nephropathy (MN)

3.5.3.1 Introduction

Membranous nephropathy (membranous glomerulopathy) is a common cause of nephrotic syndrome in adults. It occurs as primary (idiopathic, IMN) or secondary disease. Pediatric MN is rare, accounting for <1.5 % of all children with nephrotic syndrome (up to 5 % of children with glucocorticoid-resistant nephrotic syndrome), compared with 25 % of adults with nephrotic syndrome. The disease is defined by the presence of subepithelial deposits which leads to thickening of the glomerular basement membrane.

3.5.3.2 Etiology and Pathogenesis

- Membranous nephropathy in children is usually secondary to a systemic disease (>75 %), particularly due to hepatitis B or SLE. Other causes are HCV infection, malaria, schistosomiasis and syphilis, drugs or, with advanced age, malignancies (see Table 3.17).
- MN is characterized by subepithelial deposits consisting of immunoglobulins and complement components that result in characteristic, progressive changes of the GBM and in podocyte cytoskeletal abnormalities leading to proteinuria.
- Genetic factors are not well defined. Up to 70 % of (adult) patients with IMN have antibodies to the M-type phospholipase A2 receptor (PLA2R).

3.5.3.3 Clinical Features

- MN occurs at any age from newborn to young adults.
- Male preponderance has been reported by some centers.

Table 3.17 Causes of membranous nephropathy in children

Infections
Hepatitis B, congenital syphilis, hepatitis C, tuberculosis, malaria (Plasmodium malariae), filariasis, schistosomiasis, leprosy
Autoimmune disease
SLE, rheumatoid arthritis, mixed connective tissue disease, Grave's disease, Hashimoto's thyroiditis, primary biliary cirrhosis
Drugs
NSAID, penicillamine, captopril, gold, lithium, mercury
Others
Sarcoidosis, sickle cell disease, sclerosing cholangitis

- Typical presentation as nephrotic syndrome, but up to 20 % have only mild to moderate proteinuria.
- Microscopic hematuria is common; gross hematuria is rare.
- Hypertension in <25 %.

3.5.3.4 Laboratory Investigations

- Urine analysis, 24-h urine protein excretion or at spot Upc, renal function, serum albumin, C3, C4, CH50 and C5b-9 (where available), and renal biopsy
- Rule out secondary forms: hepatitis B surface antigen, IgM to hepatitis C and/or nucleic acid-based molecular assays, syphilis serology, peripheral smear for malaria, antinuclear antibody, anti-dsDNA
- Hypocomplementemia (low C3 and C4) has been reported in 15–64 % of HBV-MN, but is absent in idiopathic MN is typically found with hepatitis B

3.5.3.5 Histopathology (Table 3.18)

3.5.3.6 Therapeutic Management

- Therapy in children is extrapolated from studies in adults.
- Difficulties in the treatment of MN result from its variable course and tendency to spontaneous remission, and the unsatifactory response to existing therapeutics.
- Spontaneous remission may occur in children with non-nephrotic proteinuria. Non-specific therapy with ACE inhibitors or ARBs, reduced sodium intake ("no added salt"), and mild diuretics to control edema (beware of thrombosis risk).
- Immunosuppressive therapy is indicated in the presence of:
  - Decreased GFR at presentation or follow-up
  - Persistent nephrotic syndrome
  - Thrombosis
- High-dose prednisone (0.5–1 mg/kg per day, up to 60 mg daily) can be tried, with or without three daily pulses of IV methylprednisolone (10–20 mg/kg or up to 600 mg/m^2 per dose). Note: Children with nephrotic MN will already have received prednisone prior to biopsy. Failure to respond to 2–3 months glucocorticoids justifies the addition of a second-line agent.

Table 3.18 Histopathological features in membranous nephropathy

Light microscopy	May be normal in early stages Pathognomonic feature is thickening of the capillary loops due to subepithelial deposits and deposition of new membrane Silver stain shows characteristic spikes indicating basement membrane between deposits Normal cellularity of the glomerulus Presence of inflammatory cells or mesangial proliferation suggests secondary forms of MN
Immunofluorescence	Fine granular deposits of IgG (IgG4) in subepithelial space Less pronounced staining of IgA and IgM is common, except in SLE-MN. C3 of low intensity is found in up to 95 %; C4 and C1q are typically absent
Electron microscopy	Subepithelial immune deposits Thickening of the basement membrane Effacement of foot processes of podocytes

  - Oral cyclophosphamide (2 mg/kg daily for 8–12 weeks), or
  - Cyclosporine (4–5 mg/kg) or tacrolimus (0.1–0.15 mg/kg per day, divided in 2 doses; initial target trough levels 5–8 ng/ml)
- Rituximab 375 mg/m^2 weekly × 4 doses has shown efficacy in adult IMN with minimal degree of tubulo-interstitial injury.
- Treatment of secondary membranous nephropathy targets the underlying cause.

3.5.3.7 Prognosis

- Asymptomatic proteinuria portends good clinical outcome
- High spontaneous remission rate in younger children, usually within 12–18 months
- CKD risk in pediatric MN <25 %
- Poor prognostic factors are nephrotic-range proteinuria, renal dysfunction and hypertension at onset and biopsy showing glomerulosclerosis and/or tubulointerstitial fibrosis

3.5.4 C1q Nephropathy

3.5.4.1 Definition

C1q nephropathy (C1qN) is a glomerular disorder characterized immunohistochemically by prominent mesangial C1q containing immune deposits. Earlier authors emphasized the exclusion of SLE as a prerequisite for the diagnosis of C1qN. Some pathologists do not recognize C1qN as a distinct disease entity.

3.5.4.2 Etiology and Pathogenesis

The etiology of C1qN remains unclear. The pathogenesis and the clinical importance of C1q immune deposits are still to be elucidated.

3.5.4.3 Clinical Signs and Symptoms

- Initial presentation ranges from microscopic hematuria with or without proteinuria to gross hematuria and nephritis or a mixed nephritic–nephrotic picture.
- More than 50 % of pediatric patients present with nephrotic syndrome.

3.5.4.4 Investigations

- The diagnosis depends on the demonstration of dominant or codominant immune staining for C1q and the presence of mesangial or paramesangial immune deposits by electron microscopy.
- Histopathological features associated with C1qN include minimal lesions, mesangial proliferation, focal segmental or global sclerosis, and membranous nephropathy.
- Where studied, serum C3 and C4 concentrations were found to be normal or elevated.

3.5.4.5 Approach and Management

- Diagnostic and treatment are guided by the degree of proteinuria and disease complications.
- Children with nephrotic-range proteinuria and hypoalbuminemia are treated as outlined in Sect. 3.3.1.6 for children with idiopathic nephrotic syndrome.
- Treatment goals for patients with C1qN are remission (or reduction) of proteinuria and preservation or restoration of renal function, independent of the persistence or resolution of C1q deposits.

3.5.4.6 Prognosis and Outcome

- Outcome appears favorable in patients presenting with low-grade proteinuria and minimal tubulo-interstitial or glomerular sclerosis.
- More than 50 % of patients presenting with nephrotic syndrome will experience frequent relapses or glucocorticoid dependence, and about 30 % of these may become glucocorticoid resistant.
- Overall, <15 % of patients with C1qN may progress to chronic kidney disease and ESRD.
- Outcome is poor in patients with C1qN collapsing glomerulopathy.

3.6 Systemic Vasculitis Affecting the Kidney

3.6.1 Abstract

This section describes a diverse group of systemic inflammatory blood vessel diseases (vasculitides) with variable degrees of kidney involvement. Individual diseases are detailed according to their importance and frequency in the pediatric age group including Schönlein-Henoch nephritis (SHN), anti-neutrophil cytoplasmic antibody (ANCA) mediated vasculitis (AAV) and pauci-immune glomerulonephritis, lupus nephritis (LN) and rarer vasculitides.

3.6.2 Definitions

Currently used classifications of childhood vasculitides are derived from the 2012 Chapel Hill Consensuses Conference and the related European League against Rheumatism/Paediatric Rheumatology European Society (EULAR/PRES) classification from 2010 that are based on the size of the predominantly affected blood vessels, as shown in Box 3.9 (see also Fig. 3.10).

Box 3.9 Classification of Childhood Vasculitis[a]

Childhood vasculitis can be classified based on the size of the blood vessel affected:

1. Large vessel vasculitis (LVV)
    (a) Takayasu arteritis TAK, (see Sect. 3.6.5.1)
    (b) Giant cell arteritis (GCA)
2. Medium-sized vessel vasculitis
    (a) Childhood polyarteritis nodosa (cPAN) (see Sect. 3.6.5.2)
    (b) Kawasaki disease (KD) (see Sect. 3.6.5.3)
3. Small vessel vasculitis (SVV)
    (a) Pauci-immune vasculitis/ANCA-associated vasculitis (AAV) (see Sect. 3.6.3)
        (i) Microscopic polyangiitis (MPA) (see Sect. 3.6.3.4)
        (ii) Granulomatosis with polyangiitis (GPA, formerly Wegener's granulomatosis) (see Sect. 3.6.3.5)
        (iii) Eosinophilic granulomatosis with polyangiitis (EGPA; formerly Churg-Strauss syndrome) (see Sect. 3.6.3.6)
        (iv) Renal limited vasculitis (pauci-immune necrotizing and crescentic GN (NCGN))
    (b) Immune complex vasculitis
        (i) Schönlein–Henoch purpura (SHP)/Schönlein–Henoch nephritis (SHN or IgA vasculitis, IgAV) (see Sect. 3.6.2)
        (ii) Cryoglobulinemic vasculitis (CV)
        (iii) Anti-glomerular basement membrane (anti-GBM) disease (see Table 3.12)
4. Vasculitis associated with systemic disease
    (a) Lupus vasculitis (lupus nephritis, LN) (see Sect. 3.6.4)
    (b) Vasculitis associated with chronic juvenile arthritis, mixed connective tissue disease and overlap syndromes
5. Vasculitis associated with probable etiology
    (a) Vasculitides associated with infections, malignancy, drugs, hypersensitivity

[a]Based on the 2012 Chapel Hill Consensus Conference (CHCC 2012)

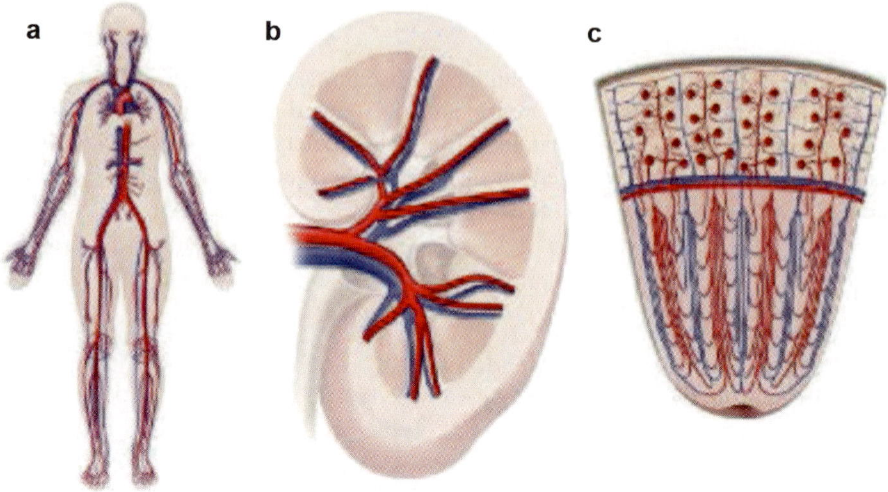

Fig. 3.10 Types of vessels that are defined as large vessels (**a**), medium vessels (**b**), and small vessels (**c**) in the Chapel Hill Consensus Conference nomenclature system. The kidney is used to exemplify medium and small vessels. Large vessels are the aorta and its major branches and the analogous veins. Medium vessels are the main visceral arteries and veins and their initial branches. Small vessels are intraparenchymal arteries, arterioles, capillaries, venules, and veins (With permission from Jennette et al. 2012)

3.6.3 Schönlein–Henoch Purpura Nephritis

3.6.3.1 Abstract

- Schönlein–Henoch purpura (SHP) is the most common vasculitis in children. Manifestations in addition to purpura and/or petechiae (with normal thrombocyte numbers), predominantly of the lower limbs, are abdominal pain (associated with submucosal vasculitis), joint involvement (nondeforming arthritis/arthralgia), and nephritis.
- SHP vasculitis is characterized by granulocytic infiltrates in the walls of small arterioles and venules (leukocytoclastic vasculitis) with immunoglobulin A (IgA) deposits, hence the name IgA vasulitis or IgAV (see Box 3.9).
- About 80 % of children with SHP will develop microscopic and occasionally macroscopic hematuria. One-third of patients with SHP present with abnormal urinalysis (mostly hematuria with or without proteinuria), less than 10 % develop nephritic and/or nephrotic syndrome. Proteinuria is mild and transient in most instances, and both hematuria and proteinuria are expected to resolve within 1–3 months of onset of the purpura.
- In contrast, nephrotic syndrome, severe histopathological changes by kidney biopsy and rapid rise of creatinine (rapidly progressive glomerulonephritis, RPGN) are ominous signs associated with an increased risk of chronic (CKD) or end-stage kidney disease (ESRD).

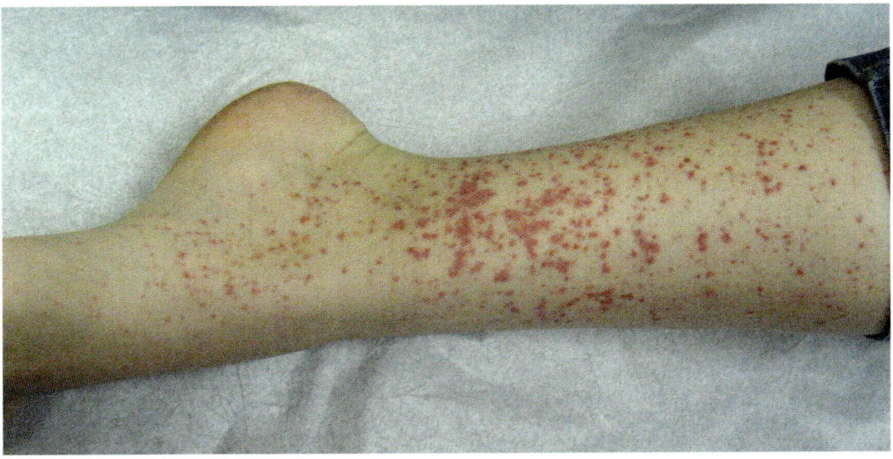

Fig. 3.11 Typical lower limb purpura in a teenage patient with recurrent Schönlein–Henoch purpura and mild SHP nephritis

- The majority of patients with SHP do not require medical therapy. Patients suffering from severe abdominal pain or arthritis benefit from glucocorticoids or nonsteroidal anti-inflammatory drugs. Glucocorticoids during the acute presentation of SHP (e.g., RPGN) do not prevent the occurrence of GN or affect long-term outcome.
- SHP is an acute, self-limited disease lasting about 4 weeks. Fifteen to 60 % of patients experience one or more purpura recurrences. The long-term prognosis is determined by the severity of the associated glomerulonephritis.

3.6.3.2 Definition

- In accordance with the European League against Rheumatism/Paediatric Rheumatology European Society (EULAR/PRES) criteria, the diagnosis of SHP is based on the appearance of a palpable purpura and/or petechiae predominantly on the lower limbs (Fig. 3.11) and at least one of the following features: diffuse abdominal pain, biopsy (skin, kidney) showing predominant IgA deposition, arthritis or arthralgia, and renal involvement (any hematuria or proteinuria).
- The EULAR/PRES classification provides a sensitivity of 100 %, a specificity of 87 %, and accuracy (area under the receiver operating characteristic curve (AUC)) of 93.5 %.
- SHP nephritis (SHN) is characterized by acute or chronic recurrent nephritis episodes (hematuria, proteinuria) with histological changes of kidney indiscernible from IgA nephropathy (see Sect. 3.5.2, Table 3.16) with mesangial hypercellularity and dominant (mesangial) IgA deposits.

3.6.3.3 Etiology and Pathogenesis

- SHP vasculitis affects small vessels (arterioles and venules) and is mediated by the deposition of IgA-containing immune complexes.

- SHP, similar to IgA nephropathy (IgAN), can be triggered by mucosal infections of the upper respiratory or gastrointestinal tract. No single eliciting antigen has been identified.
- Both SHP/SHN and IgAN have been linked to defective sialylation and galactosylation of IgA1 which may result in circulating (defective) IgA mixed IgA1/IgG immune complex formation.
- Persisting IgA1 containing aggregates can induce a local inflammatory response in glomerular mesangial cells.

3.6.3.4 Clinical Features of SHN

- Manifestations of SHN include isolated microhematuria or gross (macroscopic) hematuria.
- Mild transient proteinuria to nephrotic syndrome.
- Arterial hypertension is rare at presentation and may occur with minimal urinary abnormalities.
- Acute kidney injury (AKI), RPGN (rare).
- Nephrotic syndrome, clinically important hypertension, and progressive kidney failure are rare (<3 %).

3.6.3.5 Laboratory Investigations (see Table 3.19)

3.6.3.6 Renal Histopathology

- Indications for kidney biopsy in SHP/SHN are rising serum creatinine, nephrotic-range or persistent proteinuria (e.g., >20 mg/m^2/h or >0.5 g/m^2/day).

Table 3.19 Basic investigation and interpretation of laboratory findings in patients with SHP

Material	Test	Expected results and comments
Blood sample	Creatinine	Usually normal. Elevated creatinine may indicate acute or chronic kidney injury. Close follow-up and referral to nephrologist
	Complete blood cell count (CBC) and blood smear	Normal, with or without mild neutrophilia If anemia or pancytopenia, schistocytosis, and/or thrombocytopenia are present, consider SLE, HUS, or related autoimmune disorder
	C3, C4	Normal or elevated (acute phase reactant) If C3 is reduced, consider APIGN If C3 and C4 are reduced, consider SLE
	Albumin (total protein)	Normal. Reduced in SHP with nephrotic syndrome
Urinalysis	Blood, protein	Blood positive in 34 % (range 20–55 %), with or without proteinuria. Follow-up as per algorithm (Fig. 3.12). In 80 %, renal manifestations are present within 4 weeks of SHP onset
	Microscopy	Presence of erythrocyte or mixed cellular casts indicate nephritic syndrome
	Upc	Simple quantitation (and follow-up) of urine protein excretion when urinalysis (Albustix) is positive

- Although severe inflammatory changes and crescents are more frequently found in patients with clinically severe nephritis, no single biopsy classification scheme for the long-term outcome of SHN has been widely accepted or independently validated.
- Tubulointerstitial changes (interstitial mononuclear infiltrate, interstitial edema, tubular injury) and signs of chronicity (interstitial fibrosis and tubular atrophy, fibrous crescents, global sclerosis, and vascular hyalinosis and intimal hyperplasia) – in association with clinical findings (rising creatinine, large proteinuria) – indicate disease progression with poor outcome.

3.6.3.7 Treatment

Patient Monitoring

- Proteinuria usually appears during the first week, but <3 % of patients will develop chronic kidney disease.
- Eighty percent of patients with SHN demonstrate proteinuria within the first 4 weeks and all within 3 months of onset.
- The algorithm (Fig. 3.12) attempts to balance benefit (or risk) with feasibility and costs of monitoring.
- Urine protein monitoring can be done by a nurse or trained parent/family member, provided results are reported back to a physician.
- Patient is discharged from surveillance if free of proteinuria and recurrences by 6 months.
- Follow-up beyond 6 months of patients with persistent SHN/proteinuria.
- Worsening proteinuria or declining renal function should prompt referral to nephrologist for kidney biopsy.

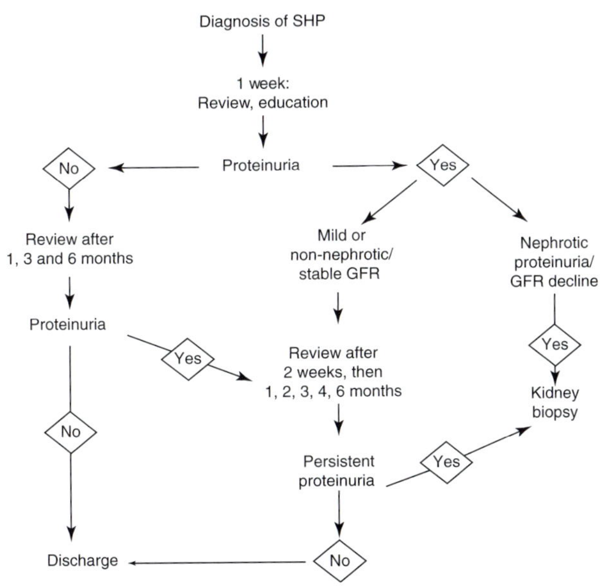

Fig. 3.12 Algorithm for the monitoring for SHP nephritis and indication for kidney biopsy

Medication Therapy of SHP/SHN

- Treatment of SHP is symptomatic and consists of pain medication (usually non-steroidal anti-inflammatory drugs, e.g., naproxen) for arthralgia.
- Severe abdominal pain and arthritis responded to a short course of glucocorticoids.
- In a recently published randomized controlled trial from Finland, prednisone at a dose of 1 mg/kg daily for 2 weeks, followed by a 2-week taper, reduced the severity and duration of abdominal and joint pain.
- Prednisone at this dose was not effective in treating the purpura, preventing nephritis, shortening disease duration or preventing recurrences.
- The 2012 KDIGO Clinical Practice Guideline for Glomerulonephritis suggests that children with SHN and persistent proteinuria >0.5–1 g/day/1.73 m^2 (0.3–0.6 g/day/m^2) be treated with ACE inhibitor or ARB.
- Treatment of patients with significant renal involvement is controversial.
- Immunosuppressive regimens include glucocorticoids (methylprednisolone pulses [followed by oral prednisone]), cyclophosphamide, plasma exchange, cyclosporine A (CSA)/tacrolimus, or azathioprine.
- CSA or mycophenolate mofetil (MMF) appear to be as effective as glucocorticoid therapy to achieve freedom from proteinuria and maintain long-term renal function.
- A practical regimen for patients with SHN with nephrotic syndrome is prednisone at a dose of 60 mg/m^2/day (2 mg/kg/day) for 1 month (maximum 60 mg/m^2/day), followed by 40 mg/m^2 every 2 days (max 40 mg/dose) followed by 0.5 mg/kg every other day (total duration up to 6 months). ACE inhibitors or ARBs can be added for prolonged proteinuria.
- Cyclophosphamide PO or IV has been used for severe disease.
- Alternatively, CSA (starting dose 5 mg/kg/day), tacrolimus (0.1–0.2 mg/kg/day divided in 2 doses; target trough level 4–6 ng/ml), or MMF (600–900 mg/m^2/day divided BID) may be initiated for 6 months (to avoid cyclophosphamide-associated adverse effects).

3.6.3.8 Prognosis and Outcome

- The renal outcome of SHP glomerulonephritis is favorable.
- Among patients, who developed CKD following SHN, >50 % presented with a nephrotic–nephritic syndrome, 40 % with nephrotic syndrome, and 15 % with a nephritic syndrome and/or heavy, non-nephrotic proteinuria. Less than 5 % of children with CKD had only hematuria or minimal proteinuria.
- Of patients who developed ESRD during follow-up, all had nephrotic proteinuria at onset and decreased GFR <70 mg/min/1.73 m^2 at 3 years. Conversely, less than 20 % of children with nephrotic proteinuria and severe histopathological changes and none with crescentic GN (>50 % crescents) is expected to recover normal kidney function if left untreated.
- The relative risk of progression (doubling of serum creatinine) was estimated to be 1.77 for each 1 g/day of proteinuria. The relative risk rises to 3.8 and 4.7 with impaired GFR (versus normal GFR) and nephrotic-range versus mild proteinuria at onset, respectively.
- Recurrence of non-renal symptoms (purpura) does not correlate with renal outcome.

3.6.4 ANCA-Associated Vasculitis (AAV)

Antineutrophil cytoplasmic antibody (ANCA)-mediated vasculitis, also called pauci-immune vasculitis, is characterized by absence of immune deposits in tissue biopsies by immunofluorescence. It is an important differential diagnosis for rapidly progressive glomerulonephritis (RPGN) in children (see Sect. 3.4.3).

3.6.4.1 Definitions

AAV typically involves small vessels with a predisposition for small arteries, arterioles, capillaries, and postcapillary venules, including small renal vessels (Box 3.9). ANCA (see Box 3.10) are detected in 90 % of patients with small vessel vascultitis. The characteristic glomerular lesions are paucimmune (immunofluorescence-negative) focal and segmental necrotizing and crescentic glomerulonephritis (NCGN). The latter may also occur as renal-limited disease.

3.6.4.2 Clinical Presentation of AAV

- Systemic vasculitides affect a variety of tissues, including upper and lower respiratory tract, central nervous system, eyes, skin and kidney.
- Acute nephritis with microscopic hematuria, dysmorphic RBCs and RBC casts.
- Usually moderate proteinuria <1 g/m^2 per day.

Box 3.10 Anti-Neutrophil Cytoplasmic Antibodies (ANCA)

- An indirect immunofluorescence assay on ethanol fixed neutrophils is traditionally used to screen for ANCA
- Sera from patients with ANCA-associated vasculitis (AAV) produce distinct pattern of immunofluorescence:
  - Staining around the nucleus is known as perinuclear (pANCA). It is generally associated with antibodies against the enzyme myeloperoxidase (MPO)
  - Diffuse granular staining of the neutrophil cytoplasm is termed as cytoplasmic (cANCA). It corresponds to specificity for the enzyme proteinase 3 (PR3)
- ANCA bind to antigens in the primary granules of neutrophils and peroxidase-positive lysosomes of monocytes
- Another proposed target for ANCA is lysosomal-associated membrane protein 2 (LAMP2)
- ANCA are an important serological marker for pauci-immune vasculitides and glomerulonephritides
- There is evidence that ANCA activate activated neutrophils (and monocytes) and that ANCA-reactive neutrophils activate complement via the alternative pathway
- Testing for ANCA should include an enzyme-linked immunoassay (ELISA) with selective antigen specificity for MPO and PR3

- Rapidly progressive GN with declining kidey function over days to weeks.
- 10 % of patients with AAV and necrotizing crescentic GN (NCGN) suffer severe (diffuse) pulmonary hemorrhage associated with high death rates.
- Minority of patients presents with mild or asymptomatic disease.

3.6.4.3 Microscopic Polyangiitis (MPA)

- MPA is a necrotizing vasculitis with few or no immune deposits and no granulomatous inflammation involving small vessels.
- Extrarenal manifestations:
  - Pulmonary: hemoptysis, pulmonary hemorrhage
  - Upper respiratory: chronic sinusitis, otitis media, nasal passage ulcers
  - Skin: purpuric rashes, leukocytoclastic vasculitis
  - Constitutional: fever, malaise, weight loss, anorexia
- Investigations:
  - Anemia, leukocytosis, thrombocytosis, elevated ESR and C-reactive protein (CRP)
  - C3 and C4 serum complement (normal)
  - ANCA: 65 % of patients are pANCA (anti-MPO) and 10 % cANCA (anti-PR3) positive
  - Chest X-ray, CT chest (pulmonary hemorrhage, pneumonia)
  - Renal biopsy

3.6.4.4 Granulomatosis with Polyangiitis (GPA, Wegener's Granulomatosis)

- Triad of GPA: necrotizing granulomatous inflammation of upper or lower respiratory tract, vasculitis involving small to medium-sized vessels, and necrotizing glomerulonephritis
- Extrarenal manifestations:
  - Upper respiratory tract: sinusitis, epistaxis
  - Lower respiratory tract: pulmonary infiltrates, pulmonary hemorrhage, hemoptysis, pulmonary nodules
  - Constitutional features: fever, weight loss, arthralgia/arthritis, rash
  - Neurological: mononeuritis multiplex, stroke
  - Cardiovascular: pericarditis, myocardial infarction
- Investigations:
  - Anemia, leukocytosis, thrombocytosis, elevated ESR
  - Normal serum levels of C3 and C4
  - ANCA: 80–90 % of patients are cANCA (anti-PR3) positive
  - Chest X-ray, CT chest (granuloma, penumonia, hemorrhage)
  - Renal biopsy
  - Lung/sinus biopsy (granuloma)

3.6.4.5 Eosinophilic Granulomatosis with Polyangiitis (EGPA; former Churg–Strauss Syndrome)

- EGPA is rare in children.
- Characterized by eosinophil-rich and necrotizing granulomatous inflammation involving the respiratory tract.

- Granulomatous and non-granulomatous extravascular inflammation is common.
- Associated with eosinophilia and asthma.

3.6.4.6 Renal Histopathology of ANCA-Associated Vasculitis

- Renal manifestations are similar in MPA and GPA, and in renal-limited (pauci-immune) NCGN (see also Sect. 3.4, Table 3.12).
- Light microscopy: The hallmark finding is necrotizing injury of the glomerular tuft and crescent formation (necrotizing and crescentic glomerulonephritis). Segmental fibrinoid necrosis, neutrophilic infiltration, karyorrhexis; vasculitis involving interlobular arteries with or without crescents. Late changes are (diffuse) glomerulosclerosis and nephron loss.
- Immunofluorescence: no or minimal deposits with occasional weak positivity for C3. Invariable presence of fibrin deposition.
- Electron microscopy: Display of glomerular endothelial injury (swelling, GBM detachment), gaps in GBM and Bowman's capsule.

3.6.4.7 Treatment of ANCA Vasculitis

- AAV treatment, particularly of MPA and GPA, is similar.
- *Induction therapy*: Glucocorticoids and cyclophosphamide.
- Alternatively, glucocorticoids and rituximab may be used as initial treatment in patients with milder disease (absence of pulmonary hemorrhage and preserved kidney function).
- Methylprednisolone IV (3–6) doses (10 mg/kg per dose or 500 mg/1.73 m^2), followed by oral prednisolone (or prednisone) 2 mg/kg per day up to 60 mg per day. Prednisolone is given for 4 weeks and then tapered to alternate-day dosing.
- IV cyclophosphamide (500–750 mg/m^2/dose) is given every 4 weeks for 6 months; it is stopped after 3 months, if patient remains dialysis-dependent.
- When oral cyclophosphamide is used, give 1.5–2 mg/kg/day (reduce oral dose for GFR <20 ml/1.73m^2). Adjust daily dose to keep WBC >3/nl.
- Rituximab is dosed 375 mg/m^2 every week × 4 doses.
- *Maintenance therapy, once remission is achieved*:
  - Oral azathioprine 1–2 mg/kg/day or mycophenolate mofetil (MMF) up to 1 g/1.73 m^2 twice daily.
  - Methotrexate (0.3 mg/kg per week, not exceeding 25 mg/week) if patient is intolerant to azathioprine and MMF, and if GFR is >60 ml/min/1.73 m^2.
  - Trimethoprim sulfamethoxazole has been tried in patients with upper respiratory tract disease.
- Maintenance therapy is continued for at least 18 months, if patient remains in remission.
- *Plasmapheresis* is indicated in children with rapidly rising serum creatinine or requiring dialysis, diffuse pulmonary hemorrhage, or poor response to induction therapy.
- All patients with systemic disease should receive immunosuppressive therapy, regardless of kidney function.
- Careful judgement is needed when patients with severe NCGN have already reached ESRD. Immunosuppressants may not be appropriate in the absence of systemic disease.

3.6.4.8 Outcome

- Five-year survival is >80 %.
- About 30 % of patients progress to ESRD.
- Untreated ANCA-associated NCGN has a poor prognosis. Immunosuppressive treatment has dramatically improved short- and long-term survival.
- Histological criteria affecting renal outcome are the percentage of glomeruli with crescents or globally sclerosed glomeruli. The prognosis is favorable in the presence of limited injury (e.g. focal GN, crescents in <50 %) and poor with diffuse (>50 %) global glomerulosclerosis.
- Patients may experience recurrence of AAV or NCGN after kidney transplantation.

3.6.5 Lupus Nephritis (LN)

Systemic lupus erythematosus (SLE) is a multisystemic inflammatory disease associated with autoantibodies to different cell components. The clinical manifestations can be varied depending on the type and extent of organ system involvement. It is a chronic disease characterized by remissions and relapses. The peak incidence in children is around puberty. Ethnicity affects prevalence and severity of SLE and LN. Both are 2–3 times higher in East Asian and Southeast Asian and in native North American children compared with European children. High rates are likewise found among people of African ancestry.

3.6.5.1 Definition

The American Rheumatology Association (ARA, changed in 1988 to "American College of Rheumatology" (ACR)) has put forth the ARA criteria for the diagnosis of SLE. At least 4 of the 11 criteria should be positive to diagnose SLE. Renal manifestations are a part of the diagnostic criteria for SLE. However, some of these manifestations may occur in isolation or may not present early in the disease course (Box 3.11). Lupus nephritis is an important determinant for the survival of patients with SLE. The updated 2012 guideline recommendations of the American College of Rheumatology for the diagnosis and treatment of LN are summarized in Box 3.12.

3.6.5.2 Pathogenesis

Autoantibodies, immune complexes, complement activation, and T lymphocytes are responsible for mediating the damage to various organ systems. Alteration in regulatory T cells increases autoreactive T lymphocytes. Autoantibodies are produced against various components of the cell, especially nuclear components. Dendritic cells play a role in activation of self-reactive T and B cells resulting in the production of autoantibodies.

3.6.5.3 Clinical Features

Extrarenal

- Systemic features: weight loss, loss of appetite, fever
- Skin manifestations: malar rash, discoid rash, photosensitivity, Reynaud's phenomenon, oral ulcers
- Musculoskeletal: arthralgia, arthritis, tendinitis, myositis

Box 3.11 American Rheumatology Association Criteria for SLE (1982)[a]

- Malar rash
- Discoid rash
- Photosensitivity
- Oral ulcers
- Arthritis
- Serositis – pleuritis or pericarditis
- Renal abnormalities – persistent proteinuria >0.5 g/day/1.73m^2 or >3+ or cellular casts in urine
- Neurologic disorder – seizures or psychosis
- Hematologic disorder – hemolytic anemia, leukopenia 4 × 10^9/l (<4,000/mm^3) or lymphopenia 1.5 × 10^9/l (<1,500/mm^3) or thrombocytopenia 100 × 10^9/l (<100,000/mm^3) (on two or more occasions)
- Immunologic disorder – abnormal anti-dsDNA titer, or presence of anti-Sm antigen
- Antinuclear antibody – abnormal titer of antinuclear antibody

[a]Four or more criteria, definite SLE; 3 criteria, probable SLE; 2 criteria, possible SLE

Box 3.12 American College of Rheumatology Guideline Recommendations for the Diagnosis and Treatment of Lupus Nephritis

Diagnostic

- Renal biopsy for all SLE patients with active LN

Therapy

- Induction therapy with MMF or Euro-Lupus cyclophosphamide for active LN class III/IV
- No modification of the induction therapy before 6 months of treatment
- Maintenance therapy with MMF or azathioprine
- Rituximab or calcineurin inhibitor optionally for refractory LN

Adjunctive therapy

- Hydroxychloroquine for all patients with LN
- Blood-pressure control
- Hyperlipidemia treatment with statins
- Angiotensin inhibition for all patients with proteinuria of >0.5 g/1.73 m^2 per day
- Counseling on suitable contraception and pregnancy risks for all female patients of child-bearing potential

- Hematological: anemia, bleeding manifestation, thrombosis, Coombs test positivity with or without hemolytic anemia, lymphadenopathy, hepatosplenomegaly
- Pulmonary: pneumonitis, pleuritis, pulmonary hemorrhage
- Cardiovascular: myocarditis, pericarditis, (Libman–Sacks) endocarditis
- Neuropsychiatric: headache, chorea, cranial nerve palsy, hemiparesis, seizures

Renal

- Renal manifestations are seen in up to 80 % of patients with SLE, usually within the first 6 months.
- Asymptomatic proteinuria, hematuria, acute nephritis, nephrotic syndrome, rapidly progressive glomerulonephritis, chronic kidney disease, hypertension.
- Hypertension and/or decreased renal function in 40–50 % of patients.

3.6.5.4 Laboratory Investigations

- Urinanalysis: proteinuria from mild to nephrotic range, RBC, WBC, RBC casts
- Renal function tests
- Complement: serum C3, C4, CH50 (all typically reduced)
- Serological tests:
  1. Antinuclear antibodies (ANA): highly sensitive (95–98 %), but non-specific
  2. Anti-dsDNA: highly specific for SLE (90–95 %)
  3. Antibodies to ribonucleoprotein, anti-Sm antibody (100 % specific), anti-histone antibodies, and antiphospholipid antibodies may be present
- Skin biopsy, renal biopsy

3.6.5.5 Renal Histopathology

- Histological changes in LN comprise vascular, glomerular and tubulointerstitial lesions. The glomerular lesions are described in terms of mesangial, endothelial and epithelial patterns of injury.
- The WHO morphological classification is widely used to grade the severity of lupus nephritis (Box 3.13). Its latest modification by the International Society of Nephrology/Renal Pathology Society (ISN/RPS) from 2003 is shown in (Boxes 3.14 and 3.15).

3.6.5.6 Treatment

- The treatment is based on the severity of renal and extrarenal disease and renal histopathology (Table 3.20).
- Fig. 3.13 depicts the practical ACR consensus algorithm for adult patients with LN emphasizing the shift from IVCY to MMF.
- Further changes in the medical management of juvenile LN are expected following current trials with biological agents aimed at reducing adverse events associated with exposure to high-dose, long-term glucocorticoids and to cytotoxic agents.

3.6.5.7 Prognosis

- The prognosis of SLE has improved with aggressive therapy.
- Complete or partial remission is usually achieved by 18–24 months.
- Deaths are due to infections, thrombotic, or neurological complications.
- With current treatment regimens, most patients have stable renal functions at 10 years after onset of disease.
- Complications: infections, atherosclerosis, cardiovascular morbidity.

Box 3.13 WHO Morphologic Classification of Lupus Nephritis (Modified in 1982)

Class I Normal glomeruli
(a) Nil (by all techniques)
(b) Normal by light microscopy but deposits by electron or immunofluorescence microscopy
Class II Pure mesangial alterations (mesangiopathy)
(a) Mesangial widening and/or mild hypercellularity (+)
(b) Moderate hypercellularity (++)
Class III Focal segmental glomerulonephritis (associated with mild or moderate mesangial alterations)
(a) With "active" necrotizing lesions
(b) With "active" and sclerosing lesions
(c) With sclerosing lesions
Class IV Diffuse glomerulonephritis (severe mesangial, endocapillary, or mesangiocapillary proliferation and/or extensive subendothelial deposits)
(a) Without segmental lesions
(b) With "active" necrotizing lesions
(c) With "active" and sclerosing lesions
(d) With sclerosing lesions
Class V Diffuse membranous glomerulonephritis
(a) Pure membranous glomerulonephritis
(b) Associated with lesions of category II (a or b)
(c) Associated with lesions of category III (a–c)
(d) Associated with lesions of category IV (a–d)
Class VI Advanced sclerosing glomerulonephritis

Box 3.14 International Society of Nephrology/Renal Pathology Society (ISN/RPS) Classification of Lupus Nephritis (2003)[a]

Class I Minimal mesangial lupus nephritis
Class II Mesangial proliferative lupus nephritis
Class III Focal lupus nephritis[a]
Class IV Diffuse segmental (IV-S) or global (IV-G) lupus nephritis[a]
Class V Membranous lupus nephritis[b]
Class VI Advanced sclerosing lupus nephritis[c]

[a]Class III and IV are further characterized as *A* active, *C* chronic, and *A/C* active and chronic lesions (the activity and chronicity indices are listed in Box 3.15)

[b]Class V can occur in combination with class II, III or IV, in which case both will be noted (e.g., "lupus nephritis class II and V")

[c]Designates biopsy with >90 % global glomerulosclerosis attributed to lupus nephritis without evidence of active glomerular disease

Box 3.15 Active and Chronic Glomerular Lesions as Defined in the ISN/RPS 2003 Classification of Lupus Nephritis

Active lesions[a]
Endocapillary hypercellularity with or without leukocyte infiltration and with substantial luminal reduction
Karyorrhexis
Fibrinoid necrosis
Rupture of glomerular basement membrane
Crescents – cellular or fibro-cellular
Subendothelial deposits identifiable by light microscopy (wire loops)
Intraluminal immune aggregates (hyaline thrombi)
Chronic lesions[b]
Glomerular sclerosis (segmental, global)
Fibrous adhesions
Fibrous crescents
Interstitial fibrosis
Tubular atrophy

[a]Active lesions graded as 0–3 (necrosis and cellular crescents graded 0–6); max. activity score, 24
[b]chronic lesions, maximum score 10

Poor Prognostic Factors

- Clinical: younger age, males, African origin, hypertension, renal dysfunction at onset, delay in treatment, response to treatment in the first year
- Class IV lupus nephritis, extensive crescents, necrotizing glomerular lesions

3.6.5.8 Renal Transplantation

- Renal transplant should be deferred until disease activity and the serological markers are quiescent. The duration of quiescence is not well defined but generally accepted as 1–2 years.
- Risk of recurrence of LN in the graft is low.

3.6.6 Other Vasculitides

3.6.6.1 Takayasu Arteritis

- Granulomatous vasculitis involving the aorta and its major branches. Hypertension is the most common manifestation due to either narrowing of the aorta or due to renal artery stenosis.
- Common cause of renovascular hypertension in some Asian countries.
- Weak peripheral unequal pulses, claudications, bruit over the aorta or its branches.
- Angiography shows stenosis or occlusion of affected blood vessels.
- Glucocorticoids may be used during acute phase; reconstructive vascular surgery may be required later.

Table 3.20 Therapeutic regimens for lupus nephritis[a]

Disease	Induction	Maintenance
Class II or mild disease	PRED (0.5–1.0 mg/kg/day for 4–6 weeks)	Tapering PRED for 2–3years after remission AZA (1–2 mg/kg/day) may be considered if no response by 3 months or switch to protocol for moderate disease
Class III or moderate disease	PRED (1.0–1.5 mg/kg/day for 4–6weeks) AZA 1–2 mg/kg/day, or MMF (900–1,200 mg/m^2/day, or IVCY monthly pulses 0.5–1.0 g/m^2/dose × 6 doses	Tapering PRED for 2–3years after remission AZA to continue, MMF may be reduced to 750 mg/m^2/day or IVCY quarterly pulses for 18 months
Class IV or severe disease	IV methylprednisolone pulses 20–25 mg/kg/dose (max 1 g) × 3 pulses followed by PRED PO 1.0–1.5 mg/kg/day and IVCY monthly × 6 doses 0.5–1.0 mg/m^2/dose or MMF 1,200 mg/m^2/day × 6 months If treatment-refractory: RTX, PLEX, IVIG	Tapering PRED for up to 5 years after remission IVCY quarterly pulses for 18 months or MMF 750–1,000 mg/m^2/day or AZA 1–2 mg/kg/day
Class V	High-dose PRED (1.0–1.5 mg/kg/day) with ACE inhibition, or May combine with CSA 3–5 mg/kg/day or MMF, or RTX	CSA/ACEi ? Low-dose PRED or repeat RTX (if effective)

[a]All patients with LN should also be treated with hydroxychloroquin and antiproteinuric agents (ACE inhibition) if appropriate

ACEi angiotensin-converting enzyme inhibitor, *AZA* azathioprine, *CSA* cyclosporine A (or tacrolimus 0.1–0.2 mg/kg/day), *CYP* cyclophosphamide, *IV* intravenous, *IVIG* intravenous immunoglobulin, *MMF* mycophenolate mofetil, *PLEX* plasma exchange, *PRED* prednisone or prednisolone, *RTX* rituximab (1 g/m^2 × 2, two weeks apart)

3.6.6.2 Childhood Polyarteritis Nodosa (cPAN)

- PAN is a necrotizing vasculitis associated with aneurismal nodules along the walls of *medium size* arteries of skin, peripheral nerves, muscles, gastrointestinal tract, and kidneys.
- It does not affect renal arterioles and capillaries and is not associated with ANCA.
- Rare in children.
- Renal manifestations: asymptomatic hematuria, proteinuria, acute nephritis, nephrotic syndrome, hypertension.
- Extrarenal manifestations: fever, malaise, weight loss, myalgia, arthralgia, abdominal pain, visual loss, focal neurological deficits, mononeuritis multiplex, testicular pain and occasionally, cardiac or respiratory manifestations.
- It can be associated with hepatitis B.
- Renal biopsy and renal angiogram may be required for evaluation of renal disease.

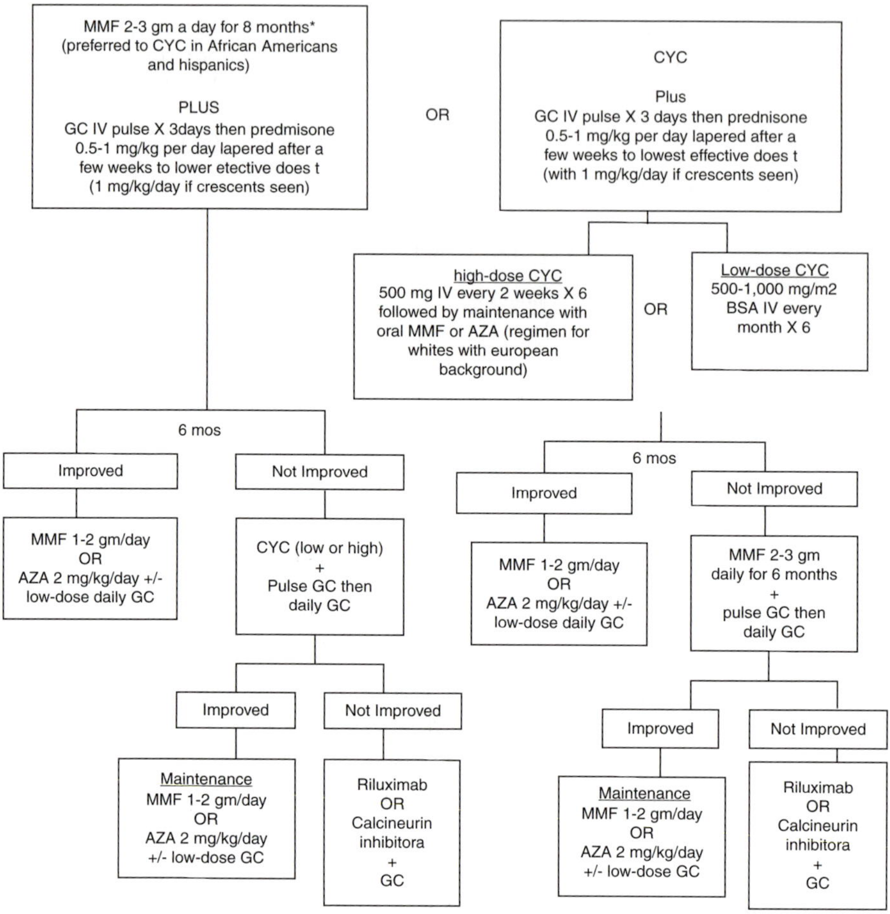

Fig. 3.13 Lupus nephritis class III/IV induction therapy. *The Task Force Panel discussed their preference of MMF over cyclophosphamide (CYC) in patients who desire to preserve fertility; †recommended background therapies for most patients are discussed in section III in the publication. *AZA* azathioprine, *BSA* body surface area, *GC* glucocorticoids, *IV* intravenous, *MMF* mycophenolate mofetil (With permission from Hahn et al. 2012)

- Renal medium-sized vessel aneurysms, perfusion defects, collaterals, and delayed emptying of small vessels may be seen on angiography.
- Glucocorticoids and cyclophosphamide are the mainstay of treatment.

3.6.6.3 Kawasaki Disease (KD)

- KD is the commonest pediatric vasculitis (after SHP). Incidence per 100,000 <5 years is 138 in Japan and <18 in Europe and North America.
- Affects infants and young children under 5 years of age.
- Five of 6 diagnostic criteria have to be fulfilled: fever persisting more than 5 days (mandatory), palmar erythema, polymorphous exanthema, bilateral conjunctival injection/congestion, strawberry tongue/red lips and acute, non-purulent cervical lymphadenopathy. Coronary aneurysms may occur.

- Renal involvement may occur with hematuria and proteinuria.
- Treated with aspirin and intravenous immunoglobulin with or without glucocorticoid and (if accessible) infliximab.

3.7 Hemolytic Uremic Syndrome/Thrombotic Microangiopathies

3.7.1 Introduction and Definitions

Hemolytic uremic syndrome (HUS) is defined clinically by the triad of microangiopathic hemolytic anemia, thrombocytopenia and renal involvement/acute kidney injury (AKI). Based on common pathomorphological features, HUS and clinically similar, but etiologically heterogenous disorders, such as thrombotic thrombocytopenic purpura (TTP), are often referred to as thrombotic microangiopathies (TMA) (see Box 3.16).

TTP is traditionally defined by the added features of neurological involvement and fever. However, the latter two may also be present in HUS and do therefore not distinguish between the two syndromes.

The term "typical" (or "classical") HUS is reserved for HUS induced by Shiga toxin-producing bacteria (STPB, predominantly Shiga toxin-producing *Escherichia coli* (STEC); STEC HUS). "Atypical" initially referred to all non-STEC HUS, but is now commonly applied to HUS related to the dysregulation of the alternative pathway (AP) of complement (aHUS; Box 3.16, Fig. 3.14).

Despite substantial progress in this field over the past decade, no etiological diagnosis is found in about 40 % of patients with atypical forms of HUS.

3.7.2 Approach to a Patient with HUS

- Children with HUS may present at any age, often, but not exclusively, in the context of an infection.
- In more than 70 %, HUS is proceeded by diarrhea, often as colitis with abdominal cramps and frequent discharge of bloody stools (generally indicative of Shiga toxin-induced HUS).
- For prognostic and therapeutic reasons, presumptive classification of the type of HUS or thrombotic microangiopathy and rapid etiological diagnosis are warranted in each case.
- The pathophysiological and genetic workup can be time consuming or remain unsuccessful. In many settings, appropriate laboratories or resources may be lacking.
- The correct etiological diagnosis of aHUS is complex and may involve more than one gene mutation.
- Box 3.17 lists a set of *six key questions* at the time of presentation that help narrow down the possible etiology of the HUS.
- A rationale approach for the diagnosis and initial management of HUS/TMA is provided in Fig. 3.15. The diagram is based on the recommendations of the "European Paediatric Study Group for HUS" from 2009.

Box 3.16 Thrombotic Microangiopathies (TMA)

A. Etiologically recognized forms of HUS and TTP

1. *Infection induced HUS*

1.1 Shiga toxin-producing bacteria (STPB):

Enterohemorrhagic *Escherichia coli* (STEC/EHEC) O157:H7 (worldwide most commonly associated with Shiga toxin-mediated HUS), *Shigella dysenteriae* type 1, *Citrobacter freundii*

1.2 Neuraminidase-producing organisms:

Streptococcus pneumoniae, *Clostridium perfringens*, influenza virus

1.3 Human immunodeficiency virus (HIV)

2. *HUS due to disorders of complement regulation* (mostly alternative pathway)

2.1 Inherited:

2.1.1 Haploinsufficiency

Soluble (plasma) factors: Factor H (CFH), factor I (CFI), factor H related proteins 1 (CFHR1) and 5 (CFHR5)

Membrane-bound regulators: membrane cofactor (MCP, CD46)

Other proteins interacting with the complement pathway: thrombomodulin (THBD)

2.1.2 Copy number variations:

e.g., CHFR 1/3 deletion, CFH/CHFR1 hybrid

2.1.3 Activating (heterozygous) mutations: CFB, C3

2.2 Acquired:

Anti-factor H (CFH) autoantibody (may be associated with CFHR1/3 deletion)

3. *ADAMTS13 (von Willebrand factor-cleaving protease) deficiency (TTP)* (*a d*isintegrin *a*nd *m*etalloproteinase with a *t*hrombo*s*pondin type 1 motif, member *13*)

3.1 Inherited:

Upshaw-Schulman syndrome (autosomal recessive)

3.2 Acquired:

ADAMTS13 autoantibody

4. *Metabolic deficiencies (not directly complement-related)*

4.1 Defective cobalamin metabolism:

Cobalamin processing deficiency of the cblC type (mutations in *MMACHC* [methylmalonic aciduria and homocystinuria, cblC type], autosomal recessive)

4.2 Diacylglycerol kinase-epsilon (DGKE) (autosomal recessive)

5. *Drug induced:*

Quinine, mitomycin C, ticlopidine, calcineurin inhibitors

B. Speculative/unknown etiology

1. Pregnancy-associated HUS, HELLP syndrome, oral contraceptives
2. Bone marrow/stem cell transplantation (CFHR1/3 deletion?)
3. Superimposed on preexisting disorders/secondary forms:

SLE, antiphospholipid antibody syndrome, malignancy, ionizing radiation

[a]Generally heterozygous mutation leading to reduced expression of functional proteins. Few cases of homozygous deficiencies of CFH and MCP have been described (with severe phenotype)

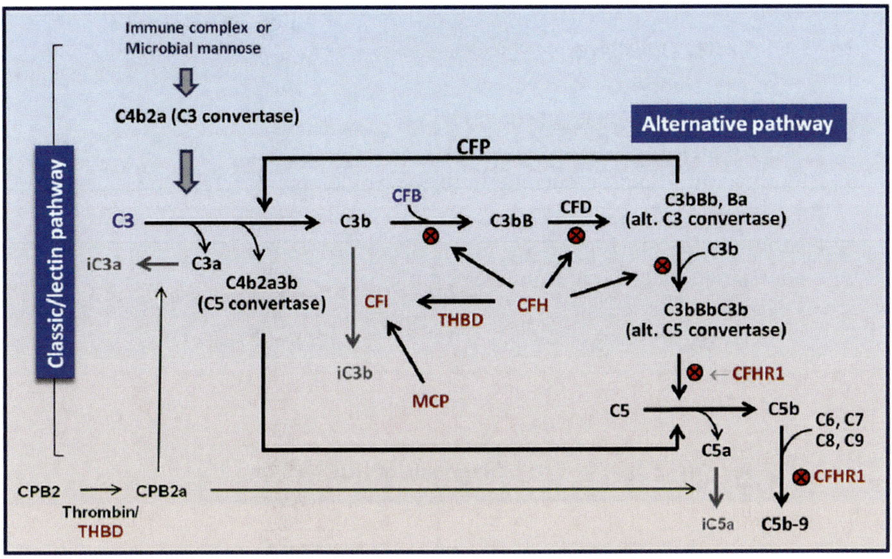

Fig. 3.14 Schematic Diagram of the Major Complement Activation Pathway and their Regulators. Depicted are the soluble regulators CFH (complement factor H) and CFI (complement factor I) who interact with cell bound MCP (membrane cofactor protein) and with THBD (thrombomodulin) to cleave activated C3 (C3b) into inactive iC3 thus preventing uncontrolled (alternative pathway) C3 convertase (C3bBb) and C5 convertase (C3bBbC3b) formation. CFHR-1 (CFH-related protein 1) may regulate C5 convertase and terminal C5b-9 "membrane attack complex" (MAC) assembly. Below-threshold concentrations or inactivating mutations of CFH, CFI, MCP and THBD as well as activating (gain-of-function) mutations of CFB (complement factor B) and C3 have all been associated with a HUS susceptibility due to excessive AP complement activation and MAC formation (With permission from Tsai 2013)

3.7.3 Typical (Enteropathic/STEC) HUS

- Generally preceded by diarrhea or (bloody) colitis.
- HUS risk 8–15 % after *E. coli* O157:H7 colitis, variable with other STEC serotypes/STPB.
- At rare occasions, diarrhea cannot be elicited.
- HUS due to urinary tract infection by STEC has been described.
- Accounts for 70–90 % HUS in preschool children (peak age group 1–5 years).
- STEC transmission with contaminated foods or drinking water, animal contact (Petting Zoo) or person to person.
- Antimotility drugs and certain antibiotics during STEC diarrhea increase the risk of developing HUS.
- Seasonal peak late summer/early fall, but sporadic or epidemic cases are seen year-round.
- Clinical Features

Box 3.17 Six Key Questions

1. Age at presentation?
2. Rapid or insidious onset/chronic HUS?
3. First presentation or recurrence of HUS?
4. Bloody colitis and/or current outbreak/epidemic of STEC infection or shigellosis?
5. Past family history for HUS?
6. Underlying renal or autoimmune disorder?

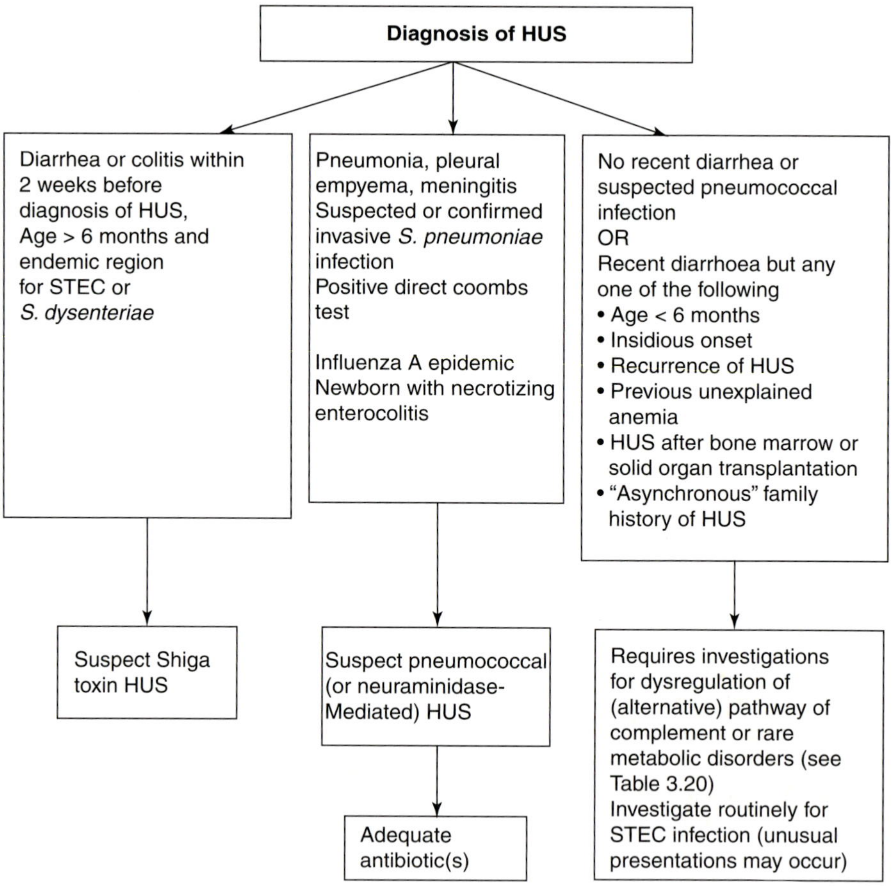

Fig. 3.15 Approach to a patient with HUS

  - Triad: acute kidney injury, microangiopathic hemolytic anemia (Coombs negative, schizocytes on peripheral smear), thrombocytopenia; partial or limited HUS refers to the absence of one of the features of the triad.
  - Diarrhea is typically frequent and bloody with abdominal cramps.
  - Onset of STEC HUS is characterized by sudden clincal deterioration 3–7 (–10) days after begin of diarrhea.
  - Moderate extracellular volume depletion. Hypovolemic shock is rare.
  - Renal manifestations range from mild hematuria and proteinuria to severe AKI with renal cortical necrosis due to renal (thrombotic) ischemia.
  - Other organ systems may be involved, including the gastrointestinal tract (ischemic colitis, perforation, rectal prolapse, intussusception, toxic megacolon, colonic strictures, gallstones), pancreatitis with amylase/lipase elevation or transient, occasionally lasting insulin-dependent diabetes mellitus, CNS (lethargy, irritability, seizures, paresis, coma, cerebral edema, cranial nerve palsy), retinal blindness, and myocardial ischemia or cardiomyopathy.
- Baseline Investigations
  - Complete blood count (anemia, thrombocytopenia) with a peripheral smear (schistocytes), reticulocyte count and LDH (both increased), serum haptoglobin (depleted)
  - Renal function
  - Serum lipase and amylase
  - Coagulation profile
  - Blood group typing and crossmatch
  - Urinalysis and urine culture
  - Stool culture for Shiga toxin producing bacteria and common enteropathogens
  - Fecal Shiga toxin (Vero cell assay, immunological detection); PCR for Shiga toxin and EHEC genes; serotyping of identified coliform organism; serological response to locally relevant O serotypes (Western blot, ELISA)
- Other Investigations (see also Table 3.21)
  - Direct Coombs test
  - Abdominal ultrasonography to rule out underlying structural renal abnormality/pancreatitis/gall stones, appendicitis, gangrenous or perforating colitis
  - CT abdomen if pancreatitis is suspected
  - ECG in case of dyselectrolytemia
  - Echocardiography in case of suspected pericardial perfusion or cardiac failure
  - MRI brain (or CT) in case of focal or complicated seizures, progressive lethargy or (axial) hypotonia
  - Renal biopsy (if doubtful diagnosis or delay in renal recovery): does not reliably differentiate between typical (STEC-mediated) and other forms of HUS/TMA, but useful to assess chronic renal injury/extent of cortical necrosis and renal prognosis
- Treatment
  - Pre-HUS (STEC colitis)
    - Intravenous volume expansion with isotonic saline (start within 4 days of diarrhea onset, if STEC infection suspected or proven)
    - Avoidance of antimotility agents and antibiotics (except *S. dysenteriae*)

Table 3.21 Investigations for HUS and other thrombotic microangiopathies (TMA)

HUS/TMA	Investigations[a]	Comments
STEC/STPB infection (*"Typical" of STEC HUS*)	Stool or rectal swab culture Free fecal toxin assay PCR for *stx* gene and STPB virulence markers in stool or bacterial isolates Anti-LPS IgM antibodies against select serotypes, anti-Stx antibodies (in serum)	Consider complement regulator defect in children with severe or unusual course STEC HUS
Infection by *S. pneumoniae* or other NANAse producing pathogen (*"Pneumococcal" HUS*)	Bacterial culture (blood, CSF, pleural fluid) Respiratory viral antigen/PCR/culture Direct Coombs test Thomson-Friedenreich (TF) antigen detection on RBCs (peanut lectin *Arachis hypogea*)	Invasive pneumococcal infection Influenza A virus infection *C. perfringens* colitis/necrotizing enterocolitis
Complement regulator deficiency (*"Atypical" or complement regulator HUS*) Inherited Acquired: anti-CFH auto-antibody	Plasma/serum C3, C4 (CH50, SC5b-9) Factor H (CFH) and factor I (CFI) serum protein level, MCP (CD46) leukocyte surface expression (FACS) Anti-factor H antibody Extended genetic workup for CFH, MCP, CFI, CFB, C3, and THBD mutations and CFHR1/3 deletion	Note that 30 % of a HUS may be triggered by diarrhea Normal plasma concentrations of factors do not exclude diagnosis of a HUS or mutation HUS risk conferred by reduced plasma concentrations or surface expression (MCP), or activating mutations (C3, CFB). Most cases related to heterozygous mutations. More than one complement component can be mutated. CFHR1/3 deletion is associated with anti-CFH antibodies
ADAMTS13 (vWF protease) deficiency (*TTP*) Inherited: Upshaw-Schulman syndrome Acquired: anti-ADAMS13 auto-antibody	Plasma ADAMTS13 (protease) activity (<10 % of normal) and protein level If low, test for ADAMTS13 autoantibody (inhibitor) Genetic mutation screen when no inhibitor found	Measure pre-treatment and after recovery
Defective cobalamin metabolism (*Cbl-C disorder/cHUS*)	Increased plasma and urine methylmalonic (MMA) and homocystein concentrations and hypomethioninemia *MMACHC* mutation (autosomal recessive) or mutation of other proteins affecting cobalamin metabolism	Manifestation in newborn period, but also anytime later in life

(continued)

Table 3.21 (continued)

HUS/TMA	Investigations[a]	Comments
HIV infection	Serology Viral PCR	
Pregnancy, HELLP syndrome	Pregnancy test, liver enzymes	Investigate (also) for complement dysregulation and ADAMTS13 activity In teenage girl with HUS or TTP always consider pregnancy
Miscellaneous	Antinuclear or anti-DNA antibodies, lupus anticoagulant/ antiphospholipid antibody	Exclude secondary TMA/HUS due to SLE, antiphospholipid syndrome

[a]Genetic and some functional assays require access to specialized laboratories

*ADAMTS13 a d*isintegrin *a*nd *m*etalloproteinase with a *t*hrombo*s*pondin type 1 motif, member 13 (von Willebrand factor protease; physiologically cleaves and degrades large vW multimers decreasing their activity), *CFB* complement factor B, *Cbl-C* cobalamin C, *HELLP* hemolysis, elevated liver enzymes, low platelet count, *MCP* membrane cofactor protein, *FACS* fluorescence-activated cell sorter, *MMACHC* methylmalonic aciduria and homocystinuria type C protein, *NANAse* neuraminidase, *STEC* Shiga toxin-producing *Escherichia coli*, *STPB* Shiga toxin-producing bacteria, *TTP* thrombotic thrombocytopenic purpura

- Acute kidney injury
  - Fluid an electrolyte management
  - Antihypertensive therapy
  - Initiation of renal replacement therapy (1/3 to 2/3 of patients with STEC HUS require temporary dialysis)
- Management of extrarenal manifestations
- Blood Products
  - Packed red cell transfusion for anemia when Hb <60 g/l (6 g/dl) or when symptomatic (tachypnea, tachycardia, shock). Be mindful of volume overload.
  - Platelet transfusion is rarely indicated unless for active bleeding or invasive surgery.
- Plasma Exchange
  - Practiced in some centers for children with neurological involvement in analogy to treatment of TTP. No evidence base. However, PLEX or anti-complement therapy may be indicated if atypical HUS is suspected.
- Newer therapies on the horizon (experimental)
  - Synsorb Pk – diatomaceous silicon diamide compound linked to an oligosaccharide chain: binds and neutralizes Shiga toxin (negative trial results).
  - Starfish/Daisy – action similar to Synsorb, but several logs higher toxin binding capacity. Not yet trialed in humans.
  - Monoclonal antibodies specific for A subunit of Shiga toxin 2 or to Shiga toxin 1 and 2 combined. Antibodies well tolerated in phase 2 trials, but not yet available for therapeutic use.
  - Vaccination against O157 LPS or Shiga toxin (not yet available).

- Prognosis
  - Acute mortality rate 1–5 %.
  - 5–10 % may develop CKD.
  - After >15 years of follow-up, 20–60 % of patients may have (mild) proteinuria and/or hypertension and/or (mild) renal dysfunction despite full initial recovery.
- Poor Renal Prognostic Factors
  - Very young age
  - Neutrophilia $>20\times10^9$/l
  - Severe ischemic injury/hypovolemic shock during the acute phase
  - Anuria >2 weeks
  - Catasrophic CNS disease
  - Gangrenous colitis
  - Severe cortical necrosis on renal biopsy

3.7.4 Pneumococcal (Neuraminidase-Induced) HUS (pnHUS)

- Pneumococcal infections account for one third to one half of all non-enteropathic (non-STEC) HUS.
- Peak age 6–18 months.
- More than 2/3 of pnHUS patients present with pneumonia, often with pleural empyema, and 1/3 with pneumococcal meningitis, bacteremia and other invasive *S. pneumoniae* infections. Prognosis is considered poor.
- Presumed pathological principle is (excess) neuraminidase production.
- Laboratory diagnosis (see Table 3.22).
- Influenza virus A and has also associated with this form of HUS (to be differentiated from aHUS in patients with complement regulator defect).
- Treatment consists of antibiotics, management of pleural empyema or meningitis and transfusion of PRBC as needed.
- Plasma therapy (PLEX), IVIG infusion and blood exchange transfusion (in young infants) have been used.

3.7.5 Atypical (Complement-Induced) HUS (aHUS)

- HUS due to disordered complement regulation can arise at any age.
- Atypical HUS may begin insidiously and follow a fluctuating course. This contrasts with the usually rapid onset of Shiga toxin- and neuraminidase-induced (pneumoccal) HUS.
- Specific regulator defects associated with aHUS and their role in the alternative pathway of complement activation are depicted schematically in Fig. 3.14.
- Serum C3 and C4 concentrations are unreliable to differentiate between atypical and other forms of HUS.

- Familial occurrence of HUS may be synchronous, due to a common source of STEC infection (epidemic HUS or person-to-person transmission), or asynchronous, raising the suspicion of an inherited susceptibility for HUS.
- Mutations of genes encoding complement factors are generally heterozygous mutations leading to reduced protein expression or function (except aHUS-associated mutations of C3 and factor B) (see Box 3.16 and Table 3.21).
- The differential diagnosis of post-kidney transplant HUS includes recurrence of an atypical, inherited form, calcineurin inhibitor-induced HUS or TMA due to antibody-mediated rejection.
- Specific Investigations for select, atypical forms of HUS are detailed in Table 3.21.

3.7.6 Treatment of Atypical HUS

3.7.6.1 Plasma Therapy

- Referral to experienced (pediatric) center is advised due to the complexities of treatment and laboratory workup.
- Current standard of care for first presentation of aHUS is rapid initiation of plasma exchange therapy (PLEX) against (fresh) frozen plasma (Fig. 3.16)
- Rationale for PLEX
  - In case of autoantibodies to factor H (or ADAMTS13), plasma exchange removes the autoantibody and provides additional factor H
  - Mutated C3 or factor B that permits excessive complement activation is removed

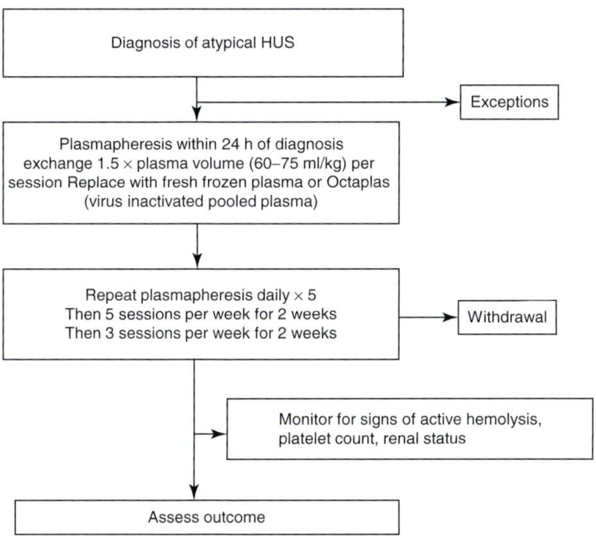

Fig. 3.16 Treatment recommendations for atypical HUS (With permission from Ariceta et al. 2009)

- Where access to PLEX is limited due to lack of expertise or resources, plasma infusions (10–20 ml/kg) may be tried, initially daily, via a peripheral vein.
- Intense plasma infusion therapy may lead to improvement in some patients with CFH or CFI mutation or (genetic) ADAMTS13 deficiency.
- In contrast, patients with (heterozygous) MCP mutation may recover spontaneously within a week. Furthermore, up to 40 % of children with aHUS will not have an identifiable complement regulator defect and/or may not benefit from plasma therapy.

Exceptions from PLEX Initiation Recommendations

- HUS in a sibling of a patient with congenital ADAMTS13 deficiency is likely to have the same diagnosis and might be expected to respond to plasma infusion 10 ml/kg/day every 2–3 weeks.
- Clinical presentation suggestive of early onset cobalamin-C disorder (feeding difficulty, failure to thrive, hypotonia, lethargy, leukopenia, thrombocytopenia, gastrointestinal bleeding, metabolic acidosis, and megaloblastic anemia) which is treated by 5 mg/day of hydroxocobalamin associated with betaine.

Withdrawal from PLEX Therapy

- Alternative diagnosis where the condition is not expected to respond to plasma therapy, for example, cobalamin-C disorder.
- Diagnosis of congenital ADAMTS13 deficiency is made, in which case plasma infusion may help.
- Hematological remission is achieved.

Rationale for Plasma Exchange

1. In case of autoantibodies to factor H, plasma exchange removes the autoantibody and provides additional factor H.
2. Mutated factor B that permits excessive complement activation is removed by plasma exchange.

3.7.6.2 Alternative Treatment Strategies

- Human plasma-derived complement factor H concentrate (not yet available)
- Synthetic (recombinant) complement blockers (not yet available)
- Monoclonal antibodies against activating components of complement such as eculizumab (against C5)
- Glucocorticoids, cyclophosphamide, immunoglobulins, rituximab (mainly for autoantibody induced HUS and TTP, in combination with PLEX or anti-complement agents)

3.7.6.3 Anti-C5 Monoclonal Antibody Therapy

- A complement (C5) blocking monoclonal antibody (mAb), eculizumab, initially developed for treatment of paroxysmal nocturnal hematuria (PNH), has now been approved in several jurisdictions for treatment of aHUS.
- mAb infusions replace or complement PLEX therapy.

- Precautions needed to prevent infections by encapsulated (complement-dependent) bacteria (*Neisseria spp.*, *S. pneumoniae*, *H. influenzae*).
- Treatment should be restricted to experienced centers.

3.7.7 Renal Transplantation in HUS

- STEC (enteropathic) HUS: risk of graft failure is <1 %, living donor possible, provided family history is negative for aHUS.
- Atypical HUS due to complement regulator deficiency or persistent autoantibody: recurrence risk is high (except for isolated MCP mutation).
- In case of anti-Factor H or anti-ADAMTS13 autoantibodies, transplant may be tried after disappearance of antibodies and clinical quiescence for at least one year. Precautions should be made to treat with PLEX in case of TMA in the graft.
- Combined kidney/liver transplantation has been advocated for patients with genetic factor deficiency. Measures include aggressive peritransplant treatment with plasma exchange and/or complement inhibition.

3.8 Other Inherited Glomerular Diseases

3.8.1 Alport Syndrome

3.8.1.1 Introduction

Alport syndrome is an inherited glomerular disease caused by mutations in genes coding for type IV collagen. It is a progressive form of glomerular disease often associated with sensori-neural deafness and ocular abnormalities.

3.8.1.2 Etiopathogenesis

- The alpha (α) 3, 4, and 5 trimers of type IV collagen are found in the glomerular basement membrane, cochlea, and eye.
- The most common form of Alport syndrome is a mutation in COL4A5 genes located on the X chromosome coding for the alpha 5 chain and accounts for about 80 % of patients with Alport syndrome.

Table 3.22 Renal histopathological changes in Alport syndrome

Light microscopy	Mesangial hypercellularity, matrix expansion, presence of lipid-laden foam cells, irregular thickening of capillary walls, glomerulosclerosis in late stages
Immunofluorescence	No immune deposits IF for collagen type IV α 3,4, and 5 is negative in GBM, depending on inheritance
Electron microscopy	Pathognomonic. Diffuse attenuation of the GBM, splitting, splintering, and "basket weave" pattern of lamina densa, intramembranous vesicles or electron-dense granulations

- Males are severely affected, whereas most females have only hematuria; however, some female carriers may develop renal failure.
- Approximately 15 % of patients with Alport syndrome have autosomal recessive inheritance. They have mutation in either the COL4A3 or COL4A4 genes carried on chromosome 2 coding for alpha 3 or alpha 4 chains.
- The remaining patients are heterozygotes for a mutation in the COL4A3 or COLA4 gene yet may have progressive renal disease.

3.8.1.3 Clinical Features

- The phenotype depends on the genotype and the gender of the patient.
- X linked: persistent microscopic hematuria is seen in almost all patients, both males and females. Gross hematuria is common. Proteinuria and hypertension occur in second decade and progress. End-stage renal disease usually occurs in males by the end of adolescence or early adulthood. Though progression to ESRD is less common and later in females, proteinuria and sensorineural deafness are risk factors for progression.
- Hearing defects: though normal at birth, bilateral symmetric high frequency sensorineural hearing loss occurs in second decade. Hearing loss is less common and later in females.
- Ocular: anterior lenticonus, cataracts, and retinal pigmentation are known associations.
- Rarely: males with X-linked Alport syndrome and female carriers can develop leiomyomas of the esophagus, and female carriers can develop leiomyomas of the genitalia. Platelets with an abnormal number and size have been reported.
- Autosomal recessive: renal manifestations including progression to ESRD are similar to that in X-linked disease. Hearing defects are also known. Males and females are equally affected.
- Family history of hematuria, deafness, and end-stage renal disease should always be asked. Typically mother's male relatives are affected. In about 15 % of cases, there is no family history because the case represents a new COL4A5 mutation or is an autosomal recessive form of Alport syndrome.

3.8.1.4 Laboratory Evaluation

- Urine analysis: proteinuria – usually non-nephrotic range, RBC, RBC casts.
- Serum creatinine, evaluation of renal functions.
- Complement levels – to rule out other diseases.
- Pure tone audiometry and ophthalmological evaluation.
- Renal biopsy: the diagnosis is usually made by a renal biopsy showing thin GBMs with a laminated appearance. This can be confirmed by staining the GBM for the components of type IV collagen. The alpha 5 chain is also present in the epidermal basement membrane. Its absence in a skin biopsy from a male or a mosaic expression in a female by immunostaining with an antibody against the alpha 5 chain is also diagnostic of X-linked Alport syndrome. However, skin basement membrane stains positively in 20 % of affected males. Hence, a positive result does not exclude a diagnosis of Alport syndrome.

- Genetic mutation analysis.
- Family screening.

3.8.1.5 Histopathology

See Table 3.22.

3.8.1.6 Treatment

- ACE inhibitors: currently recommended to preserve renal function in patients with hypertension and/or proteinuria.
- Cyclosporin: calcineurin inhibitors have been tried in few cases aiming to slow progression of renal disease.
- Renal transplantation: First-degree relatives at risk for end-stage renal disease should not be accepted as donors. Alport syndrome does not recur in the graft, but 3–4 % of transplant recipients develop anti-GBM antibodies and a crescentic glomerulonephritis.

3.8.2 Thin Basement Membrane Disease

- Thin basement membrane disease is a histopathological term which includes sporadic and familial cases of hematuria associated with the thinning of basement membrane on electron microscopy.
- The terms thin basement membrane nephropathy and benign familial hematuria are used to describe an autosomal dominant condition with familial microscopic hematuria.
- Heterozygous mutations in the genes COL4A3 or COL4A4 are seen in 40 % cases.
- There is no evidence of proteinuria, hypertension, and progression of renal disease.
- There is no sensorineural hearing loss or ocular defects.
- Renal biopsy: electron microscopy shows diffuse attenuation of the GBM (<200–250 nm) especially at lamina densa.
- No specific treatment is required. Prognosis is excellent. Regular follow-up should be done to detect occurrence of significant proteinuria or hypertension.

Suggested Reading

Ariceta G et al (2009) European Paediatric Study Group for HUS. Guideline for the investigation and initial therapy of diarrhea-negative hemolytic uremic syndrome. Pediatr Nephrol 24:687–696

Benbassat J, Gergawi M, Offringa M, Drukker A (1996) Symptomless microhaematuria in schoolchildren: causes for variable management strategies. QJM 89:845–854

Bergstein J, Leiser J, Andreoli S (2005) The clinical significance of asymptomatic gross and microscopic hematuria in children. Arch Pediatr Adolesc Med 159:353–355

Bolton WK (2000) Treatment of RPGN. Semin Nephrol 3:244–255

Cattran D (2005) Management of membranous nephropathy. When and what for treatment. JASN 16(5):1188–1194

Coppo R, Troyanov S, Camilla R et al (2010) The Oxford IgA nephropathy clinic-pathological classification is valid for children as well as adults. Kidney Int 77:921–927

Dillon MJ, Elefhtheriou D, Brogan PA (2010) Medium vessel vasculitis. PediatrNephrol 25:1641–1652

EdströmHalling S, Söderberg MP, Berg UB (2012) Predictors of outcome in paediatric IgA nephropathy with regard to clinical and histopathological variables (Oxford classification). Nephrol Dial Transplant 27:715–722

Gbadegesin R, Lavin P, Foreman J, Winn M (2011) Pathogenesis and therapy of focal segmental glomerulosclerosis: an update. Pediatr Nephrol 26(7):1001–1015

Gipson DS, Massengill SF, Yao L, Nagaraj S, Smoyer WE, Mahan JD, Wigfall D, Miles P, Powell L, Lin JJ, Trachtman H, Greenbaum LA (2009) Management of childhood onset nephrotic syndrome. Pediatrics 124:747–757

Glassock RJ (2003) Diagnosis of membranous nephropathy. Semin Nephrol 23(4):324–332

Hahn BH et al (2012) American College of Rheumatology guidelines for screening, treatment, and management of lupus nephritis. Arthritis Care Res 64:797–808

Jauhola O, Ronkainen J, Autio-Harmainen H, Koskimies O, Ala-Houhala M, Arikoski P, Hölttä T, Jahnukainen T, Rajantie J, Ormälä T, Nuutinen M (2011) Cyclosporine A vs. methylprednisolone for Henoch-Schönlein nephritis: a randomized trial. Pediatr Nephrol 26:2159–2166

Jauhola O, Ronkainen J, Koskimies O, Ala-Houhala M, Arikoski P, Hölttä T, Jahnukainen T, Rajantie J, Örmälä T, Nuutinen M (2012) Outcome of Henoch-Schönlein purpura 8 years after treatment with a placebo or prednisone at disease onset. Pediatr Nephrol 27:933–939

Jennette JC et al (2012) Revised International Chapel Hill Consensus Conference Nomenclature of Vasculitides. Arthritis Rheumat 2013; 65:1–11

Kanjanabuch T, Kittikowit W, Eiam-Ong S (2009) An update on acute postinfectious glomerulonephritis worldwide. Nat Rev Nephrol 5:259–269

Kashtan C, Ding J, Gregory M, Heidet L, Knebelman B, Rheault M, Licht C (2013) Clinical practice recommendations for the treatment of Alport syndrome: a statement of the Alport Syndrome Research Collaborative. Pediatr Nephrol 28(1):5–11

Kidney Disease: Improving Global Outcomes (2012) KDIGO practice guideline for glomerulonephritis. Kidney Int Suppl 2:

Lombel RM, Gipson DS, Hodson EM (2013a) Treatment of steroid-sensitive nephrotic syndrome: new guidelines from KDIGO. Pediatr Nephrol 28(3):415–426

Lombel RM, Hodson EM, Gipson DS (2013b) Treatment of steroid-resistant nephrotic syndrome in children: new guidelines from KDIGO. Pediatr Nephrol 28(3):409–414

Nakopoulou L (2001) Membranoproliferative glomerulonephritis. Nephrol Dial Transplan 16(6):71–73

Ozen S et al (2010) Paediatric Rheumatology International Trials Organisation (PRINTO). EULAR/PRINTO/PRES criteria for Henoch-Schönlein purpura, childhood polyarteritis nodosa, childhood Wegener granulomatosis and childhood Takayasu arteritis: Ankara 2008. Part II: Final classification criteria. Ann Rheum Dis 69:798–806

Pallan L, Savage CO, Harper L (2009) ANCA associated vasculitis: From bench research to novel treatments. Nat Rev Nephrol 5:278–286

Plank C, Kalb V, Hinkes B, Hildebrandt F, Gefeller O, Rascher W (2008) For Arbeitsgemeinschaft für Pädiatrische Nephrologie. Cyclosporin A is superior to cyclophosphamide in children with steroid-resistant nephrotic syndrome—a randomized controlled multicentre trial by the Arbeitsgemeinschaft für Pädiatrische Nephrologie. Pediatr Nephrol 23:1483–1493

Quigley R (2008) Evaluation of hematuria and proteinuria: how should a pediatrician proceed? Curr Opin Pediatr 20:140–144

Ren P, Han F, Chen L, Xu Y, Wang Y, Chen J (2012) The Combination of Mycophenolate Mofetil with Corticosteroids Induces Remission of Henoch-Schönlein Purpura Nephritis. Am J Nephrol 36:271–277

Tsai HM (2013) Thrombotic thrombocytopenic purpura and the atypical hemolytic uremic syndrome - an update. Hematol Oncol Clin N Am 27:565–584

Tumlin JA, Lohavichan V, Hennigar R (2003) Crescentic, proliferative IgA nephropathy: clinical and histological response to methylprednisolone and intravenous cyclophosphamide. Nephrol Dial Transplant 18:1321–1329

Tune BM, Lieberman E, Mendoza SA (1996) Steroid-resistant nephrotic focal segmental glomerulosclerosis: a treatable disease. Pediatr Nephrol 10:772–778

van Husen M, Kemper MJ (2011) New therapies in steroid-sensitive and steroid-resistant idiopathic nephrotic syndrome. Pediatr Nephrol 26(6):881–892

Weening JJ, D'Agati VD, Schwartz MM, Seshan SV, Alpers CE, Appel GB, Balow JE, Bruijn JA, Cook T, Ferrario F, Fogo AB, Ginzler EM, Hebert L, Hill G, Hill P, Jennette JC, Kong NC, Lesavre P, Lockshin M, Looi LM, Makino H, Moura LA, Nagata M, International Society of Nephrology Working Group on the Classification of Lupus Nephritis, Renal Pathology Society Working Group on the Classification of Lupus Nephritis (2004) The classification of glomerulonephritis in systemic lupus erythematosus revisited. Kidney Int 65:521–530

Wenderfer SE, Swinford RD, Braun MC (2010) C1q nephropathy in the pediatric population: pathology and pathogenesis. Pediatr Nephrol 25:1385–1396

Wong CS, Fink CA, Baechle J, Harris AA, Staples AO, Brandt JR (2009) C1q nephropathy and minimal change nephrotic syndrome. Pediatr Nephrol 24:761–767

Tubular Disorders

4

Paul Goodyer

4.1 An Approach to Renal Tubulopathies

Most renal tubulopathies cause polyuria (>5 mL/kg/h), polydipsia, and failure to thrive in infancy. The excessive urine volume (number of diapers/day) and thirst are often recognized by the parents, especially when they have had unaffected children for comparison. However, urine volumes may decrease when the child is chronically dehydrated and many infants come to attention because of recurrent episodes of vomiting and unexplained fever.

Infants who present with polyuria and growth failure should be investigated for one of the inborn renal tubulopathies that interfere with salt and/or water reabsorption. However, tubular damage secondary to obstructive uropathy, renal dysplasia, acquired tubulointerstitial nephritis, or nephrotoxins should always be considered.

A first-line approach at the time of a clinic visit includes:

1. Urinalysis to rule out pyuria associated with infection or interstitial nephritis
2. Ultrasonography, serum creatinine to rule out urinary tract obstruction, renal dysplasia
3. Obtaining a urine specimen prior to fluid intake in the morning; if osmolality is above 500 mOsm/L or specific gravity is >1.020, the child is unlikely to have tubulopathy causing major loss of solutes and water
4. Taking careful family history (draw pedigree) including prematurity and polyhydramnios
5. Examining child for signs of dehydration, wasting, and rickets
6. Blood and urine samples to check one or more functions in each renal tubular segment, as given below

P. Goodyer
Division of Pediatric Nephrology, Montreal Children's Hospital,
McGill University, 2300, rue Tupper, Montreal, QC H3H 1P3, Canada
e-mail: paul.goodyer@mcgill.ca

K. Phadke et al. (eds.), *Manual of Pediatric Nephrology*,
DOI 10.1007/978-3-642-12483-9_4, © Springer-Verlag Berlin Heidelberg 2014

Proximal tubule dysfunction:
- Generalized amino aciduria
- Proximal renal tubular acidosis
- Phosphaturia (TRP <85 %) when serum phosphate is normal
- Potassium wasting (TTKG >12)
- Low molecular weight proteinuria (e.g., β2-microglobulin)
- Glucosuria (with normal serum glucose)

Thick ascending limb of the loop of Henle:
- FENa >1 %
- Increased plasma renin
- Hypercalciuria

Distal convoluted tubule:
- FENa >1 %
- Increased plasma renin
- Hypocalciuria

Cortical collecting duct Na/H+ exchange:
- Normal anion gap acidosis (serum bicarbonate <21 mmol/L)
- Urine pH > 6 in the face of acidosis
- Positive urine anion gap in the face of acidosis

Cortical collecting duct Na+/K+ exchange:
- Trans-tubular potassium gradient (TTKG > 12 = potassium wasting)

Medullary collecting duct water reabsorption:
- Urine osmolality <150 mOsm/L after 6 h water deprivation

4.2 An Approach to Polyuria

4.2.1 Causes of Polyuria

4.2.1.1 Acquired Dysfunction of Salt/Water Reabsorption

- Obstructive uropathy
- Osmotic diuresis: diabetes mellitus (glucose), mannitol
- Diuretic phase of ATN
- Psychogenic polydipsia
- Tubulointerstitial damage – pyelonephritis, nephronophthisis, sickle cell

4.2.1.2 Hereditary Tubulopathies Affecting Salt Reabsorption

- Cystinosis
- Bartter syndrome
- Gitelman syndrome
- Pseudohypoaldosteronism
- Congenital adrenal hyperplasia
- Renal tubular acidosis

4.2.1.3 Abnormal Production of ADH or Resistance to ADH

- Central diabetes insipidus – deficiency of ADH production
- Nephrogenic diabetes insipidus – genetic mutations of V2 receptors or aquaporin channels; acquired causes (see Sect. 4.3)

4.2.2 Clinical Features

- In the antenatal period, presence of polyhydramnios may be an indicator of fetal polyuria especially in salt-losing states like Bartter syndrome.
- In the neonate and infant, recurrent episodes of fever, dehydration, constipation are common. Failure to thrive is generally seen. Normal urine output in the presence of dehydration is an important clue. Typical facial features may be seen in Bartter syndrome. Rickets may be seen in RTA and chronic kidney disease. Salt craving may be seen in salt-losing states.
- History of nocturia and nocturnal enuresis may be present. Secondary nocturnal enuresis may be seen in conditions like juvenile nephronophthisis. Presence of polyphagia and recent weight loss may give clue to diabetes mellitus.
- Psychogenic polydipsia and diuretic abuse are rare in children.

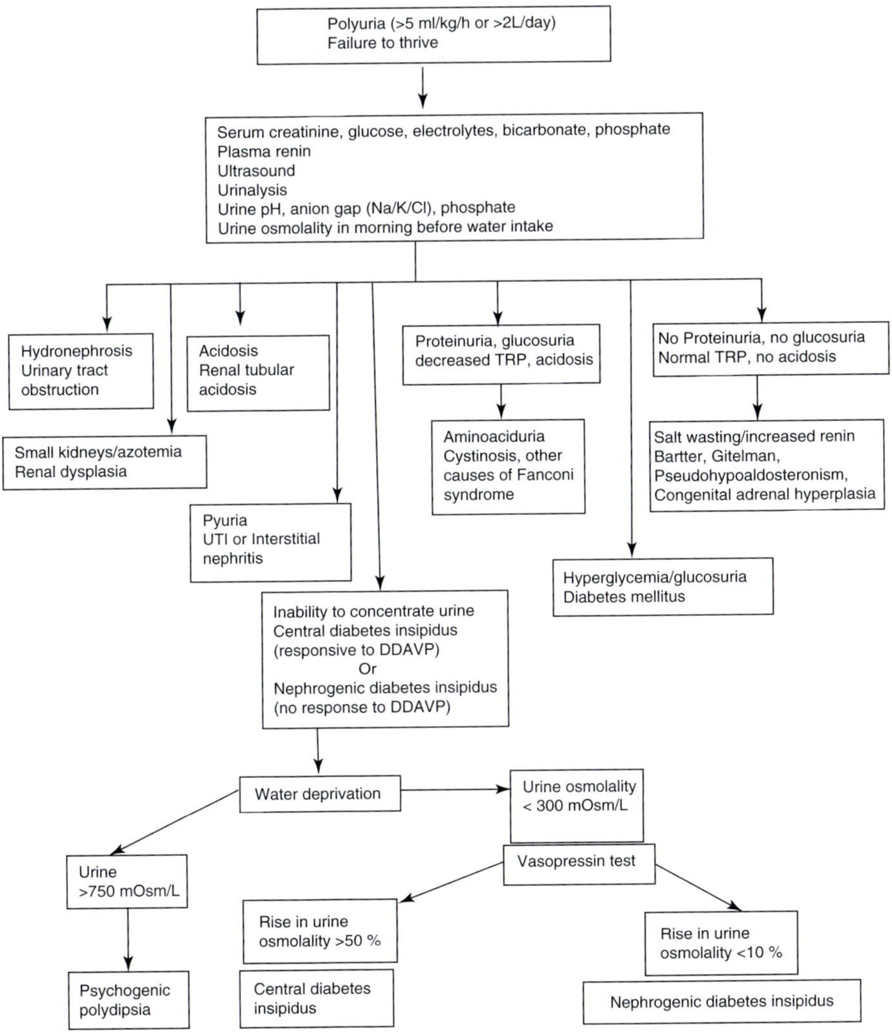

4.3 Diabetes Insipidus

Diabetes insipidus can occur due to

- Deficiency of vasopressin production or release – central diabetes insipidus (DI)
- Resistance to the action of vasopressin at the renal collecting duct – nephrogenic DI

4.3.1 Nephrogenic DI (NDI)

4.3.1.1 Etiology

1. Congenital: more common in children. X-linked recessive inheritance of vasopressin 2 receptor (AVP2) mutations accounts for 90 % of congenital NDI. 10 % may be due to autosomal recessive and autosomal dominant inheritance of mutations in aquaporin 2 receptors.
2. Acquired: the common causes are obstructive uropathy, chronic renal failure, nephrocalcinosis/ hypercalcemia, uric acid nephropathy, sickle cell anemia, analgesic nephropathy, chronic pyelonephritis, chronic hypokalemia, amyloidosis, drugs – lithium, tetracycline.

4.3.1.2 Clinical Presentation

(a) Neonates and infants: recurrent fevers, episodes of dehydration, irritability, seizures, recurrent vomiting, constipation, failure to thrive. Breast-fed infants are less symptomatic as a result of reduced osmolar load. Antenatal polyhydramnios is not a typical feature as the concentrating ability of the fetal kidney is rather immature.

(b) Older children: present with polyuria, polydipsia, nocturia, and enuresis. Hyperactivity, mental retardation, intracranial calcifications (secondary to intracranial bleed due to episodes of hypernatremia) may be seen in severe cases.

(c) Hydroureteronephrosis and megacystis may be seen due to persistent polyuria.

4.3.1.3 Diagnosis

(a) Clinical clues: polyuria despite dehydration is a clue to the diagnosis.

(b) Serum electrolytes: hypernatremia, hyperchloremia, high serum osmolality

(c) Urine osmolality <500 mOsm/kg in a dehydrated child.

(d) Water deprivation and DDAVP test: inability to concentrate urine when subjected to dehydration by water deprivation suggests diabetes insipidus. Failure to increase urine osmolality after intranasal or intravenous administration of DDAVP is typical of NDI (see Sects. 1.5 and 2.2.4).

4.3.1.4 Treatment

(a) Ensure adequate fluid intake.

(b) Low salt diet – to reduce the osmotic load on the tubules. Low protein diet is not recommended in children as it compromises growth.

(c) Hydrochlorothiazide: despite being widely used as a diuretic, thiazides paradoxically reduce polyuria in NDI. Thiazides induce volume contraction by inhibiting distal tubular reabsorption of sodium and hence water. This results in increased proximal reabsorption of sodium and water and reduction in urine output.
Usual dose – 1–2 mg/kg/day in 2 divided doses. Prominent side effects are hypokalemia, hyperlipidemia, hyperuricemia, and hyperglycemia. Amiloride may be concurrently used to reduce hypokalemia.
(d) Indomethacin: inhibits prostaglandins and increases water reabsorption by reducing GFR and by increasing response to vasopressin. Dose 1–3 mg/kg/day in 3–4 divided doses. Common side effects are GI intolerance, bleeding tendency, and deterioration of renal function.
(e) Combination of thiazides, indomethacin, and amiloride is most effective. Close monitoring is required for side effects.

4.3.2 Central Diabetes Insipidus (CDI)

CDI occurs due to absence or deficiency of vasopressin secretion and release. CDI may be seen in critical care unit patients who are brain dead.

4.3.2.1 Etiology

- Genetic – autosomal dominant; syndromic: –associated with holoprosencephaly, septo-optic dysplasia
- Acquired – trauma, following neurosurgery; congenital malformations, tumors – craniopharyngioma, pinealoma, leukemia; infiltrative disorders – tuberculosis, histiocytosis; drugs – phenytoin, opiate antagonists, halothane.
- Brain-dead patient, being worked up for organ donation.

Treatment:

- Desmopressin – vasopressin analogue, available as oral or intranasal preparations
- Following surgery, continuous administration of vasopressin intravenously 1–1.5 mU/kg/h

4.4 Renal Tubular Acidosis

Renal tubular acidosis is a group of disorders resulting from defective reabsorption of bicarbonate or secretion of hydrogen ions or both. Biochemically, it is characterized by hyperchloremia, normal anion gap metabolic acidosis, bicarbonaturia, reduced urinary excretion of titrable acid and ammonia, and elevated urinary pH.

4.4.1 Classification of RTA

(a) Type I: Distal RTA – defect in net H+ excretion
(b) Type II: Proximal RTA – defect in proximal tubular reabsorption of bicarbonate

(c) Type III: A combination of type I and II
(d) Type IV: Secondary to true or apparent hypoaldosteronism

4.4.2 Etiology

4.4.2.1 Distal RTA

- Inability to secrete H+ (secretory defect)
  - Primary
  - Secondary to hypercalciuria, medullary cystic disease, sickle-cell anemia, autoimmune diseases like chronic active hepatitis, SLE; drugs – amphotericin B, analgesics, lithium, mercury; obstructive uropathy, pyelonephritis
- Exchange defect (functional RTA)
  - Hyponatremic states – nephrotic syndrome, cirrhosis, volume depletion
- Gradient defect
  - Amphotericin B
- Voltage defect – also termed as hyperkalemic type 1 RTA

4.4.2.2 Proximal RTA

- Primary – may be autosomal dominant or recessive; associated with mitochondrial myopathies
- Secondary
  - Fanconi syndrome – multiple proximal tubular dysfunctions. Seen in inborn errors of metabolism such as cystinosis, galactosemia, glycogen storage disorder, hereditary fructose intolerance, tyrosinemia, Wilson's disease. Drugs – valproate, ifosfamide, outdated tetracycline, heavy metals
  - Metabolic disorders – Lowe syndrome, osteopetrosis, hyperparathyroidism
  - Miscellaneous – cyanotic heart disease, amyloidosis

4.4.2.3 Type IV RTA

- Primary
- Secondary
  - Aldosterone deficiency – primary – Addison disease, congenital adrenal hyperplasia, pyelonephritis, interstitial nephritis
  - Resistance to action of aldosterone – pseudohypoaldosteronism, chronic tubulointerstitial nephritis, obstructive uropathy; drugs – spironolactone, heparin, NSAIDS, captopril, cyclosporine, tacrolimus

4.4.3 Clinical Features

- Failure to thrive, polyuria, polydipsia, salt craving, refractory rickets are the features common to all types of RTA.
- Hyperchloremic metabolic acidosis with normal GFR, hypokalemia, normal anion gap is seen in proximal and distal RTA. Type IV RTA may have hyperkalemia.
- Severe rickets, severe failure to thrive, organomegaly, cataracts, cystine crystal deposits in the corneas are clues to proximal RTA.

- Nephrocalcinosis and nephrolithiasis are more commonly seen with distal RTA
- May present with muscle weakness, especially involving proximal muscles as a result of hypokalemia.

4.4.4 Investigations

Details of various tests described below are given in Sect. 1.5. Please refer to the algorithm describing an approach to RTA at the end of this chapter

- Urine anion gap: used to differentiate between RTA and diarrhea, both of which cause normal anion gap metabolic acidosis. Urinary anion gap indicates urinary excretion of ammonium. UAG = Na + K − Cl. Normally, it is positive, so also in RTA. It is negative in diarrhea.
- Urine pH: performed on a fresh sample of urine using pH meter. In proximal RTA as the distal acidification is intact, urine pH can be reduced to <5.5. However, in distal RTA, urine pH remains >5.5 despite severe metabolic acidosis.
- Fractional excretion of bicarbonate: >15 % indicates proximal tubular dysfunction resulting in bicarbonaturia.
- Urine to blood CO_2 gradient: In classical distal RTA, as there is a defective urinary excretion of H+, there is a decrease in urinary CO_2 resulting in decreased gradient.
- Acid load test may be used with caution to induce metabolic acidosis in mild cases and then assess the urinary acidification
- Hypocitraturia is typically seen in distal RTA
- TTKG helps in diagnosis of type IV RTA. TTKG <7 in presence of hyperkalemia suggests defective potassium secretion
- Bicarbonate loading test: In the presence of acidosis caused by proximal RTA, the distal tubule can acidify urine to a pH below 5.5 after bicarbonate loading.

4.4.5 Treatment

- Alkali therapy
  - Sodium bicarbonate as tablet (4 meq/tablet) or Shohl solution (1 meq/mL) is administered. The dosage varies from 2 to 4 meq/kg/day in distal RTA to 15–20 meq/kg/day in proximal RTA (see Chap. 17). The dose should maintain serum bicarbonate of 20–22 mmol/L.
  - Citrate may be used as an alkali in the form of potassium citrate in distal RTA
- Potassium supplements may be required in some cases (dose of 1–2 meq/kg/day, preferably as potassium citrate).
- Correction of hypokalemia takes precedence over correction of acidosis.
- In type IV RTA, treatment of hyperkalemia is required. In select cases, mineralocorticoid replacement may be required.
- Regular monitoring of serum bicarbonate, serum potassium as well of growth is required.
- Bony deformities despite correction of metabolic abnormalities may require surgical correction.
- Generally, the treatment of RTA is life long, but the dosage of medications may reduce with increasing age.

4.4.6 Fanconi Syndrome

Disorder is characterized by multiple proximal tubular dysfunctions resulting in hyperchloremic metabolic acidosis, bicarbonaturia, phosphaturia, tubular proteinuria, glycosuria, generalized aminoaciduria.

4.4.6.1 Etiology

Congenital Causes

- Galactosemia, tyrosinemia, mitochondrial myopathies, hereditary fructose intolerance, cystinosis, Lowe syndrome, Fanconi–Bickel syndrome, Dent's disease, Wilson's disease

Acquired Causes

- Drugs: ifosfamide, aminoglycosides, outdated tetracycline, antiretroviral drugs (adefovir, tenofovir), valproate, and toluene
- Heavy metals: lead, cadmium
- Tubulointerstitial nephritis

A description of some conditions such as nephropathic cystinosis appears later in subsequent chapters.

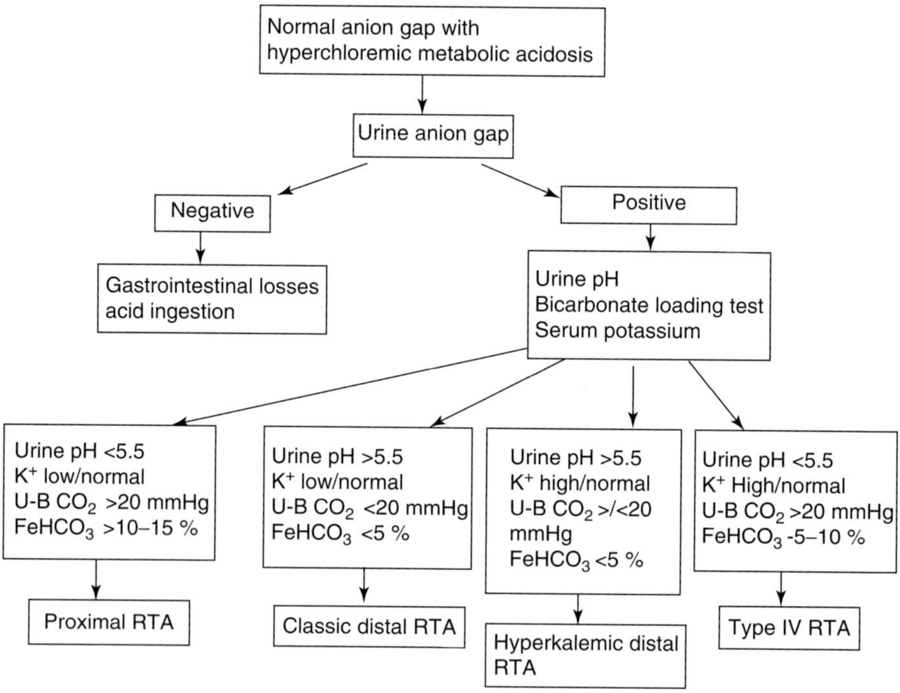

4.5 Bartter and Gitelman Syndrome

4.5.1 Bartter Syndrome

Bartter syndrome is an autosomal recessive disorder characterized by hypokalemic metabolic alkalosis; polyuria; hyperreninemia; hyperaldosteronism; normal blood pressure; urinary wasting of Na^+, K^+, Cl^-; and elevated urinary prostaglandin levels.

Classification of Bartter syndrome and the genetic defects associated are given in Table 4.1.

4.5.1.1 Pathophysiology

Table 4.1 Classification of Bartter syndrome

Disorder	Gene defect	Clinical presentation
Bartter syndrome type I	NKCC2	Perinatal presentation, polyhydramnios, prematurity, hypercalciuria, nephrocalcinosis
Bartter syndrome type II	ROMK	Perinatal presentation, polyhydramnios, prematurity, hypercalciuria, nephrocalcinosis, hyperkalemia in the initial stages
Bartter syndrome type III	ClC–Kb	Onset 0–5 years, failure to thrive, polyuria, polydipsia, salt craving, recurrent dehydration
Bartter syndrome type IV	Barttin	Perinatal presentation, polyhydramnios, prematurity, sensorineural deafness
Bartter syndrome type V	CaSR	Perinatal presentation, polyhydramnios, prematurity, and sensorineural deafness, hypocalcemia

(a) Impaired sodium reabsorption at the TAL/DCT/cortical and medullary collecting duct (TAL, thick ascending limb; DCT, thick convoluted tubule)

(b) TAL: NKCC is a luminal channel responsible for reabsorption of sodium along with chloride and potassium. ROMK is also a luminal channel which recycles the absorbed potassium from the cell back into the lumen. ClC–Ka and Kb are basolateral channels which facilitate the exit of chloride from the cell into the blood. The β subunit of the ClC–K channels is termed Barttin.

(c) Bartter syndrome type V is an autosomal dominant disorder with gain-of-function mutation in the calcium-sensing receptors resulting in hypocalcemia with renal salt wasting.

(d) Digenic mutations of ClC–Ka and ClC–Kb cause perinatal presentation and deafness.

4.5.1.2 Presentation

Characteristic facial features noted are thin triangular face, prominent forehead, protruding eyes, protruding ears.

(a) Features of Bartter syndrome mimic furosemide administration. Hypokalemia is the most prominent feature. Metabolic alkalosis and hypochloremia are the other salient features. These biochemical abnormalities usually present

by 3–6 weeks of age. During early neonatal period, metabolic alkalosis and hypokalemia may not be present, making the diagnosis difficult.
(b) Hypercalciuria and nephrocalcinosis may be seen.
(c) Fractional excretion of Na, K, and Cl is increased. Urinary prostaglandin (PGE2) excretion is also increased. Increased amniotic fluid chloride levels give a clue to the diagnosis in the fetus.
(d) Hyperreninemia and increase in aldosterone levels are seen.
(e) Screening for sensorineural deafness must be performed in all cases.
(f) Genetic analysis: for identification of gene defect and genetic counseling

4.5.1.3 Treatment

(a) Correction of dehydration and electrolyte abnormalities.
(b) Prostaglandin synthesis inhibitors: Indomethacin is generally used. The drug is started at a dose of 0.05 mg/kg/day and gradually increased to 2 mg/kg/day in 3–4 divided doses. Common side effects are GI intolerance, bleeding tendency, and deterioration of renal function. Selective COX2 inhibitors may be used to reduce the side effects. It requires close monitoring for side effects.
(c) Potassium supplements are required to maintain normal serum potassium levels.
Prognosis: Prognosis is poor in neonatal onset type and in those associated with deafness, as there is poor response to therapy and progression to chronic kidney disease.

4.5.2 Gitelman Syndrome

- It is an autosomal recessive disorder with mutation in the gene coding for thiazide-sensitive NaCl cotransporter in the distal convoluted tubule.
- Clinical presentation: age of onset 5–10 years. Features mimic chronic thiazide administration. Usually present with muscle weakness, tetany, polyuria, polydipsia, muscle cramps, salt craving. The clinical presentation is mild compared to Bartter syndrome.
- Biochemical abnormalities include hypokalemia, metabolic alkalosis, hypomagnesemia. Hyperreninism and high aldosterone levels are found.
- Hypomagnesemia, increased urinary magnesium excretion, hypocalciuria, normal urinary excretion of prostaglandins are the features that differentiate it from Bartter syndrome.
- Treatment: magnesium supplements given in the form of magnesium chloride. Rarely, potassium supplements and prostaglandin inhibitors are required.
- Prognosis is good and chronic kidney disease is extremely rare.

4.6 Nephropathic Cystinosis

- It is autosomal recessive disorder characterized by defective lysosomal transport of cystine leading to accumulation of cystine within the lysosomes. Cystine crystals get deposited in cornea, conjunctiva, bone marrow, leucocytes, thyroid, pancreas, and other organs. The cystinosis gene, on chromosome 17p, encodes for a lysosomal protein, cystinosin, presumed to be the cystine transporter. Tubular handling of cystine is normal; there is no cystinuria.

- Usually normal at birth, symptoms begin after 6 months of age. The predominant symptoms are failure to thrive, vomiting, constipation, recurrent dehydration, polyuria, polydipsia, vitamin D-resistant rickets (features of Fanconi syndrome).
- They have no dysmorphic features, but the patients are generally short, have blond hair, fair skin, frontal bossing, and signs of rickets.
- Severe stunting is universal; hypothyroidism is seen in 50 % of patients. Insulin resistance and diabetes develop in 50 % by second decade; delayed puberty is seen.
- Neurological manifestations include bradykinesia, tremors, rigidity, weakness, dysarthria, and dysphagia. There is no mental retardation.
- Visual acuity is normal in young adults. Gradually, haziness, photophobia, corneal erosions, and revascularization result in diminution of vision. Cystine crystal deposits in the cornea. Slit lamp examination confirms the diagnosis. Fundus shows hypopigmented areas.
- Cystine crystals may also be seen on bone marrow or lymph node biopsy. The diagnosis is confirmed by elevated levels of cystine in leucocytes.
- Neutrophils in patients with cystinosis have 50–100 times the normal levels 3–23 nmol half-cystine/mg protein (normal, <0.2). Units of half-cystine are used, because early assays did not distinguish cystine from cysteine. The values in heterozygotes are generally less than 1 nmol half-cystine/mg protein.
- Natural history of disease: progressive renal dysfunction leading to ESRD by end of first decade.
- Treatment: Cysteamine is the specific treatment. It converts cystine to a disulfide and allows transport across lysosomes. It delays progression of renal disease, reduces cystine deposits in organs as well. Cysteamine eye drops prevent the progression of ocular manifestations. Usual dose is 1.3 g/m^2/day in 4 divided doses. The dosage is titrated with the levels of half-cystine. Bad taste and non-compliance to medications are frequently encountered.
- For management of various manifestations of Fanconi syndrome, please refer to Sect. 4.4
- Renal transplantation does not correct the systemic disorder. Postrenal transplantation, cystine continues to accumulate in nonrenal tissues (hypothyroidism, diabetes mellitus, myopathy, cerebral calcifications). Cysteamine treatment needs to be continued to prevent deposits in various organs.

4.7 Hypophosphatemic Rickets

Hypophosphatemia may result as a part of multiple tubular defects affecting proximal renal tubule (as a part of Fanconi syndrome) or due to an isolated tubular defect in phosphate handling. Inherited forms of hypophosphatemic rickets will be described here. The Fanconi syndrome has been discussed in Sect. 4.4.

4.7.1 X-Linked Hypophosphatemic (XLH) Rickets

- X-linked dominant transmission with mutations in the PHEX gene located to region Xp22.1.
- The age of onset is usually after 6–12 months when the child starts walking; lower limb deformities are more prominent. Dental anomalies are typically present.
- Urinary phosphate excretion is high; TMP/GFR is low.
- Serum calcium is low. Inappropriately low levels of 1, 25(OH)$_2$D$_3$ suggest deranges response of renal 1-alpha-hydroxylase to a low phosphate signal. PTH levels are normal. On treatment with phosphates alone (without vitamin D$_3$), PTH values may increase.
- Oral phosphates (30–50 mg/kg/day – 1–3 g elemental phosphorus) divided into 4–6 doses are given in the form of Joules' solution or as neutral phosphate tablets. A higher dose may produce diarrhea. Vitamin D therapy is needed to prevent hyperparathyroidism. Alfacalcidol or 1:25 dihydroxycholecalciferol is given at a dose of 30–70 ng/kg/day (maximum 3 ug/day), monitoring the dose with periodic spot urine calcium creatinine ratios, to prevent hypervitaminosis D. Renal ultrasound should be done periodically and/or PTH to avoid vitamin D excess.
- Patients with inadequate height gain despite good healing of rickets may benefit from growth hormone therapy.

4.7.2 Other Hereditary Forms of Hypophosphatemic Rickets

1. Autosomal dominant: The underlying defect is a mutation in the gene for FGF 23 (fibroblast growth factor).
2. Autosomal recessive: Mutations in DMP1 (dentin matrix protein) result in this form.
3. Hereditary hypophosphatemic rickets with hypercalciuria (HHRH): Mutations in the gene SLC34A3; 1, 25(OH)$_2$D$_3$ levels are high resulting in hypercalciuria and nephrocalcinosis. Phosphate supplements are given; vitamin D should not be used.
4. Dent's disease: Mutations in CLCN5, low molecular weight tubular proteinuria, phosphaturia, hypercalciuria, nephrocalcinosis, progressive worsening of renal functions, X-linked recessive transmission.

4.8 Primary Hyperoxaluria (PH)

Primary hyperoxaluria is characterized by increased urinary excretion of oxalates that results in renal stone disease as well as extrarenal manifestations

4.8.1 Primary Hyperoxaluria (PH) Type 1

An autosomal recessive disorder caused by a defect in hepatic peroxisomal pyridoxal phosphate-dependent enzyme alanine glyoxylate aminotransferase (AGT).

- Most common type (80–90 %) of primary hyperoxaluria.
- Clinical presentation
  - Infantile: early nephrocalcinosis, rapid development of renal failure
  - Childhood onset: usual onset by the age of 5 years
  - Adult onset: present with recurrent renal calculi
  - Recurrence in transplanted kidney
- Renal manifestations: loin pain, hematuria, urinary tract infection, renal calculi, nephrocalcinosis, chronic kidney disease
- Renal failure occurs by the third decade, except in infantile onset, where it may be seen in 80 % by 3 years of age.
- Extrarenal manifestations (oxalosis): Extrarenal deposition begins when GFR reduces and urinary excretion of oxalate decreases. Affects bone (bone pains, oxalate deposits in the bones appear as dense metaphyseal bands, erythropoietin-resistant anemia), joints (pain, synovitis), heart (cardiomyopathy, arrhythmias), nerves (polyneuritis), skin (calcinosis cutis, gangrene).
- Diagnosis
  - Clinical presentation, family history
  - Stone analysis: calcium oxalate monohydrate
  - 24-h urine analysis for oxalates
  - Freshly frozen liver biopsy for assessment of AGT activity
  - Sequencing of AGXT gene
- Management
  - Adequate hydration to keep the urine concentration of calcium and oxalate low
  - Inhibitors of crystallization: urinary alkalinization using citrate, sodium bicarbonate aiming at urine pH >7
  - Reduced intake of oxalate-rich foods like roots, spinach, peanuts, coffee, cocoa
  - In patients responsive to pyridoxine, high doses (2–5 mg/kg/day) may delay progression to ESRD
  - Dialysis: oxalate clearance is poor by conventional dialysis; hence, daily dialysis with high flux membrane may be ideal
  - Transplantation- isolated renal transplantation is not recommended as it carries high risk of graft loss due to recurrence of disease. Combined liver and renal transplantation is the treatment of choice.

4.8.2 Type 2 Hyperoxaluria

- Characterized by the absence of glyoxylate reductase, hydroxypyruvate reductase, and d-glycerate dehydrogenase activity

- Normal AGT activity
- Autosomal recessive
- Clinical features: onset by 1–2 years, presents with recurrent calculi, hematuria, obstruction. Less severe than type 1 hyperoxaluria
- Progresses to ESRD by fourth to fifth decade.
- Treatment is the same as for type 1 hyperoxaluria. There is no role for the use of pyridoxine.

4.9 Miscellaneous Tubular Disorders

4.9.1 Pseudohypoaldosteronism

- A disorder characterized by renal tubular unresponsiveness to aldosterone.
- Hyponatremia, hyperkalemia, metabolic acidosis, and high aldosterone levels are the characteristic metabolic abnormalities. A close differential diagnosis is congenital adrenal hyperplasia.
- High urine sodium and low urine potassium are common to all types.
- Systemic type 1 PHA is refractory to salt supplementation and carries a poor prognosis (Table 4.2).

4.9.2 Cystinuria

Cystinuria is due to a genetic defect in the transporter for cystine, ornithine, arginine and lysine in the renal proximal tubule and small intestine.

- Genetics: Recessive mutations of SLC3A1(Ucystine normal in parents) or incompletely dominant mutations of SLC7A9 (Ucystine moderately elevated in parents).
- Low solubility of cystine in acidic urine results in stone formation
- Clinical features: Present in first to third decade with renal calculi, colic, UTI, obstruction.
- Diagnosis: stones are radiopaque, may be staghorn. Urine shows flat hexagonal crystals which precipitate by acidification. Cyanide nitroprusside test may be a screening test and confirmation requires chromatography.
- Treatment includes good hydration, oral alkali therapy – citrate or bicarbonate. Reduction of oral intake of methionine (precursor of cystine) is not recommended in children.
- L-Glutamine (oral or intravenous), D-penicillamine, mercaptopropionyl glycine can be tried in severe cases but require close follow-up for complications.

Table 4.2 Types of Pseudohypoaldosteronism

Types	Mode of inheritance and mutation	Clinical features	Investigations	Treatment
Renal limited type 1	Autosomal dominant Mineralocorticoid receptor mutation	Most common. Infantile onset: failure to thrive, polyuria, dehydration, vomiting	High renin and aldosterone levels	Salt supplements
Systemic type 1	Autosomal recessive Loss of function mutation of epithelial sodium channels	Severe salt wasting, recurrent lung infections	Similar to above	Salt supplements, potassium binding resins
Type 2 Gordon syndrome	Autosomal dominant Gene for WNK1&4	Present with short stature, hypertension	Low renin, normal/low aldosterone	Furosemide, thiazides
Type 3	Acquired: reflux nephropathy, sickle cell disease, amyloidosis	Failure to thrive, salt wasting	High renin, high aldosterone	Salt supplements

4.9.3 Lowe Syndrome

Also known as oculocerebrorenal syndrome (OCRL). It is characterized by facial dysmorphism, ocular abnormalities (cataract, strabismus, and glaucoma), neurological involvement (hypotonia, hyporeflexia, psychomotor retardation, behavioral abnormalities), and renal involvement. Fanconi syndrome is noted during early infancy. Low molecular weight proteinuria is often severe and may cause nephrotic syndrome. Renal function deteriorates in second decade of life. It is transmitted as X-linked recessive, caused by a mutation in the gene OCRL1, and located on chromosome Xq26.1. Treatment is symptomatic.

4.10 Tubulointerstitial Nephritis

Tubulointerstitial nephritis is characterized by inflammation of the tubulointerstitium without significant glomerular or vascular involvement. It may be acute or chronic.

4.10.1 Acute Tubulointerstitial Nephritis (Acute TIN)

4.10.1.1 Etiology

1. Drug induced: due to β lactam antibiotics, sulfonamides, fluoroquinolones, rifampicin, NSAIDs, diuretics, proton pump inhibitors
2. Infection: Bacterial – *Leptospira*, *Mycobacteria*, *Streptococci*, *Salmonella typhi*, *Mycoplasma*
   Viral – Epstein Barr virus, Hepatitis B virus, HIV, cytomegalovirus, measles, Hanta virus, BK polyoma virus
   Rickettsiae, fungi, parasites are also implicated.
3. Immune mediated:
   (i) Associated with glomerulonephritis – IgA nephropathy, membranous nephritis, lupus nephritis
   (ii) Not associated with glomerular disease – Allograft rejection, TINU (tubulointerstitial nephritis with uveitis) syndrome – may be seen in SLE, sarcoidosis, Sjogren syndrome, Wegener's granulomatosis, Behcet's disease
   (iii) Infections (tuberculosis, brucellosis, toxoplasmosis, EBV, HIV, chlamydia)
4. Idiopathic

4.10.1.2 Clinical Presentation

(a) Renal manifestations. Variable degree of renal dysfunction may be present.
   - Acute kidney injury: The period of onset is variable, ranging from few days to 2 months. The absence of oliguria, significant edema, significant proteinuria, RBC casts, and hypertension helps to differentiate from acute glomerulonephritis.
   - Tubulopathy: Hyperchloremic metabolic acidosis, glycosuria, phosphaturia, proteinuria, hypokalemia suggest proximal tubular dysfunction; polyuria,

hyperkalemia, hypomagnesemia suggest distal tubular dysfunction; polyuria with hypernatremia suggests collecting duct dysfunction

(b) Extrarenal manifestations
- Fever, rash, arthralgia, anorexia, flank pain, vomiting are nonspecific symptoms.
- Systemic features relevant to the infection or immunological disorder.
- Signs of uveitis in patients with TINU syndrome.

4.10.1.3 Investigations

(a) Urinalysis: Proteinuria (<1 g/day), RBC, WBC. Eosinophiluria (urine eosinophils >1 % by Wright/Hansel stain) is seen typically in drug-induced TIN. Granular, hyaline, and WBC casts may be seen. RBC casts are rare.
(b) Tubular dysfunction if present: hyposthenuria, glycosuria, aminoaciduria, bicarbonaturia, phosphaturia, and magnesium loss.
(c) Normocytic, normochromic anemia, leucocytosis, peripheral eosinophilia, high ESR, elevated liver enzymes may be seen with drug-induced TIN.
(d) Ultrasound may show normal or enlarged kidneys with increased echogenicity.
(e) Increased gallium uptake is a sensitive test
(f) Histopathological evaluation by renal biopsy showing mononuclear infiltration (eosinophils in drug-induced ATN) in the interstitium with edema confirms the diagnosis.
(g) Typical features which may help in diagnosis of NSAID-induced tubule interstitial nephritis: onset within days to months, edema, nephrotic range proteinuria, urine eosinophils >1 %.

4.10.1.4 Treatment

(a) Supportive treatment: Stopping the suspected causative drug, treatment of the associated systemic infection is the first step in treatment.
(b) Use of corticosteroids – prednisolone 2 mg/kg/day rapidly tapered over 2–4 weeks, pulses of methylprednisolone followed by oral steroids have been used. However, there are no studies or recommendations which show a proven benefit with the use of steroids.
(c) Dialysis may be indicated in severe cases.

4.10.1.5 Prognosis

Recovery of renal function is excellent. Poor prognostic factors are presence of severe interstitial inflammation on biopsy, duration of acute kidney injury, and peak serum creatinine levels.

4.10.2 Chronic Tubulointerstitial Nephritis

4.10.2.1 Etiology

(a) Inherited renal disease: nephronophthisis, cystic renal disease, cystinosis, oxalosis, Alport syndrome, sickle cell disease, Wilson's disease

(b) Drugs and toxins: heavy metals such as lead, arsenic, cadmium, mercury; drugs such as NSAIDs, lithium, calcineurin inhibitors, cisplatin
(c) Structural renal disease: reflux nephropathy, renal dysplasia, obstructive uropathy
(d) Metabolic: hypercalciuria, hyperuricemia, hypokalemia, hyperoxaluria
(e) Immune mediated:
    1. Associated with glomerulonephritis – SLE, anti-GBM antibody disease, polyarteritis nodosa, Wegener's granulomatosis
    2. Not associated with glomerulonephritis – allograft rejection, chronic active hepatitis
(f) Radiation induced

4.10.2.2 Clinical Features

Nonspecific symptoms – weight loss, anorexia, nausea, vomiting, growth failure, occasionally polyuria and polydipsia. Hypertension may be present but is less pronounced than in glomerular disease. Anemia and bone disease may be disproportionate to the degree of renal dysfunction.

4.10.2.3 Treatment and Prognosis

- Conservative treatment of chronic kidney disease (described in Chapter 9).
- Treatment of the primary illness.
- Prognosis depends on presence of comorbidities such as hypertension, anemia, obesity, and dyslipidemia.

Suggested Reading

Brinkert F, Ganschow R, Helmke K, Harps E, Fischer L, Nashan B, Hoppe B, Kulke S, Müller-Wiefel DE, Kemper MJ (2009) Transplantation procedures in children with primary hyperoxaluria type 1: outcome and longitudinal growth. Transplantation 87:1415–1421

Cochat P, Liutkus A, Fargue S, Basmaison O, Ranchin B, Rolland MO (2006) Primary hyperoxaluria type 1: still challenging! Pediatr Nephrol 21:1075–1081

Kleta R, Bockenhauer D (2006) Bartter syndromes and other salt-losing tubulopathies. Nephron Physiol 104:73–80

Nesterova G, Gahl WA (2013) Cystinosis: the evolution of a treatable disease. Pediatr Nephrol 28:51–59

Wilmer MJ, Schoeber JP, van den Heuvel LP, Levtchenko EN (2011) Cystinosis: practical tools for diagnosis and treatment. Pediatr Nephrol 26:205–215

Cystic Renal Diseases

5

Indra Gupta and Martin Bitzan

5.1 Definitions

- A cyst is an epithelium-lined cavity filled with fluid. Cysts in the kidney may be inherited or acquired.
- Most true renal cysts originate from tubules.
- Genetically characterized forms of cystic kidney disease all involve mutations in a critical organelle for maintenance of epithelial cell polarity, the cilium.
- Primary cilia are (usually) nonmotile and serve as sensory organelles.
- Proteins mutated in renal cystic diseases are localized to primary cilia, basal bodies (the anchor for the cilium), or centrosomes (organelle that functions as microtubule organizing center and regulator of cell cycle progression).

5.2 Introduction

Renal cysts are found in varied congenital, hereditary, and acquired kidney diseases and occur with physiological aging. It is important to differentiate between simple unilateral or bilateral renal cysts; nonfunctioning, multicystic, dysplastic kidneys; and cystic diseases that lead to progressive deterioration of

I. Gupta (✉) • M. Bitzan
Division of Pediatric Nephrology,
Montreal Children's Hospital,
McGill University,
2300, rue Tupper, Montreal,
QC H3H 1P3, Canada
e-mail: indra.gupta@muhc.mcgill.ca; martin.bitzan@mcgill.ca

K. Phadke et al. (eds.), *Manual of Pediatric Nephrology*,
DOI 10.1007/978-3-642-12483-9_5, © Springer-Verlag Berlin Heidelberg 2014

kidney function and eventual end-stage renal failure (ESRD) due to loss of functional renal tissue (polycystic kidney diseases) or as part of multisystem disorders or syndromes with important nonrenal manifestations. A classification of cystic renal diseases is given in Table 5.1. Medically important cystic kidney diseases are those that progress to ESRD. The term glomerulocystic kidney (GCK), referring primarily to significant dilatations of Bowman's capsule, is used for a wide variety of conditions, including forms of PKD, hereditary forms, and various obstructive, vascular, and unilateral or bilateral malformations. See Fig. 5.1 for a general diagnostic approach to cystic renal disease. The remainder of the chapter discusses important forms of cystic renal diseases in childhood and adolescence.

Table 5.1 Classification of renal cystic diseases

Heredity	Mode of inheritance	Disease
Hereditary	Autosomal dominant	ADPKD
		Tuberous sclerosis
		Von Hippel-Lindau disease
		Renal cysts and diabetes syndrome (RCAD)
		Medullary cystic disease
	Autosomal recessive	ARPKD
		Nephronophthisis
		Meckel-Gruber syndrome
		Bardet-Biedl syndrome
		Zellweger syndrome
	X-linked	Orofaciodigital syndrome
	Chromosomal abnormalities	Aneuploidy
Nonhereditary	Acquired	Simple cysts
		Acquired renal cysts (chronic renal failure)
		Hypokalemia
	Congenital (without known genetic association)	Multicystic dysplasia
		Medullary sponge kidney

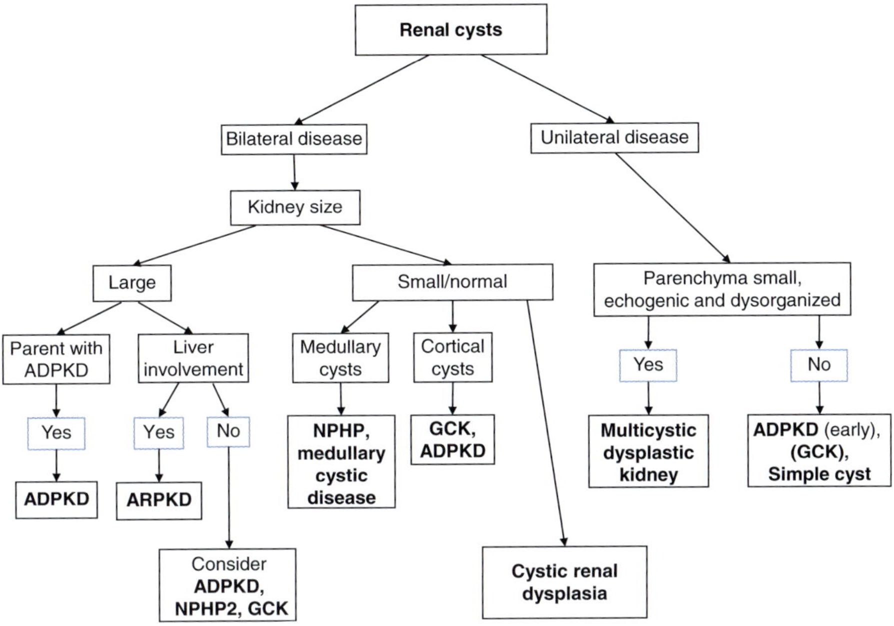

Fig. 5.1 Algorithmic approach to the diagnosis of cystic kidney diseases, based on ultrasound imaging. *Abbreviations*: *ADPKD* autosomal dominant polycystic kidney disease, *ARPKD* autosomal recessive polycystic kidney disease, *GCK* glomerulocystic kidney, *NPHP* nephronophthisis

5.3 Autosomal Dominant Polycystic Kidney Disease (ADPKD)

- Most common inherited kidney disease.
- Incidence – 1 in 1,000.
- Mutations in *PKD1* (85 %) and *PKD2* (15 %) on chromosomes 16p13.3-p13.12 and 4q21-q23, respectively, encoding polycystin 1 (PC1) and 2 (PC2).
- PC1 senses nephron and collecting duct urine flow via the N-terminus of the protein, and PC2 responds to urine flow by generating calcium influx via the cilium of the renal tubular epithelial cell.
- Cysts arise from any segment of the nephron.
- Variable phenotype – even within a family:
  - Antenatal ultrasound – large kidneys with or without cysts.
  - In children, ADPKD may be detected incidentally or because of screening at any age including neonates. Symptoms are rare during childhood. Occasionally, patients may present with abdominal/flank pain, palpable abdominal mass, gross/microscopic hematuria, a urine concentrating defect, urinary tract infections (UTI), hypertension, or nephrolithiasis.

- Adults may be asymptomatic, with cysts being incidentally detected by ultrasound.
- Chronic kidney failure occurs in 60–70 %, usually by the sixth decade of life.

5.3.1 Extrarenal Manifestations

- Commonly seen in adults.
- Cerebral aneurysms; cysts in liver, pancreas, and ovary; cardiac valvular disease (mitral valve prolapse); and colonic diverticula, abdominal wall and inguinal hernias are commonly associated.
- A ruptured cerebral aneurysm is the most serious extrarenal complication.
- The use of routine screening for cerebral aneurysm is controversial but may be indicated for those patients with a previous rupture, a family history of intracranial aneurysm, or overt warning symptoms such as a severe headache.

5.3.2 Diagnosis

- Diagnosis is relatively straightforward in the symptomatic patient with a positive family history (Table 5.2).
- Clinical criteria to differentiate between ADPKD and ARPKD are listed in Table 5.3.
- Ultrasound typically shows enlarged kidneys with multiple bilateral cysts (Fig. 5.2, panels **b** and **d**).

Table 5.2 Diagnostic criteria for ADPKD

Positive family history with autosomal dominant pattern
Ultrasound screening of parents may be positive
Enlarged kidneys with multiple bilateral renal cysts (ultrasound or CT scan) and a positive family history
Age <30 years
≥2 renal cysts (unilateral/bilateral)
Age 30–59 years
≥2 renal cysts in each kidney
Age >60 years
≥4 renal cysts in each kidney

Table 5.3 Differentiation between ARPKD and ADPKD (see also Fig. 5.2)

Features suggesting ARPKD	Features suggesting ADPKD
Neonatal onset	Asymptomatic presentation
Progression to ESRD in childhood	Unilateral/bilateral presentation
Hepatosplenomegaly	Hematuria, UTI
Portal hypertension	Extrarenal cysts
Negative family history	Positive family history

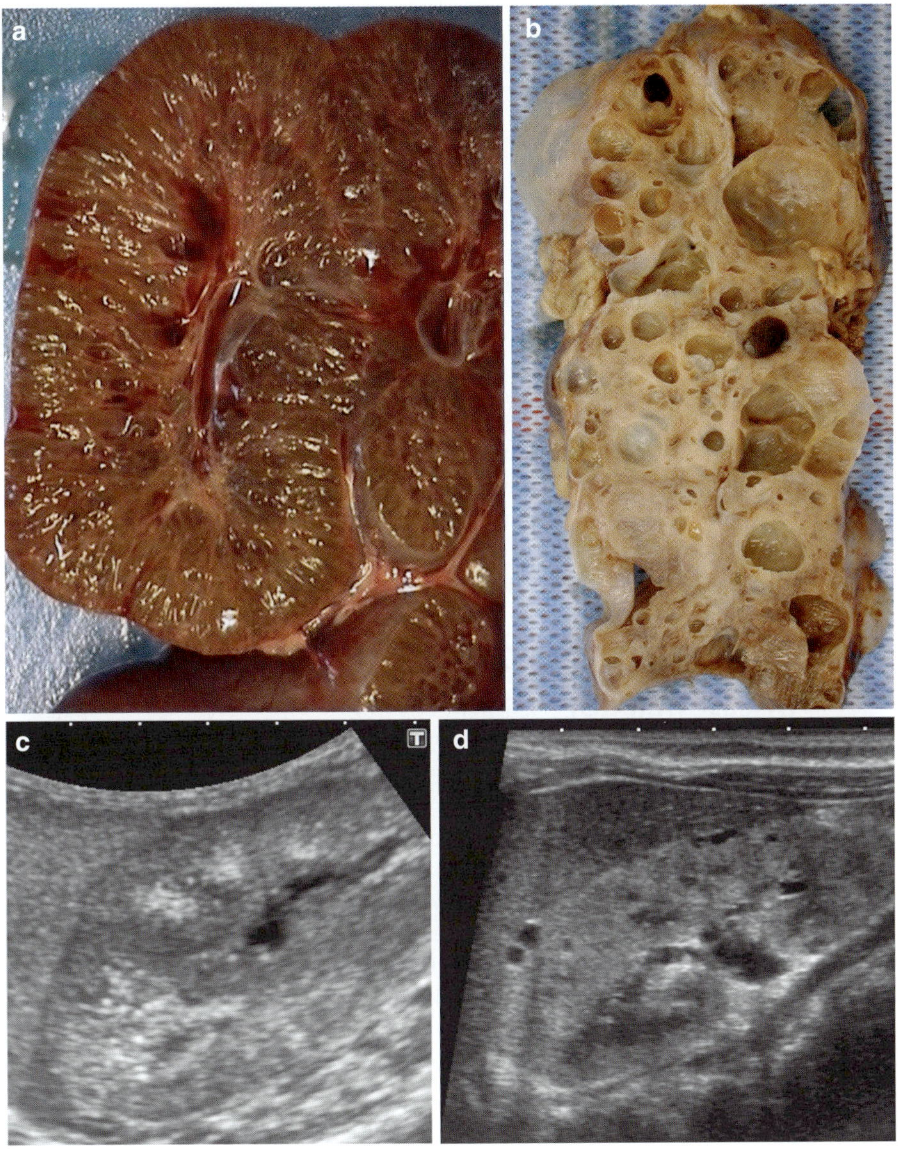

Fig. 5.2 ARPKD (**a**, **c**) and infantile ADPKD (**b**, **d**) – pathology and ultrasound comparison. (c) Ultrasound of the right kidney of a 3-day-old infant with ARPKD (for details see Fig. 5.3). (d) Ultrasound of the right kidney of a 1-month-old infant with suspected congenital ADPKD (bilaterally increased echogenicity with partially preserved corticomedullary differentiation. Numerous parenchymal cysts in the cortex and some in the medulla, measuring 1–5 mm. Kidney length was 5.4 cm on the right and 6.1 cm on the left). Scale bar (cm) on top of the ultrasound images

- Without positive family history, there is no age or cyst number threshold to rule in or rule out the disease.
- Negative ultrasound results do not exclude ADPKD until the fourth decade of life.

5.3.3 Family Screening

- Screening of parents of index case or grandparents, if parents younger than 30 years.

5.3.4 Patient Monitoring

- If asymptomatic, US screening every 5 years; more frequently once symptomatic.
- Annual BP and urinalysis (proteinuria).
- Routine screening for intracranial aneurysms is not recommended.

5.3.5 Treatment

- No specific treatment. Vasopressin 2 receptor antagonists (e.g., tolvaptan) and mTOR inhibitors (mammalian inhibitors of rapamycin) have shown minor or disappointing effects in clinical trials.
- ACE inhibitors or ARB for hypertension and proteinuria.
- Consider generous water intake to suppress systemic and local levels of vasopressin; vasopressin is believed to contribute to cyst formation.

5.4 Autosomal Recessive Polycystic Kidney Disease (ARPKD)

- Incidence: 1 in 10,000–40,000.
- Genetic defect in *PKHD1* (on chromosome 6p21) encoding fibrocystin.
- Cysts usually arise from the collecting duct.
- Clinical presentation is variable (Tables 5.3 and 5.4).
  - Neonatal onset: majority of patients with ARPKD present in infancy. Antenatal ultrasound may show enlarged kidneys with loss of corticomedullary differentiation and oligohydramnios. Newborns may have a Potter phenotype with large palpable flank masses and pulmonary hypoplasia, renal insufficiency, and severe hypertension.
  - Death in neonatal period usually due to pulmonary complications as opposed to renal insufficiency.
  - Older children may present with hypertension, polyuria, renal dysfunction, and recurrent UTI.

Table 5.4 Diagnostic criteria for ARPKD

Ultrasound features
Enlarged, echogenic kidneys with poor corticomedullary differentiation. Cysts are usually small and only visualized by high-resolution ultrasound (Figs. 5.2 and 5.3)
One or more of the following
(a) Absence of renal cysts in both parents if evaluated after 30 years of age
(b) Clinical, laboratory, or radiographic evidence of hepatic fibrosis
(c) Hepatic pathology demonstrating characteristic ductal plate abnormality
(d) Previous affected sibling with pathologically confirmed disease
(e) Parental consanguinity suggestive of autosomal recessive inheritance

– Chronic renal failure occurs early. Patients who are diagnosed later in life are more likely to present with signs and symptoms of liver/biliary tract disease: hepatosplenomegaly, hypersplenism, variceal bleeding, and cholangitis (Table 5.4).

5.4.1 Extrarenal Manifestations

- Liver involvement is overt in 50–60 %. Microscopic abnormalities are detected by liver biopsy in 100 %. Congenital hepatic fibrosis may present with hepatomegaly and portal hypertension. Histopathology shows ductal plate abnormalities.
- Choledochal cysts. Subset of patients with overt biliary duct dilatation (Caroli's disease; see Fig. 5.3b).
- Hypersplenism, esophageal varices, and cholangitis may complicate liver disease.

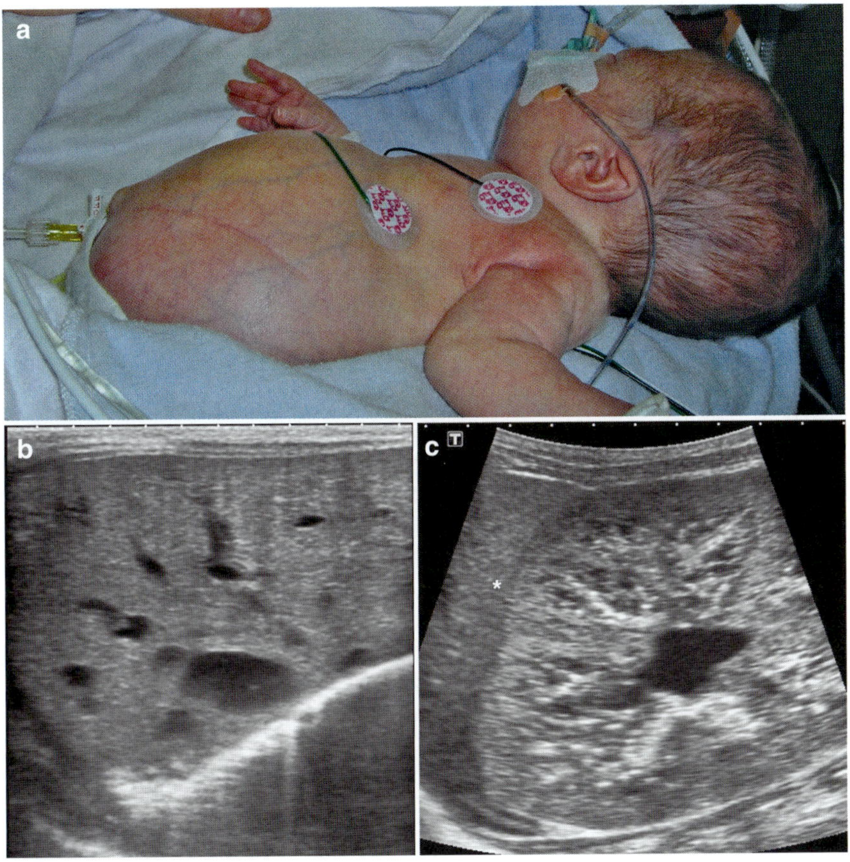

Fig. 5.3 Infant with ARPKD. (**a**) Protruding abdomen due to hugely enlarged kidneys. Ultrasound images on the third day of life. (**b**) Liver shows dilatation of the intrahepatic biliary tree with cystic components (Caroli type of appearance). (**c**) Right kidney: bilateral loss of corticomedullary differentiation; the renal parenchymal echogenicity exceeds that of the liver located cephalad (to the *left*) of the kidney (*); multiple tiny cysts of 1–2 mm diameter are seen throughout the renal parenchyma. The right kidney measured 7.4 cm and the left kidney 8.1 cm. Scale bar at the top of the ultrasound images (dots at 1 cm intervals)

5.4.2 Treatment

- No specific treatment. Vasopressin receptor antagonists, tyrosine kinase inhibitors, rapamycin, and octreotide hold some promise.
- Control of hypertension.

5.4.3 Monitoring

- Yearly ultrasound for hepatic and splenic size
- Endoscopic evaluation of esophageal varices
- Monitoring of hematological parameters

5.5 Nephronophthisis (NPHP)

- NPHP is the most common genetic cause of ESRD during childhood and adolescence.
- It is related to mutations in at least 13 genes (Table 5.5).
- All NPHP genes express proteins related to the function or structure of ubiquitously expressed cilia, hence the multiorgan involvement of NPHP-related diseases.
- The range of disease manifestations and severity is related to gene locus heterogeneity, allelism, and the impact of modifier genes.
- Inheritance, including NPHP variants with extrarenal abnormalities, is autosomal recessive.
- NPHP is caused by genetic defects in *NPHP1* (nephrocystin-1), *NPHP2* (inversin), or *NPHP3* which encode the nephrocystin family of proteins.
- Classified as infantile NPHP (NPHP type 2; ESRD usually occurs between 1 and 3 years of age), juvenile NPHP (NPHP type 1; ESRD around 13 years of age), and adolescent NPHP (NPHP type 3; ESRD around 19 years *of age*).
- Infantile, juvenile and adolescent forms are commonly due to mutations in *NPHP2*, *NPHP1* and *NPHP3* respectively. Juvenile onset is the most common.
- The clinical spectrum of NPHP includes the syndromic cerebello-ocular-renal disorders like Senior-Løken syndrome (NPHP types 4, 5, or 6), Joubert syndrome (NPHP types 6 and 8), Bardet-Biedl syndrome, and Meckel-Gruber syndrome (NPHP types 6 and 8) (Table 5.5).
- The frequencies of mutations identified in a worldwide cohort study of >1,000 patients with NPHP were 21 % for *NPHP1*, 3 % for *NPHP5*, and 2 % or less for the remainder, including *NPHP2* (1 %). No mutations were identified in 70 %.
- Genetic testing:
  - Juvenile NPHP (type 1) can generally be diagnosed clinically, including age of renal function impairment and ultrasound morphology.
  - Figure 5.4 describes a targeted approach to genotyping for patients with suspected NPHP.
  - Laboratories and available genetic testing are found in the GeneTest™ website: http://www.ncbi.nlm.nih.gov/sites/GeneTests/review/disease/nephronophthisis?db=genetests&search_param=contains

Table 5.5 Association between nephronophthisis types, gene mutations, ESRD onset, and extrarenal manifestations

NPHP type	Gene (gene product)	Median age at onset of ESRD (years)	Extrarenal manifestations
Type 1 (juvenile)	*NPHP1* NPHP1, nephrocystin-1	13	Subsets with SLS, OMA, JS, MKS
Type 2 (infantile)	*NPHP9/INVERSIN* NPHP2, inversin	1–3	SLS, VSD, situs inversus
Type 3 (adolescent)	*NPHP3* NPHP3, nephrocystin-3	19	SL, liver fibrosis[a]
Type 4	*NPHP4* NPHP4, nephroretinin	20	SLS
Type 5 (early onset SL)	*NPHP5/IQCB1* Nephrocystin 5/IQ motif containing B1[b]	13	SLS
Type 6	*NPHP6/CEP290* NPHP6, centrosomal protein 290 (Cep290)	<13	SLS, JS, MKS
Type 7	*NPHP7/GLIS2* GLI-similar family zinc finger 2	17	ND
Type 8	*NPHP8/RPGRIP1L* NPHP8, RPGRIP1-like	<13	JS, MKS
Type 9	*NPHP9/NEK8* NPHP9-(NIIMA-) related kinase	13	ND
Type 10	*NPHP10*	Juvenile	Renal and eye, occasional additional organ involvement (CNS, obesity, hypogenitalism)
Type 11 NPHP with liver fibrosis	*MKS3/TMEM67* Meckelin, transmembrane protein 67	9 (<14)	JS, ocular involvement[c]
Type 12	*AHI1/JBTS3* Jouberin	Juvenile	JS with or without NPHP
Type 13	*CC2D2A/JBTS9* Coiled coil and C2 domain containing 2A	ND	Dysplastic renal phenotypes, including infantile NPHP; CNS, liver, and bone involvement

Modified from Hurd TW and Hildebrandt F: Mechanisms of nephronophthisis and related ciliopathies. Nephron Exp Nephrol 2011; 118: e9–e14; and Salomon R et al. Nephronophthisis. Pediatr Nephrol 2009; 24: 2333–2344

Abbreviations: *ESRD* end-stage renal disease, *JS* Joubert syndrome, *MKS* Meckel-Gruber syndrome, *OMA* oculomotor apraxia-type Cogan, *SLS* Senior-Løken syndrome: juvenile NPHP with Leber amaurosis, *ND* not defined/unknown. *MKS*, *JS*, and *NPHP* (can be caused by mutations in the same gene locus)

[a]NPHP3 mutations can cause a broad clinical spectrum of early embryonic patterning defects comprising situs inversus, polydactyly, central nervous system malformations, structural heart defects, preauricular fistulas, and a wide range of congenital anomalies of the kidney and urinary tract (CAKUT)

[b]NPHP5 is in complex with retinitis pigmentosa GTPase regulator (RPGR) and localized in connecting cilia of photoreceptors and in primary cilia of renal epithelial cells

[c]Retinal coloboma, retinal degeneration, oculomotor disorders

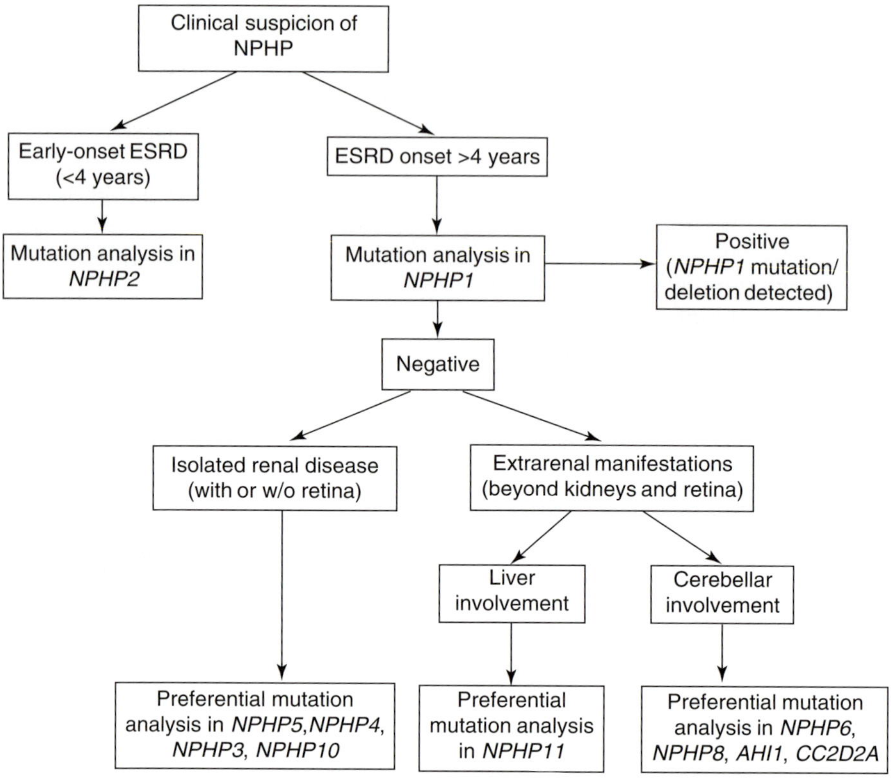

Fig. 5.4 Algorithm for genotyping in NPHP (Modified from Chaki M et al. Kidney Int 2011; 80: 1239–1245)

5.5.1 NPHP Type 1

- Most common type of nephronophthisis
- Clinical features of NPHP type 1:
  - Insidious onset of chronic kidney disease leading to ESRD by the second decade.
  - Polyuria, polydipsia, secondary enuresis are common.
  - Failure to thrive, growth failure.
  - Severe anemia.
  - Hypertension is rare.
  - Ultrasound shows normal-sized kidneys which are echogenic with small cortical cysts.
- Renal biopsy
  - Characteristic, but nonspecific findings: glomerular sclerosis, tubular atrophy, marked interstitial fibrosis, dilation primarily of distal tubules and collecting ducts, often containing Tamm-Horsfall protein, tubular basement membrane alterations

- Extrarenal manifestations
  - Associated with retinitis pigmentosa in Senior-Løken syndrome
  - Congenital amaurosis
  - Oculomotor apraxia
  - Congenital hepatic fibrosis
  - Aplasia of cerebellar vermis in Joubert syndrome
  - Situs inversus
  - Mental retardation
  - Urinary tract malformations
  - Encephalocele
  - Cleft lip/palate
  - Postaxial polydactyly
  - Heart malformations
  - Anomalies of the distal limb
  - Obesity
  - Male hypogenitalism

5.5.2 NPHP Type 2 (Infantile Form)

- Distinct from other forms of NPHP
  - Early loss of kidney function (ESRD generally by age 3 years)
  - Enlarged kidneys
  - Microcysts in the cortex (absent in the medulla)
  - Changes in the tubular basement membrane, typical for juvenile NPHP, are usually absent
- Associated with situs inversus in some patients
- Commonly severe hypertension

5.6 Medullary Cystic Kidney Disease (MCKD)

- Autosomal dominant.
- Mutations in MCKD 1 and 2. The MCKD 2 gene encodes for the urinary protein uromodulin (Tamm-Horsfall protein) – its relationship to cyst formation is not understood.
- Presents in early adulthood.
- Ultrasound shows normal-sized kidneys which are echogenic with small cysts at the corticomedullary junction.
- Associated with hyperuricemia.
- Hypertension.
- Can present with polyuria from concentrating defect; renal lesion can resemble chronic interstitial nephritis.
- Typically have normal urinalysis, no hematuria or proteinuria.
- Not associated with syndromes.

5.7 Multicystic Dysplastic Kidneys (MCDK)

- Incidence of unilateral MCDK is one in 2,200–4,300 live births in unselected populations.
- Bilateral MCDK is rare and presents with newborn renal failure and pulmonary hypoplasia which may not permit survival.
- Unilateral MCDK may be diagnosed antenatally as cystic mass and in the neonate as palpable kidney.
- Characterized by the presence of multiple noncommunicating cysts (differential diagnosis is large hydronephrosis from utero-pelvic junction (UPJ) obstruction) and disorganized, small parenchyma.
- Involved kidneys are nonfunctional with an atretic ureter. Lack of function can be confirmed by DMSA or MAG3 scan.
- If tracer uptake or excretion is demonstrated, consider severe PUJ obstruction as part of the differential diagnosis.
- Contralateral kidney abnormalities are found in up to 20 % consisting of vesicoureteral reflux (80 % of abnormalities), UPJ obstruction (20 %), renal dysplasia (20–30 %), or renal positional abnormalities.
- Malformations of the ipsilateral internal genitalia in up to 15 %, e.g., seminal cysts and Gartner duct in boys even with involuted MDCK.
- The dysplastic kidney fails to grow and often shrinks in size. Twenty to 25 % of multicystic kidneys involute by 2 years of age. Those >7 cm in length rarely involute (Fig. 5.5).
- Hypertension due to MCDK in 0.1 % of cases.
- Malignancy: Wilms tumor and renal cell carcinoma were thought to be associated with MCDK. However, there are no data to confirm an increased risk of malignancies. Nephrectomy is rarely indicated.
- Management: Observation, longitudinal monitoring of the size of both kidneys. Routine antibiotic prophylaxis is not recommended.
- Monitoring: Ultrasound postnatally and at 1 year of age, then in yearly or greater intervals, depending on the size of the multicystic kidney, its rate of involution, and compensatory growth or abnormalities of the ipsi- or contralateral kidney and urinary tract (Table 5.6).
- Routine BP measurement and urinalysis with follow-up visits.

5.8 Simple Renal Cysts

- Incidence of simple renal cysts appears to increase with the increasing use of imaging, but is rare in children and adolescents (<1 %).
- May be solitary or multiple and bilateral.
- Not associated with other renal or extrarenal problems.
- Usually no substantial growth in size.
- Most common site is upper pole of right kidney.

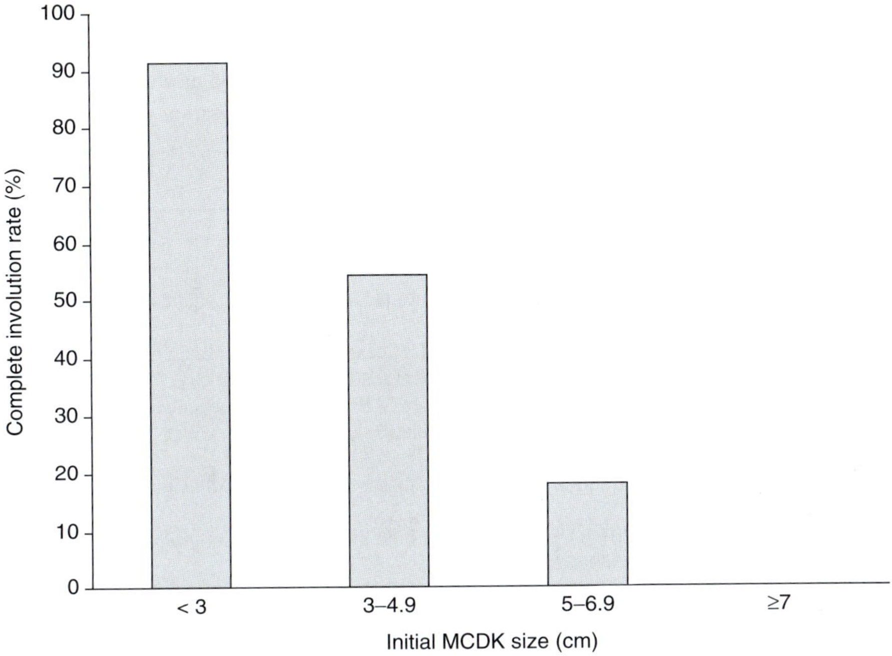

Fig. 5.5 Involution of multicystic dysplastic kidney (MCDK) at the 5-year follow-up based on initial size (From Hayes WN et al. Pediatr Nephrol 2012; 27: 1335–1340)

Table 5.6 Management of infants/children with multicystic dysplastic kidney

Prenatally	Prenatal imaging, differential diagnosis, counselling
Postnatally	Ultrasound DMSA (or MAG3) renal scan between 6 weeks and 3 months ±VCUG (MCU), e.g., in case of ureteral dilatation by ultrasound (rule out higher grade vesicoureteral reflux)
Monitoring	Ultrasound years 1, 2, 5, 10, and 15 until involution of the MCKD and compensatory growth of contralateral kidney have been documented[a] Continued monitoring until end of puberty in boys with ipsilateral malformation of internal genitalia BP and urinalysis at each of these visits

[a]Adjust frequency of visits/studies in case of clinically important (additional) abnormalities of the ipsi- and contralateral kidney and urinary tract

- Usually asymptomatic; rarely presenting with pain, e.g., due to (mainly spontaneous) rupture and hemorrhage.
- Repeat ultrasound after 6–12 months. Frequency of further follow-up depends on rate of change of the cyst size and character.

- In adults, the prevalence of simple cysts increases sevenfold from 5 % in the fourth decade to 36 % in the eighth decade.
- The Bosniak classification of renal cysts was initially created as a diagnostic and management tool to recognize cysts associated with malignancy (categories III and IV). This is a rare concern in children.

Suggested Reading

Arts HH, Knoers NVAM (2013) Current insights into renal ciliopathies: what can genetics teach us? Pediatr Nephrol 28:863–874

Avni FE, Garel C, Cassart M, D'Haene ND, Hall M, Riccabona M (2012) Imaging and classification of congenital cystic renal diseases. Am J Roentgenol 198:1004–1013

Chaki M, Hoefele J, Allen SJ, Ramaswami G, Janssen S, Bergmann C, Heckenlively JR, Otto EA, Hildebrandt F (2011) Genotype-phenotype correlation in 440 patients with NPHP-related ciliopathies. Kidney Int 80:1239–1245

Dell KM (2011) The spectrum of polycystic kidney disease in children. Adv Chronic Kidney Dis 18:339–347

Deltas C, Papagregoriou G (2010) Cystic diseases of the kidney: molecular biology and genetics. Arch Pathol Lab Med 134:569–582

Hayes WN, Watson AR, Trent & Anglia MCDK Study Group (2012) Unilateral multicystic dysplastic kidney: does initial size matter? Pediatr Nephrol 27:1335–1340

Lennerz JK, Spence DC, Iskandar SS, Dehner LP, Liapis H (2010) Glomerulocystic kidney: one hundred-year perspective. Arch Pathol Lab Med 134:583–605

Parisi M, Glass I Joubert syndrome and related disorders. In: Pagon RA, Bird TD, Dolan CR, Stephens K, Adam MP, (eds). GeneReviews™ (updated 14 Jun 2012). http://www.ncbi.nlm.nih.gov/books/NBK1325/

Sweeney WE Jr, Avner ED (2011) Diagnosis and management of childhood polycystic kidney disease. Pediatr Nephrol 26:675–692

Wolf MT, Hildebrandt F (2011) Nephronophthisis. Pediatr Nephrol 26:181–194

Issues Related to Pediatric Urology

6

Arpana A. Iyengar, John-Paul Capolicchio,
Mohamed El-Sherbiny, Roman Jednak,
and Konrad M. Szymanski

6.1 Antenatal Diagnosis of Renal Diseases

Antenatally detected renal abnormalities are the most common abnormalities seen on maternal ultrasonography and include renal injury due to obstruction (obstructive nephropathy), renal insufficiency from abnormal development (renal dysgenesis), and abnormalities of position. Paramount to elucidating the fetal diagnosis and prognosticating postnatal kidney functions is an understanding of nephrogenesis and fetal urine production.

6.1.1 Fetal Urine Production

- Urine production begins at 8–10 weeks gestation.
- By 16–18 weeks most amniotic fluid is urine; therefore, oligohydramnios in the second half of gestation is indicative of impaired renal function. Intrauterine growth retardation is another common cause for oligohydramnios.
- Normal rate of fetal urine production may approach 50 ml/h (i.e., 50-fold that of the newborn, which explains why half of antenatal hydronephrosis resolves or improves postnatally).

A.A. Iyengar (✉)
Department of Pediatric Nephrology,
St John's Medical College Hospital,
Bangalore, Karnataka 560034, India
e-mail: arpanaiyengar@gmail.com

J.-P. Capolicchio • M. El-Sherbiny • R. Jednak • K.S. Konrad
Division of Pediatric Urology,
Montreal Children's Hospital, McGill University,
2300, rue Tupper, Montreal, QC H3H 1P3, Canada
e-mail: jp.capolicchio@muhc.mcgill.ca; mohamed.el-sherbiny@muhc.mcgill.ca; roman.jednak@muhc.mcgill.ca; szymanski.konrad@gmail.com

K. Phadke et al. (eds.), *Manual of Pediatric Nephrology*,
DOI 10.1007/978-3-642-12483-9_6, © Springer-Verlag Berlin Heidelberg 2014

6.1.2 Nephrogenesis

- Begins at 8 weeks gestation.
- At 20 weeks gestation 43 % of nephrogenesis is complete.
- Maximum nephron number is fully attained at 36 weeks gestation. No new nephrons are formed later.
- Renal urinary obstruction in the first 20 weeks gestation causes renal dysplasia.
- Renal dysplasia is an embryonic maldevelopment of the kidney characterized histologically by persistent primitive renal tubules.
- Renal urinary obstruction in the second half of gestation will cause hydronephrosis or obstructive nephropathy, but not dysplasia.

6.1.3 Imaging the Fetal Urinary Tract

- Amniotic fluid can be detected as early as 10 weeks.
- Fetal bladder can be visualized by 15 weeks.
- Fetal kidneys can be identified by 11 weeks on transvaginal ultrasound and by 12–17 weeks by transabdominal ultrasound.
- Markedly dilated collecting systems can be seen by 12–14 weeks.
- Normal kidney grows by 1.1 mm per gestational week.
- Kidneys appear as echoic as liver in the first trimester. The echogenicity diminishes by the third trimester.
- Genitalia can be visualized by 16 weeks.
- By 20 weeks the genital anatomy can be reliably imaged.
- Normal renal pelvic anteroposterior diameter is less than 5 mm at 32 weeks gestation.
- Renal pelviectasia greater than 7 mm in the third trimester is predictive of mild postnatal pathology, greater than 10 mm is moderate, and greater than 15 mm is most likely to require surgical intervention.
- Ultrasonographic criteria of significance include caliectasia, worsening hydronephrosis, cortical echogenicity, cortical cysts, oligohydramnios, and dilated or persistently filled bladder.
- For a nomogram of fetal renal growth expressed in length and parenchymal area derived from ultrasound images, please refer to Shin et al *2007*.
- Fetal bladder sagittal length (FBSL) = gestational age(GA) (weeks) – 5 mm; thus, dilated bladder ≥ GA + 2 mm (Maizels et al 1995).

6.1.4 Fetal Genitourinary Ultrasound Assessment

- Assessment of fetal size and maturity
- Amniotic fluid volume evaluation
- Identification of gender

- Localization and characterization of urinary tract abnormalities
- Identification of associated abnormalities
- Monitoring detected lesions

Obstructive nephropathy is identified by the presence of hydronephrosis, whereas renal impairment from obstruction or renal dysgenesis is identified by the presence of oligohydramnios.

6.1.5 When to Refer Antenatally?

- High-grade bilateral hydronephrosis
- High-grade hydronephrosis in a solitary kidney or *functionally solitary* kidney
- Persistently distended bladder
- Oligohydramnios
- Congenital anomalies of the kidney and the urinary tract.

6.1.6 Why Refer Antenatally?

- For counseling, further evaluation, and planning of the postnatal referral.
- In select cases, fetal intervention in utero may be possible at tertiary care referral centers.
- Fetal urine biochemistry obtained from vesicocentesis (similar to amniocentesis) can predict renal dysplasia (pathologic, if sodium >100 mmol/dl, calcium >2 mmol/l, osmolality >200 mOsm/l, total protein >200 mg/l (>20 mg/dl)).
- Fetal vesicocentesis should be repeated with 2-day intervals so as to obtain the most representative, third sample.

6.1.7 When to Evaluate Hydronephrosis Postnatally?

- Most centers use 7 mm renal pelvic diameter (RPD) in the third trimester as a cutoff for postnatal screening (see Table 6.1).
- RPD greater than 15 mm is warrants further evaluation.

Table 6.1 Prenatal interpretation of renal pelvic diameter

Diagnosis	Prenatal RPD (mean ± SD)
Normal	8 ± 2 mm
Non-obstructive hydronephrosis	11 ± 7 mm
Vesicoureteric reflux	13 ± 7 mm
Obstruction	22 ± 12 mm

Adapted from Coplen et al., *J Urol* (2006), 176: 724

6.1.8 Recommendations for Postnatal Referral

- Bilateral or solitary hydronephrosis.
- Megacystis, oligohydramnios.
- Unequal size kidneys and congenital anomalies of the kidney and the urinary tract.

6.1.9 Ultrasound Findings Suggestive of Renal Disease

6.1.9.1 Number of Kidneys

- Bilateral renal agenesis – diagnosed on the basis of absent renal structure, absent bladder, and severe oligohydramnios. It is incompatible with life. It may be a part of syndromes like TAR (thrombocytopenia with absent radius) and Fraser syndrome.
- Unilateral renal agenesis – occurs 1 in 500 pregnancies.

6.1.9.2 Renal Position

Ectopic kidneys – may be due to abnormal location of kidneys in the pelvis, horseshoe kidney or cross fused kidney. They may be small in size and dysplastic and have associated ureteric anomalies.

6.1.9.3 Echogenicity of Kidneys

- Hyperechoic fetal kidneys: Normal fetal kidneys are hypoechoic when compared to the liver in the third trimester.
- Common conditions associated with hyperechoic kidneys are dysplastic kidneys, polycystic kidneys, and Bardet-Biedl and Beckwith-Wiedemann syndromes.
- In case of hyperechoic kidneys, look for size of kidneys, macrocysts, dilatation of collecting system, and amniotic fluid volume.

6.1.9.4 Size of Kidneys

- Small size – suggestive of hypoplastic/dysplastic kidneys
- Large size – may be due to hydronephrosis, inborn errors of metabolism, polycystic kidney disease, and tumors

6.1.9.5 Antenatal Hydronephrosis

- Hydronephrosis is a common abnormality seen on ultrasound.
- Accounts for 2/3 of all anomalies detected on antenatal scan.
- 1 in 100–500 pregnancies.
- Anteroposterior diameter of renal pelvis >10 mm is considered significant after 28 weeks of gestation.
- False-positive rate as confirmed by postnatal ultrasound is 9–22 % when the pelvic diameter cutoff is >10 mm and 6 % when diameter is >15 mm.
- Ultrasound must be repeated every 6–8 weeks till delivery.
- Pelviureteric junction (PUJ) obstruction (PUJO) is the most common cause of antenatal hydronephrosis.
- The grading for antenatal hydronephrosis is given in Table 6.2.

Table 6.2 Grading of antenatal hydronephrosis – Society for Fetal Urology

Grade	Central renal complex (intrarenal pelvis, calyces)	Parenchymal thickness
0	Intact	Normal
1	Slight splitting	Normal
2	Evident splitting, confined within renal border	Normal
3	Wide split, pelvis dilated outside renal border	Normal
4	Further dilatation of pelvis and calyces	Thin

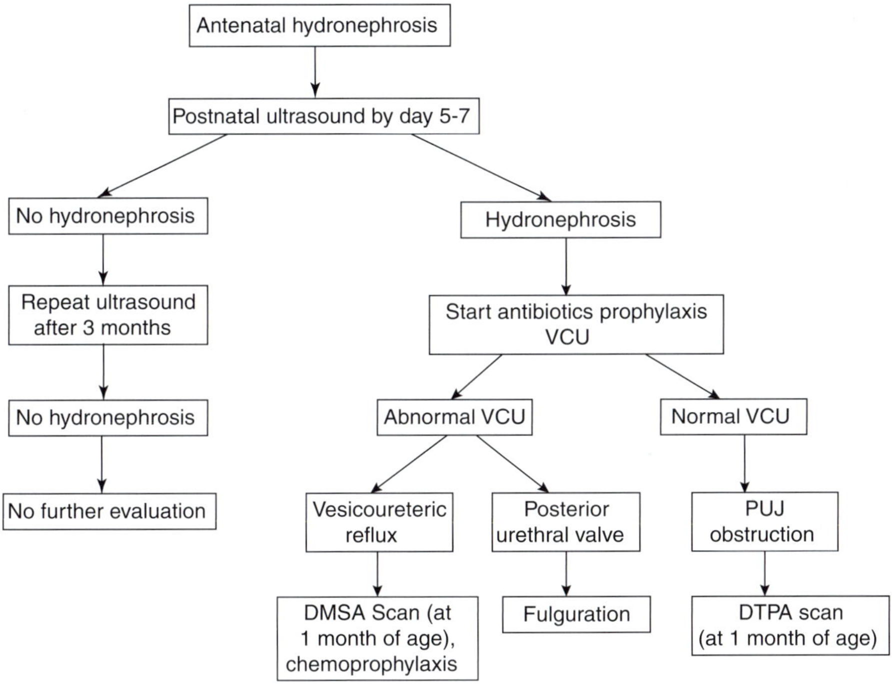

Fig. 6.1 An approach to antenatally diagnosed hydronephrosis

Postnatal Evaluation of Antenatal Hydronephrosis

- More than 50 % of antenatally detected hydronephroses disappear spontaneously and are not seen on postnatal ultrasound.
- 50–60 % of neonatal hydronnephroses are due to PUJ obstruction and 20–30 % are due to vesicoureteric reflux (VUR).
- Clinical evaluation for palpable abdominal mass, urine stream, palpable bladder, and the presence of urinary ascites.
- For details on postnatal evaluation, algorithm, and management, refer to Fig. 6.1 and Sect. 6.2 .
- The predictors of poor function in postnatal period are given in Table 6.3.

Table 6.3 Antenatal hydronephrosis: predictors of poor function in the postnatal period

(a) Pelvic dilatation visualized before 24 weeks of gestation
(b) Moderate to severe hydronephrosis – pelvic diameter >20 mm
(c) Thickened bladder wall
(d) Oligohydramnios
(e) Ultrasonographic evidence of renal dysplasia – echogenic cortex, microcysts

6.1.9.6 Renal Cysts

- Most common causes of renal cysts on the antenatal scan are renal dysplasia (with or without obstruction) and multicystic dysplastic kidneys.
- Rarely, ADPKD presents with perinatally evident renal cysts (see Chap. 5, Sect. 5.3 and Fig. 5.2).

Cystic kidneys must alert the physician to the presence of several syndromes – Bardet-Biedl, Beckwith-Wiedemann, tuberous sclerosis, trisomy 13, and trisomy 18.

6.1.9.7 Renal Tumors

- Renal tumors are rare in the fetus.
- The most common congenital tumor is mesoblastic nephroma – usually appears as a large, solitary retroperitoneal mass, which is in continuity with the kidney.
- Usually solid, but may have a cystic component.
- Other rare tumors are Wilms and nephroblastomatosis.
- Adrenal neuroblastoma may be mistaken for a renal tumor.

6.1.9.8 Ureteric Dilatation

- Ureteric dilatation is detected at the level of the bladder, in transverse view.
- Suggestive of obstructive uropathy or vesicoureteric reflux.

6.1.9.9 Bladder Abnormalities

- Non-visualization of bladder with severe oligohydramnios suggests bilateral severe renal impairment.
- Enlarged bladder: >3 cm in second trimester and >6 cm in third trimester suggest bladder outlet obstruction, secondary to posterior urethral valve and urethral atresia/stenosis.
- Intravesical cyst: ureterocele.
- "Key hole bladder": due to dilated posterior urethra.

6.1.9.10 Miscellaneous

- Urinoma – suggests a "pop-off" mechanism secondary to increase in bladder pressure due to bladder outlet obstruction.
- Ascites – urinary ascites due to bladder outlet obstruction is the most common cause of abdominal fluid collection in the fetus.
- Spinal defects – meningomyelocele.

- Duplex renal systems: have been described with a long list of malformations and syndromes. Look for anomalies of the cardiovascular and gastrointestinal system.

6.2 Congenital Hydronephrosis and Hydroureter

6.2.1 Definitions

Hydronephrosis (HN) – dilation of the renal collecting system
Pyelectasia – dilation of the renal pelvis
Caliectasia – dilation of the calyces; termed hydrocalyx if only one calyx is dilated
Hydroureter – dilation of the ureter, also known as megaureter
Obstruction – an impediment to urinary flow, which if uncorrected will limit the ultimate functional potential of a kidney

6.2.2 Postnatal Evaluation of Hydronephrosis

- Ultrasound (U/S) abdomen/pelvis – after day 3 of life in order to avoid "downgrading" of the HN due to (physiological) volume depletion; important to assess the bladder, both full and post-void.
- Voiding cystourethrogram (VCU or VCUG) – indicated in grade 3 and 4 hydronephrosis to distinguish reflux-related dilation from obstruction; of no proven benefit in grade 0, 1, and 2 hydronephrosis.
- MAG3 diuretic renogram – indicated in grade 3 and 4 HN. It serves as a baseline for comparison with serial studies, hence no benefit in delaying the first study to 6 weeks of life when the glomerular filtration rate (GFR) has matured.
- Serum creatinine – indicated if significant bilateral disease or solitary kidney. Creatinine concentration should decrease from maternal level after day 3 of life.

6.2.3 VCUG: Common Pitfalls

- Foley instead of feeding tube (the Foley balloon will mimic or obscure a ureterocele, in addition to potentially obstructing the bladder outlet during micturition)
- No scout film (urolithiasis or foreign bodies can be missed)
- Inadequate bladder filling (false-negative study for vesicoureteric reflux if the bladder is not fully distended)
- No voiding views of the urethra (will miss posterior urethral valves in males or the spin top deformity of voiding dysfunction in girls)
- No post-void views (inadequate assessment of the post-void residual, an indicator of bladder function)
- No delayed views (especially helpful to rule out concomitant ureteropelvic junction obstruction in the setting of high-grade vesicoureteric reflux)

6.2.4 MAG3-Furosemide Renogram (Diuretic Renogram)

Currently used radiotracers for dynamic renal scintigraphy are ^{99m}Tc-DTPA and ^{99m}Tc-MAG3 (see Sect. 1.7.6). A standardized protocol is recommended which permits comparison between serial studies (Conway and Maizels *1992*). The importance of patient hydration and the placement of a bladder catheter in non-toilet-trained children is emphasized. Contrary to a common misconception MAG3 renography can (and should) be performed in the newborn, despite an immature GFR, in cases with high-grade hydronephrosis that would benefit from early surgical intervention.

The cortical phase measures the cortical transit time (CTT) and the split renal function or differential renal function (DRF). The CTT represents the time for the radiotracer to traverse from the glomerulus to the renal collecting system. Values <5 min indicate significant renal dysfunction. The DRF is measured at 1–2 min and reflects the relative contribution of each kidney to total renal function. The normal distribution is 50 ± 5 %.

The drainage phase measures the T-half (represents the time needed for half of the radiotracer in the renal pelvis to be cleared), the total drainage over time and the shape of the drainage curve (Fig. 6.2).

6.2.5 Ancillary Tests (Not Routinely Indicated)

- Intravenous pyelogram (IVP)
- Percutaneous antegrade pyelography
- Endoscopic retrograde pyelography
- Cystoscopy
- Computed tomography (CT), magnetic resonance imaging (MRI)
- Whitaker pressure-flow urodynamics

6.3 Congenital Malformations of the Kidney and Urinary Tract

Malformations of the kidney and urinary tract consist of a broad range of disorders that result from abnormal development of these during intrauterine life. Hence, these malformations are by definition congenital.

Malformations of the kidney can be classified as:

1. Aplasia (agenesis) – defined as congenital absence of kidney tissue
2. Hypoplasia – renal length <2 SD below the mean for age or body height. Normal renal architecture, reduced number of nephrons
3. Dysplasia with or without cysts – malformation of tissue elements
4. Isolated dilation of collecting system
5. Anomalies of position – ectopic, fused, including horseshoe kidney

Anomalies of the kidney are associated with structural anomalies of the lower urinary tract in about 50 % of affected patients. Reno-urinary tract malformations have been grouped by some under the term CAKUT (congenital anomalies of the

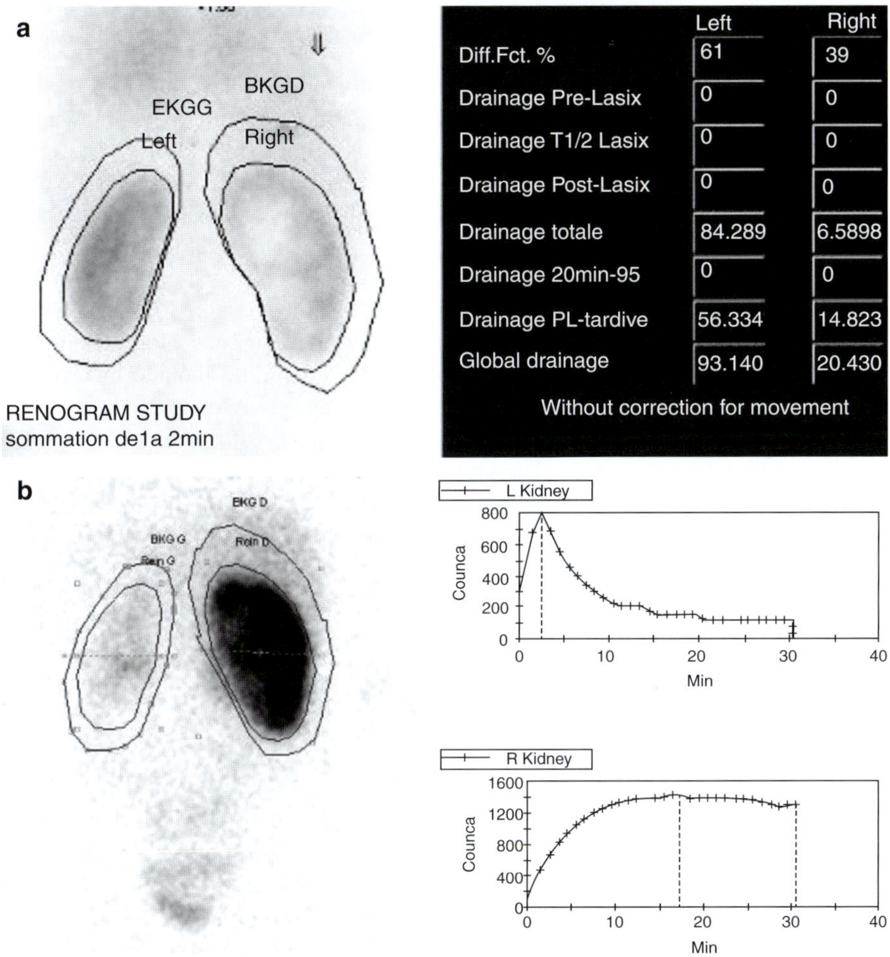

Fig. 6.2 (**a**) The DRF of the hydronephrotic right kidney is measured as 39 %. (**b**) This same right kidney demonstrates a delayed drainage time as shown by the prolonged drainage curve compared to the normal left kidney

kidney and urinary tract). They may be associated with anorectal malformations and/or genital abnormalities. In about 30 % of cases, the malformations occur as a part of a genetic syndrome, a chromosomal disorder, or an inborn error of metabolism. Environmental factors, implicated in CAKUT, include exposure to teratogens. Prenatal exposure to ACEI (angiotensin converting enzyme inhibitors) and ARBs (angiotensin II receptor blockers) are associated with renal tubular genesis (RTD), a severe perinatal disorder with poor prognosis.

This section describes duplex kidneys (duplication), ureteroceles, and some anomalies of lower urinary tract, especially epispadias and hypospadias. Congenital hydronephrosis and hydroureter have been described in Sect. 6.2. Posterior urethral valves and prune belly syndrome will be detailed in Sect. 6.4.

6.3.1 Duplex Kidneys

- Unilateral duplication is more common than bilateral duplication.
- Girls are more frequently affected than boys. Familial occurrence in known.
- The most common form of fusion anomaly is a horseshoe kidney. The lower poles of both kidneys unite across the midline. Due to failure of ascent, the renal blood supply may be derived from other vessels such as iliac arteries. One third of cases may have vesicoureteric reflux. Other associated urological abnormalities include ureteral duplication, ectopic ureter, and retrocaval ureter. Since it is placed anteriorly, the horseshoe kidney is susceptible to trauma. This is seen in children with Turner syndrome, trisomy 18, and the Laurence-Moon-Biedl syndrome. Long-term follow-up is recommended and should include intermittent radiological and laboratory assessment.
- Duplex kidney has two distinct pelvicalyceal systems with incomplete or complete duplication of ureters. The ureter draining the upper moiety may have an ectopic vesical opening with a ureterocele. The ureter draining the lower pole has an abnormal insertion into the bladder with vesicoureteric reflux. Some cases may require surgical intervention – endoscopic ureterocele incision, ureterocele excision with reimplantation, and upper pole heminephrectomy for a nonfunctioning upper pole.

6.3.2 Ureterocele

- Ureterocele is a cystic dilatation of the terminal segment of the ureter.
- Single system ureterocele is more common in boys than girls. They lie within the bladder (orthotopic ureterocele) or may be associated with an ectopic ureter. It may be asymptomatic or it may present with urinary tract infection or occasionally with bladder outflow obstruction. It is managed by endoscopic incision or ureterocele excision with ureteric reimplantation.
- Uteroceles may be associated with duplex kidneys.

6.3.3 Anomalies of the Lower Urinary Tract

I. Congenital Anomalies of the Bladder
   1. Anomalies of bladder formation – agenesis of bladder, hypoplastic bladder
   2. Anomalies of bladder compartmentalization – duplication of bladder, septate bladder, hourglass bladder, and bladder diverticulae
   3. Megacystis – congenital megacystis, megacystis-megaureter syndrome, and megacystis-microcolon-hypoperistalsis syndrome
   4. Urachal abnormalities – patent urachus, urachal cyst, urachal sinus, and urachal diverticulum
   5. Bladder exstrophy and epispadias complex

II. Cloacal exstrophy
III. Urogenital sinus and cloacal abnormalities
IV. Hypospadias

These are rare anomalies. Clinical presentation ranges from a stillborn to urinary incontinence, hydronephrosis or renal dysplasia, urinary tract infections, and renal failure. Small primary bladder diverticula may remain asymptomatic. Associated genital and other system anomalies are frequent. Most will require reconstruction of the bladder.

6.3.3.1 Bladder Exstrophy-Epispadias Complex

The exposed bladder and urethral plates are anteriorly displaced and appear as a diamond-shaped area bound by the umbilicus, anus, and rectus muscles. Pubic diastasis is characteristic. Exposure of the bladder mucosa to air results in inflammation and polypoid appearance. In epispadias the bladder is closed and the urethral plate remains open and anteriorly displaced. The urethral meatus in most patients with epispadias is at the penopubic junction. The penis is short and wide with dorsal curvature. In girls, the clitoris is bifid and the urethra is patulous. Upper tract is usually normal. Vesicoureteral reflux occurs because the ureters enter the bladder with almost no tunnel.

Incidence

Bladder exstrophy: 1/20,000–40,000 live births. The exstrophy risk for subsequent children is 3.6 %. The male to female ratio is between 1.5 and 2:1. Epispadias: 1/40,000 live births. The male to female ratio is 3.5:1.

Clinical Presentations

Prenatal ultrasound findings in bladder exstrophy are absence of bladder filling, low-set umbilicus, widened pubis rami, and diminutive genitalia. Anterior abdominal mass suggests bladder exstrophy, omphalocele, or gastroschisis. The changes can be seen as early as 20th week of gestation.

After birth – obvious exposed bladder with associated abnormalities in the abdomen and perineum, the urinary tract, the genitalia, and the bony pelvis.

Immediate Management

The umbilical cord is preferably tied with 2-0 silk close to the abdominal wall so that the umbilical clamp does not traumatize the delicate bladder mucosa. The bladder can be covered with a nonadherent film of plastic wrap to prevent sticking of the bladder mucosa to diapers. The plastic wrap is regularly changed and the bladder surface is irrigated with saline. Antibiotic prophylaxis is initiated.

Management

- Objectives: (1) secure abdominal wall closure, (2) urinary continence, (3) preserving renal function, and (4) creation of functionally and cosmetically acceptable external genitalia.
- Approaches: modern staged repair of exstrophy (MSRE) and complete primary repair (CPRE). The choice mainly depends on the surgical experience and training.

Staged approach includes bladder and posterior urethral closure shortly after birth. Epispadias repair in males is performed between 6 and 12 months. Bladder neck reconstruction (BNR) is performed at 3.5–5 years when adequate bladder capacity is obtained and the child is motivated to be dry. CPRE involves simultaneous bladder closure and epispadias repair without an attempt to narrow bladder neck.

- Complications: dehiscence, urinary tract infections, hydronephrosis, bladder stones and perforations, fistulas, and hypospadias.
- Continence: the published rates of continence vary from 37 to 90 %. Up to 70 % of patients void spontaneously without augmentation or CIC. Successful initial bladder closure is an important factor for achieving continence. There appears to be a higher continence rate in female versus male patients.
- Renal function: the loss of renal function can be due to hydronephrosis and recurrent pyelonephritis with renal scarring. Recent series have shown improved rates of renal preservation (80–87 %) compared to older series where intestinal augmentation or ureterosigmoidostomy was employed. Renal cortical defects and hydronephrosis were seen in 20 %. Longitudinal evaluation that includes serial renal nuclear scans and ultrasounds, and renal functional studies are essential part of follow-up in bladder exstrophy patient.
- Sexual function: 60 % of male patients reported a straight penis following reconstruction. Infertility may be due to retrograde ejaculation or duct obstruction from scarring. Substantially higher fertility rates have been achieved in female following reconstruction after reconstruction than in males.

6.3.3.2 Hypospadias

Hypospadias occurs in 1 of 300 male children. The urethral meatus opens on the ventral (under) side of the penis proximal to the tip of the glans penis.

Classification

According to meatal location: (1) glandular – opening on the ventral aspect of the glans penis, (2) coronal – opening at the coronal sulcus, (3) penile shaft, (4) penoscrotal, and (5) perineal

About 70 % of all cases of hypospadias are distal penile or coronal.

Clinical Findings

- Hooded appearance of the penis, caused by deficient or absent ventral foreskin.
- Difficulty directing the urinary stream, stream spraying.
- Variable degree of penile curvature (chordee) causes ventral bending and bowing of the penile shaft, which can prevent sexual intercourse.
- Proximal forms of hypospadias in adults can be the cause of infertility.
- Undescended testicles or inguinal hernia may be present.

Indications for Intersex Work-Up

1. Penoscrotal and perineal hypospadias.
2. Any degree of hypospadias with undescended testis (palpable or non-palpable).

3. Hypospadias with bilaterally non-palpable testes needs urgent work-up to rule out masculinized female with congenital adrenal hyperplasia.

Work-up includes abdominal and pelvis ultrasound, karyotyping, genitogram, urethroscopy, and cystoscopy.

Management

Newborns with hypospadias should not be circumcised, because the preputial skin may be useful for future reconstruction. Surgical repair is preferred between 6 and 18 months of age for psychological reasons. Severe forms may be repaired in two stages. Surgical reconstruction aims at achieving a straight penis and creation of a normally located cosmetically acceptable urethral meatus.

Prognosis

After corrective surgery, most patients are able to void in the standing position as well as to deposit semen into the vagina.

6.4 Posterior Urethral Valves (PUV)

- The most common cause of bladder outlet obstruction.
- PUV accounts for 10 % of cases of hydronephrosis in a neonate and 2/3 of all cases of lower urinary tract obstruction.
- PUV described in about 1/5,000 live births in Caucasian population and up to 2-fold higher in economically deprived and select non-European populations.
- The most commonn form consists of obstructing membranous folds within the lumen of the prostatic (posterior) urethra.
- The traditional classification into 3 types appears to be artifactual and is now obsolete. Currently, only 2 embryologically distinct forms of obstruction in the posterior urethra are recognized (1) congenital obstructive posterior urethral membrane (COPUM; used by some instead of the classic term PUV), an oblique membrane intimately associated with the distal verumontanum and (2) a more distal bulbar anomaly (Cobb's collar), a transverse membrane that is unrelated to the verumontanum and may be the remnant of the urogenital diaphragm.

6.4.1 Clinical Presentations

- Antenatal – hydroureteronephrosis, oligohydramnios, and its consequences in severe cases: pulmonary hypoplasia and postural defects (congenital dislocation of hip, talipes, receding jaw (Potter sequence))
- Postnatal – recurrent urinary tract infections, dribbling of urine, poor urinary stream, straining during micturition, failure to pass urine in the first 24 h of life, palpable bladder, respiratory distress (secondary to pulmonary hypoplasia as a result of oligohydramnios or due to spontaneous pneumothorax), sepsis, azotemia, failure to thrive, abdominal distension, and urinary incontinence

6.4.2 Effects on the Urinary Tract and Kidneys

- Urethra – posterior urethral dilatation and distortion of bladder neck
- Bladder – thickened wall, trabeculated, and noncompliant
- Ureters – Ureterectasis, hydroureters, vesicoureteric reflux, and in some cases VUJ (vesicoureteric junction) obstruction
- Kidneys – pelvicaliectasis, parenchymal thinning, renal dysplasia, hydronephrosis, and tubular damage (hyponatremia/metabolic acidosis)
- Others – retroperitoneal urinoma and urinary ascites

6.4.3 Pop-Off Mechanisms to Relieve Bladder Pressure

- Vesicoureteric reflux – most common; VURD syndrome (valves, unilateral reflux, renal dysplasia) may lead to preservation of contralateral renal function in patients with "unilateral reflux into a nonfunctioning kidney."
- A large bladder diverticulum.
- Renal urinary extravasation – urinoma and urinary ascites.

6.4.4 Evaluation

- Renal ultrasound.
- VCU – gold standard investigation for diagnosis. Findings – posterior urethral dilatation, trabeculated bladder, and vesicoureteric reflux.
- Urine microscopy and culture.
- Serum electrolytes – hyponatremia and metabolic acidosis can occur due to tubular damage.
- Renal function tests – serial monitoring to assess the degree of – prognostically important – residual renal dysfunction.
- DMSA or MAG3 scintigraphy – performed at 1 month of age to know the degree of renal dysplasia and measure the differential (split) renal function.
- Urodynamic studies – in cases where incontinence persists even after the age of 5 years and as a part of pre-transplant work-up.

6.4.5 Differential Diagnosis of the Dilated Bladder on Ultrasound

6.4.5.1 Bladder Level Causes

- Neurogenic bladder dysfunction
- Prune belly syndrome
- Megacystis-megaureter syndrome
- Bladder diverticulum
- Pelvic tumor (e.g., ovarian or sacrococcygeal teratoma)
- Urogenital sinus (UGS) or cloacal anomaly

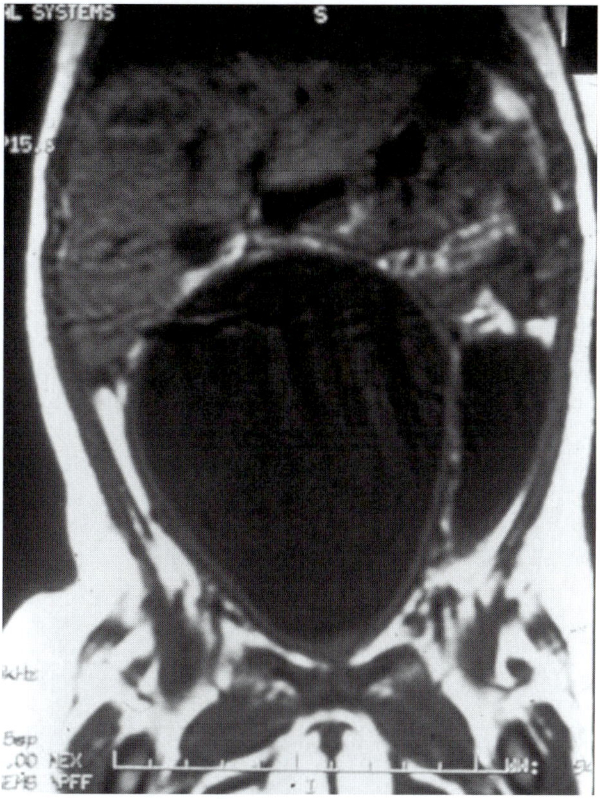

Fig. 6.3 MRI demonstrates large hydrocolpos in a girl with UGS anomaly, causing bladder outlet obstruction and bilateral hydronephrosis

- Hydrocolpos
- Ectopic multicystic dysplastic kidney
- Megacystis-microcolon intestinal hypoperistalsis syndrome (MMIHS) (Figs. 6.3 and 6.4)

6.4.5.2 Urethral Level Causes

- Posterior urethral valves Fig. 6.5
- Urethral atresia
- Anterior urethral valves (band of tissue on the ventral aspect of the urethra with or without a proximal diverticulum)
- Urethral diverticulum
- Pseudovagina (enlarged male utricle)
- Seminal vesicle cyst

6.4.6 Management

- Hemodynamic stabilization of the child – achieve fluid and electrolyte balance.
- Immediate bladder decompression by urethral catheter placement is of paramount importance. Catheter placement can be difficult due to the tortuous urethra and

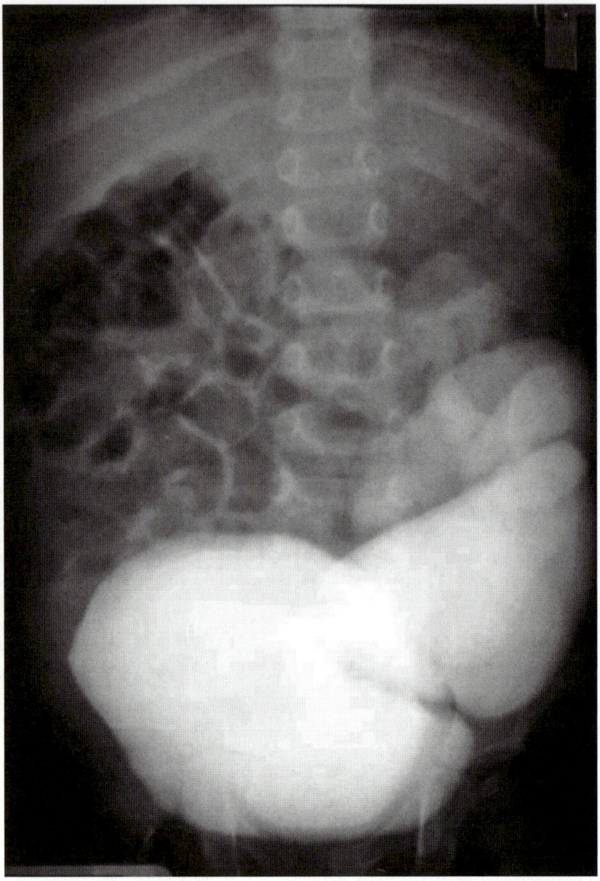

Fig. 6.4 Large bladder with massive left VUR in a boy with prune belly (VCUG)

bladder neck. Confirmation of placement within the bladder is prudent. An infant feeding tube is preferred over a Foley catheter (balloon can fall back into the dilated posterior urethra).

- Once the ventilation and metabolic changes have stabilized, a definitive surgical treatment is performed.
- The surgical options include endoscopic valve ablation, cutaneous vesicostomy, and rarely supravesical diversion by ureterostomy.
- Cystoscopic ablation of the valves is the treatment of choice. Primary valve ablation involves transurethral incision of the PUV during first few days of life. Current infant resectoscopes are available in size 8F and smaller. The valves can be incised at the 12, 5, and 7 o'clock positions with either a cold knife or electrocautery.
- Temporary urinary diversion (vesicostomy/bilateral ureterostomies) should be considered if primary ablation is not possible either due to small caliber of the urethra preventing endoscopic ablation or due to hemodynamic instability or severe renal dysfunction.

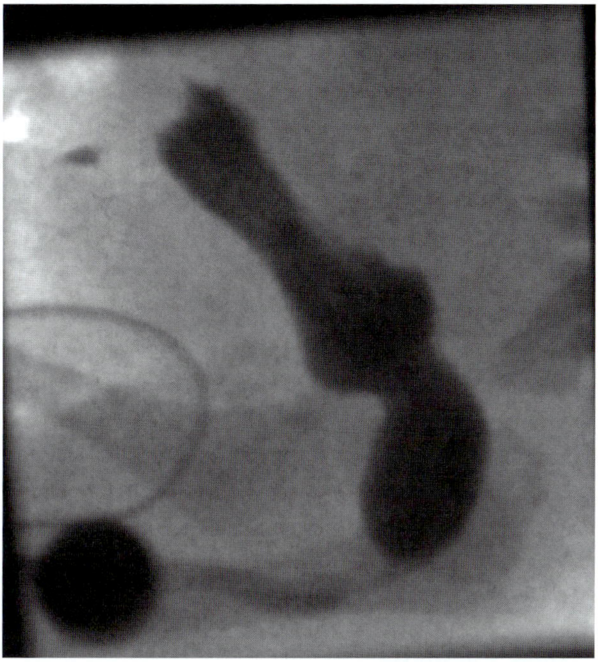

Fig. 6.5 Posterior urethral valves on VCUG, including classic hypertrophied detrusor, bladder neck hypertrophy, dilated posterior urethra, and distal pooling in phimosis

- Prophylactic antibiotics before the initial catheter insertion and as a part of uroprophylaxis in case of VUR.
- Regular follow-ups are mandatory to assess renal functions, proteinuria, electrolyte and acid base status, blood pressure, and growth. Serial ultrasounds, DMSA scans and VCU, urinary flow rates, and urodynamic studies are done during follow-ups, as indicated.
- Prenatal intervention is essentially experimental and is limited to a few centers. Options include percutaneous placement of a vesicoamniotic shunt, open fetal surgery, and fetal cystoscopic ablation. Significant complications may occur, resulting in maternal or fetal morbidity as well as fetal loss.

6.4.7 Complications of PUV

- Short term – dyselectrolytemia, metabolic acidosis, acute kidney injury, and dehydration (due to diuresis following relief of lower urinary tract obstruction).
- Long term – hypertension and chronic kidney disease (CKD). Progression of CKD is determined by underlying dysplasia, urinary tract infections, the presence of high bladder pressures, and compliance for follow-ups. Rapid worsening of renal functions may occur at the time of puberty due to the increased metabolic workload placed on the kidneys during that time.

- Valve bladder syndrome – loss of bladder compliance, urinary incontinence, deterioration of renal functions, and poor renal concentrating ability.

6.4.8 Why Does PUV Lead to Chronic Kidney Disease?

- Inherent renal dysplasia
- Obstruction with back pressure
- Recurrent urinary tract infections
- Superimposed focal segmental glomerulosclerosis
- Hypertension

6.4.9 Predictors of a Poor Renal Function

6.4.9.1 Antenatal

- Maternal oligohydramnios, regardless of gestational age
- Early detection on antenatal ultrasound of bright kidneys and pelvicalyceal dilatation

6.4.9.2 Postnatal

- Presentation in the first 12 months of life (if undetected prenatally)
- Bilateral vesicoureteric reflux
- Infants with severe renal function impairment (GFR <30 ml/min/m^2)
- Serum creatinine >100 μmol/l (>1.2 mg/dL) at 12 months of age
- Proteinuria/albuminuria
- Impaired urinary continence at 5 years of age upwards

6.4.10 Prune Belly Syndrome (PBS)

- There are three components to prune belly syndrome – bilateral undescended testes, absence of muscles of the anterior abdominal wall, and variable functional and anatomical anomalies of the urinary tract (kidney and bladder findings are similar to those in posterior urethral valves).
- Rarely, patients may have megalourethra.
- Extra-genitourinary anomalies are frequently found, including orthopedic (e.g., club feet, pectus excavatum), gastrointestinal (malrotation), and cardiopulmonary.
- Incomplete forms of the triad with only the abdominal wall laxity, or pseudo prune belly syndrome due to other forms of abdominal wall defect, and female PBS have been rarely described.
- VCU will demonstrate characteristic findings. The crucial difference between PBS and PUV in the VCU is the widely patulous bladder neck seen in PBS versus the narrow hypertrophied bladder neck seen with PUV. In addition, the bladder is usually smooth walled in PBS as opposed to the trabeculated bladder of PUV.

- The surgical options for PBS are similar to PUV; though the most important question is whether any surgery is indicated to address "bladder voiding efficiency (BVE)." BVE is best determined by urodynamic studies and serial imaging. Intervention is indicated for proven obstruction or intractable infection.
- PBS also requires surgical management of the cryptorchid testes and frequently the abdominal wall laxity. Abdominoplasty can improve constipation, stabilize gait, and improve cosmesis.

6.5 Urinary Tract Infections

6.5.1 Introduction

Urinary tract infections (UTI) are common bacterial infections in infants and children. The risk of having a UTI before the age of 14 years is approximately 1–3 % in boys and 3–10 % in girls. The incidence of symptomatic UTI in term neonates is approximately 1 % and is 3 % in preterm neonates. During the first year of life, the male to female ratio is 3–5:1. Beyond 1–2 years, there is female preponderance with male to female ratio of 1:10. Since the symptomatology varies with age and is most often nonspecific, the diagnosis of UTI can be challenging. A major concern with UTI is its potential to lead to significant renal injury. Physicians have witnessed important turning points of the traditional approach to diagnosis and management of UTI in children, based on clinical and biological evidence, but also on societal discomfort with invasive procedures and exposure to ionizing radiation, especially in Western countries. However, existing challenges and priorities in regions with limited resources, such as easy access to medical care and advanced diagnostic technologies, make it difficult for clinicians in emerging countries to abide by western protocols. A needs-based approach prevails taking into account the lack of follow-up, equipment and trained personnel as well as medical insurance. This chapter tries to avoid controversies in management of UTI and to give a simplified, practical approach. See Box 6.1 for UTI-related definition.

Box 6.1 Urinary tract infection (UTI) definitions

Significant bacteriuria	Colony count of $>10^5$/ml of a single species in a mid-stream clean catch sample
Asymptomatic bacteriuria	Significant bacteriuria in absence of symptoms of UTI
Recurrent infection	Second episode of UTI, usually within 6 months
Complicated UTI	Presence of fever >39 °C, systemic toxicity, persistent vomiting, dehydration, renal angle tenderness, and raised creatinine
Simple UTI	UTI with low-grade fever, dysuria, frequency, urgency; none of the symptoms of complicated UTI

6.5.2 Etiopathogenesis

Organisms: *Escherichia coli* remains the predominant uropathogen. Other organisms such as *klebsiella*, *proteus* and *enterobacter species*, staphylococci, and *Streptococcus faecalis* are encountered in children with recurrent UTI, prolonged urinary catheterization, and in nosocomial settings.

Hematogenous spread is common in newborns and infants in contrast to ascending infection in older children.

6.5.3 Clinical Features

- Newborns/infants: Symptoms of UTI are nonspecific like fever, irritability, poor feeding, vomiting, prolonged jaundice, diarrhea, and lethargy. UTI should be suspected in younger children who present with fever without apparent focus.
- Older children: Urinary symptoms such as burning, urgency, frequency, flank pain, turbid odorous urine, and recent onset of enuresis are common (Box 6.1).
- Specific signs on examination: Urinary stream, spine abnormalities, phimosis, labial adhesions, anal tone, palpable bladder, and abdominal masses (faecaliths, palpable kidneys) should be specifically looked for.

6.5.4 Diagnosis

The gold standard for diagnosis of UTI is the urine culture. The urine sample needs to be appropriately collected and evaluated for bacterial growth (Table 6.4). The presence of >5 white blood cells/high power field (HPF) in a centrifuged sample and 10 white cells/HPF in an uncentrifuged sample of urine is seen in the majority of patients with UTI.

6.5.5 Tests That Help Improve the Predictive Value of UTI

- *Nitrate reductase test*: The principle behind this test is reduction of nitrate to nitrite by nitrate reductase enzyme present in bacteria. This test has a sensitivity of 53 % and specificity of 98 % in detecting UTI.
- *Leukocyte esterase test*: This test has 83 % sensitivity and a specificity of 78 % to detect UTI.
- The combination of leukocyte esterase and nitrite tests has a sensitivity of 72 % and specificity of 96 % for diagnosing UTI.

Table 6.4 Urinary Tract Infection: Diagnostic criteria

Method of collection	Colony count	Probability of infection (%)
Suprapubic aspiration	Any number of pathogens	99
Urethral catheterization	$>5 \times 10^4$ CFU/ml	95
Midstream clean catch	$>10^5$ CFU/ml	90–95

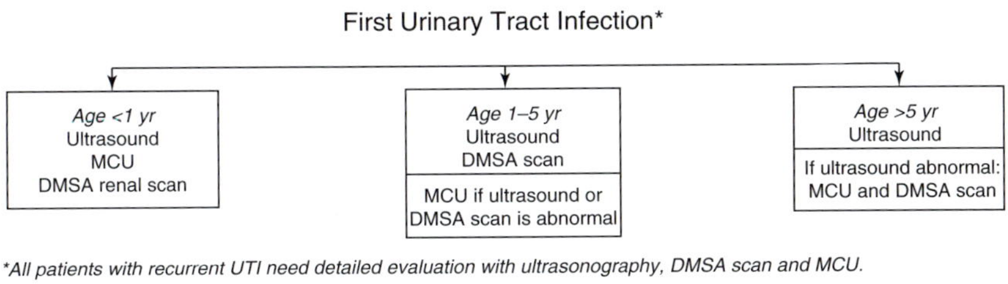

Fig. 6.6 Evaluation following initial urinary tract infection – Guideline of the Indian Society of Pediatric Nephrology. Reproduced from: Vijayakumar et al. (2011) (with permission). *MCU* miction cysturethrogram

6.5.6 Imaging

When to image and which imaging modality for a child with UTI remains controversial. A relevant issue is the importance attributed to a vesico-ureteral reflux (VUR) in the etiology of renal scarring. Imaging following a documented UTI is aimed at identifying underlying urologic anomalies and renal scarring. Primary imaging modalities are renal and pelvic ultrasound, voiding cystourethrogram (VCUG), and DMSA scan.

Simplified, practical protocols for imaging after the first episode of UTI, based on the recently revised practice guidelines of the Indian Society of Pediatric Nephrology (Fig. 6.6) and the American Academy of Pediatrics (Fig. 6.7), are shown as examples.

6.5.7 Management

The management of UTI consists of the adequate treatment of the properly diagnosed infection, and prevention of scarring and its complications. Parenteral antibiotics are indicated in complicated UTI and are given for the first 2–3 days followed by orally administered antibiotics for 7–14 days as per the culture sensitivity report (Table 6.5).

6.5.8 Recurrent UTI

Recurrence is seen in 30–50 % of children following the first episode of UTI.

The risk factors for recurrent UTI are:

- Girls
- Age <6 months
- Phimosis/labial adhesions

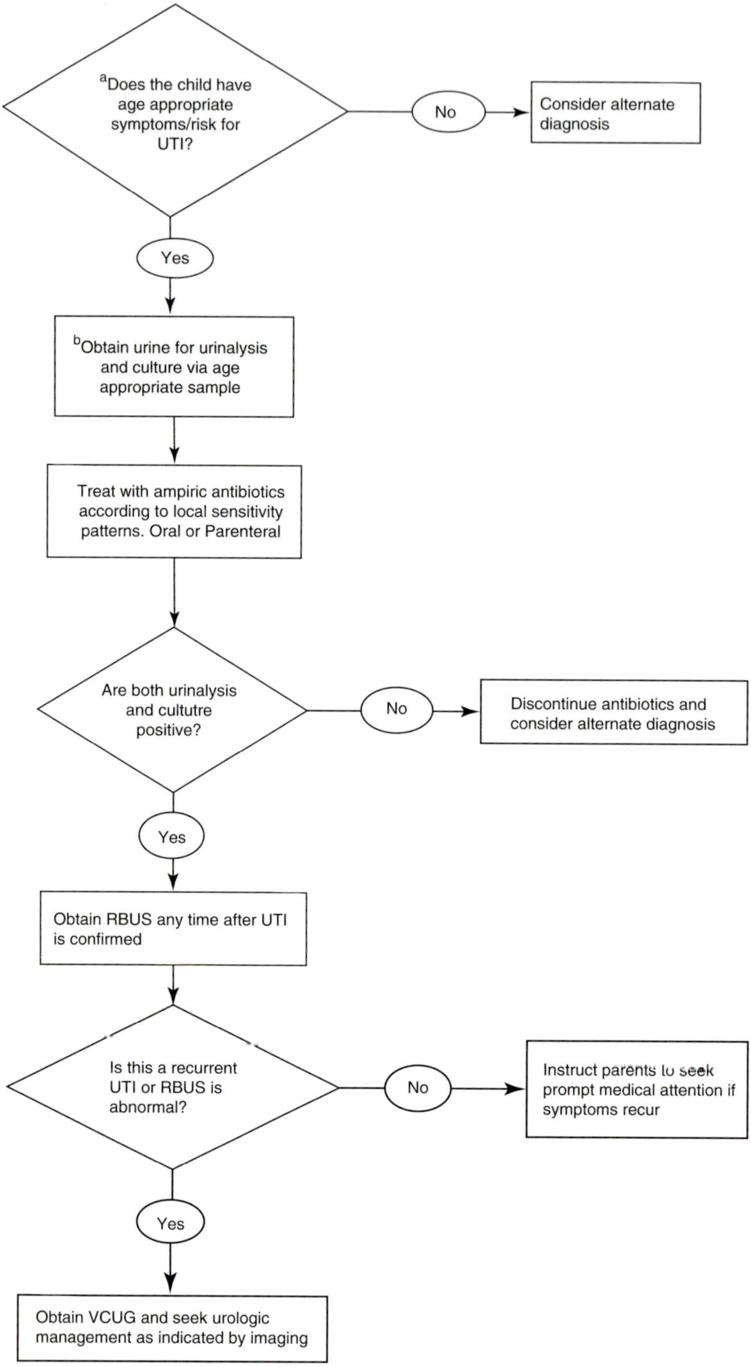

Fig. 6.7 Management of infants and young children with the first documented UTI, based on the Revised American Academy or Pediatrics (AAP) Clinical Practice Guideline algorithm. Reproduced from: Paintsil (2013) (with permission). *RBUS* renal bladder ultrasonograpy

Table 6.5 Antimicrobials for Treatment of UTI

Antibiotic	Dose (mg/kg/day)[a]
Parenteral	
Ceftriaxone	75–100, in 1–2 divided doses IV
Cefotaxime	100–150, in 2–3 divided doses IV
Amikacin	10–15, single dose IV or IM
Gentamicin	5–6, single dose IV or IM
Co-amoxiclav (amoxicillin + clavulanate)	30–35 of amoxicillin, in 2 divided doses IV
Oral	
Cefixime	8, in 2 divided doses (or once daily)
Co-amoxiclav	30–35 of amoxicillin, in 2 divided doses
Ciprofloxacin	10–20, in 2 divided doses
Ofloxacin	15–20, in 2 divided doses
Cephalexin	50–70, in 2–3 divided doses

[a]Dose adjustments for children with reduced GFR (see Chap. 17, Sect. 17.4.1)

- Obstructive uropathy
- Voiding dysfunction
- Constipation
- High-grade vesico-ureteral reflux (VUR)

6.5.9 Chemoprophylaxis for Urinary Tract Infections

- Preventing recurrence of infection and its complications is the crux of the debate on UTI management. Ten to 30 % of children with UTI will have at least one more episode of infection. The majority of recurrences will occur within the first 12 months after the primary infection. The risks for renal damage include age less than 6 months at the initial UTI, the presence of dilating VUR, and renal damage (scarring) detected at the time of initial UTI which may be congenital in origin.
- Growing evidence over the last 10 years showed that prophylactic antibiotic therapy has a limited role in UTI. Adequately powered, well-designed, placebo-controlled trials of long-term antibiotics for the prevention of urinary tract infection in children are lacking. The wide-spread clinical practice of routine antimicrobial prophylaxis is now being questioned.
- There is a concern that common urinary tract pathogens become resistant to traditional agents used for treating UTI.

6.5.9.1 The Evidence Base for Chemoprophylaxis

1. Chemoprophylaxis after the first UTI:

   There is a questionable role of using chemoprophylaxis in all children diagnosed with the first UTI. The evidence to support use of prophylactic antibiotics cannot be generalized to all children experiencing their first UTI. Early diagnosis and prompt treatment of urinary tract infection and predisposing factors are likely to go a long way towards preventing long-term renal damage.

Table 6.6 Antibiotic UTI Prophylaxis

Drug	mg/kg/day	Remarks
Cotrimoxazole	1–2 (trimethoprim)	Avoid in infants <3 months age and G6PD deficiency
Nitrofurantoin	1–2	Gastrointestinal upset; avoid in infants <3 months age, G6PD deficiency and renal insufficiency
Cephalexin	10	Drug of choice in first 3 months of life
Cefixime	2	In select circumstances only

2. Antibiotic prophylaxis in recurrent UTI with or without VUR:
   The evidence that prophylactic antibiotics prevent recurrent UTI in children without VUR is weak. Guidelines from the American Academy of Pediatrics, American Urological Association, and Swedish Medical Research Council recommend using long-term antibiotic prophylaxis (Table 6.6) and yet at the same time acknowledge a lack of evidence for this recommendation.

   Antibiotic prophylaxis may not be warranted in children with low-grade (grade I–II) VUR. We feel that antibiotic prophylaxis may have a role in grade III–V VUR, especially in children <5 years of age.
3. Chemoprophylaxis (medical management) versus surgical management in VUR:
   - Present evidence reveals that renal growth, UTI recurrence, somatic growth, and renal function do not differ between children receiving chemoprophylaxis and those who have surgical intervention.
   - However, surgical intervention can be considered over antibiotic prophylaxis alone in:
     - Grade IV/V (unilateral or bilateral) reflux in children 1–5 years of age
     - Progressive scarring with any grade of VUR
     - Single kidney with grade IV–V reflux
   - Antibiotic prophylaxis is continued for up to 6 months after surgical correction of VUR.
4. Chemoprophylaxis in antenatal hydronephrosis:
   All infants diagnosed with (higher grade) antenatal hydronephrosis should receive antibiotic prophylaxis until they are further evaluated with imaging studies.
5. Chemoprophylaxis in transplantation:
   All children post renal transplantation with features of UTI or evidence of hydronephrosis in the transplanted kidney should receive prophylactic antibiotics. However, there is no convincing evidence that UTI post transplantation is always associated with poor graft outcomes in children.
6. Chemoprophylaxis is not indicated in:
   - Asymptomatic bacteriuria
   - Sibling of children with VUR
   - Children on clean intermittent catheterization
   - Urinary tract obstruction
   - Urolithiasis
   - Neurogenic bladder dysfunction

7. Breakthrough UTI in children receiving antibiotic prophylaxis:
   Recurrences can occur due to infections caused by bacteria that are resistant to the antibiotic used for prophylaxis or by sensitive bacteria (due to poor compliance, inadequate or infrequent dosing). Poor bladder emptying also predisposes to breakthrough infections. Breakthrough UTI should be treated with appropriate antibiotics. Change of the prophhylactic antibiotic after breakthrough infection is not usually required. There is no role for "cyclic" therapy, where the antibiotic used for prophylaxis is changed every 6–8 weeks. Patients suffering breakthrough infections may benefit from double prophylaxis with cotrimoxazole and nitrofurantoin.
8. Choice of antibiotics used for prophylaxis:
   Nitrofurantoin has a lower rate of recurrence of UTI and causes fewer emergences of resistant bacteria compared to trimethoprim and sulfamethoxazole (Table 6.6).

6.5.9.2 Long-Term Follow-Up

Questions remain about the duration of antimicrobial prophylaxis and the need and frequency of urine cultures. After infancy, boys experience far fewer recurrences of UTI than girls. In general, new scarring does not occur after the age of 5 to 7 years. Note that scars can develop in the absence of VUR. Children with renal scarring should receive continued care once or twice a year through adulthood. Patients are monitored for physical growth and blood pressure. Investigations include urinalysis for proteinuria. Children with CKD and progressive loss of renal function may need more frequent visits and comprehensive renal care including regular blood tests. Urine should be promptly cultured in patients having features suggestive of UTI. Yearly ultrasound examinations are done to monitor renal growth.

6.6 Vesicoureteral Reflux

Vesicoureteral reflux (VUR) is seen in 40–50 % infants and 30–50 % children with UTI. Its severity is graded using the International Study Classification, from grades I to V, based on the morphological appearance of the urinary tract on VCUG (Fig. 6.8 and see Sect. 6.6.1). Lower grades of reflux (grades I–III) are more likely to resolve

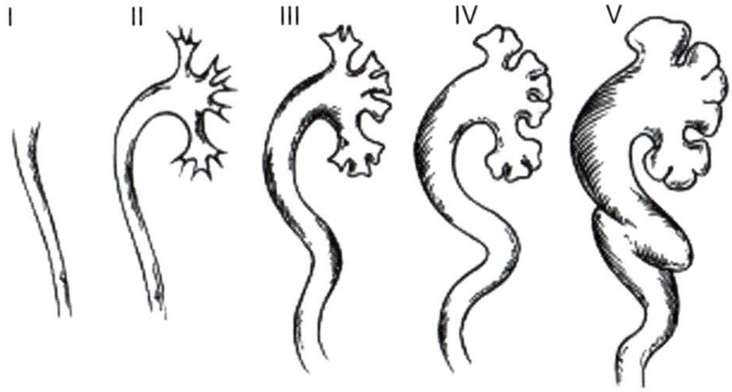

Fig. 6.8 Grading of VUR on VCUG

than higher grades. VUR may be primary or secondary to bladder outflow obstruction (e.g., posterior urethral valves), neurogenic bladder dysfunction, or functional voiding disorder.

The presence of moderate to severe VUR is an important risk factor for pyelonephritis and renal scarring, with subsequent risk of hypertension, albuminuria, and progressive kidney disease. The risk of scarring is highest in the first year of life. The presence of intrauterine VUR has been associated with renal hypoplasia and/or dysplasia.

6.6.1 Grading of VUR

Grade 1: Reflux of urine in a non dilated ureter
Grade 2: Reflux into renal pelvis and calyces without dilatation
Grade 3: Mild dilatation of ureter, pelvis, and calyces with blunting of fornices
Grade 4: Dilatation of ureter, pelvis, and calyces and blunting of fornices
Grade 5: Ureteral tortuosity, gross dilatation of ureter and calyces, and loss of papillary impressions (Fig. 6.8)

Conventional therapy for VUR includes antibiotic prophylaxis and surgical intervention. A recent systematic review on patients with dilating reflux concluded that the outcomes following surgical repair versus prophylaxis were similar in terms of the number of breakthrough UTI and risk of renal scarring. The management of patients with VUR depends on the patient age, grade of reflux, and whether there are any breakthrough infections (Table 6.7).

6.6.1.1 Indications for Surgical Treatment

- Persistent grade IV/V reflux
- High-grade reflux in a single functioning kidney
- Deterioration of renal function due to UTI while on chemoprophylaxis

6.6.2 Screening for VUR in the Sibling

The risk for a sibling to have VUR is 44 % at <2 years age and 9 % at >6 years. Female siblings of a female proband and monozygotic twins have a higher risk. One-third of these may be asymptomatic. Two-thirds have a low-grade reflux which

Table 6.7 Management of VUR[a]

VUR grade	Management
Grades II	Antibiotic prophylaxis until 1 year old Restart antibiotic prophylaxis if breakthrough febrile UTI
Grades III–V	Antibiotic prophylaxis up to 5 years of age Consider surgery if breakthrough febrile UTI Beyond 5 years: prophylaxis continued in children with bowel bladder dysfunction

[a]Derived from the revised Indian Society of Pediatric Nephrology 2011 guidelines

is unilateral in 50 % of cases. A renal ultrasound to screen asymptomatic siblings for VUR is not generally recommended.

6.6.3 VUR and Circumcision

Circumcision reduces the risk of recurrent UTI in high-grade VUR. The indications for circumcision include neonatal VUR, high-grade VUR, and VUR associated with multicystic dysplastic kidneys/renal agenesis.

6.6.4 Newer Interventions for VUR

Conventional, open ureteric reimplantation is increasingly replaced by alternative techniques:

- Subureteric transurethral injection ("STING") of dextranomer/hyaluronic acid copolymer (Dx/HA) (or "Deflux" procedure)
  - The advantages are that it is economical, patient friendly, technically easy, and FDA approved, with cure rates greater than 80 %; needs experience; chances of recurrence of VUR.
- Laparoscopic procedures
  Intra and extra-vesical techniques, shorter hospitalization, limited experience, only short-term follow-ups are available
- Robot-assisted procedures

6.6.5 Outcome

It is not (only) the grade of reflux that predicts the risk of recurrent, febrile UTI and long-term renal outcome, and hence management, but the combination of medical history, presenting symptoms, elimination dysfunction, likelihood of VUR resolution and renal status (Table 6.8). However, genetic factors, the social environment, deprivation, and lack of access to qualified renal care may be the more important determinants of adverse renal outcome.

Table 6.8 Differences in VUR diagnosed while evaluating antenatally diagnosed hydronephrosis versus VUR diagnosed while evaluating urinary tract infection

Feature	Antenatal VUR	Post UTI VUR
Gender, age	Male, infant	Female, older child
Severity	High grade	Low grade
Associated anomalies of kidney and urinary tract	Frequent	Rare
Renal dysplasia	Severe, global	Mild, focal
Urodynamic studies	High voiding pressures, detrusor sphincter dyssynergia	Overactive bladder

6.7 Neurogenic Bladder Dysfunction

The management and evaluation of patients with neurogenic lower urinary tract dysfunction is an essential part of any pediatric urologic practice. Common causes in children are listed in Box 6.2.

6.7.1 Sacral Agenesis

- Complete or partial absence of sacral vertebral bodies.
- Seen in infants of diabetic mothers, in genetic defects of chromosome 7.
- May be associated with presacral mass and anorectal malformations (Currarino triad).
- May be asymptomatic in neonatal period; later incontinence and repeated urinary infections.
- Absence of gluteal cleft; flat buttocks are a clue to underlying defect.
- A lateral X-ray of spine will show a partial or complete absence of sacral vertebrae.
- MRI may be done to confirm the diagnosis and look for associated abnormalities.
- Urodynamic studies may show dyssynergy or complete denervation of bladder and sphincter resulting in recurrent UTI and incontinence, respectively.
- Patients may benefit from clean intermittent catheterization (CIC) and anticholinergic medications, such as oxybutynin or tolterodin for detrusor dyssynergy and surgical correction for incontinence.

6.7.2 Anorectal Malformation

- Failure of canalization of the lower part of colon and rectum usually associated with fistula.
- Renal associations as a part of VACTERL association – unilateral renal agenesis, vesicoureteric reflux, and tethered cord with neurogenic bladder changes.
- Bladder sphincter dyssynergy and denervation of bladder resulting in incontinence can be seen.

Box 6.2 Causes of neurogenic bladder dysfunction in children

Spinal dysraphism (myelomeningocele, lipomyelomeningocele)
Tethered cord
Sacral agenesis
Cerebral palsy
Transverse myelitis
Spinal cord injuries

Note: Daily maternal folate supplementation at a dose of 400 μg can reduce the incidence of spinal dysraphism by as much as 50 %

6.7.3 Cerebral Palsy

- Usually presents with an upper motor neuron (UMN) bladder dysfunction with detrusor overreactivity, rarely with bladder sphincter dyssynergy. Lower motor neuron (LMN) lesion with complete denervation of the bladder can also be seen.
- Incontinence, UTI, and VUR are rarely present.

6.7.4 Spinal Injury

- During the acute phase of the injury, the bladder has reduced contractility and the urethral sphincter is nonreactive.
- Over a variable period of time, detrusor contractility and sphincter reactivity return as spinal cord edema subsides.
- With return of function, an overactive detrusor and bladder sphincter dyssynergy may develop.
- When the lesion affects the cauda equina, there is little to no return of bladder or sphincter function.
- The predominant urodynamic pattern in patients with a thoracic-level lesion is an overactive detrusor with sphincter dyssynergy, high voiding pressures, eventual hydronephrosis, and vesicoureteral reflux.

6.7.5 Spinal Dysraphism

- May be seen as an occult dysraphism or open meningomyelocele with varying degrees of spinal cord damage.
- Myelomeningocele (MMC) accounts for 90 % of open spinal dysraphisms, most commonly seen in the lumbar region.
- 85 % of children with MMC have associated Arnold-Chiari malformation with herniation of the cerebellar tonsils and hydrocephalus.
- The neurologic lesion is variable and cannot be predicted by the level of spinal lesion.
- Assessment in the newborn: urgent renal ultrasound and post-void residue, renal function tests and urine analysis. The closure of the spinal defect takes precedence over assessment. Urodynamic evaluation is done later.
- 5–10 % of neonates have hydronephrosis on renal ultrasound.
- Urodynamic studies (UDS) allow to diagnose (and differentiate): (a) synergy between bladder and external urethral sphincter, (b) dyssynergia with or without bladder hypertonicity, and (c) complete denervation of external sphincter.
- Dyssynergia and bladder pressure >40 cm H_2O have higher risk of urinary tract deterioration and need to be treated and followed up closely.
- The bladder may become hypertrophied assuming "Christmas tree" appearance.
- If bladder sphincter dyssynergy, elevated voiding pressures, or reflux > grade 3 are present, clean intermittent catheterization (CIC) must be initiated.

- Addition of anticholinergic medications like oxybutynin helps reduce the detrusor pressure.
- If a significant post-void residue is present, Credé maneuver or clean intermittent catheterization (CIC) may be used to ensure bladder emptying. Credé maneuver is less effective than CIC and not recommended in routine practice.
- Urodynamic studies may be repeated after 6 weeks to see the improvement in bladder function. Ultrasound is recommended every 6 months and VCU yearly.

6.7.5.1 Occult Spinal Dysraphism

- This includes spina bifida occulta, tethered cord, intraspinal lipoma, neuroenteric cyst, and diastematomyelia.
- The presence of a midline defect like sinus, dermal vascular malformation, hypertrichosis, dimpling of skin, and skin tag in the lower back region may give a clue to underlying spinal abnormality.
- These children are usually asymptomatic at birth and manifest during growth, especially puberty due to traction and cephalad displacement of the cord.
- They may present with new onset incontinence, altered voiding habits, urinary tract infections, or fecal soiling. Lower limb neuromuscular changes and back pain may also develop.
- Investigations: renal function tests, urine examination, ultrasound, and urodynamic studies. VCU may be required to diagnose the presence of VUR.
- Bladder sphincter dyssynergy is common in younger children and denervation of bladder in older children.
- Treatment: de-tethering of cord is done in case of tethered cord. The bladder management is the same as in myelomeningocele (Box 6.3).

6.7.6 Approach to a Child with Neurogenic Bladder Dysfunction

- Neonatal period: mass in the lower back region and abnormal anal opening may be present.
- Older children: incontinence, recurrent UTI, continuous dribbling, constipation, and gait abnormalities.
- Examination: look for spinal defects, sinus, tuft of hair, lipoma, and vascular malformations in the lumbosacral area. Look for a palpable bladder, kidneys, perineal sensations, urine stream, anal reflex, gait, high-arched feet, hammer toes, limb length discrepancy, deep tendon reflexes and tone of lower limbs, and hypertension.
- Investigations: renal function tests, urine routine examination, and culture as required.
- Ultrasonography: to look for renal size, the presence of hydroureteronephrosis, bladder volume, wall thickness, trabeculations, and post-void residue.

Box 6.3 Spinal dysraphism – initial assessment of the newborn

1. Physical examination
   - A critical point to remember is that the level of the vertebral defect cannot be reliably used to predict the degree of neurological impairment
   - Emphasis placed on tone and function of abdominal wall, lower extremities, and anal sphincter
   - The presence or absence of the bulbocavernosus reflex should be noted
   - Abdominal exam to assess for bladder distension and renal size
   - Attempt to characterize voiding pattern:
     - Stream with dry intervals
     - Continuous dribbling
2. Laboratory investigation
   - Serum electrolytes
   - Blood urea nitrogen and creatinine
     - Creatinine reflects that of the mother initially and should be repeated in a few days
   - Urinalysis
3. Radiologic investigations
   - At the time of initial investigation, 15 % can have abnormal upper tract findings
   - Ultrasound to evaluate renal size, assess for associated renal anomalies and hydronephrosis, and determine bladder wall thickness
   - Voiding cystourethrogram to assess for vesicoureteral reflux, bladder diverticulae, bladder wall contours and irregularities, and the bladder neck
   - Radionuclide imaging is not initially required unless renal function or obstruction is a concern
4. Urodynamic investigations
   - Performed as soon as child has recovered from spinal shock
   - Should assess bladder capacity and storage pressure
   - Bladder pressure at the time of leaking should be noted (leak point pressure)
   - Sphincteric function classified as dyssynergic (increased activity), synergic (relaxation), or denervated (absence of activity)
   - Dyssynergic sphincter activity creates a significant risk for upper tract deterioration in the first years of life
   - Upper urinary tract deterioration is also a concern for children with storage pressures of 35–40 cm H_2O or more
   - It is important to remember that bladder dynamics can change with time and regular testing should be performed to assess for deterioration

- VCU may be required to confirm and grade VUR.
- Urodynamic study to assess bladder function and bladder sphincter synergy.
- Spinal MRI to know the cause and extent of spinal injury.
- Antenatally spinal dysraphism can be detected by ultrasound and raised amniotic fluid alpha-fetoprotein levels.

6.7.7 Management

6.7.7.1 Anticholinergic Medications and Clean Intermittent Catheterization (CIC)

- Tailored according to the urodynamic evaluation.
- Goals are to maintain a compliant low-pressure reservoir that can be emptied regularly to protect the kidneys and to achieve urinary continence.
- Children with satisfactory bladder emptying associated with synergic or weak sphincter function can be observed without catheterization.
- CIC should be instituted in patients with a flaccid bladder that does not empty.
- Latex catheters should be avoided to minimize the risk of developing a latex allergy.
- CIC ensures regular, complete emptying of bladder. Reusable catheters may be cleaned and stored in a clean container and discarded after 2–4 weeks. Catheterization is typically performed at 3–4 h (intervals 5–6 times during the day and 2–3 times during the night). Parents or children >6 years old can be trained.
- Combination of CIC with an anticholinergic medication (oxybutynin, tolterodine) is indicated for poorly compliant or unstable bladders and for detrusor sphincter dyssynergia.
- Anticholinergic agents increase the bladder capacity and decrease the magnitude of uninhibited contractions. Oxybutynin is given 2–3 times per day at a dose of 0.3–0.6 mg/kg/day. The medication can be safely used even in the neonatal period. Common anticholinergic side effects are dry mouth, constipation, flushing of the skin, blurred vision, and hyperactivity. Intravesical high doses of oxybutynin (0.9 mg/kg/day) have been used in some patients.

6.7.7.2 Cutaneous Vesicostomy

- Cutaneous vesicostomy is a useful form of temporary urinary diversion in the neonatal period.

6.7.7.3 Botulinum Toxin-A

- Involves injecting the toxin at multiple sites within the bladder detrusor.
- Effects typically last for 6–9 months, thus making repeat injections necessary.

6.7.7.4 Bladder Augmentation

The primary goal of bladder augmentation is to create a low-pressure storage reservoir of adequate capacity to preserve upper urinary tract function and maintain or establish urinary continence when medical therapy has failed (Box 6.4).

Management Issues Following Augmentation

Electrolyte abnormalities are a potential problem when gastrointestinal segments are introduced into the urinary tract. Hyperchloremic metabolic acidosis can develop with ileum or colon and hyperkalemic, hypochloremic metabolic alkalosis can occur

Box 6.4 Techniques for bladder augmentation

1. Techniques without urothelial preservation
   (a) Ileo- and colocystoplasty
   (b) Gastrocystoplasty
2. Techniques with urothelial preservation
   (a) Ureterocystoplasty
   (b) Autoaugmentation
   (c) Seromuscular enterocystoplasty

with stomach. Serum creatinine and electrolytes including bicarbonate, chloride, potassium, phosphorus, calcium, and magnesium should be checked at regular intervals. Excess mucus may be a problem with ileum and colon and these patients may benefit from a program of daily bladder irrigation. Bacteriuria is common and should not be treated unless there are signs of infection (e.g., incontinence, abdominal pain, hematuria, and foul-smelling urine). The risk of malignancy following enterocystoplasty is well recognized. Annual surveillance cystoscopy starting 10 years following augmentation has been recommended. Patients should be made aware of the possibility of bladder perforation, a potentially life-threatening complication following augmentation.

6.7.7.5 Continent Catheterizable Conduits

Anatomic factors or physical restrictions sometimes make urethral catheterization difficult. Under these circumstances fashioning an alternative conduit for catheterization in a more accessible location is indicated. Most commonly the appendix or reconfigured ileum or colon is used to construct a tube. The proximal end of the tube is implanted into the bladder and the distal end is brought out on the abdominal wall as a cutaneous stoma. If possible, it is concealed within the umbilicus; otherwise, it is placed in the lower abdominal quadrant.

6.7.7.6 Bladder Outlet Management (Continence Procedures)

Please see Box 6.5 for various options for management of bladder neck.

Box 6.5 Options for management of the bladder neck

1. Medications to increase bladder outlet resistance

   Alpha agonists (ephedrine, pseudoephedrine) can produce an increase in bladder neck tone and outlet resistance

   Clinical results are often less than satisfactory

(continued)

Box 6.5 (continued)

2. Periurethral injection of bulking agents
   Used to facilitate mucosal coaptation and continence
   Include agents such as collagen, Teflon, and dextranomer/hyaluronic acid
   Continence rates are 5–55 %
3. Urethral lengthening procedures
   Increase bladder outlet resistance by using a portion of the anterior bladder to create a one-way valve to prevent leakage
   Commit the patient to intermittent catheterization
   Often need to be performed with bladder augmentation to improve success
4. Bladder neck suspension and fascial sling procedures
   Fascial slings improve outlet resistance by compression of the urethra
   Bladder augmentation is often needed to improve continence
   Intermittent catheterization is often required
   More successful outcomes in girls
5. Artificial urinary sphincter
   Continence is achieved by bladder neck compression with an inflatable cuff
   Excellent chance of not needing catheterization if it was not required before surgery
   Should monitor for postoperative changes in bladder compliance
   Significant chance of subsequent revision (25 %)
   Continence rates of over 90 % have been achieved

6.7.8 Other Associated Issues in Spinal Dysraphism

Please see Box 6.6 below.

Box 6.6 Associated issues in children with spinal dysraphism

1. Vesicoureteral reflux
   Occurs in 3–5 % of newborns and may develop in up to 40 % with time
   Children with poor compliance and dyssynergia are at particular risk
   Resolution rates of up to 50 % are possible with medical management
   Vesicostomy is an option for infants who respond poorly to medial management
   Reimplantation should be performed at the time of any bladder outlet procedure
   The need to correct low-grade reflux at the time of bladder augmentation remains controversial

Box 6.6 (continued)

2. Urinary tract infection
   - Bacteriuria is common in children performing intermittent catheterization
   - Antibiotic prophylaxis has not been shown to be of benefit
   - Two modifiable factors that have been shown to promote bacteriuria are high catheterization volumes and low catheterization frequency
   - Bacteriuria should be treated when clinical symptoms develop (e.g., fever, abdominal pain, new onset incontinence)
3. Fecal continence
   - The goal to eliminate diapers requires fecal and urinary continence be achieved
   - A bowel regimen should be instituted early
   - Evacuation may be achieved through manual stimulation, suppositories, or enemas
   - Children refractory to medical management may benefit from an antegrade continence enema procedure which creates a continent catheterizable conduit between the skin and the colon that can be used to administer enemas and promote evacuation
4. Sexuality
   - Females typically have more positive experiences with sexual relationships
   - 70 % of females may go on to have children but vaginal delivery may be difficult
   - Sexual satisfaction of males hampered by erection problems, ejaculatory dysfunction, and poor semen quality
   - Fecal and urinary continence can affect the chances of achieving a satisfying sexual relationship
5. Latex allergies
   - Up to 40 % of children with spinal dysraphism become sensitized to latex due to repeated exposure
   - Anaphylactic reactions are almost exclusively intraoperative events
   - Latex exposure should be minimized with the use of latex-free products

6.8 Voiding Dysfunction

6.8.1 Lower Urinary Tract Symptoms

The International Children's Continence Society has standardized the terminology used in children with lower urinary tract symptoms.

The symptoms in the storage phase of the bladder are:

(a) Daytime frequency: applicable in children >5 years of age. Frequency >8 times during the day is considered increased and <3 times per day decreased.
(b) Incontinence: uncontrollable leakage of urine; intermittent or continuous.
(c) Enuresis: intermittent incontinence during sleep.
(d) Urgency: the sudden unexpected urge to void – applicable after 5 years of age.
(e) Nocturia: child has to wake up at night to void.

The symptoms in the voiding phase are:

(a) Hesitancy: difficulty in initiating the stream of urine. Used in children older than 5 years of age.
(b) Straining: the child needs to use abdominal wall muscles to void. Relevant at all ages
(c) Weak stream: urine stream which has no force. Applicable after infancy.
(d) Intermittency: Interruption in the stream of urine.

Other symptoms:

(a) Holding maneuvers: standing on tiptoes, crossing legs, and squatting with the heel pressing on the perineum to hold urine (Vincent's curtsy sign)
(b) Feeling of incomplete emptying
(c) Post-micturition dribble: involuntary leakage of urine after voiding
(d) Pain while passing urine

6.8.2 Investigations for Evaluation of Functional Bladder Abnormalities

6.8.2.1 Elimination Diary

The following details must be recorded. It is relevant in children aged more than 5 years.

(a) Voiding: timing and volumes for at least 48 h, including nighttime voids
(b) Nocturia episodes, daytime incontinence, enuresis episodes, enuresis volumes, bedtime and wake-up time, other symptoms, bowel movements, and encopresis for at least 14 days
(c) Fluid intake for 48 h
(d) Record of bowel habits

6.8.2.2 Measurement of Urine Flow and Residual Urine

This should be performed in a well-hydrated child.

(a) Measurement of urine flow: If the square of the maximum flow rate equals the volume of urine, it is considered normal.
(b) The flow curve will be smooth and bell shaped.
(c) The residual urine is measured by ultrasound examination – Up to 5 ml of urine in the bladder is considered normal; 5–20 ml may suggest incomplete emptying; >20 ml on repeated evaluation is suggestive of significant residue (Box 6.7).

Box 6.7 Bladder calculations

Expected bladder capacity: This is calculated using the following formula up to 12 years of age EBC = 30 + (age in years × 30) ml
The maximum voided volume is considered increased or decreased if it is >150 % or <65 % of the EBC respectively
Residual urine: >20 ml on repeated evaluation is considered significant

6.8.2.3 Urodynamic Studies (UDS)/Cystometry

This is used to determine the following:

Filling Phase

(a) Bladder sensation: can be described only by older children. May be reduced or absent in children with detrusor underactivity or lazy bladder syndrome.
(b) Detrusor activity: normal detrusor activity allows bladder filling without increase in pressure and without involuntary contractions.
(c) Bladder compliance: bladder compliance is the change in unit pressure in the bladder per unit change in bladder volume.
(d) Bladder capacity (see Box 6.7).
(e) Urethral function during filling cystometry.

Voiding Phase

(a) Detrusor underactivity is contraction of reduced strength and/or duration, resulting in prolonged bladder emptying and/or a failure to achieve complete bladder emptying within a normal time span.
(b) Dysfunctional voiding is characterized by an intermittent and/or fluctuating uroflow rate due to involuntary intermittent contractions of the striated muscle of the external urethral sphincter or pelvic floor during voiding.
(c) Detrusor sphincter dyssynergia is the cystometric observation of a detrusor voiding contraction concurrent with an involuntary contraction of the urethral and/or periurethral striated muscle.

Procedure

- The child is catheterized with a triple-lumen catheter after a small amount of liquid lidocaine (1 %) has been injected into the urethra.
- Intravesical pressure is recorded and the bladder is drained and the residual urine carefully measured.
- A small balloon catheter is passed into the rectum to measure intra-abdominal pressure during the cystometrogram to identify artifacts of motion and monitor increases in abdominal pressure during the filling and emptying phases of the study.
- The side-hole port of the urethral pressure channel is positioned at the highest point of resistance in the urethra and kept in place, measuring this resistance throughout bladder filling and emptying to determine the leak point pressure.
- External urethral sphincter electromyography (EMG) is performed using a 24-gauge concentric needle electrode inserted perineally in boys or paraurethrally in girls and advanced into the skeletal muscle component of the sphincter until individual motor unit action potentials are seen or heard on a standard EMG recorder.
- The characteristics of the individual motor unit potentials at rest and in response to various sacral reflexes (i.e., bulbocavernosus, anocutaneous, and Valsalva and Credé maneuvers), bladder filling, and emptying are recorded to detect degrees of denervation.
- The bladder is filled through the second port, while intravesical pressure is monitored via the third port of the tri-lumen urodynamic catheter.

- The rate of filling is set at 10 % of expected capacity for age [age (in years) $+30\times30=$expected capacity in ml].
- Detrusor pressure measurements are continuously recorded throughout filling to calculate compliance and during voiding or leaking to denote emptying pressure.
- Detrusor overactivity is defined as any short-lived pressure rise of >15 cm H_2O from baseline before capacity is reached.
- The child urinates or leaks and the "voiding" pressure is measured.
- The normal end filling pressure should be <10 cm H_2O, while the normal voiding pressure varies from 55 to 80 cm H_2O in boys and from 30 to 65 cm H_2O in girls.
- Detrusor overactivity is considered an abnormal finding at any time.
- The examination findings are considered normal when there is an appropriate capacity; good compliant bladder, with no overactivity; and normal innervation of the sphincter with normal sacral reflexes and an increase in sphincter activity during filling and complete silencing during emptying.
- An upper motor neuron lesion is present when there is detrusor overactivity and/or hyperactive EMG responses to sacral reflexes and/or a failure of the sphincter muscle on EMG to relax (either partially or completely) with a bladder contraction or leaking at capacity.
- A lower motor neuron lesion is noted when there are no contractions of the detrusor muscle and/or there is a degree of denervation, either partial or complete, in the sphincter muscle, with characteristic EMG changes in the motor units or no motor unit activity at all and little or no response in the sphincter to sacral reflexes and/or bladder filling or emptying.

6.8.3 Various Presentations of "Voiding Dysfunction"

(a) Overactive bladder/urge incontinence: usually present with urgency or incontinence associated with urgency.
(b) Voiding postponement: habitually postpone micturition and use holding maneuvers frequently. They may have incontinence due to full bladder.
(c) Underactive bladder/lazy bladder: have a low voiding frequency and use abdominal muscles and strain to achieve bladder emptying.
(d) Dysfunctional voiding: habitually contracts the urethral sphincter during voiding – leads to a staccato pattern on uroflow study.
(e) Stress incontinence: leakage of small amount of urine due to rise in intra-abdominal pressure.
(f) Vaginal reflux: leakage of small amounts of urine about 20 min after voiding.
(g) Giggle incontinence: leakage of small amounts of urine during laughing.

6.8.3.1 Associated Symptoms

(a) Constipation and encopresis
(b) Recurrent urinary tract infections
(c) Sleep disorders

6.8.4 Different Types of Voiding Dysfunction (Non-neurogenic Disorders of Voiding)

1. Transient detrusor sphincter discoordination:
   - Seen in children <2 years
   - Interrupted voiding
   - May present with UTI
   - UDS: DSD, interrupted voiding, high voiding pressure, and good emptying
   - Usually resolves with toilet training
2. Detrusor overactivity (overactive bladder):
   - Presents with frequency, urgency, urge incontinence, holding maneuvers, constipation
   - UDS: unstable detrusor contractions during filling
   - Anticholinergics help
3. Stress incontinence:
   - Leak of small amounts of urine during coughing, straining
   - Rare in children
4. Giggle incontinence:
   - Usually seen in girls
   - Incomplete/complete emptying of bladder while giggling
   - Pelvic floor rehabilitation needed
5. Post-void dribbling:
   - Leakage of urine after voiding and on standing
   - Due to urine trapped in the vagina during voiding
6. Dysfunctional voiding:
   - A urodynamic entity with daytime symptoms.
   - UDS: staccato pattern, fractionated voiding, detrusor sphincter dyssynergia, pelvic floor activity during voiding, and incomplete voiding.
   - More common in girls.
   - Secondary VUR may develop as a result of repetitive episodes of abnormally high intravesical pressure consequent to a combination of detrusor overactivity and detrusor sphincter dyssynergia.
7. Infrequent voider (Lazy bladder syndrome):
   - Diminished urge sensation with overflow incontinence, UTI
   - UDS: poor detrusor contractility, poor emptying, increased capacity, and high compliance
   - Toilet training and timed voiding
8. Hinman syndrome:
   - Also termed as non-neurogenic neurogenic bladder.
   - Present typically at 5–8 years with UTI, poor bladder emptying, incontinence, and constipation.
   - No evident neurologic abnormality.
   - Children grossly overuse their external urethral sphincter to counteract unstable detrusor contractions in an attempt to stay dry. This leads to excessive intravesical pressures, to detrusor hypertrophy, and ultimately to detrusor noncompliance with consequent secondary upper renal tract complications.

- VCU: sacculation and elongation of bladder (fir tree bladder).
- UDS: excessive sphincter activity and dyssynergy.
- Treatment: similar to neurogenic bladder – CIC and anticholinergic medications.

6.8.5 Treatment Options for Voiding Dysfunction

General measures

- Prevent and treat UTI.
- Avoid constipation – use of laxatives and high-fiber diet.
- Maintaining an "elimination diary" should be encouraged to note changes in bowel and bladder patterns.

Behavioral therapy

- Encourage to void every 2–3 h
- Correct posture during voiding

Drugs

- Drugs are selected depending on the pattern of UDS.
- Detrusor antispasmodics – oxybutynin may be used to relax the detrusor during filling. Slow release oxybutynin may be more effective in some than the conventional preparation. Tolterodine is another option.
- Alpha adrenergic blockers: to relax the external sphincter during voiding.

Nonconventional therapies – Botulinum toxin injections are given into the bladder at about 30 sites using a rigid cystoscope under general anesthesia.

Biofeedback

6.9 Enuresis

6.9.1 Introduction

Enuresis is a common condition affecting 5–10 % children. The problem may persist into teenage and, rarely, adulthood. Boys are more commonly affected than girls and the condition tends to run in families.

6.9.2 Terminologies

(As per the International Children's Continence Society (ICCS) guidelines)
Incontinence: Wetting at an inappropriate time and place in a child aged 5 years or older. Incontinence can be continuous or intermittent.

Intermittent enuresis is further classified as daytime and nocturnal incontinence ("enuresis").

Nocturnal enuresis can be categorized as monosymptomatic nocturnal enuresis and non-monosymptomatic nocturnal enuresis.

Monosymptomatic enuresis (MNE) is characterized by bed-wetting for >6 months, symptoms only during nighttime, without lower urinary tract symptoms like urgency, frequency, or dysuria. It is caused by a disparity between bladder capacity and nocturnal urine production and the child's failure to awaken in response to a full bladder. It is termed "primary" when bladder control was never achieved and "secondary" when enuresis manifests after more than 6 months of continence.

6.9.3 Guidelines to Approach

- A checklist for history:
  - Timeframe: primary/secondary enuresis?
  - Bladder: daytime bladder symptoms? voiding frequency?
  - Bowel symptoms: constipation? fecal incontinence?
  - Behavior: problems at home or at school? distressed by enuresis?
  - Previous treatment: which strategies have been used?
  - Family history: enuresis in the family?
  - Difficult to arouse from sleep?
- Evaluation:
  - Tonsillar adenoid hypertrophy: obstructive sleep apnea
  - Abdomen: palpable bladder, kidneys, and fecal masses
  - Genitalia: hypospadias, meatal stenosis, and labial adhesions
  - Neurologic exam: gait, muscle tone, power, perianal/perineal sensation, and rectal sphincter tone
  - Examination of spine: evidence for spina bifida
- Investigations:
  - Urine analysis: dipstick test for glucose, leukocytes, protein, blood, and bacteria.
  - Blood tests, radiology, and urodynamic studies are not routinely indicated in uncomplicated MNE.
  - Bladder diary/voiding charts: strongly recommended.
- Warning signs that do *not* indicate monosymptomatic enuresis
  - Enuresis in a previously dry child
  - Daytime incontinence
  - Weak stream, straining to void, and interrupted micturition
  - Weight loss, excessive thirst, and nausea
  - Glycosuria and proteinuria

6.9.4 Management

6.9.4.1 Counseling

- Children to take control of:
  - Good voiding practices: void regularly during the day and always at bedtime and on awakening
  - Bowel habits
  - Fluid intake
  - No caffeine intake before bedtime

- Parents to be reassured and counseled about:
  - Child's physical and emotional health
  - No blame game
  - Positive reinforcement for *desired behavior* – the use of star charts
  - Waking child at a particular time is a onetime benefit
  - Regular follow-up to sustain the effect

6.9.4.2 First-Line Therapy: Alarm Device Therapy (Level of Evidence 1)

- Enuresis resolves in two thirds of children during use and 50 % of them remain dry.
- Use until either 14 consecutive dry nights or 2–3 months.
- Children who do well with an alarm:
  - A cooperative family
  - No coexisting emotional and behavioral problems
- Frequent bed-wetting (≥4 times/week).
- Drawback: requires time, motivation, and hard work.
- Alarm *clock:* simple and inexpensive – effective in 60–75 %; relapse rates 3 months after completion of treatment same as with "enuresis alarm."

6.9.4.3 First-Line Therapy: Desmopressin Therapy (Level of Evidence 1)

- Assets: easy to use, quick effect, and harmless if not combined with excessive fluid intake (see Box 6.8)
- Drawback: low curative potential
- Practicalities:
  - Dosage: oral tablets 0.2–0.4 mg taken 30–60 min before sleep (may be used as an intranasal spray as well).
  - Keep evening fluid intake below 200 ml and no nighttime drinking.

Box 6.8 Stepwise management of enuresis

First line
New attempt with the alarm if incorrectly used
Combine alarm and desmopressin
Exclude/treat constipation if present
Consider correction of airway obstruction in heavy snorers
New attempt with the alarm approximately every second year

Second line (level I evidence)
Anticholinergics, with or without desmopressin
(Exclude residual urine and/or constipation)

Third line (level I evidence)
Imipramine, with or without desmopressin
(Cardiotoxic if overdosed)

  - Stop treatment if no effect within 2 weeks.
  - Continuous treatment or "on important nights only" may be the alternatives.

6.9.4.4 Therapy-Resistant Enuresis

These children should see a pediatric nephrologist/pediatric urologist. The following issues need to be addressed:

- Case history
  Was the alarm correctly used?
  Exclude occult constipation. Is there heavy snoring?
- Additional evaluation
  - Voiding charts (if not already performed)
  - Measurement of nocturnal urine production
  - Ultrasound (increased bladder wall thickness, distended rectum)
  - Uroflowmetry with measurement of residual urine (recommended)
  - Psychiatric/psychological evaluation

6.9.4.5 Summary of Evidence-Based Management

- Enuresis alarm versus no treatment:
  - Alarms more effective than no treatment
  - Insufficient evidence to compare types of alarms
- Enuresis alarm versus desmopressin therapy:
  - Alarms and desmopressin equally effective.
  - Desmopressin has more immediate effect than alarm.
  - The alarm has more prolonged effect than desmopressin.
- Desmopressin versus no treatment:
  - Desmopressin more effective than no treatment
- Behavioral therapy:
  - Rewards and lifting and waking up the child work better than no treatment.
  - Not as effective as alarm training.
  - Goes a long way as an "added on therapy," added to other interventions.

6.9.5 Conclusion

Enuresis in children needs prompt evaluation to avoid the risk of psychosocial comorbidity. Monosymptomatic enuresis does not warrant extensive investigations. Alarm device and desmopressin in addition to behavioral interventions form the mainstay of therapy for monosymptomatic enuresis.

6.10 Stone Disease (Urolithiasis)

6.10.1 Introduction

The incidence and prevalence of childhood calculi (stone disease) has been increasing over the last decade with considerable regional variability and is referred to as the "stone wave." The pattern of stone composition and localization has also changed. The frequency of calcium oxalate and calcium phosphate has progressively increased while ammonium urate stones that are typically associated with recurrent urinary tract infections and obstructive uropathy have become less common, even in developing countries. The frequency of calculi in bladder has decreased as compared to upper urinary tract calculi. Metabolic factors as the cause for calculi are more likely to be identified in children as compared to adults. The modality of treatment is individualized based on the age of the patient; the size, number, and location of calculi; and the presence of risk factors.

6.10.2 Epidemiology

There is a paucity of data on the burden of urolithiasis in children. The prevalence of calculi in the tropics ranges from 4 to 20 %. In North America, a fivefold increase in the prevalence of calculi in children has been observed in the last decade. Arab countries and South Asia have reported increased prevalence of stone disease. Caucasian population is more commonly affected by stones blacks. Children between 14 and 18 years are 10 times more likely to have urolithiasis compared to children between 0 and 13 years.

6.10.3 Etiology and Risk Factors

6.10.3.1 Metabolic Factors

Metabolic factors are identified in 20–50 % of children with urolithiasis. Younger children are more likely to have an identifiable metabolic risk factor. Hypercalciuria and hypocitraturia are detected in 30–50 % of stone-forming children. The reported prevalence for cystinuria is 1–5 % of all patients with urolithiasis. The prevalence of stones is twice as high in boys as in girls. A geographical "stone belt" extending from the Balkan across Turkey, the Middle East, and Pakistan to northern India is characterized by a high incidence of endemic bladder stones.

6.10.3.2 Dietary Factors

Studies suggest that change in dietary habits has significantly contributed to the increasing prevalence of urolithiasis. Malnutrition and obesity are associated with an increased risk of urolithiasis. Consumption of animal protein is closely linked to the increasing prevalence of stone disease. The high purine content in animal protein results in increased uric acid excretion. The animal proteins contain amino acids containing sulfur, such as cystine and methionine which generate an acid load thereby aggravating calcium mobilization from bones. High protein load augments glomerular filtration resulting in increased excretion of calcium and oxalates. Diet low in animal protein, calcium, and phosphorous but high in cereals results in an acidic urine leading to the development of bladder stones composed of ammonium urate, as seen in children with malnutrition. High sodium intake increases the risk of urolithiasis as high urinary sodium excretion is associated with hypercalciuria and decreased excretion of citrates. Carbohydrate consumption also induces increased urinary calcium excretion. Potassium- and magnesium-rich foods lower the risk of stone formation.

6.10.3.3 Urinary Tract Infection

Urinary tract infection by urease-producing bacteria (e.g., Proteus, Pseudomonas) results in increased ammonia production. This results in formation of struvite and carbonate apatite stones.

6.10.3.4 Genetic Factors

Genetic factors are recognized to play an important role in urolithiasis. The mode of inheritance is predominantly polygenic. Single gene defects and autosomal inheritance are responsible for cystinuria, primary hyperoxaluria, and in few diseases associated with hypercalciuria (e.g., Dent's disease, Bartter syndrome). Two-thirds of patients with idiopathic hypercalciuria may have positive family history of stones. Common environmental and dietary factors may result in familial recurrences and hence a family history of stone disease does not always indicate a genetic cause.

6.10.3.5 Other Factors

People in regions with hot climates have an increased prevalence of stone disease that is related to increased urine concentration secondary to a combination of dehydration and low fluid intake.

Melamine contamination of infant milk formula has been associated with urolithiasis in young children.

An increase in antibiotic use has been postulated as a contributor to urolithiasis by reducing normal gut flora that ordinarily inhibits the absorption of lithogenic substances (Table 6.9).

Table 6.9 Causes of urolithiasis in children

Hypercalcemia with hypercalciuria Vitamin D overdose Hyperparathyroidism Prolonged immobilization William's syndrome	*Hyperoxaluria* Primary hyperoxaluria, type I, Primary hyperoxaluria type II, Secondary hyperoxaluria (e.g., malabsorption syndrome, chronic diarrheal disease, small bowel resection, cystic fibrosis)
Normal serum calcium with hypercalciuria Idiopathic hypercalciuria, familial hypophosphatemia with hypercalciuria, Dent's disease, Bartter syndrome, autosomal dominant hypocalcemia with hypercalciuria, familial hypomagnesemia, Lowe syndrome	*Hyperuricemia* Lesch-Nyhan syndrome, partial HPRT deficiency, glycogenosis type 1a and type 1b, xanthinuria, lymphoproliferative disorders, salicylates
Hypocitraturia Distal renal tubular acidosis	*Miscellaneous* Cystinuria Melamine toxicity Drugs – indinavir, steroid excess, furosemide, topiramate

HPRT hypoxanthine-guanine phosphoribosyltransferase

6.10.4 Pathogenesis

Stone formation is a multifactorial process. The key event in the initiation and growth of calculi is urinary supersaturation of the concerned ions. Supersaturation reflects the ratio of an ion's concentration in urine to its solubility which determines the likelihood of formation of crystals. Supersaturation is influenced by urine pH, flow volume, and concentration of stone-forming ions and the balance between inhibitors and promoters of crystallization in urine. Low urine volume increases the ion concentration. Cystine and uric acid are more likely to precipitate in acidic urine, while calcium phosphate is more like to aggregate in alkaline urine. The aggregation of calcium oxalate is primarily determined by the concentrations of calcium and oxalate in urine. Uric acid in urine also promotes calcium oxalate precipitation. Urine citrate is an important inhibitor of calcium oxalate and phosphate stone formation. Other inhibitors in urine are magnesium, pyrophosphate, and Tamm-Horsfall protein.

6.10.5 Clinical Features

The clinical presentation of stones in children is heterogeneous. Acute severe flank pain that radiates to the groin is usually seen in older children. It is rare in children <5 years. Younger children may present with nonspecific pain involving the whole abdomen or localized to the flanks or suprapubic region which may be confused with a colic. Macroscopic or microscopic hematuria can occur in up to 90 % of children with urolithiasis. Dysuria and increased frequency may be the presenting manifestation in a subset of children with urolithiasis. Symptoms of urinary tract infection as the presenting feature are not uncommon. Urethral stone may cause acute urinary obstruction and strangury. Renal stones may be incidentally detected during evaluation of children who present with features of tubular disorders or chronic kidney disease.

6.10.6 Evaluation

6.10.6.1 History and Examination

A good medical history and a thorough examination will help in establishing an accurate diagnosis:

- Family history of hematuria, renal failure, and urolithiasis suggest an underlying metabolic or genetic condition (e.g., primary hyperoxaluria, Dent's disease).
- A dietary history with a focus on fluid and salt consumption.
- History of drug intake (e.g., furosemide, protease inhibitors, topiramate) could provide clues to the underlying etiology.
- Children with history of recurrent UTIs, symptoms of intestinal malabsorption (secondary hyperoxaluria), and prolonged immobilization are at risk of urolithiasis. Polyuria, failure to thrive, and rickets suggest renal tubular acidosis. Carpopedal spasms indicate defect in calcium metabolism, while features of gout suggest underlying enzyme defect in uric acid metabolism.

6.10.6.2 Imaging

- Ultrasonography (US) is the initial study of choice in the assessment of calculi in children as it is noninvasive and avoids radiation. Majority of calculi confined to the kidney can be detected by US. However, ureteral calculi and smaller calculi (<5 mm) may be missed by US.
- Plain abdominal radiography will pick up radiopaque stones (e.g., calcium oxalate, calcium phosphate, struvite stones), while radiolucent calculi may be missed (e.g., uric acid, cystine, xanthine, indinavir).
- Noncontrast computed tomography is the gold standard and is indicated in children with persistent symptoms of urolithiasis and a normal US.

6.10.6.3 Metabolic Tests

All children presenting with urolithiasis should undergo a complete metabolic evaluation:

- Blood tests include serum creatinine, calcium, phosphorous, bicarbonate, uric acid, and magnesium. Serum electrolytes will be indicated in children with tubular disorders. 25-hydroxyvitamin D and parathormone (PTH) should be estimated in children with hypercalcemia.
- Fresh urine sample should be examined for crystals (e.g., rhomboid- or rosette-shaped uric acid crystals, coffin-lid-shaped triple phosphate crystals, hexagonal cystine crystals; for images, see Chap. 1, Sect. 1.3.3.4). The presence of low molecular weight protein (β2 microglobulin) in urine may suggest Dent's disease.
- Twenty-four hour urine collection is used for estimation of calcium, oxalate, citrate, uric acid, and sodium. The adequacy of urine collection is confirmed with measurement of urinary creatinine excretion (0.13–0.22 mmol or 15–25 mg/kg/day).
- Random urine sample may be obtained for measuring ratio of calcium, citrate, oxalate, and uric acid to creatinine in infants and young children who are not toilet trained. The normal values of the urinary solutes are given in Sect. 17.1.
- Urine culture is advised if a concomitant UTI is suspected.

6.10.6.4 Stone Analysis

Stones (passed in the urine or surgically removed) can be analyzed with infrared spectroscopy or radiograph diffraction.

6.10.7 Treatment

6.10.7.1 Medical Therapy

Acute Management

Renal colic is often severe and should be treated promptly with oral or parenteral analgesics. Oral or intravenous hydration at 1.5–2 times maintenance to maintain a high urine flow rate is recommended in acute symptomatic patients. Although studies in children are limited, some drugs (e.g., tamsulosin) have been used which may aid in the passage of stones. Antibiotic therapy is initiated if UTI is suspected.

Diet and Fluids

- Liberal fluid intake is an important component of stone prevention by effectively reducing the concentration of lithogenic factors. Increased fluid intake may be required during summer or in situations of increased insensible fluid losses. Fluids that increase urinary pH and citrate excretion such as fruit juices like orange, lime water, and coconut water are suggested.
- A low-salt diet corresponding to less than 2–3 mmol (mEq)/kg/day is generally recommended for those with calcium containing stones.
- Children with calculi should consume 100 % of the daily recommended protein allowance for age but should not eat excessive animal protein (meat, poultry, and fish).
- Calcium restriction is not recommended.
- Fruits and vegetables contain large amounts of potassium and citrate and inhibit crystallization in urine.
- Children with hyperoxaluria should avoid high-oxalate food like spinach, soy beans, tofu, rhubarb, beets, sweet potatoes, nuts (almonds, peanuts, and cashews), and chocolates.

Medications

- Alkalinization of urine with potassium citrate (2–4 mmol (mEq)/kg/day) prevents calcium oxalate stone formation by increasing urinary citrate levels. It is also useful in children with hyperoxaluria, uric acid stones, and cystinuria (goal is to keep urine pH >7). Overtreatment with alkali may increase the risk of calcium phosphate stone formation.
- Thiazide diuretic is often indicated for children with hypercalciuria who do not respond to dietary measures.
- Allopurinol (4–10 mg/kg/day) is the therapy of choice for children with uric acid calculi in combination with high urine flow rate and alkalinization of the urine.
- One third of children with primary hyperoxaluria type I are responsive to pharmacological doses of pyridoxine (vitamin B6). The treatment is initiated with 2–5 mg/kg/day; the dose is gradually increased to 8–10 mg/kg/day.

6.10.7.2 Surgical Treatment

- Surgical intervention is reserved for children with uncontrolled pain, who present with acute urinary obstruction, or who have large stones in the urinary tract that will not spontaneously pass.
- Surgical approaches are extracorporeal shockwave lithotripsy (ESWL), ureteroscopy, percutaneous nephrolithotomy, and open surgery. The choice of modality will depend on the child's size, urinary tract anatomy, location, and number and size of stones.
- ESWL is a first-line treatment option for most pediatric upper tract urinary calculi. Routine ureteral stenting may not be required during ESWL. Stents before ESWL may be indicated in sepsis, obstruction, and solitary kidney. ESWL

is not effective in children with calcium monohydrate or calcium phosphate or cystine stones, due to their hardness. Overall stone-free rates for ESWL in children range from as low as 44 % after a single session to 95 %. Retreatment may be required in 10–54 % of cases.

- Ureterorenoscopy (URS) using ureteroscopic endoscopes is ideally suited for calculi in the mid and distal ureter but also has been used for removing calculi in the proximal ureter or kidney. Success rates range from 50 to 97 % for a single session.
- Percutaneous nephrolithotomy (PCNL) is indicated in children with anatomic abnormalities, infected stones, and stones resistant to ESWL. Stone-free rates for PCNL range from 70 to 90 %.
- Open surgery is preferred for removing stones that are large (e.g., staghorn calculi) or associated with anatomical abnormalities.

6.11 Kidney Trauma

6.11.1 Natural Protection and Predisposition

- The kidney is protected by heavy lumbar muscles, vertebral bodies, and ribs.
- Existing pathology such as hydronephrosis or tumors are more readily ruptured from mild trauma.

6.11.2 Etiology and Mechanism of Injury

- Blunt trauma (90 %), e.g., motor vehicle accidents, fights, falls, and speed sports, is the most common mechanism. Rapid deceleration injuries may cause major vascular avulsion, thrombosis or ureteropelvic junction avulsion. Surgical exploration rate in blunt trauma is less than 2 %.
- Penetrating injuries (10 %) results from gunshot and stab wounds. Associated abdominal visceral injuries are present in 80 %.

6.11.3 Complications

- *Urinoma*: Persistent urinary extravasation may cause hydronephrosis and abscess formation.
- *Hydronephrosis*: Large retroperitoneal hematomas may result in perinephric fibrosis engulfing the ureteropelvic junction, causing hydronephrosis.
- *Arteriovenous Fistula*: May occur after penetrating injuries.
- *Renal Vascular Hypertension*: 1–7 % of cases. It may be due to ischemic renal tissue or constriction of the renal artery by fibrosis during healing. Rarely, hypertension occurs as a result of arteriovenous fistula.

6.11.4 Clinical Findings

6.11.4.1 Symptoms

- Visible evidence of abdominal trauma.
- Flank or abdominal pain.
- Large retroperitoneal hematoma may cause paralytic ileus, nausea, and vomiting.
- Evidence of associated injuries

6.11.4.2 Signs

- Shock or signs of a large loss of blood may be noted.
- A resolving retroperitoneal hematoma may cause slight fever (38.3 °C), but higher temperatures suggest infection.
- Ecchymosis in the flank or upper quadrants of the abdomen.
- Palpable large retroperitoneal hematoma or urinoma. The size and expansion of palpable masses must be carefully marked for monitoring.
- Acute abdomen with absent intestinal sounds if intraperitoneal bleeding occurs.

6.11.5 Laboratory Findings

- Microscopic or gross hematuria indicates injury to the urinary tract:
  - The degree of renal injury does not correspond to the degree of hematuria. It may be absent with significant injuries: renal vascular injury, rapid deceleration accidents.
  - Significant microscopic hematuria is defined as greater than 50 RBC/HPF in blunt trauma and greater than 5 RBC/HPF in penetrating injuries.
- The hematocrit may be initially normal, but a drop greater than 3.0 units indicates persistent bleeding.

6.11.6 Imaging Findings

6.11.6.1 Indications

- Children with positive findings on clinical examination for abdominal, flank or pelvic pain, or ecchymosis
- Significant microscopic hematuria or gross hematuria
- Rapid deceleration injury

6.11.6.2 Modalities

- Abdominal CT scan is the most direct and effective means of staging renal injuries. It clearly defines parenchymal lacerations and urinary extravasation, shows the extent of the retroperitoneal hematoma, identifies nonviable tissue, and outlines injuries to surrounding organs.
- Ultrasonography is of little use initially but can be used for follow-up of hematoma/urinoma size.

6.11.7 Grading of Renal Trauma

- Grade 1 (90 %): Contusion or subcapsular hematoma, nonexpanding without parenchymal laceration. Microscopic hematuria is common, but gross hematuria is rare.
- Grade 2: Parenchymal laceration less than 1.0 cm in depth without extravasation. Nonexpanding hematoma and perirenal hematoma confined to renal retroperitoneum.
- Grade 3: Parenchymal laceration more than 1.0 cm in depth without collecting system rupture or urinary extravasation. Bleeding can be significant.
- Grade 4: Parenchymal laceration extending through renal cortex, medulla, and collecting system with urinary extravasation or laceration at a segmental vessel or vascular thrombosis of segmental renal artery.
- Grade 5: Multiple grade 4 parenchymal lacerations resulting in a shattered kidney, thrombosis of the main renal artery, and renal pedicle avulsion.

6.11.8 Treatment

- Initial treatment: Prompt treatment of shock and hemorrhage, complete resuscitation, and evaluation of associated injuries.
- Children with hemodynamic instability or those with penetrating intra-abdominal trauma should undergo immediate abdominal exploratory laparotomy. These patients can be staged intraoperatively with one-shot excretory urography.
- Children with blunt trauma who were hemodynamically stable are managed according to the stage:
  - Grade I injury without gross hematuria: Safely discharged home to be followed with urinalysis.
  - Grades I to III with gross hematuria: Hospital admission, strict bed rest, and observation until gross hematuria clears with no additional laboratory studies or imaging necessary. After hematuria resolves, the patient may begin ambulation and can be discharged home.
  - Grade IV and V: ICU admission, strict bed rest, and clinical monitoring, serial hematocrit, and repeat imaging at 48 h or earlier if clinically prompted:
    - Worsening hematoma with hemodynamic instability or unresponsiveness to up to 3 units of packed RBC transfusions necessitates renal exploration.
    - Worsening hematoma with hemodynamic stability and evidence of aneurysm may necessitate angioembolization.
    - Worsening extravasation on serial CT: percutaneous drainage of the collecting system with or without ureteral stent.
    - After the critical window of the first 48 h has passed and repeat imaging confirms successful conservative management, the child can be transferred from the ICU, remaining on bed rest until the resolution of gross hematuria. Then, he or she may be discharged home with strict instructions to avoid all strenuous activity for 1 month.

6.11.9 Prognosis and Follow-Up

- Most renal injuries have an excellent prognosis, with spontaneous healing and return of renal function. Heavy late bleeding may occur 1–4 weeks after injury.
- Careful monitoring of blood pressure for several months is necessary.
- At 3–6 months, a follow-up CT scan and/or ultrasound and DMSA scan should be obtained to asses healing and to rule out hydronephrosis.

Suggested Reading

American Academy of Pediatrics, Committee on Quality Improvement Subcommittee on Urinary Tract Infections (2011) Practice parameters: the diagnosis treatment and evaluation of the initial urinary tract infections in febrile infants and young children. Pediatrics 128(3):595–610

Conway JJ, Maizels M (1992) The "well tempered" diuretic renogram: a standard method to examine the asymptomatic neonate with hydronephrosis or hydroureteronephrosis. A report from combined meetings of The Society for Fetal Urology and members of The Pediatric Nuclear Medicine Council – The Society of Nuclear Medicine. J Nucl Med 33(11):2047–2051

Fernbach (1993) Ultrasound grading of hydronephrosis: introduction to the system used by the Society for Fetal Urology. Pediatr Radiol 23:478

Fonseca FF, Tanno FY, Nguyen HT (2012) Current options in the management of primary vesicoureteral reflux in children. Pediatr Clin North Am 59:819–834

Frimberger D, Cheng E, Kropp BP (2012) The current management of the neurogenic bladder in children with spina bifida. Pediatr Clin North Am 59(4):757–767

Hodson EM, Wheeler DM, Smith GH, Craig JC, Vimalachandra D (2007) Interventions for primary vesicoureteric reflux. Cochrane Database Syst Rev 3: CD001532

Indian Pediatric Nephrology Group. Consensus statement on management of urinary tract infections. Indian Pediatr 48:709–717. 2011, Indian Pediatric Nephrology Group (2011) Consensus statement on management of urinary tract infections. Indian Pediatr 48:709–717

Lopez M, Hoppe B (2010) History, epidemiology and regional diversities of urolithiasis. Pediatr Nephrol 25:49–59

Maizels et al (2004) Fetal bladder sagittal length: a simple monitor to assess normal and enlarged fetal bladder size, and forecast clinical outcome. J Urol 172:1995

Mourtzinos A, Stoffel JT (2010) Management goals for the spina bifida neurogenic bladder: a review form infancy to adulthood. Urol Clin N Am 37:527–535

Nevéus T, von Gontard A, Hoebeke P, Hjälmås K, Bauer S, Bower W, Jørgensen TM, Rittig S, Vande Walle J, Yeung CK, Djurhuus JC (2006) The standardization of terminology of lower urinary tract function in children and adolescents: report from the standardisation committee of the International Children's Continence Society (ICCS). J Urol 176:314–324

Shin JS et al (2007) Nomogram of fetal renal growth expressed in length and parenchymal area derived from ultrasound images. J Urol 178:2150

Song R, Yosypiv IV (2011) Genetics of congenital anomalies of the kidney and urinary tract. Pediatr Nephrol 26:353–364

Yamaçake KG, Nguyen HT (2012) Current management of antenatal hydronephrosis. Pediatr Nephrol 28(2):237–243

Yeung CK, Sihoe JDY, Bauer SB (2007) Chapt. 123: Voiding dysfunction in children: non-neurogenic and neurogenic. In: Wein AJ, Kavoussi LR, Novick AC, Partin AW, Peters CA (eds) Campbell-Walsh urology, vol 4, 9th edn. W.B. Saunders, Philadelphia, pp 3604–3655

Hypertension 7

Martin Bitzan

7.1 Introduction

Blood pressure (BP) measurement should be part of routine pediatric health care. The wide application of normative BP values for children and adolescents revealed that mild elevations in BP during childhood are more common than previously recognized, particularly in adolescents.

- During childhood and adolescence, systolic and diastolic BP increases with age and body growth. It tends to "track" within a narrow percentile range into adulthood.
- Based on cross-sectional studies from various societies, 2–5 % of school children are hypertensive and about 16 % have prehypertension. Hypertension (HTN) is third on the list of chronic pediatric diseases (after asthma and obesity).
- Factors that increase the likelihood for (pediatric) HTN include family history, ethnic background, birth weight, weight percentile and body mass index (BMI), nutritional sodium intake, physical activity, insulin resistance, and sympathetic nervous system activation. Many of the latter variables are amenable to modification.
- HTN in childhood is a risk factor for adult hypertension, accelerated atherosclerosis, and premature cardiovascular complications.
- HTN has become a significant public health problem worldwide, affecting 20–25 % of adults. Poor BP control is the # 1 attributable risk for death. It is the cause of 60 % of cerebrovascular disease (CVD) and almost 50 % of heart disease. HTN and related CVD consume >15 % of all health-care costs.
- Early intervention may impact on adult HTN and the risk of cardiovascular and renal morbidity.

M. Bitzan
Division of Pediatric Nephrology, Montreal Children's Hospital,
McGill University, 2300, rue Tupper, Montreal, QC H3H 1P3, Canada
e-mail: martin.bitzan@mcgill.ca

K. Phadke et al. (eds.), *Manual of Pediatric Nephrology*,
DOI 10.1007/978-3-642-12483-9_7, © Springer-Verlag Berlin Heidelberg 2014

7.2 Definitions

- Definitions of HTN in adult and pediatric populations differ conceptually.
- HTN in adults was defined by the Joint National Committees (JNC7) (Chobanian et al. 2003). Threshold values for adults have been validated by association with outcome (morbidity and mortality). A single set of values is used.
- In contrast, the definition of "normal" BP in children is statistical: <95th percentile for age, gender, and height. Consequently, HTN is defined as a systolic or diastolic BP ≥95th percentile for age, gender, and height on at least three separate occasions (Box 7.1). However, there is limited validation of BP boundaries.

Box 7.1 Definitions: Pediatric Hypertension

Hypertension in children is defined by systolic or diastolic blood pressure (BP) consistently >95th percentile for age, gender, and height on at least three separate occasions

Stages of Hypertension

Normal	BP <90th percentile
Prehypertension ("high-normal")	BP ≥90th to <95th percentile
Prehypertension in adolescents	BP ≥120/80 mmHg, even if <90th percentile
Stage 1 hypertension	BP 95th to 99th percentile plus 5 mmHg
Stage 2 hypertension	BP >99th percentile plus 5 mmHg

Primary hypertension

Hypertension for which a single underlying cause cannot be identified

Dominant form of hypertension above age 12 years, but also found in younger children

>90 % of adults with significantly increased BP have primary hypertension

Secondary hypertension

Hypertension for which a cause can be identified

Children requiring antihypertensive therapy have to a large part secondary hypertension

80–90 % of children with severe secondary hypertension have underlying renal disease

Hypertensive emergency

Symptomatic, often acute BP >99th percentile for age, height, and gender with *evidence of target-organ injury* that requires prompt treatment to prevent further damage or death

Hypertensive urgency

Symptomatic BP elevation >99th percentile *with no current evidence of secondary organ injury*. If left untreated, target-organ injury may result imminently

Hypertensive encephalopathy

Serious complication of severe hypertension due to impaired autoregulation of cerebral blood flow that leads to cerebral hypoperfusion

- Current recommendations are summarized in several documents, such as the *Fourth Report on the Diagnosis, Evaluation, and Treatment of High Blood Pressure in Children and Adolescents* from the National High Blood Pressure Education Program (NHBPEP) Working Group on Children and Adolescents (2004) and the Guidelines of the European Society of Hypertension (Lurbe et al. 2009).
- The nomograms for BP percentiles recommended for day-to-day practice are given in the Appendix.

7.3 Etiology of Hypertension

Differentiation between primary and secondary HTN has important implications for the extent of investigations and treatment. The term "essential" HTN is not used anymore.

Primary Hypertension

- For the majority of older children and adolescents with HTN, an etiology cannot be identified currently (primary hypertension).
- Children with primary HTN are more often obese, have hyperinsulinism or insulin resistance, and ingest more sodium salt than normotensive subjects.

Secondary Hypertension (Hypertension with Definable Cause)

- HTN can be caused by a variety of acute or chronic diseases, often involving the kidneys; structural, genetic, and/or metabolic abnormalities; and extrinsic causes (secondary hypertension).
- Frequent causes of secondary HTN in a primary care setting are coarctation of the aorta, renal parenchymal disease (e.g., glomerulonephritis, scars), and renovascular (e.g., renal artery stenosis) and endocrinological disorders (e.g., hyper- or hypothyroidism).
- Causes and clinical presentation or secondary HTN are listed in Table 7.1.

Causes of Hypertension in the Newborn

- Acute urinary obstruction
- Renal vascular (venous, arterial) thrombosis
- Renal artery stenosis
- Coarctation of aorta
- Renal failure
- Congenital renal anomalies (e.g., ARPKD)
- Bronchopulmonary dysplasia
- Drugs (glucocorticoids, aminophylline)

Monogenic (Mendelian) Forms of Hypertension

All forms of monogenic HTN so far identified share two principles: excessive (unregulated) sodium reabsorption, generally via the epithelial sodium channel (ENaC) in the distal nephron (distal tubule or collecting duct) as a functional consequence of a genetic mutation, and the invariable suppression of plasma renin

Table 7.1 Causes and presentation of secondary hypertension

Causes of hypertension	Specific diagnoses and associated conditions	Diagnostic clues and clinical and laboratory findings
Drug mediated	Glucocorticoids, calcineurin inhibitors, sympathomimetics, oral contraceptives, stimulants (e.g., methylphenidate), ephedrine, erythropoietin, NSAIDs Caffeine, tobacco, ethanol Cocaine, amphetamines (MDMA, ecstasy)	History, drug screen
Renal parenchymal disease	Renal scars	History of UTI, abnormal upper or lower urinary tract imaging
	Acute postinfectious GN	Gross hematuria, edema, preceding infection, low C3
	Henoch-Schönlein purpura nephritis	Purpuric rash, hematuria, proteinuria
	Hemolytic uremic syndrome	Hemolytic anemia, thrombocytopenia, hematuria, renal failure
	Acute tubulointerstitial nephritis	Sterile pyuria, dysuria, fatigue
	Idiopathic nephrotic syndrome/FSGS	(Large) proteinuria
	Chronic glomerulonephritis (MPGN, IgA nephropathy, SLE)	Proteinuria, hematuria, elevated serum creatinine, specific laboratory tests
	Other forms of chronic kidney disease (CKD)	Elevated serum creatinine, proteinuria Laboratory and metabolic changes related to CKD
		Abnormal urinary tract imaging
Traumatic injury	(Vascular) renal trauma	History, gross hematuria
	Orthopedic procedure with bone traction	Medical history
Acute urinary obstruction		Flank pain, renal mass, urinary retention
Renovascular disease	Renal artery stenosis (Fibromuscular dysplasia, NF1, Williams syndrome [Williams-Beuren syndrome, WBS])	Neurofibromata, café au lait (NF), hypercalcemia (WBS)
	Arteritis (Kawasaki, Takayasu, Moyamoya)	
	Renal arterial or venous thrombosis	Gross hematuria, renal mass

Table 7.1 (continued)

Causes of hypertension	Specific diagnoses and associated conditions	Diagnostic clues and clinical and laboratory findings
Cardiovascular	Coarctation of the aorta, hypoplastic abdominal aorta (middle aortic) syndrome	Pulse difference, systolic murmur; cardiac echocardiography, angiography
Polycystic disease	ARPKD, ADPKD	Renal mass, family history
Neurological causes	Increased intracranial pressure	Head trauma, intracranial bleed, meningitis
	Spinal injury, Guillain-Barre syndrome	History of trauma Paralysis, loss of bladder/bowel control
Tumor	Wilms tumor (nephroblastoma), sarcoma	Gross hematuria, renal mass, loss of bladder or bowel control, (other) neurological signs
Neuroendocrine	Pheochromocytoma	Flushing, palpitations, headache
Mendelian forms of hypertension	See table at the end of the chapter (Table 7.8)	See Fig. 7.1

activity (PRA) secondary to sodium retention and extracellular fluid volume expansion. HTN can be associated with excessive or suppressed aldosterone secretion. Rationale therapies are available to prevent long-term morbidity and death.

- Mutations in at least eight different genes have been identified that lead to hypertension.
- Suspect monogenic causes in patients with a family history of early-onset severe hypertension or death from premature cerebral vascular accidents and heart failure.
- Hypokalemia is a common feature of the majority of low-renin hypertension states with the exception of Gordon's syndrome.
- Aldosterone levels are dependent on the effect of the gene mutation: they are high in Gordon's syndrome, GRE, and FHII.
- Monogenic hypertension can be divided into distal nephron and adrenal disorders based on the tissue where the mutated gene is primarily expressed (see table at the end of the chapter).
- Figure 7.1 outlines a rational, physiological approach to diagnostic and genetic work-up.
- Baseline evaluation for suspected monogenic (hereditary) hypertension includes serum and urine electrolytes (Na^+, K^+) and PRA and aldosterone.
- Important points to remember:
  - Family history can be misleading due to the high prevalence of primary HTN even in adolescents.
  - A child with severe HTN is more likely to have one of the inherited disorders, but many individuals with inherited HTN have only mild or moderate HTN. Likewise, classical serum potassium changes may be modest and not fall outside normal laboratory ranges.
- The definitive diagnosis often requires genetic testing.

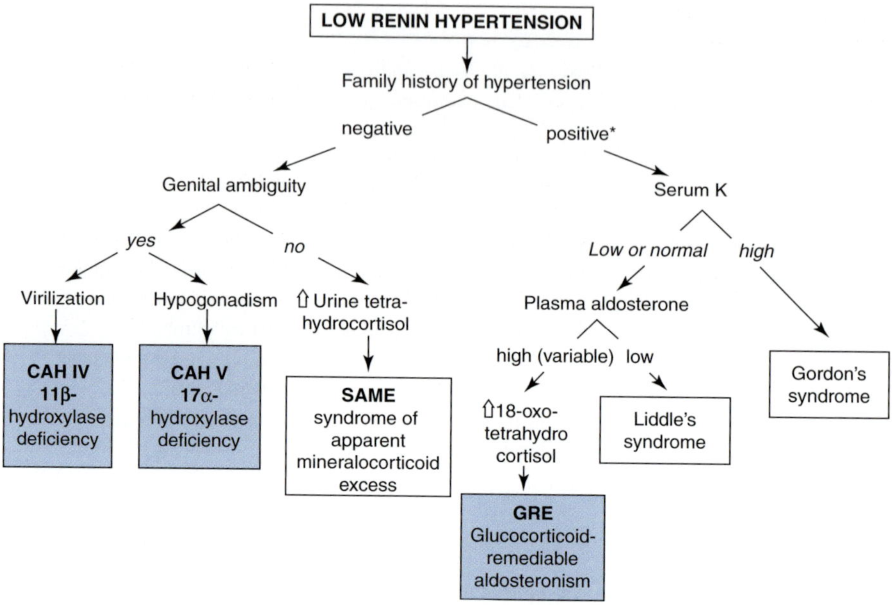

Fig. 7.1 Simplified decision tree for the rational diagnosis of defined, monogenic low-renin hypertension syndromes, limited to those presenting during childhood or adolescence. For details and abbreviations, see Table 7.8. *White boxes*, distal tubular disorders; *shaded boxes*, adrenal disorders; *, "positive" family history may be misleading in view of the high prevalence of primary hypertension

7.4 Clinical Signs and Symptoms

- *Primary hypertension* in children is usually mild or moderate (stage 1 or less) with insidious onset. Detection is often incidental during routine medical appointment.
- Childhood hypertension is not silent. Studies showed significantly higher rates of headache, difficulty falling asleep and daytime fatigue, and chest and abdominal pain compared with matched controls – all of which improved after BP normalization.
- Severe hypertension can present with headache, vomiting, visual disturbances, altered sensorium, epistaxis, palpitations, or flushes.
- *Secondary hypertension* may present with mild to severe symptoms and target-organ injury, but may also be asymptomatic.
- Patients with *Mendelian* (*monogenic*) *forms of hypertension* are diagnosed during infancy or later childhood. Search for early-onset severe hypertension or death from premature cerebral vascular accidents or myocardial infarction in the family.
- Important findings in history and physical examination are listed in Table 7.2.

Table 7.2 Important points in history and physical examination

History and physical examination	Findings	Associated disorders
Family history	Hypertension, cardiovascular disease, cerebral infarction in the family	Primary hypertension, monogenic hypertension
Social history	Weight gain, diet, sedentary lifestyle, sleep apnea	Primary hypertension
	Excessive muscle building, exercise	Glucocorticoids, growth hormone, erythropoietin abuse
	Caffeine, tobacco, alcohol, street drugs	Adverse effect to drugs (e.g., ecstasy, methylphenidate) versus unrelated HTN
Medication history	Glucocorticoids, calcineurin inhibitor, sympathomimetics (salbutamol, aminophylline) growth hormone, decongestants, stimulants, antidepressants, hormonal contraceptives	Adverse drug effects
Previous medical history	Umbilical catheterization	Renovascular disease, renal venous or large vein thrombosis
	Perinatal complications/asphyxia	Renal atrophy, renal venous thrombosis, CKD
	Urinary tract infections	Renal scars, atrophic kidneys
	Hematuria, edema, rash, purpura	Vasculitis, renal parenchymal disease
Physical findings	Palpable kidneys, abdominal masses	Polycystic kidney disease, renal tumor, severe hydronephrosis
	Abdominal bruit	Examine for cranial and neck bruit
	Neurofibroma	Vascular disease, renal artery stenosis, Williams syndrome, NF1
	Hypercalcemia	
	Radio-femoral delay, unequal BP, and/or weak pulses in limbs	Vascular diseases, including coarctation, mid-aortic syndrome, Takayasu arteritis
	Cushingoid features	Endocrine causes, glucocorticoid use
	Goiter	Thyroid disorder (hyper-/hypothyroidism)
	Ambiguous genitalia	17-α-hydroxylase pathway disturbance
	Overgrowth syndromes	
Genetic syndromes	Turner	Coarctation of aorta, aortic root dilatation with bicuspid aortic valve
	Williams (Beuren), syndrome	Aortic stenosis, prerenal failure, hypercalcemia
	Neurofibromatosis 1	Renal artery stenosis

7.5 Approach to the Child and Adolescent with Hypertension

Normal BP boundaries are based on standardized measurements. Correct BP measurement is critical. Reliable readings are difficult to obtain in infants and may require Doppler devices.

7.5.1 Standardized BP Measurement and Confirmation of Hypertension

- Recommendations stipulate that casual BP be measured at least once a year at the time of a medical encounter. However, office BP measurements have a low yield in asymptomatic patients and in children or adolescents with unrelated complaints.
- Current normative values are based on "casual" sphygmomanometric measurements (mercury or aneroid devices).
- Aneroid manometers need regular calibration.
- Reliable BP measurements require standardized conditions to avoid falsely high readings.
  - Child should rest at least 3 min, sitting if possible, right arm supported, and cubital fossa at heart level.
  - Cuff bladder length should be 80–100 % of the circumference of the arm; the width should be 40 % of the arm circumference midway between the olecranon and acromion.
  - Three cuff sizes cover needs for most children, 4×8, 6×12, and 10×24 cm, and thigh cuff for obese teenagers (Table 7.3).
  - If cuff is too small, BP recordings are falsely high. Use the next larger cuff.
  - Systolic BP is taken as K1 Korotkoff sound. Disappearance of the K5 sound corresponds to the diastolic BP. If K5 is unreliable, use K4 (muffling of sounds).
- Oscillometric devices measure the mean arterial BP; systolic and diastolic values are calculated values and often higher than sphygmomanometric measurements.
- Oscillometrically derived BPs can be used for screening purpose; if elevated, confirm by sphygmomanometry.
- Noninvasive (oscillometric) monitoring is useful to document blood pressure trends.
- Intra-arterial ("on-line") BP monitoring is indicated in critically ill patients, usually in the intensive care unit. Nitroprusside drips for hypertensive emergencies are a relative indication for invasive BP monitoring.
- Doppler BP is useful in newborns and infants, when sphygmomanometric measurement is technically not feasible. The "flush method" is not reliable.

Table 7.3 Recommended blood pressure cuff dimension for pediatric age groups

Age range	Width (cm)	Length (cm)	Maximum arm circumference (cm)[a]
Newborn	4	8	10
Infant	6	12	15
Child	9	18	22
Small adult	10	24	26
Adult	13	30	34
Large adult	16	38	44
Thigh	20	42	52

From National High Blood Pressure Education Program Working Group on High Blood Pressure in Children and Adolescents (2004)
[a]Circumference calculated so that the largest arm would still allow bladder to encircle it by ≥80 %

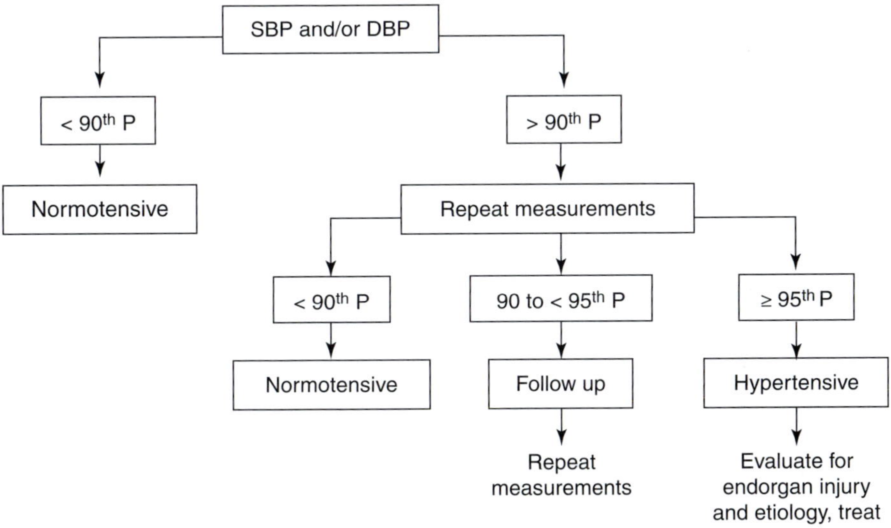

Fig. 7.2 Diagnostic algorithm of hypertension in children and adolescents. *P* percentile (Modified from Lurbe et al. 2009)

- Ambulatory BP measuring is a good method to confirm or rule out true hypertension under "real-life" circumstances (see below under "Ambulatory Blood Pressure Monitoring").
- Elevated blood pressure has to be confirmed by (sphygmomanometric) measurements at three separate occasions.
- Diagnosis of hypertension is made if all three measurements are above the 95th percentile (see Box 7.1).
- Initial hypertensive BP readings >95th percentile "normalize" under subsequent observation in up to 40 % of cases.
- Figure 7.2 describes steps to confirm "true" hypertension.

7.5.2 Evaluate for End-Organ Injury

- Fundoscopy to rule out papilledema and hypertensive retinopathy
  - Up to 50 % of children with hypertension may display retinal abnormalities, detectable by direct ophthalmoscopy. In one study, each 10-mmHg increase in SBP was associated with 1.43–2.08-mm narrowing of retinal arterioles detected by analyzing digital retinal photographs.
  - Despite a definite correlation between retinal findings and arterial (systemic) HTN, fundoscopic examination is limited due to interobserver and intra-observer variation and high rates of misclassification and uncertainty regarding the added value of fundoscopy in the management of HTN. This may change with the more recent introduction of digital imaging and software-aided analysis.
  - The European guidelines stipulate that routine fundoscopy be restricted to evaluating hypertensive encephalopathy or malignant hypertension.
- Cardiac echo to rule out left ventricular hypertrophy (LVH)
  - The fourth report recommends echocardiography in children with hypertension.
  - LVH is an independent risk factor for cardiovascular complications in hypertensive adults. In the absence of similar epidemiological data in children and adolescents, identification of LVH as a surrogate marker and indication for treatment appears prudent for the prevention of future cardiovascular disease.
  - LVH is defined as left ventricular mass (LVM) exceeding the 95th percentile (expressed in $g/m^{2.7}$, Devereux equation).
  - Increased LV mass indexed to height (LVMI) correlates with SBP and systolic ambulatory BP (SABP), high pulse pressure (SBP-DBP difference), and lack of nighttime "dipping" (see "Home and Ambulatory BP Monitoring").
  - LVH has been found in ≈15–40 % of children and adolescents with primary hypertension.
  - Presence of LVH is an indication to initiate or intensify antihypertensive therapy.
  - EKG is a simple but insensitive technique to diagnose mild-to-moderate LVH in children.
- Renal function and urinalysis to rule out secondary renal injury
  - Serum creatinine elevation (decreased GFR) and/or proteinuria suggest underlying renal disease.
  - Microalbuminuria: Urine albumin >30 mg/L or albumin-to-creatinine ratio (Uac) 2–30 mg/mmol creatinine (20–300 μg/g creatinine) has been shown to predict diabetic nephropathy. It also correlates with LVH and may be associated with long-term cardiovascular risk. Overt albuminuria (>300 mg/24 h in adults, corresponding to 7 $mg/h/m^2$) indicates presence of renal parenchymal injury.
- CNS complication due to HTN
  - Seizures, stroke, visual impairment, and renal vasculature damage

   - Diagnostic procedures in addition to neurologic and ophthalmological evaluation including EEG and CT (to rule out hemorrhage) and MRI (improved sensitivity for small brain infarcts or bleeds and white matter lesions)

7.5.3 Differentiate Between Primary and Secondary Hypertension

Identifying a cause of hypertension (secondary hypertension) can provide an opportunity for causal or definitive therapy.

Clinical and Laboratory Clues

- Prepubertal children have more often secondary hypertension compared with adolescents.
- A recent study of 220 children with confirmed HTN demonstrated that absence of clinical signs and symptoms, normal serum creatinine concentration, family history of HTN, and overweight/obesity were associated with primary HTN.
- Systemic signs, such as abnormal urinalysis, serum electrolyte disturbance, edema and tachycardia or flushing, and elevated serum creatinine, are suggestive of secondary hypertension.
- Severe (stage 2) hypertension is generally secondary. Primary hypertension is usually milder (not exceeding stage 1).
- Incidence of diastolic and nocturnal hypertension is higher in secondary than in primary hypertension.

7.5.4 When to Suspect Monogenic Hypertension

- Positive family history of hypertension in *young age*
- Member of kindreds with known monogenic hypertensive disease
- Hypokalemia in hypertensive children and their first-degree relatives (except in Gordon's syndrome)
- Low PRA (in contrast to renovascular hypertension)
- For details, see Fig. 7.1 and Table 7.8

7.6 Investigations

The diagnostic yield of commonly recommended laboratory and imaging studies in patients with mild and moderate hypertension (pre- and stage 1 HTN) is low, and detailed work-up is usually not urgent. In contrast, patients with moderate-to-severe (stage 2) HTN warrant thorough evaluation of the underlying etiology and presence of end-organ injury. A reasonable approach for a stepwise work-up is outlined in Box 7.2.

7.6.1 Investigations for Mild-to-Moderate Hypertension

- This pertains to elevated BP from pre- to stage 1 HTN.
- In one survey, abnormal urinalysis and blood biochemistry results were found in <5 % of patients with "mild-to-moderate" HTN.
- Less than 15 % of these patients had abnormal renal abdominal US findings; important abnormalities were reported in <5 %.
- In contrast, fasting lipid profile was abnormal in ~40 % (total cholesterol determination was sufficient to detect >80 % of those with lipid abnormalities).
- Ambulatory blood pressure monitoring (ABPM, see below) is useful to confirm the presence of hypertension, quantitate BP "load," and monitor the effect of therapy.
- Basic work-up is shown in Box 7.2, Step 1.1. Step 1.2 is indicated if secondary hypertension is suspected.

7.6.2 Investigations for Moderate-to-Severe (Stage 2) Hypertension

- Complete work-up is mandatory for patients with severe (sustained) HTN. The yield of abnormal laboratory or imaging findings is >80 %.
- Box 7.2, Step 2 is aimed at the timely detection of target-organ injury.
- Box 7.2, Step 3 suggests specialized tests based on suspected etiology and differential diagnosis. Details for the choice of tests are listed in Table 7.4.

7.6.3 Diagnose Underlying Cause for Secondary Hypertension

- Secondary hypertension may be suspected in patients with severe HTN or hypertensive urgency and emergency.
- An etiology is more likely to be present in infants and young children than in older children and adolescents with HTN.
- Renal and extrarenal disorders leading to secondary hypertension are listed in Table 7.4.
- Specific tests, indicated for patients with suspected secondary hypertension, are found in Box 7.2 and Table 7.4.

7.7 Home (HBPM) and Ambulatory BP Monitoring (ABPM)

- ABPM has become indispensable for the diagnosis and management of hypertension.
- BP measurements may be elevated in the office setting due to anxiety, lack of time to have child calm down and rested, etc.

Box 7.2 Investigations in Children and Adolescents with Hypertension

Step 1: Baseline diagnostic

1.1 *Patients with mild-to-moderate hypertension (Pre- to stage 1 hypertension)*

- Ambulatory (ABPM, if available) or home BP monitoring (HBPM)
- Fasting serum cholesterol (or lipid profile) in overweight patients
- Echocardiography

1.2 *Differentiation between primary and secondary hypertension*

- Serum creatinine, Na^+, K^+, CBC, uric acid
- Urinalysis and microscopy
- Abdominal ultrasound

Step 2: Advanced diagnostic

Diagnostic evaluation of children and adolescents with moderate and severe hypertension, including search for end-organ damage

- Urine protein (albumin/creatinine [Uac])
- Fasting blood glucose and lipid profile, uric acid, plasma renin activity (and aldosterone)
- Echocardiography, EKG, chest X-ray
- Fundoscopy

Step 3: Specific tests, based on working diagnosis or previous findings

Imaging studies

- DMSA scan
- Captopril DTPA renogram (for renal artery stenosis)
- Voiding cystourethrogram (in the presence of dilated ureters and/or bladder abnormality)
- Angiography, CT angio, MR angio, digital subtraction angiography (DSA)
- Abdominal CT/MRI, MIBG scan (for pheochromocytoma)

Laboratory studies

- Serum cortisol (or stimulation test), urine corticoid metabolites
- Urine catecholamine metabolites (Vanillylmandelic acid [VMA], homovanillic acid [HVA], and metanephrines)
- Molecular studies (see Tables 7.4 and 7.8, Fig. 7.1)

- Documentation of home BPs, if done properly, will help to overcome this limitation.
- 24-h ABPM allows frequent measurements, statistical evaluation, a permanent record, and analysis of diurnal/nocturnal differences (nighttime dipping).
- Home measurements (HBPM) allow BP assessment where ABPM is not available and for follow-up.

Table 7.4 Investigations for secondary hypertension

Suspected etiology (Clues from patient's or family history)	Select investigations	Remarks and specific diagnoses
Drug induced	Urine drug screen Therapeutic drug monitoring	See Table 7.1
Endocrine diseases: Thyroid, Cushing's, primary aldosteronism	TSH, free thyroxin (T4), cortisol profile/stimulation, renin, aldosterone	
Glomerulonephritis	C3, C4, ASOT, ANCA, anti-GBM antibodies, ANA Kidney biopsy	Details see Chap. 3, glomerular diseases
CAKUT, reflux nephropathy (*History of UTI*)	Abdominal ultrasound (US) DMSA scan Renal function	VCUG indicated in the presence of dilated lower urinary tract or bladder abnormalities per US
Renovascular disease	Doppler US (abdomen) Angiography, CT angio, MR angio Plasma renin activity	Fibromuscular dysplasia (majority of cases of renovascular disease). Search for stenosis in other arterial beds NF1 (stenosis often at root of renal artery at aorta)
Pheochromocytoma	Ambulatory BP monitoring (ABPM) Urine metanephrines Abdominal US, CT scan, or MRI	
Neuroblastoma	Vanillylmandelic acid (VMA), homovanillic acid (HVA) ^{123}I Metaiodobenzylguanidine (MIBG) scintigraphy MRI Bone marrow biopsy	
Suspected monogenic disorders (*Family history of premature hypertension or myocardial infarction*)	Urine and plasma Na^+, K^+, renin, aldosterone Urine cortisol/cortisone (confirm) Genetic testing	See Table 7.8, Fig. 7.1
Polycystic kidney disease (*Family history of parent with ADPKD or ESRD*)	Family history US/CT/MRI Genetic testing	
Vascular disease/ atherosclerosis (*Family history of hyperlipidemia, premature myocardial infarction*)	Fasting lipid profile	
Chronic kidney disease (CKD)	Proteinuria (Upc, Uac), casts Abdominal US	

7.7.1 How to Perform ABPM?

- Selection of equipment: lightweight monitor, able to tolerate movements without excessive error readings, pediatric cuff sizes. Most centers use oscillometric monitors.
- Few monitors have been validated in children. A list of independently tested monitors is maintained at www.dableducational.org.
- Software is generally adapted to enter the 95th percentiles reported by Soergel et al. (2004) or the cut points from the LMS-transformed data of Wühl et al. (2001) (see also Chap. 17).
- Cuff of appropriate size is fitted to the nondominant arm, unless contraindicated (e.g., AV fistula) and connected to the device which is worn on the belt or with a shoulder strap. The cuff inflates automatically in preset intervals (usually every 20 or 30 min during daytime and 30–60 min at night), and BP and heart rate are recorded with the manufacturer's propriety software.
- Patients are requested to keep a diary of their activities and sleeping hours for correlation with the automated recordings.
- An example of ABPM results and interpretation is shown in Fig. 7.3.

7.7.2 Interpretation of ABPM Studies, Calculations, and Nocturnal Dipping

- Mean SBP and DBP are calculated by an interactive analysis program.
- It allows users to define parameters such as wake and sleep times and to calculate average BPs for selected day and/or night periods and blood pressure "load" and to visualize outliers.
- Editing may also include the removal of a 2-h window around bedtime and awakening, to check for technical problems, outliers (to be discarded), aborted measurements, etc.
- Circadian BP variations include the physiological "dipping" of SBP and DBP during sleep time, which corresponds to a decrease of mean systolic and diastolic BP by ≥7 and 14 %, respectively.
- While the long-term effect of blunted nocturnal dipping is debated, it is often noted in patients with parenchymal (native) renal disease and in kidney transplant recipients.
- "BP load" is defined as the percentage of ABPM exceeding the upper limit of normal for age, height, and period of day. BP load is related to target-organ damage. Loads of 25 % or more indicate hypertension.

7.7.3 Indications for ABPM Studies

- Confirmation of diagnosis of hypertension
- Assessing nighttime dipping in patients at risk for end-organ injury
- Evaluation of the efficacy of antihypertensive therapy
- Rule out white coat HTN and masked HTN

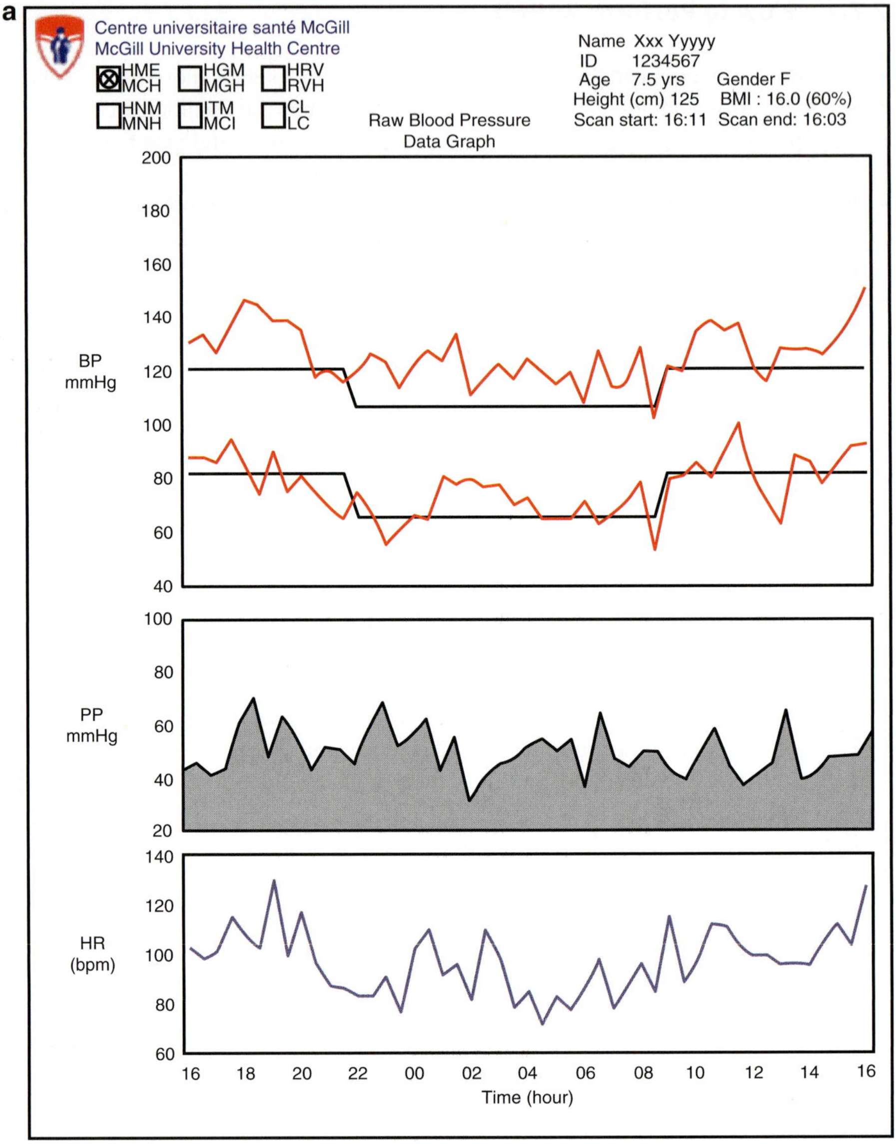

Fig. 7.3 24-h ambulatory BP monitoring of a 7-year-old girl with CKD stage 2 due to juvenile nephronophthisis. *Panel a* depicts the computer software-generated curves of SBP and DBP (*red lines*) above the corresponding upper reference values for wake and sleep periods, based on age and height stratified nomograms published by Wühl, Soergel et al. (1997; 2002). In addition, concomitant pulse pressure (difference between SBP and DBP) and heart rates are displayed. *Panel b* shows the numerical calculations, including blood pressure "loads," i.e., percentage of readings above the age- and height-adjusted reference range (95th percentiles). In the depicted case, systolic and diastolic BP loads were significantly elevated during the wake and sleep periods with preserved nocturnal "dipping" (physiological drop from daytime BP)

b

Centre universitaire santé McGill
McGill University Health Centre

☒ HME MCH ☐ HGM MGH ☐ HRV RVH
☐ HNM MNH ☐ ITM MCI ☐ CL LC

Name	Xxxx	Yyyy		
ID	1234567			
Age ABPM	7			
Age (calc.)	7.5 yrs			
DOB	####-##-##			
Gender	F			
Height (cm)	125	BMI :	16.0 (60%)	
Weight (Kg)	25			
Race	Other Race			
Print date	2011-03-25			

Date init:	Wed 2011-03-09 11:13
Serial Number?	0
Number of studies:	56
Failed Readings:	7
Successful readings:	49 (94)%
Wake readings:	27
Sleep readings:	22
Scan start:	Fri 2011-03-11 16:11
Scan end:	Sat 2011-03-12 16:03
Duration:	23:52:0

Overall Summary

	Min			AVG	MAX			STD		Dipping
Systolic	103	Sat 12:33	2x	126	151	Sat 16:03	1x	10.38	mmHg	11.3%
Diastolic	53	Sat 13:03	1x	77	101	Sat 11:33	1x	10.77	mmHg	19.8%
MAP	73			94	113			9.85	mmHg	6.2%
Pulse Pressure	31			50	71			8.98	mmHg	
Heart Rate	71			97	130			13.25	bpm	

	Limits	Readings		SDS for Ht	Centile (Z-Score)
Percent of SBP >	115.6 mmHg	42 of 49:	86%	+3.25	100%
Percent of DBP >	72.8 mmHg	31 of 49:	63%	+2.69	100%

Wake Period **09:00 – 22:00**

	Min			AVG	MAX			STD	
Systolic	116	Sat 12:33	2x	132	151	Sat 16:03	1x	9.50	mmHg
Diastolic	63	Sat 13:03	1x	83	101	Sat 11:33	1x	9.23	mmHg
MAP	83			99	113			7.43	mmHg
Pulse Pressure	37			49	71			8.98	mmHg
Heart Rate	86			104	130			11.01	bpm

	Limits	Readings		SDS for Ht	Centile (Z-Score)
Percent of SBP >	121.3 mmHg	22 of 27:	81%	+3.36	100%
Percent of DBP >	81.8 mmHg	14 of 27:	52%	+1.78	96%

Sleep Period **22:00 – 09:00**

	Min			AVG	MAX			STD	
Systolic	103	Sat 08:33	1x	120	134	Sat 01:33	1x	7.47	mmHg
Diastolic	53	Sat 08:33	1x	69	81	Sat 01:33	1x	7.77	mmHg
MAP	73			87	106			8.09	mmHg
Pulse Pressure	31			51	69			9.13	mmHg
Heart Rate	71			88	110			10.82	bpm

	Limits	Readings		SDS for Ht	Centile (Z-Score)
Percent of SBP >	106.9 mmHg	21 of 22:	95%	+3.65	100%
Percent of DBP >	65.5 mmHg	14 of 22:	64%	+2.30	99%

Auto edit limits Max:	189 / 117 mmHg
Auto edit limits Min:	63 / 39 mmHg
BP readings deleted:	0

DateID	Hour	SBP	DBP	MAP	PP	HR	Reason for deletion

Fig. 7.3 (continued)

7.7.4 White Coat Hypertension (WCH) and Masked Hypertension (MH)

- Home BP monitoring (HBPM) and ABPM have revealed two "new" BP states: white coat HTN (WCH), defined as elevated office BP and normal home (out-of-office) BP, and masked HTN (MH), defined as normal office BP and elevated out-of-office BP.
- MH has an estimated prevalence of 7–11 % of children and adolescents.

- In children as in adults, both WCH and masked hypertension have been associated with higher left ventricular mass (LVM) compared with normotensive individuals.
- Both WCH and MH are now believed to portend long-term cardiovascular risk comparable to sustained hypertension.

7.8 Management of Children with Hypertension

7.8.1 Treatment Indications and Goals

- Prevent or ameliorate acute BP-related complications.
- Prevent long-term complications (CVD in early adulthood, stroke, progressive loss of kidney function).
- Goal of antihypertensive therapy is to reduce elevated SBP and DBP to acceptable levels. Aim for <85th percentile (preferably <75th percentile).
- In patients with associated morbidities, aim to reduce BP to the 50th percentile. Comorbidities include diabetes mellitus, metabolic syndrome, CVD, renal impairment, and kidney transplant.
- Safe therapy: weigh risks and benefit.
  - Long-term effects of medication in children not well known.
  - Some antihypertensives are embryotoxic (e.g., RAS pathway inhibitors [ACEi, ARB]). Teenage girls and young women have to be instructed to use safe contraception and/or switch to alternative therapies.

7.8.2 Management of Hypertension Based on BP Staging

- *Prehypertension* – Lifestyle modification (weight reduction, regular physical activity, restriction of sedentary activity, dietary modification like salt restriction) and drug therapy in the presence of comorbid conditions (see above).
- *Stage I hypertension* – Lifestyle modifications. Initiate drug therapy if no response, if symptomatic, presence of comorbid conditions or presence of target-organ damage.
- *Stage II hypertension* – Always look for a cause (secondary HTN). Initiate drug therapy along with lifestyle modifications.

7.8.3 Stepwise Approach to Managing Primary Hypertension

Step 1

Maximal decrease in BP has been achieved when a weight loss program was combined with diet change and physical conditioning (see Box 7.3).

Step 2

Where diet, exercise, and behavior counseling are not effective in reducing weight and controlling BP, consider pharmacological therapy to facilitate weight reduction.

Adolescents with BMI >97th percentile and insulin resistance (and polycystic ovarian syndrome in females) may benefit from metformin 250–1,000 mg daily. Major adverse effects are flushing, anorexia, and abdominal discomfort.

Step 3

For adolescents >12 years, *orlistat* may be added. Orlistat, FDA approved for the management of obesity in individuals age 12–16 years, leads to fat malabsorption through inhibition of gastric and pancreatic lipases. The dose is 120 mg given three times daily. Major adverse effects are headache and abdominal discomfort.

An alternative agent is *sibutramine*, a serotonin reuptake inhibitor, approved for age ≥16 years. The dose is 5–15 mg daily. Major adverse effects include headache, xerostomia, constipation, nausea, and dizziness.

Step 4

If the above measures fail, consider bariatric surgery in conjunction with comprehensive multidisciplinary weight loss program (rarely offered to <16–18 year olds).

Box 7.3 Non-pharmacological Treatment of Primary Hypertension[a]

Goals

- BMI <85th percentile: maintain BMI to prevent overweight
- BMI 85th–95th percentile: weight maintenance (younger children) or gradual weight loss in adolescents to BMI <85th percentile
- BMI >95th percentile: gradual weight loss (1–2 kg/month) to 85th percentile

Practical recommendations

- Avoid/reduce intake of sugar, soft drinks, saturated fat, and sodium salt; recommend fruits, vegetables, (whole) grain products
- Moderate to vigorous physical aerobic activity 40 min, 3–5×/week; make use of stairs instead of elevators, walk where possible instead of driving, etc.
- Involve parents/families as partners in the behavioral change process
- Implement the behavioral changes tailored to individual and family characteristics
- Provide educational support and materials
- Establish realistic goals
- Develop a health-promoting reward system
- Do not limit competitive sports participation except for uncontrolled stage 2 hypertension

[a]Adapted from Lurbe et al. (2009)

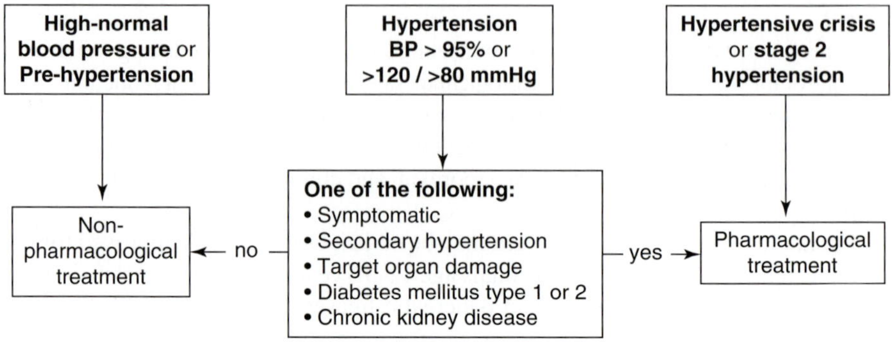

Fig. 7.4 Indications for pharmacological treatment of hypertension in children and adolescents (Based on the National High Blood Pressure Education Program Working Group on High Blood Pressure in Children and Adolescents recommendations)

7.8.4 Pharmacological Therapies of Primary and Secondary Hypertension

- While non-pharmacologic measures, specifically dietary changes, exercise, and weight loss, are considered for initial treatment of patients with primary HTN, their efficacy has been questioned due to high rates of nonadherence with prescribed lifestyle changes. These patients could benefit from pharmacological treatment.
- Prospective data or RCTs on long-term antihypertensive pharmacological treatment are scarce.
- The National High Blood Pressure Education Program Working Group on High Blood Pressure in Children and Adolescents recommends to limit pharmacological treatment to specific indications (Fig. 7.4).
  - Symptomatic HTN
  - Secondary HTN
  - Hypertensive target-organ injury
  - Diabetes types 1 and 2
  - Persistent HTN despite non-pharmacological measures
- The benefit of pharmacological treatment of hypertension has been established in children with CKD (lower blood pressure was associated with reduced CKD progression).
- Target 50th rather than 95th percentile in children and adolescents with comorbid conditions.

7.8.4.1 Principles of Antihypertensive Pharmacotherapy

- Commonly used drugs are ACE inhibitors, calcium channel blockers, vasodilators, beta-blockers, and diuretics.

- Dosages and adverse effects of commonly used antihypertensives are given in Chap. 17 (appendix).
- Monotherapy is preferred, if possible.
- If adverse effects are encountered, discontinue medication or reduce to tolerated dose and start different class agent.
- If BP is not controlled with maximum allowable dosage of the drug, a second drug is added.
- Consider drugs with complementary mechanisms of action, e.g., ACEi with diuretic or vasodilator with diuretic (or occasionally, beta-blocker).
- Recommended drug classes and contraindications for specific conditions are shown in Table 7.5.
- Approach to hypertension of CKD, dialysis and post-renal transplant, has been discussed in respective chapters. Tight control of BP in patients with CKD has a reno-protective role.
- A reasonable practical approach for long-term therapy of hypertensive children and adolescents is the "ACD" strategy.

7.8.4.2 "ACD" Strategy

- Focus on drug with daily dosing (long half-life).
- *"A" drugs* interfere with the renin-angiotensin (aldosterone) system (RAAS) activation, ACE inhibitors (ACEi), and angiotensin receptor blockers (ARB).
  - Enalapril is started at a dose of 0.1 mg/kg/day (treatment range 0.2–0.5 mg/kg/day; maximum 0.6 mg/kg/day or 40 mg/day).
  - Losartan is started at 0.7 mg/kg, range up to 1.4 mg/kg (maximum 100 mg/day).
- *"C" drugs* inhibit the L-type calcium channels in vascular smooth muscle cells (calcium channel blockers, CCB). They are divided into dihydropyridines, potent vasodilators with little effect on cardiac contractility or conduction (e.g., nifedipine, amlodipine), and non-dihydropyridines that can diminish cardiac contractility and slow cardiac conduction (verapamil, diltiazem; contraindicated in patients taking beta-blockers or with severe left ventricular dysfunction or atrioventricular block).
  - Amlodipine start dose is 0.1–0.2 mg/kg/day; range, 0.1–0.3 mg/kg/day; maximum, 0.6 mg/kg or 20 mg/day.
- *"D" drugs* (diuretics: furosemide, hydrochlorothiazide [HCTZ])
  - Furosemide starting dose, 0.5 mg/kg/dose PO (range 1–4 mg/kg/day).
  - HCTZ can be prescribed alone in adolescents with primary HTN without end-organ damage (12.5 mg/day, up to 25 mg/day), but it is more frequently used to enhance the effect of other antihypertensive drugs; restrict sodium salt intake. If combined with an "A" drug, HCTZ 6.25 mg daily may suffice.

Table 7.5 Antihypertensive drug classes: recommendations and contraindications

Drug class		Examples	Indications	Contraindications	Remarks
"A" (RAS inhibitors)	ACE inhibitors	Enalapril, ramipril, lisinopril, fosinopril	Drug of choice for many patients, specifically CKD, diabetes mellitus, congestive heart failure, kidney transplant recipients	Bilateral renal artery stenosis or renal artery stenosis in solitary kidney Hyperkalemia Pregnancy	May reversibly increase S-creatinine and K^+ and cause anemia ACEi may cause cough due to increased bradykinin levels
	ARB	Losartan, candesartan			
"C" (Calcium channel blockers)	Dihydropyridines	Amlodipine Nifedipine Nicardipine	Acute or newly diagnosed hypertension while work-up pending When "A" drugs are contraindicated	Previous adverse effects (e.g., lower limb edema), congestive heart failure	
"D" (Diuretics)	Loop-acting diuretics (*thick ascending limb*)	Furosemide, bumetanide, chlorthalidone	CKD, congestive heart failure	Intravascular volume depletion (e.g., with nephrotic syndrome)	Monitor serum electrolytes and volume status May add spironolactone or triamterene
	Thiazide diuretics (*early distal tubule*)	Hydrochlorothiazide			
	Potassium-sparing ciuretics (*late distal tubule and cortical collecting auct*)	1. Amiloride, triamterene (*ENaC blocker*) 2. Spironolactone, eplerenone (*mineralo-corticoid receptor antagonists*)	Hyperaldosteronism, hypokalemia	Acute and chronic renal failure with acidosis/risk of hyperkalemia	
"B" (beta-blockers)	Beta-blockers	Atenolol, metoprolol, propanolol		Bronchial asthma	Not anymore used as first-line therapy in hypertensive children and adolescents
	Alpha-/beta-blockers	Labetalol			

- The majority of patients will need more than one drug to achieve BP goals. "A" can be combined with "C" or "D," A + C or A + D (double therapy), or A + C + D (triple therapy).
- "*B*" *drugs* (beta-blockers, e.g., propanolol or atenolol)
  - Atenolol starting dose, 1 mg/kg/dose; range 1–2 mg/kg/day; maximum 100 mg/day.
  - B drug, alone or in combination, e.g., B + D or B + C, is not recommended for the majority of hypertensive children and adolescents.
- Note that children appear to respond better to RAS blockers, in contrast to older persons and black people in North America.

7.8.5 Presentation and Management of Hypertensive Crises

7.8.5.1 Hypertensive Emergencies: Diagnosis and Treatment

- Definition: BP >99th percentile for age, height, and gender and *evidence of target-organ injury* (primarily CNS, kidneys, cardiovascular).
- Severe, symptomatic hypertension is often caused by underlying renal disease.
- Differentiate from conditions mimicking hypertensive emergencies (intracranial lesions, seizures, dysautonomia).
- Hypertensive emergencies require prompt (usually intravenous) treatment to prevent further organ injury or death (myocardial dysfunction, cerebral complications).
- Choice of medication depends on acuity and severity of BP and patient care setting (Table 7.6).
- Need continuous monitoring, usually invasive (intra-arterial), or frequent automated (oscillatory) measurements. Preferably treated in the intensive care unit.
- Monitor neurostatus, cardiac function, and vision/fundoscopy.

7.8.5.2 Hypertensive Urgencies: Diagnosis and Treatment

- Definition: symptomatic BP elevation >99th percentile *with no current evidence of secondary organ injury.*
- Typically accompanied by headache and vomiting.
- If left untreated, target-organ injury may result imminently.
- Usually require hospital admission and frequent BP monitoring.
- Prompt treatment.
- Choice of medications; see Table 7.7.
- Baseline work-up should include at least creatinine, serum electrolytes, CBC, and urinalysis.

Table 7.6 Treatment of hypertensive emergencies

Drug	Mechanism	Administration	Dose	Time-to-effect	Elimination half-life
Nicardipine[a]	Calcium channel blocker	IV bolus or continuous infusion	Start rate 0.5–1 µg/kg/min May increase every 15–30 min Max rate 4–5 µg/kg/min	Minutes	30 min (IV continuous) 3 h (single dose) (adults)
Na-nitroprusside[b]	Vasodilator (NO)	IV continuous infusion (light protected)	Start rate 0.3–1 µg/kg/min Usual rate 3–4 µg/kg/min Max rate 10 µg/kg/min (max daily dose 3 mg/kg)	Seconds	<10 min (thiocyanate 2.7–7 days)
Labetalol[c]	α- and β-blocker	IV bolus or continuous infusion	Bolus: 0.2–1 mg/kg (max 20 mg), then continuous infusion: 0.4–1 (max 3) mg/kg/h	2–5 (–10) min max effect 5–15 min	2–4 h (duration of effect)
Hydralazine[d]	Vasodilator	IV bolus q4h-12 h	Start with 0.1–0.2 mg/kg/dose May increase to 0.5 mg/kg/dose	5–20 min	2–8 h (genetic variation)
Esmolol[c]	β-blocker	IV infusion	50–300 µg/kg/min	Seconds	1–5 min (children), 9 min (adults) Duration 10–30 min

Contraindications:
[a]Advanced aortic stenosis
[b]Compensatory hypertension (aortic coarctation, AV shunting); high output hear failure; congenital optic atrophy
[c]Heart failure, asthma/bronchospasm and pulmonary edema
[d]Dissecting aortic aneurysm, mitral valve rheumatic heart disease; coronary artery disease

Table 7.7 Treatment of hypertensive urgencies[a]

Drug	Mechanism	Administration	Dose	Time-to-effect	Elimination half-life
Clonidine	Central α-agonist	PO	5–10 μg/kg/day divided every 8–12 h Gradual increase to 5–25 μg/kg/day divided every 6 h	30–60 min (PO) 10 min (IV)	6–20 h (normal GFR) 18–41 h (renal failure)
Enalaprilat[b]	ACE inhibitor	IV bolus	5–10 μg/kg/dose every 8–24 h (Adolescents/adults 0.625–1.25 mg every 6 h, max 20 mg/dose)	15 min	6–10 h (infants) 35–38 h (adults)
Fenoldopam	Dopamine 1-receptor agonist (vasodilator)	IV continuous infusion	Start with 0.2 μg/kg/min May increase every 20–30 min to 0.3–0.5 μg/kg/min (max 0.8 μg/kg/min)	10 min	3–5 min
Isradipine	Calcium channel blocker	PO	Immediate release capsule/suspension: 0.05–0.15 mg/kg/dose every 6–8 h Titrate to 0.1–0.13 mg/kg/dose every 8 h	2–3 h	8 h
Minoxidil[c]	Vasodilator	PO	<12 years 0.1–0.2 mg/kg once daily (max 5 mg/day) Increase gradually (every 3 days) to 0.25–1 mg/kg/day >12 years and adults: 5 mg daily; usual dose 10–40 mg/day divided 1–2 doses, max 100 mg/day	30 min (max effect after 2–8 h)	3.5–4.2 h (adults)

[a]And some cases of hypertensive emergency
Contraindications:
[b]Hereditary angioedema or history of angioedema with ACE inhibitor
[c]Pheochromocytoma

7.8.5.3 Complications of (Acute) Severe Hypertension

Hypertensive Encephalopathy

- Serious complication of severe HTN
- Due to impaired autoregulation of cerebral blood flow that leads to cerebral hypoperfusion
- Frequently associated with rapidly rising BP in acute renal disease
  - Acute (postinfectious) GN
  - Hemolytic uremic syndrome
- May occur with any cause of hypertension
- Diagnosis by clinical symptoms and characteristic MRI findings, "posterior reversible (leuko)encephalopathy syndrome" (PRES)

Posterior Reversible (Leuko)Encephalopathy Syndrome (PRES)

- Almost all patients demonstrate diffuse slowing by EEG.
- PRES, in 50–65 % of patients, is:
- Associated with generalized tonic-clonic seizures
- Triggered by hypertensive crisis
- Abnormal fundoscopy
- LVH
- Atypical MRI findings
- Note: Lesions may not be limited to posterior white matter and may not be completely reversible.

7.8.6 Treatment of Acute and Severe Hypertension

- Cerebral vascular autoregulatory mechanism to compensate for rapid BP changes is impaired. Reduce BP gradually.
- Best to use titratable medication with short half-life (minutes) (see Tables 7.6 and 7.7).
- Principles of BP reduction:
  - Lower BP by 25 % of planned reduction over first 8–12 h
  - Further 25 % over next 8–12 h
  - Final 50 % over the following 24 h
- If crisis is of recent onset in a patient with generally well-controlled BP, reduction can occur faster than in patients with longer duration of untreated HTN.

7.8.6.1 Approach to Hypertensive Emergencies and Urgencies Due to APIGN/APSGN

Intravascular volume expansion and renin-mediated mechanisms contribute to HTN in APIGN. Salt and fluid restriction is of paramount importance. Mild-to-moderate hypertension usually responds to treatment with oral or intravenous furosemide and sublingual or oral nifedipine. Therapy with intravenous labetalol, nicardipine, or sodium nitroprusside is recommended for patients with hypertensive emergencies. ACE inhibitors such as enalapril may be useful. Beware of hyperkalemia in azotemic individuals.

7.9 Prognosis

- Poor BP control leads to acute and chronic morbidity and is associated with increased mortality due to cardiovascular and renal disease.
- HTN accelerates progression of chronic kidney disease (CKD). Preexisting renal disease or diabetes mellitus require tight BP control, ideally <120/<80 mmHg (or <75th percentile for age and height).

Vignettes

Case 1

A 13-year-old boy is referred by his local physician for evaluation of HTN. Sphygmomanometric (manual) BPs of 130–150/80–90 mmHg have been recorded at three separate occasions at the office. Medical history is negative for serious past illnesses, including urinary tract infection. He complains of occasional headache, fatigue, and shortness of breath when exercising, but denies visual changes or nausea. The family history is remarkable for maternal HTN, obesity, and type 2 diabetes mellitus. On exam, he is overweight, without apparent malformations. The BMI is 26.6 kg/(m)^2 (>97th percentile for age). BPs are symmetric and similar on upper and lower extremities. Basic laboratory examination reveals normal urinalysis and normal serum electrolytes, glucose, creatinine, thyroid-stimulating hormone, and lipid profile. The elevated BP is confirmed by a 24-h ABPM study. Abdominal US with Doppler is unremarkable. The family is counseled about appropriate lifestyle and dietary choices. The effect of the intended measures is marginal, and the patient is prescribed treatment with a long-acting ACE inhibitor. A year later, eager to discontinue pharmacological therapy, the patient voluntarily loses 16 kg weight over 8 months (BMI 19.6; 50th percentile for age). The BP is now 115/70 mmHg (50th percentile for age and height), off any medications.

Case 2

A 15-year-old teenager presents to the emergency department because of intermittent gross hematuria during the preceding months and recent onset of headache and retro-orbital pressure. Previous medical history is otherwise unremarkable. Her height is at the 5th percentile, with normal BMI. BP on admission is 250/160 mmHg at upper and lower extremities. Urinalysis is abnormal for gross hematuria and moderate proteinuria with granular, but no RBC cast, and without evidence of acute urinary tract infection. Serum creatinine is moderately elevated to 103 μM (1.2 mg/dl; eGFR 54 mL/min/1.73 m^2). Search for end-organ injury reveals hypertensive retinopathy and left ventricular hypertrophy (by cardiac echocardiography).

The clinical presentation satisfies criteria for hypertensive emergency (Box 7.1). The patient is admitted to the intensive care unit for acute BP management. Nitroprusside IV is initiated and the BP carefully titrated to 160/90 mmHg. Diagnostic work-up demonstrates bilaterally scarred kidneys and severe right-renal atrophy (Fig. 7.5a). The renal parenchyma in the scarred but normal-sized left kidney shows impressive hypertensive injury (Fig. 7.5b, c).

The BP is subsequently controlled with an ACE inhibitor and a calcium channel blocker. LVH improved and hypertensive retinopathy resolved. Four years later, the eGFR is 50 mL/min/1.73 m^2 corresponding, to CKD stage 3.

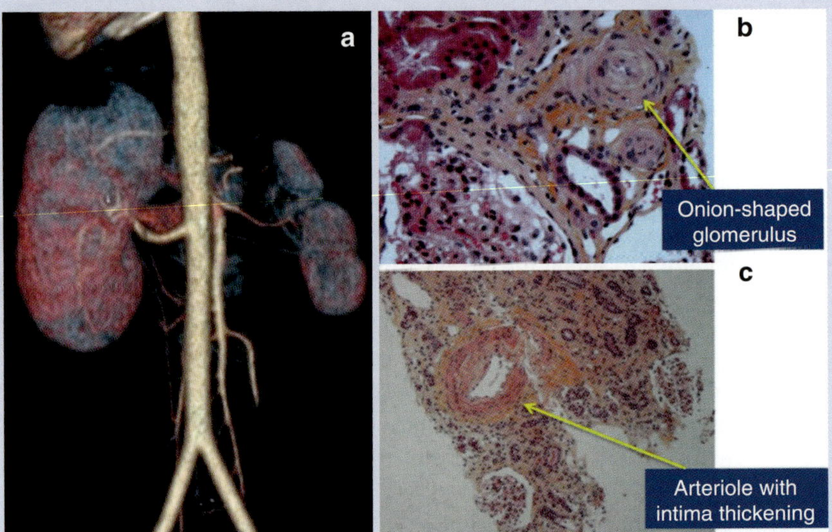

Fig. 7.5 (**a**) CT angiogram with three-dimensional reconstruction (Courtesy Department of Medical Imaging, Montreal Children's Hospital). Atrophic right kidney. Severely scarred left kidney with prominent perfusion defect of the upper pole. (**b**, **c**) Biopsy of the left kidney (Images courtesy Department of Pathology, Montreal Children's Hospital). Severe renal glomerular and parenchymal (**b**) and vascular (**c**) injury due to severe hypertension

Case 3

A 15-year-old teenager is referred for evaluation of persistent hyperkalemia between 5.3 and 6.6 mM and mild hypertension (130/80 mmHg; 90th percentile for height 122/78, 95th percentile 126/82 mmHg). She has normal kidney function and low-normal plasma bicarbonate (22 mM). She had no urinary tract infections and was never hospitalized.

Family history reveals hypertension of the patient's mother (diagnosed at age 35, medically treated), maternal grandfather, and maternal great-aunt. The maternal grandfather and his sister suffered myocardial infarctions at 55–60 years of age. The patient's father is normotensive and healthy. None of her four younger siblings is known for health problems.

Prior work-up included normal plasma ACTH and TSH levels. Urine Na is 149 and K 4.6 mmol/L. Ambulatory plasma aldosterone concentration is mildly increased (882 pmol/L; reference range, 111–861 pmol/L) and plasma renin activity undetectable (0.0 pg/mL/h).

The combination of (mild) hypertension, low plasma renin activity, and the family history suggests monogenic hypertension (see Fig. 7.1); the presence of hyperkalemia and mildly decreased serum bicarbonate led to the presumptive diagnosis of pseudohypoaldosteronism type 2, also known as familial hyperkalemic hypertension or Gordon's syndrome (see Table 7.8).

Table 7.8 Features of monogenic hypertension syndromes

Disease	Mutated protein (gene)	Inheritance	Mechanism	Treatment options	Plasma concentrations			Age	Remarks
					Aldo	K+	HCO_3^-		
Distal nephron disorders									
Liddle's syndrome (pseudohyperaldosteronism) MIM ID #177200	ENaC (β- or γ-subunit) (*SCNN1B*, *SCNN1G*)	AD (gain-of-function mutation)	Mutation impedes degradation of amiloride-sensitive luminal Na^+ channel of collecting duct principal cell (ENaC) leading to unregulated (excess) channel expression. Physiologically, ENaC is regulated by mineralocorticoids	Low-Na^+ diet Amiloride, triamterene (block Na^+ reabsorption via ENaC)	Low	Low	High	C, A	Early-onset hypertension, hypercalciuria (variable). Note: Loss-of-function mutation of epithelial Na^+ channel gene causes pseudohypoaldosteronism type 1
Gordon's syndrome (pseudohypoaldosteronism [PHA] type 2, familial hyperkalemic hypertension)	WNK4 (*WNK4*, *PHA2B*)	AR (*WNK4*, decreased function)	Pathophysiology is complex and incompletely understood. Clinical features are the opposite of Gitelman syndrome, caused by NCC loss-of-function mutation WNK4 normally reduces luminal expression of thiazide-sensitive sodium chloride cotransporter (NCC) in distal convoluted (early distal) tubule and K+channel of collecting duct. Mutation decreases inhibitory activity of WNK4, resulting in increased (unregulated) NCC activity and decreased K^+ secretion	Low-Na^+ diet, low-dose HCTZ (WNK4)	High/ normal	High	Low	C, A	Hypercalciuria, Ca-Ox stones (WNK4), hyperchloremia ("chloride shunt syndrome"), TTKG ≤4
MIM ID #145260	WNK1 (*WNK1*, *PHA2C*)	AD (*WNK1*, gain-of-function mutation)	WNK1 physiologically inhibits WNK4, prevents inhibition of NCC by WNK4, and activates ENaC. WNK1 gain-of-function mutation results in enhanced NCC activity. WNK4 and WNK1 mutations increase Cl^- reabsorption via the paracellular pathway						Furosemide worsens hypercalciuria

SAME (*AME*) [*S*yndrome of *a*pparent *m*ineralo-corticoid *e*xcess] MIM ID #218030	Hydroxysteroid (11β) dehydrogenase type 2 (*HSD11B2*)	AR (mild symptoms in heterozygote carriers)	MCR binds aldosterone and cortisol with similar affinity. 11b-HSD limits cortisol-mediated MCR activation by conversion into inactive cortisone. Mutated 11b-HSD leads to ↑ intracellular cortisol and MCR activation	Spironolactone (high dose) treats HTN, hypokalemia, and ostopenia Amiloride or triamterene is also effective Dexamethasone controls hypokalemia but not HTN Thiazide for hypercalciuria	Low	Low	High	I, C, A	Increased urinary (free) cortisol-to-cortisone ratio, prolonged cortisol half-life Symptoms (classical): low birth weight, FTT, early childhood HTN with target-organ damage, hypercalciuria, renal failure
MR$_{S810L}$ [Mineral ocorticoid receptor-activating mutation] (Hypertension exacerbated by pregnancy, H-P) MIM ID #605115	MR$_{S810L}$ (*NR3C2*, *SER810LEU*)	AD	MR mutation in hormone- binding domain resulting in nonselective MR activation, e.g., by progesterone (in females), 17-OH-progesterone (in males), and other steroids lacking 21-OH groups that are normally MR antagonists	(Spironolactone and glucocorti-coids activate mutated MR)	Low	Low or N	High	C, A	No gender difference. Severe HTN before age 20 y without gender difference, congestive heart failure Severe HTN in pregnancy (preec-lampsia without proteinuria)

(continued)

Table 7.8 (continued)

Disease	Mutated protein (gene)	Inheritance	Mechanism	Treatment options	Plasma concentrations			Age	Remarks
					Aldo	K+	HCO^-_3		
Adrenal disorders									
GRA [Glucocorticoid-remediable aldosteronism] (Familial hyperaldosteronism type I, FH I) MIM ID #103900	Chimeric 11β-hydroxy-lase/aldosterone synthase (*CYP11B1-CYP11B2* fusion)	AD	Aldosterone synthase coding sequence fused to ACTH-responsive promoter sequence of the 11β-hydroxylase gene resulting in aldosterone production that is controlled by ACTH instead of AII	HCTZ, spironolactone Glucocorticoids (low-dose GC suppress ACTH secretion and inappropriate aldosterone synthesis)	Variably elevated	Low	High	I, C	Variable degree of HTN and hypokalemia ↑ Urinary 18-oxotet-rahydro cortisol and 18-OH-cortisol-to-tetrahydroaldosterone ratio
FH II [Familial hyperaldosteronism type II][a] MIM ID #605635	Unknown (locus 7p22) [not attributable to hybrid *CYP11B1* / *CYP11B2* mutation]	AD	Hypersecretion of aldosterone associated with adrenocortical hyperplasia or aldosterone-producing adenoma, not suppressed by dexamethasone	Spironolactone Amiloride	High	Low	High	Adult	Thought to be the most common inherited type of hypertension in adults
CAH IV [Congenital adrenal hyperplasia type 4] MIM ID #202010	11β-hydroxylase (*CYP11B1*)	AR	*CYP11B1* mutation leads to disruption of conversion of 11-deoxycorticosol to cortisol. Lack of cortisol stimulates excess ACTH secretion and adrenal steroidogenesis resulting in increased androgen levels, virilization of females, precocious puberty of males	Glucocorticoids, spironolactone	Low	Low	High	I	High urinary androgens

CAH V [Congenital adrenal hyperplasia type 5] MIM ID #202110	17-α-hydroxylase/ 17,20-lyase (cytochrome P450c17) (*CYP17A1*)	AR	Ambiguous genitalia in males, amenorrhea in females due to reduced sex steroid synthesis. ACTH stimulates synthesis of precursors with mineralocorticoid effect-induced HTN and hypokalemia	Glucocorticoid and sex hormones; spironolactone	Low	Low	(high)	I	
FGR [Familial glucocorticoid resistance] MIM ID #138040	Glucocorticoid receptor mutation (*NR3C1*, *GCR*)	AR or AD	Generalized or partial target-tissue insensitivity to GC. ↑ ACTH leads to ↑ cortisol and mineralocorticoid or androgen activity without clinical hypercortisolism	Spironolactone	High	Low or N	High		Broad clinical spectrum, asymptomatic to severe hyperandrogenism, fatigue, mineralocorticoid excess ↑ Plasma cortisol, ↑ urinary free cortisol

Abbreviations: *A* adolescence, *AD* autosomal dominant, *AR* autosomal recessive, *C* childhood, *GC* glucocorticoid, *I* infancy, *MR* nuclear mineralocorticoid receptor, *N* normal

[a]Recently, a third form of familial (autosomal dominant) hyperaldosteronism has been described (FH3) with hyperreninemia, hyperaldosteronism resistant to glucocorticoids and excess 18-oxocortisol and 18-hydroxycortisol linked to mutations in the gene encoding the inwardly rectifying potassium channel KCNJ5

Suggested Reading

Chiolero A, Bovet P, Paradis G (2013) Screening for elevated blood pressure in children and adolescents: a critical appraisal. JAMA Pediatr 167:266–273

Chobanian AV, Bakris GL, Black HR, Cushman WC, Green LA, Izzo JL Jr, Jones DW, Materson BJ, Oparil S, Wright JT Jr, Roccella EJ, National Heart, Lung, and Blood Institute Joint National Committee on Prevention, Detection, Evaluation, and Treatment of High Blood Pressure, National High Blood Pressure Education Program Coordinating Committee (2003) The seventh report of the Joint National Committee on Prevention, Detection, Evaluation, and Treatment of High Blood Pressure: the JNC 7 report. JAMA 289:2560–2572

Flynn JT, Urbina EM (2012) Pediatric ambulatory blood pressure monitoring: indications and interpretations. J Clin Hypertens (Greenwich) 14:372–382

Lurbe E, Cifkova R, Cruickshank JK, Dillon MJ, Ferreira I, Invitti C, Kuznetsova T, Laurent S, Mancia G, Morales-Olivas F, Rascher W, Redon J, Schaefer F, Seeman T, Stergiou G, Wühl E, Zanchetti A, European Society of Hypertension (2009) Management of high blood pressure in children and adolescents: recommendations of the European Society of Hypertension. J Hypertens 27:1719–1742

National High Blood Pressure Education Program Working Group on High Blood Pressure in Children and Adolescents (2004) The fourth report on the diagnosis, evaluation, and treatment of high blood pressure in children and adolescents. Pediatrics 114(Suppl):555–576

Portman RJ, McNiece KL, Swinford RD, Braun MC, Samuels JA (2005) Pediatric hypertension: diagnosis, evaluation, management, and treatment for the primary care physician. Curr Probl Pediatr Adolesc Health Care 35:262–294

Redwine KM, Falkner B (2012) Progression of prehypertension to hypertension in adolescents. Curr Hypertens Rep 14:619–625

Simonetti GD, Mohaupt MG, Bianchetti MG (2012) Monogenic forms of hypertension. Eur J Pediatr 171:1433–1439

Wiesen J, Adkins M, Fortune S, Horowitz J, Pincus N, Frank R, Vento S, Hoffman C, Goilav B, Trachtman H (2008) Evaluation of pediatric patients with mild-to-moderate hypertension: yield of diagnostic testing. Pediatrics 122:e988–e993

Wühl E, Witte K, Soergel M, Mehls O, Schaefer F, German Working Group on Pediatric Hypertension (2002) Distribution of 24-h ambulatory blood pressure in children: normalized reference values and role of body dimensions. J Hypertens 20:1995–2007

Web Links

BP monitor validation: www.dableducational.org

BP percentiles calculator http://www.uptodate.com/contents/calculator-blood-pressure-percentiles-for-boys-2-to-17-years?source=see_link

http://www.uptodate.com/contents/calculator-body-mass-index-percentiles-for-girls-2-to-20-years?source=see_link

Pediatric Blood Pressure chart from the US National Institutes of Health Clinical Center http://www.cc.nih.gov/ccc/pedweb/pedsstaff/bp.html

Acute Kidney Injury

8

Indra Gupta and Martin Bitzan

8.1 Definition and Incidence

Acute kidney injury (AKI) is a common clinical problem defined by an abrupt (<48-h) increase in serum creatinine resulting from an insult that causes a functional or structural change in the kidney, with or without oliguria. Usually AKI is reversible although few cases may progress to chronic kidney disease. Children with AKI from hypoxic/ischemic insults and acute glomerulonephritis (GN) are more likely to have oliguria or anuria, while children with aminoglycoside drug toxicity, contrast-induced nephropathy, or acute interstitial nephritis are more likely to have normal or increased urine output. Mortality from AKI is reported to range from 10 to 60 %.

8.2 Classification and Staging System for AKI

Over the last decade, international efforts to define AKI and standardize the assessment of its severity have resulted in two comparable, widely accepted classification schemes, RIFLE (for *r*isk, *i*njury, *f*ailure, *l*oss, and *e*nd-stage renal disease) and AKIN (stages according to the collaborative AKI network). RIFLE "L" and "E" represent outcome variables to assess for transition to chronic kidney disease (CKD) or ESRD 3 months after the AKI episode. The RIFLE criteria were adjusted and validated in pediatric populations (pRIFLE) (Tables 8.1 and 8.2).

I. Gupta (✉) • M. Bitzan
Division of Pediatric Nephrology,
Montreal Children's Hospital, McGill University,
2300, rue Tupper, Montreal, QC H3H 1P3, Canada
e-mail: indra.gupta@muhc.mcgill.ca; martin.bitzan@mcgill.ca

K. Phadke et al. (eds.), *Manual of Pediatric Nephrology*,
DOI 10.1007/978-3-642-12483-9_8,

Table 8.1 Comparison of AKI staging by RIFLE and AKIN classification

RIFLE stage[a]	RIFLE	RIFLE and AKIN[b,c]	AKIN	AKIN stage[b]
	Serum creatinine increase from baseline (GFR decrease)	Urine output criteria	Serum creatinine increase (or fold increase from baseline)	
*R*isk	S-creatinine 1.5-fold (GFR decrease > 25 %)	<0.5 ml/kg/h over >6 h	>0.3 mg/dl [>26.4 μmol/l] ≥ 1.5 to 2-fold (150–200 %)	1
*I*njury	2-fold (>50 %)	<0.5 ml/kg/h for >12 h	>2 to 3-fold (>200–300 %)	2
*F*ailure	3-fold (>75 %)	<0.3 ml/kg/h for >24 h or anuria > 12 h	>4 mg/dl (> 354 μmol/l) or >3-fold (300 %) or acute increase of at least 0.5 mg/dl [44 μmol/l] or initiation of acute RRT	3
*L*oss	Persistent failure > 4 weeks		N/A	
*E*nd stage	End-stage renal disease > 3 months		N/A	

Definitions according to [a]Bellomo et al. (2004), and [b]Mehta et al. (2007). [c]Only one criterium needs to be fulfilled (serum creatinine/GFR or urine output)

Table 8.2 pRIFLE classifications

RIFLE	pRIFLE	
Stage	GFR-based (eCCl)	Urine output
*R*isk	GFR decrease ≥ 25 %	<0.5 ml/kg/h × 8 h
*I*njury	GFR decrease ≥ 50 %	<0.5 ml/kg/h × 16 h
*F*ailure	GFR decrease ≥75%, or <35 ml/min/1.73 m²	<0.3 ml/kg/h × 24 h or anuric for 12 h
*L*oss	Persistent failure >4 weeks	
*E*nd stage	ESRD (persistent failure >3 months)	

Based on Akcan-Arika et al. (2007)
eCCl estimated creatinine clearance

8.3 Etiology

Kidney function is dependent on the adequacy of blood supply to the kidney, the integrity of the renal parenchyma, and the patency of the urinary tract. Hence, the etiology of AKI can be divided into prerenal, intrinsic renal, or postrenal causes.

8.3.1 Prerenal Causes (Inadequate Renal Perfusion)

Represent about 60 % of AKI

8.3.1.1 Decreased True Intravascular Volume

- Gastrointestinal (GI) fluid losses: vomiting, diarrhea, and dehydration
- Renal losses: polyuria from excessive use of diuretics, salt-wasting tubulopathy, diabetes insipidus, and diabetes mellitus
- Blood losses: trauma, GI bleeding, and acute (hemorrhagic) pancreatitis
- Increased insensible losses: hyperthermia, fever, and burns

8.3.1.2 Decreased Effective Circulating Volume

- Capillary leak (sepsis, dengue hemorrhagic fever)
- Congestive heart failure
- Nephrotic syndrome
- Liver failure
- Vascular lesions: renal artery thrombosis and renal vein thrombosis

Note that prerenal insults, if prolonged and sufficiently severe, lead to (hypoxic/ischemic) acute tubular necrosis (ATN).

8.3.2 Renal Causes (Intrinsic Renal Disease)

Represent about 35 % of AKI:

- Glomerular diseases: acute glomerulonephritis, hemolytic uremic syndrome, and rapidly progressive glomerulonephritis.
- Tubular diseases: acute tubular necrosis from hypoxia/ischemia, drugs (aminoglycosides, chemotherapeutics, antimicrobials), endogenous compounds (hemoglobin, myoglobin), and exogenous compounds or toxins (ethylene glycol, methanol, snake venom, herbal toxins).
- Interstitial disease: acute interstitial nephritis (AIN; drug induced, idiopathic) and pyelonephritis.
- Uric acid nephropathy: Urate crystals may obstruct tubules, the cause of tumor lysis syndrome.
- Vascular lesions: (bilateral) renal artery thrombosis, renal vein thrombosis, and cortical necrosis.

8.3.3 Postrenal Causes

Represent about 5 % of AKI:

- Obstruction of both kidneys or of a solitary organ; it occurs at the level of pelvis, ureter, bladder or urethra.
- Causes are posterior urethral valve, bilateral ureteropelvic junction obstruction, bilateral obstructive ureteroceles, or from urolithiasis or tumors.
- Other causes: post-radiation obstruction, surgical complications following kidney transplantation, or bilateral ureteric reimplantation for severe vesicoureteral reflux.
- Neurogenic bladder dysfunction.

8.3.4 AKI in Developing Countries Versus the Developed World

The spectrum of AKI in developing countries differs from that seen in the developed world. AKI following acute gastroenteritis, sepsis, and tropical infectious diseases (see Chap. 13) are more common in resource-poor/southern countries. In the developed world, a higher proportion of patients have AKI associated with multi-organ failure, cardiac surgery, solid organ and bone marrow transplantation, and drug nephrotoxicity. Lack of access to medical care and resources leads to hospital admission with established AKI, whereas the availability of complex medical and surgical procedures increases the relative incidence of AKI in hospitalized patients.

8.4 Approach and Evaluation

8.4.1 Medical History

- Diarrhea, dysentery, vomiting, abdominal pain, fever, weight loss, and fatigue
- Fluid intake
- Decrease or increase in urine output
- Dark urine (gross hematuria, hemoglobinuria, myoglobinuria)
- Frothy urine (proteinuria)
- Edema
- Skin rash, pyoderma, sore throat, joint pain, or swelling
- Injury with internal or external blood loss
- Drug history: aminoglycosides, traditional or herbal medicines, heavy metals, ACE inhibitors, non-steroidal antiinflammatory drugs (NSAIDs)?
- Recent umbilical catheterization in newborn – arterial or venous
- Previous history of urinary tract infections
- Failure to thrive
- Family history of renal stones and kidney disease

8.4.2 Physical Examination

- Vital signs: respiration rate, heart rate and blood pressure (postural change), temperature, and weight
- Pallor, icterus, and overt bleeding
- Hydration status: features of dehydration, euvolemia, or fluid overload
- Respiratory system: respiratory distress, pulmonary edema, and pneumonia
- Cardiovascular system: tachycardia, congestive heart failure, gallop rhythm, and raised jugular venous pressure
- Ocular examination: red conjunctivae (conjunctival suffusion) – leptospirosis
- Abdominal examination: tenderness, ascites, organomegaly, renal bruit, costovertebral angle tenderness, and palpable bladder
- Neurological examination: fundi for hypertensive changes, seizure, hypertensive encephalopathy, and motor/sensory lower limb abnormalities
- Musculoskeletal system: arthritis and muscle weakness or tenderness

- Skin: rash, petechiae, and purpura
- Assessment for lymphadenopathy and hepatosplenomegaly: rule out infection and malignancy
- Evidence of spinal abnormalities: hairy patch and sacral dimple (neuropathic bladder)
- Evidence of renal osteodystrophy or rickets: suggests acute superimposed on chronic kidney disease

8.4.3 Laboratory Evaluation

Laboratory evaluation will depend on suspected underlying etiology.

8.4.3.1 Hematology

- Hemoglobin and reticulocyte count (hemolytic anemia)
- Peripheral blood smear (hemolysis, malaria, schistocytes)
- Platelet count (thrombocytopenia in sepsis, DIC, HUS, malaria, leukemia)
- Total and differential white cell count (sepsis, eosinophilia in acute interstitial nephritis)
- Coagulation profile (DIC, hepatic failure)
- Coombs' test (positive in SLE, negative in most forms of HUS)
- Blood group and cross match

8.4.3.2 Biochemistry

- Serum urea and creatinine (diagnosis of AKI, Table 8.1)
- Serum electrolytes: sodium, potassium, chloride, calcium, phosphate, magnesium, bicarbonate, and acid–base status (complications of AKI, metabolic disorder, intoxication)
- Serum glucose
- Serum albumin, proteins (nephrotic syndrome), and immunoglobulins
- Serum uric acid (raised in tumor lysis syndrome)
- Serum creatine kinase and lactate dehydrogenase (myoglobinuria, hemolysis)
- Liver injury and function tests: AST, ALT, GGT, bilirubin and prothrombin time/INR
- Serum alkaline phosphatase and parathyroid hormone (acute superimposed on chronic renal failure)
- Serum and urine osmolality
- Urine sodium and creatinine
- Serum C-reactive protein and erythrocyte sedimentation rate (ESR) (infection or inflammatory disease)

8.4.3.3 Urine Analysis

- Urine protein, blood, presence of RBC casts (hallmark of glomerulonephritis), granular and epithelial casts (ATN), pyuria with WBC and granular casts (tubulointerstitial disease, pyelonephritis), and eosinophils (may be present in acute interstitial nephritis)
- Urine for myoglobin (rhabdomyolysis)

8.4.3.4 Microbiology, Serology and Immunology

- C3 and C4 complement levels. If available, consider global complement function, CH50 and AH50 (glomerulonephritis, HUS)
- Blood culture, urine microscopy, and culture (pyelonephritis)
- Stool culture: diarrhea due to Shiga toxin-producing bacteria (*Escherichia coli* O157:H7 [STEC], other STEC serotypes, *Shigella dysenteriae*)
- Serology for leptospirosis and dengue hemorrhagic fever
- Antistreptolysin O and anti-DNAse B (acute poststreptococcal GN)
- Antinuclear antibodies (ANA), anti-double-stranded DNA, and anticardiolipin (lupus nephritis)
- Antineutrophilic cytoplasmic antibodies (ANCA)
- Antiglomerular basement membrane antibodies (anti-GBM)
- Hepatitis and HIV serology (in preparation for dialysis)

8.4.3.5 Imaging

- Chest x-ray (if respiratory or cardiac signs)
- Renal ultrasound (evaluate size and exclude obstruction)
- Renal Doppler and angiogram (renovascular event suspected)
- Renal isotope scan (selected cases)

8.4.3.6 Renal Biopsy

- Suspected rapidly progressive glomerulonephritis (RPGN)
- Unexplained renal failure (Table 8.3)

8.4.3.7 Fluid Challenge Test

- Isotonic saline is administered as a bolus of 20 ml/kg over 20 min to differentiate prerenal from intrinsic renal failure.
- If urine output does not increase, then a dose of furosemide 1–2 mg/kg/dose may be given.
- Lack of urine output despite a diuretic challenge suggests intrinsic renal failure.

Table 8.3 Urinary indices (prerenal vs. renal AKI)

Laboratory test	Prerenal	Renal
Urine osmolality (mOsm/kg)	>500, neonates >400	<500, neonates <350
Urine sodium (mmol/l)	<10, neonates <20	>30, neonates >40
Fractional excretion of sodium (FeNa = $U_{Na}/P_{Na} \times P_{Cr}/U_{Cr} \times 100$) [%]	<1, neonates <2.5	>2, neonates >3.5
Fractional excretion of urea	<35	>35
Urine/plasma creatinine ratio	>40	>40
Urine sediment	Normal, occasional hyaline or fine granular cast	Renal tubular epithelial cells, granular and muddy brown casts

8.5 Management of AKI

8.5.1 Renal-Specific Therapy (Dependent on Underlying Etiology)

- Restoration of adequate circulation and renal perfusion with appropriate fluids (isotonic saline, albumin, packed RBC)
- Glucocorticoids and/or other immunosuppressive treatment (RPGN, AIN, vasculitis)
- Prompt relief of obstruction in postrenal AKI

8.5.2 Renal Supportive Therapy

1. *Fluid management*
   - Is the patient hypovolemic, euvolemic, or hypervolemic?
   - Monitoring of weight, accurate input and output (consider urinary catheter), frequent vital signs, and neurological status.
   - Depending on diagnosis, monitor blood glucose, electrolytes, creatinine, and other relevant laboratory parameters.
   - Volume depletion (dehydration) or shock: fluid resuscitation ("fluid challenge test" where 20 ml/kg body weight of isotonic crystalloid fluid (Ringer's lactate or isotonic saline) administered rapidly over 20 min). More than one fluid bolus may be required. If more than two boluses are required, central venous pressure should be measured.
   - Commonly used formulae to calculate "maintenance" electrolyte and water replacement do not apply in the setting of AKI.
   - In AKI, a safe approach is to calculate (and replace):
     - Insensible losses (400 ml/m^2/day) + urine output + ongoing fluid losses.
     - Ongoing fluid losses refer to gastrointestinal losses, chest tube drainage, nasogastric tube losses, skin losses in high fever, etc.
   - If patient is euvolemic, then replace all losses at 100 %. If patient is fluid overloaded, restrict replacement of urine and ongoing fluid losses as appropriate in the specific clinical circumstance. Be aware of oral or gastric tube feeds and fluids given for medication administration.
   - Keep patient normoglycemic using intravenous glucose electrolyte solutions, such as 5 % dextrose with half-isotonic saline (D5W/0.45 % NaCl) for replacement of insensible losses or D5W or D10W. Provide nutrition by enteral route or intravenously, as tolerated.
   - Consider electrolyte composition of losses:
     - Urine: replace with ½ isotonic saline (0.45 % NaCl)
     - Nasogastric (NG) tube, emesis, or stool losses: replace with isotonic or ½ isotonic saline

- Replacement of potassium (e.g., from GI losses) will depend on patient's serum potassium level, acid-base status (acidemia leads to relative hyperkalemia), overall potassium depletion, and kidney function.

2. *Specific metabolic abnormalities*
   (a) Hyperkalemia $K > 6.5$ mmol/l
   - Medical emergency leading to cardiac arrhythmia: peaked T waves (earliest change), flattened P waves, increased PR interval, widened QRS on EKG.
   - Remove all potassium from IV solutions and maintain patient on low-potassium or potassium-free diet (Table 8.4).

   (b) Hyponatremia
   - Often due to extracellular fluid dilution (fluid overload) and not to sodium deficit.
   - If severe and symptomatic or serum sodium <120 mmol/l, consider administration of hypertonic saline (3 % = 0.5 mmol/ml) to correct to 125 mmol/l:
     - Formula:
     - Sodium deficit (mmol) = $(125 - [Na^+]) \times 0.6 \times$ body weight (in kg) (see Sect. 2.2.2)
   - Hypertonic (3 %) saline is infused IV over 2–4 h.
   - In the presence of anuria or if hyponatremia is persistent, may require dialysis.

   (c) Hypocalcemia
   - Hypocalcemia in patients with AKI is often secondary to hyperphosphatemia and will correct once serum phosphate levels normalize.
   - Consider IV calcium gluconate (or $CaCl_2$) for symptomatic hypocalcemia (neuromuscular irritability, numbness, muscle cramps, laryngospasm, seizures) and if bicarbonate therapy is needed to treat severe acidosis and/or hyperkalemia.

   (d) Hyperphosphatemia
   - Oral phosphate binders and dietary phosphate restriction are required.
   - Calcium carbonate can be dissolved in feeds or given as tablets before a feed.

   (e) Acidosis
   - Determine type of acidosis (metabolic/respiratory).
   - Normal or high serum anion gap metabolic acidosis (acidemia).
     - Simple anion gap calculation: $Na^+ - (Cl^- + HCO3^-) = 10 \pm 2$ (normal)
     - Elevated anion gap reflects excess endogenous or exogenous anions, e.g. lactate, keto acids, salicylate, glycols
   - If severe acidosis with pH < 7.2, sodium bicarbonate may be administered IV over 1 h (see Sect. 2.1.2).
   - Correction of acidosis can reduce ionized serum calcium concentration and cause symptomatic hypocalcemia. In the setting of hypocalcemia and acidosis, correct hypocalcemia first before correcting acidosis.

3. *Drug dosing*
   - Adjust drug dosage to renal function as determined by eCCl (estimated creatinine clearance).

Table 8.4 Treatment of symptomatic/dangerous hyperkalemia

Treatment	Dose	Onset of action and duration	Adverse effects
Calcium gluconate 10% 1 ml contains: 0.1 g Ca-gluconate 0.23 mmol (0.46 mEq) elemental Ca^{++}	0.5–1 ml/kg iv over 5–15 min Do not exceed 0.1 g (1 ml) per min	Immediate onset within min cardioprotective, but transient effect (30–60 min)	Too rapid infusion can lead to cardiac arrest, bradycardia, and arrhythmia Hypercalcemia Extravasation causes subcutaneous burns
Calcium chloride ($CaCl_2$) 10% 1 ml contains: 0.1 g $CaCl_2$ 27 mg elemental Ca^{++} 0.7 mmol (1.4 mEq) elemental Ca^{++}	0.2 ml/kg IV slowly Do not exceed 1 ml per min		
Glucose and insulin 10 % dextrose 1 ml contains: 0.1 g dextrose	0.5–1 g/kg dextrose IV over 30 min (= 5–10 ml/kg 10 % dextrose). Immediate-acting insulin 0.1–0.2 units/kg IV or SC	Peak effect after 30–60 min Persists 4–6 h	Hypoglycemia; monitor blood glucose q 15 min
Salbutamol (Albuterol)[a]	2.5 mg for <25 kg body weight, 5 mg for >25 kg By nebulizer over 10 min, may be repeated 2-hourly	Effect 5 min after inhalation; peak effect after 90 min	Tachycardia Hypertension Transient (mild) tremor Vasomotor flushing
Sodium bicarbonate 1 ml contains: 1 mmol (1 mEq) $NaHCO_3$	1–2 mmol/kg IV over 30–60 min (= 1–2 ml/kg)	Effect after 10–30 min Most effective in lowering hyperkalemia in acidotic patient; effect may last 4 h	Hypernatremia, may worsen fluid overload, reduces ionized serum calcium
Sodium polystyrene sulfonate (SPSS) (alternative: Calcium polystyrene sulfonate)	SPSS: 1 g/kg q 2–6 h per rectum (max 30–50 g/dose), or 1 g/kg q 6 h PO (max 15 g/dose)	SPSS onset of action (rectally) 30 min, and up to 12 h (PO)	Use other measures before administering polystyrene sulfonates If given orally, beware of bowel impaction Risk of necrotizing colitis in neonates

EKG changes or serum $K^+ > 6.5$ mmol/l
[a]IV salbutamol (4 mcg/kg over 20 min) is similarly effective as inhaled salbutamol

- Monitor drug levels where possible and indicated.
- Avoid nephrotoxic drugs, especially aminoglycosides, if alternatives are available.

4. *BP monitoring*
   - Aim for normal BP. Avoid rapid BP fluctuations.
   - Fluid overload may contribute to hypertension. This will require salt and water restriction, diuretics in higher doses (furosemide or bumetanide), and/or ultrafiltration (see Sect. 8.8).
   - For management of hypertensive emergency or urgency, please refer to Chap. 7, Sect. 7.8.5 and Tables 7.6 and 7.7.
5. *Treat infection*
6. *Maintain adequate nutrition*
   - High biological-value protein, low phosphorus, low-potassium diet, and sodium restriction must meet recommended calorie requirements.
   - Parenteral nutrition may be required, if enteral feeding (preferred) is not possible.
   - Infants should receive maintenance calories 120 kcal/kg/day.
   - Older children should receive appropriate maintenance calories for age.
7. *Specific clinical settings*
   - Allopurinol (if available: rasburicase): acute urate nephropathy (tumor lysis syndrome)
   - Forced diuresis and alkalinization: pigmenturia, uric acid, and methotrexate toxicity
   - N-acetylcysteine (NAC): acetaminophen toxicity
   - Dimercaprol: heavy-metal toxicity
   - Ethanol: ethylene glycol poisoning
   - Radiocontrast nephropathy: adequate hydration and oral NAC

8.5.3 Renal Replacement Therapy (RRT)

8.5.3.1 Indications for Dialysis

- *Severe fluid overload* in presence of oligoanuria
  - One suggested formula to assess fluid overload status is to calculate the difference between fluid output and fluid intake. The difference is expressed as the percentage increase above the patient's estimated dry (or admission) weight using the formula:
  - Fluid overload [%] = (fluid in – fluid out [in L])/admission weight [in kg] × 100
- *Severe electrolyte derangement* (hyperkalemia, symptomatic hyponatremia, symptomatic hypocalcemia with hyperphosphatemia) or severe metabolic acidosis that fail to respond adequately to conservative measures
- *Treatment-recalcitrant acidosis*
- *Symptomatic uremia:* Uremic encephalopathy, bleeding, pericarditis or neuropathy

- *Intoxication* (salicylates, ethylene glycol, methanol, isopropanol, metformin, valproic acid, lithium)
- *Severe hyperammonemia* >400 μmol/l – infants with inborn errors of metabolism should be rapidly hemodialyzed, once $NH4^+$ exceeds 170 μmol/l, as seen with urea cycle disorders, maple syrup urine disease and organic acidemias (these infants usually do not have AKI)
- To enable *nutritional support*
- Urea and creatinine – no absolute threshold level for dialysis initiation; decision to dialyze depends on overall clinical picture
- Early dialysis may improve the outcome in some disease conditions
- Hypercatabolic states (sepsis, burns, crush injuries) may require aggressive dialysis
- There are no absolute blood values of blood urea or serum creatinine that define the need for dialysis; overall clinical picture should be taken into consideration
- Early dialysis may improve the outcome in many disease conditions
- Hypercatabolic states (sepsis, burns, crush injuries) may require more aggressive dialysis
- Dialysis may be considered even if renal failure is not severe, when there is a need to remove fluid or give blood products or nutritional support

8.5.3.2 Choice of Various Modalities of RRT

Options are:

1. Peritoneal dialysis (PD) (Sect. 8.6)
2. Intermittent hemodialysis (HD) (Sect. 8.7)
3. Continuous renal replacement therapy (CRRT) (Sect. 8.8)

8.5.3.3 Factors Influencing the Choice of RRT Modality

- Goal of dialysis: ultrafiltration versus solute clearance versus toxin removal
- Clinical status of the child and hemodynamic stability (see Table 8.5)
- Feasibility of peritoneal or large vascular access
- Training of medical personnel, institutional preference
- Need for anticoagulation
- Cost of treatment and supplies (important consideration not only in resource-poor settings)

8.6 Acute Peritoneal Dialysis (PD)

- APD can be performed continuously or intermittently
- Technical requirements range from simple, improvised setups to programmable devices (cycler) and industry-manufactured sets of dialysate bags and tubing
- Duration of treatment, dialysate composition (specifically dextrose concentrations), exchange frequency and fill volume are adjusted to the patient's needs, anatomical limitations and hemodynamic tolerability

Table 8.5 Comparison of dialysis modalities for AKI

Dialysis modality	Technical considerations	Advantages	Disadvantages
Peritoneal dialysis (PD)	Acute catheter can be inserted at the bedside Tunneled catheter, if available, is preferred (generally inserted in the operating room) (see Appendix)	Technically easier than other forms of dialysis Gentle (continuous) fluid removal Less hemodynamic instability No anticoagulation Acute catheter can be inserted with minimal training and simple equipment	Peritoneal filling may worsen respiratory distress Fluid removal rates can vary for technical and hemodynamic reasons Less efficient solute clearance compared to HD Risk of peritonitis, impaired drainage and dialysate leak
Hemodialysis (HD)	Insertion of large vessel catheter (preferably double lumen) Tunneled catheter is preferred in case of prolonged use (e.g., >1 week)	Reliable fluid removal (if hemodynamically stable) High efficiency solute clearance Short duration of treatment session	Needs anticoagulation Fluid removal limited in hemodynamically unstable patients Risk of access site or catheter infection Needs experienced HD team
Continuous renal replacement therapy (CRRT)	Requires specific equipment, double-lumen catheter (or 2 single-lumen accesses)	Reliable fluid removal with decreased risk of hemodynamic instability High efficiency solute clearance can be achieved using dialysate, hypothetically enhanced cytokine/toxin removal	Needs anticoagulation Risk of infection and clotting/stasis from vascular access Drug dosing adjustments differ with modality (limited pharmacokinetic data) Nutritional needs on CRRT are not well-defined

- In the critical care setting, PD is often initiated as continuous, rapid cycle (1 h) procedure over 24 h, often with low fill volume (10 mL/kg) when using a freshly inserted catheter. This limits intraabdominal pressure and risk of dialysate leakage
- If fluid removal (ultrafiltration) is insufficient, try to shorten cycles to 45 or 30 min and to increase dextrose concentration or exchange volume
- Solute clearance may improve by increasing the exchange volume (if tolerated) or dwell time
- Occasionally, tidal PD (TPD) is used, where the inflow of dialysate is followed by only partial drainage and replacement of fresh dialysate, always leaving a "reserve volume" in the peritoneal cavity. TPD is designed to enhance clearance, minimize idle dialysis time (due to low catheter flow rates towards the end of complete draining) and to overcome drain pain
- PD may achieve less efficient solute removal than CRRT or HD, but advantages are relative simplicity of the setup, reduced training time and costs, and no need for anticoagulation
- PD permits other supportive measures to proceed with few limitations (e.g. enteral and parenteral nutrition) until renal function resumes. It is less effective than HD in extreme catabolic states or to rapidly improve pulmonary edema or clear toxic drug levels, low molecular weight poisons or toxins (see below)
- For more details on (acute) PD, see Chap. 10 and Sect. 17.6.5

8.6.1 Indications for Acute Peritoneal Dialysis

8.6.1.1 Renal Indications (AKI with or without Oligoanuria)

- Oliguria in hemodynamically unstable patients
- Substantial bleeding risk: Presence of bleeding diathesis or hemorrhagic conditions
- Difficulty in obtaining large-bore blood access

8.6.1.2 Non-Renal Indications (with or without AKI)

- Refractory congestive *heart failure*
- Severe *acidosis*
- Severe *hyperkalemia* not controlled otherwise
- Poisoning: Although the role of PD in the clearance of toxic drug levels and low molecular weight poisons or toxins is limited and not anymore recommended, it should be considered when HD is not feasible. Toxin removal may be enhanced by increased convective flow, e.g. by elevated dialysis dextrose concentrations, to remove larger molecular weight drugs or toxins (>10 kD)
- *Acute pancreatitis*
- *Hepatic failure*
- *Nutritional support*: PD allows improved enteral or parenteral nutrition in fluid-restricted patients; dialysate dextrose content adds nutritional calories

- Hypothermia or hyperthermia: rapid reversal by using pre-warmed or cool dialysate, respectively
  - PD permits other supportive measures to proceed without limitation until renal function resumes. However, compared to HD, it is less effective in conditions such as pulmonary edema, extreme catabolic states, some of the drug overdoses, and poisonings with low molecular weight toxins.
  - An infant's peritoneal surface is about twice that of an adult in terms of area per unit weight. This leads to more efficient clearance of urea and creatinine. But the rate of glucose absorption is also increased. This is important as to remove large fluid volumes when either higher dextrose concentrations or shorter dwell times must be used.
  - By reducing the dwell time to 30 or even 15 min, the dialysate flow rates can be increased so that more efficient dialysis is achieved in hyperkalemic and hypercatabolic states.
  - In patients with pulmonary edema, two or three consecutive exchanges with 4.25 % glucose solution and no or minimal dwell time may remove substantial fluid volume over 1 h (corresponding – in adults – to 1 L/h).
  - To increase solute clearance, increasing the exchange volume while maintaining the dwell time, is more efficient than increasing the number of exchanges with shorter dwell times.
  - Length of the session depends on the dose of the acute PD that must be delivered. A patient with oliguria or hypercatabolic states might require continuous removal of solutes and fluid with ongoing nutritional and therapeutic support.
  - For more details on acute peritoneal dialysis, see Sect. 17.6.5.

8.7 Hemodialysis (HD)

- Highly effective method to remove fluid and solutes in patients with AKI.
- Fluid removal is limited in hemodynamically unstable patient.
- Requires specialized nursing care.
- Initial treatments are of short duration (30 min to 1 h) to avoid dialysis disequilibrium; consider using mannitol if serum urea >30 mmol/l (>84 mg/l BUN). Give 0.5–1 g/kg IV (½ dose in first hour, remainder over next 2–3 h as needed).
- Requires large (usually central) vascular access to accommodate high blood flow.
- Requires efficient anticoagulation; if heparin is contraindicated, frequent saline flushes or regional citrate anticoagulation may be tried.
- *SLED* (Slow Low Efficiency Dialysis): HD modification better suitable for hemodynamically unstable patients as an alternative to CRRT. Hemodialysis machine can be used with low dialysate flows (about 200 ml/min) over prolonged (6–8 h) daily sessions.
- For details of insertion of central venous catheter and other aspects of HD, please refer to the Sects. 17.6.3 and 10.2, respectively.

8.8 Continuous Renal Replacement Therapies (CRRT)

- CRRT is a continuous from of dialysis for the management of critically ill patients with AKI. It is generally performed in intensive (critical) care units
- Although PD shares many CRRT attributes, the term is generally applied to extracorporeal forms of dialysis
- CRRT can be delivered as filtration- (solute removal by convection) or dialysis-based modality (solute removal by diffusion), or as a combination of both
- CRRT permits slower removal of solutes and fluid per unit time compared with conventional HD and is often better tolerated by hemodynamically unstable patients

8.8.1 Nomenclature for CRRT

- SCUF (Slow Continuous Ultra Filtration): used for fluid removal in volume-overloaded patients. The ultrafiltrate (UF) is not replaced. Solute clearance is insignificant. SCUF is occasionally combined with ECMO (extracorporeal membrane oxygenation) using a parallel (small-caliber) circuit (Fig. 8.1)
- CVVH (Continuous Veno-Venous Hemofiltration): filtration-based continuous treatment (solute removal by convection). A replacement fluid is infused in the circuit just before or after the hemofilter (pre- or post-dilution, see Table 8.8). Clearance of solutes is convective ("solute drag") and depends on UF rate generated by the transmembrane pressure (Fig. 8.2).

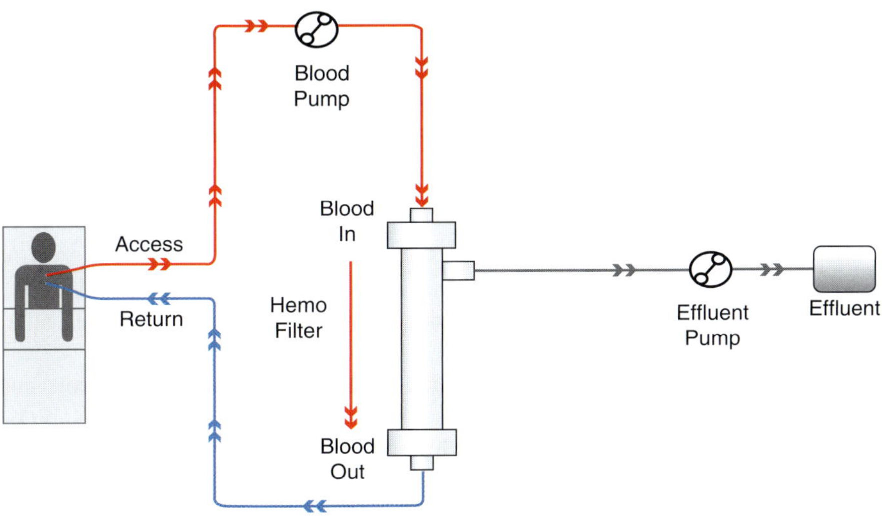

Fig. 8.1 Slow continuous ultrafiltration (SCUF). The ultrafiltrate (UF) is not replaced. Solute clearance is minimal

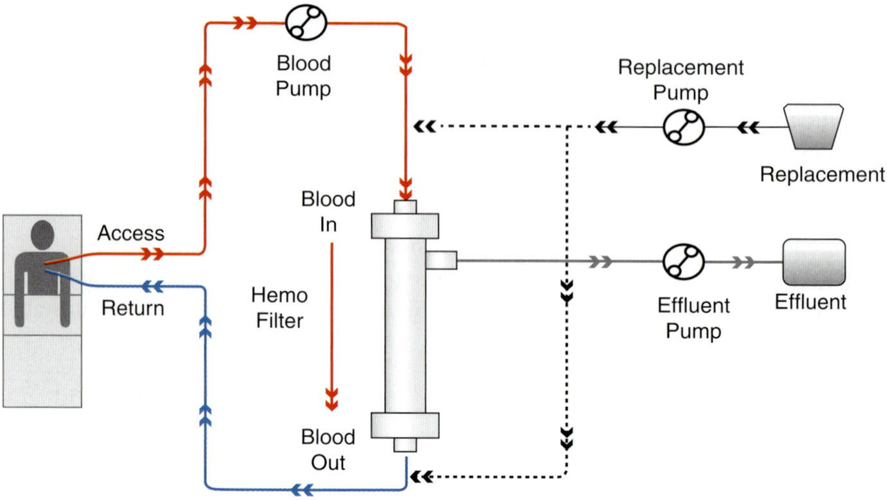

Fig. 8.2 Continuous veno-venous hemofiltration (CVVH). Filtration-based continuous treatment. A replacement fluid is infused in the circuit just before or after the hemofilter (pre- or post-dilution). Clearance of solutes is convective ("solute drag") and depends on UF rate generated by the trans-membrane pressure

- CVVHD (continuous veno-venous hemodialysis): dialysis-based treatment (solute removal by diffusion). Blood flows through the capillaries of a dialyzer; countercurrent-flow dialysate is delivered through the dialysate compartment. Replacement solution is not required. Solute clearance is mainly diffusive and limited to small molecules (Fig. 8.3)
- CVVHDF (Continuous Veno-Venous Hemodiafiltration): simultaneous removal of fluid (filtration) and solutes. Replacement solution is needed to maintain fluid balance. Solutes are cleared by convection and diffusion. CVVHDF effectively removes small and large molecules (Fig. 8.4)

8.8.2 Advantages of CRRT

- Hemodynamically unstable patients may not tolerate rapid fluid removal with (conventional) intermittent hemodialysis. CRRT is hemodynamically well tolerated. Their change in plasma osmolality is minimal.
- CRRT can help to preserve metabolic stability in critically ill patients and maintain fluid balance in oliguric patients who require IV medications, blood products or parenteral nutrition. It is highly effective in removing excess fluid.
- Episodes of hypertension are less likely to occur with CRRT than with HD, decreasing the risk of further insults to the kidneys.

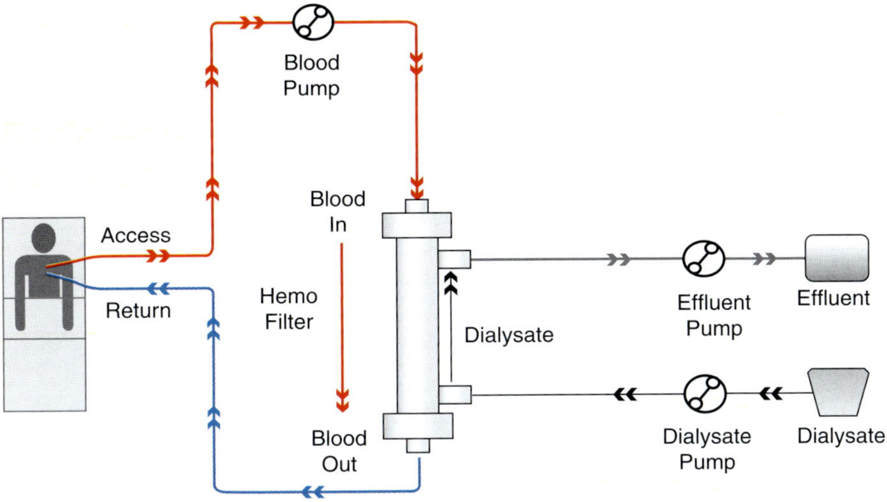

Fig. 8.3 Continuous veno-venous hemodialysis (CVVHD). Dialysis-based treatment (solute removal by diffusion). Blood flows through the capillaries of a dialyzer; countercurrent-flow dialysate is delivered through the dialysate compartment. Replacement solution is not required. Solute clearance is mainly diffusive and limited to small molecules

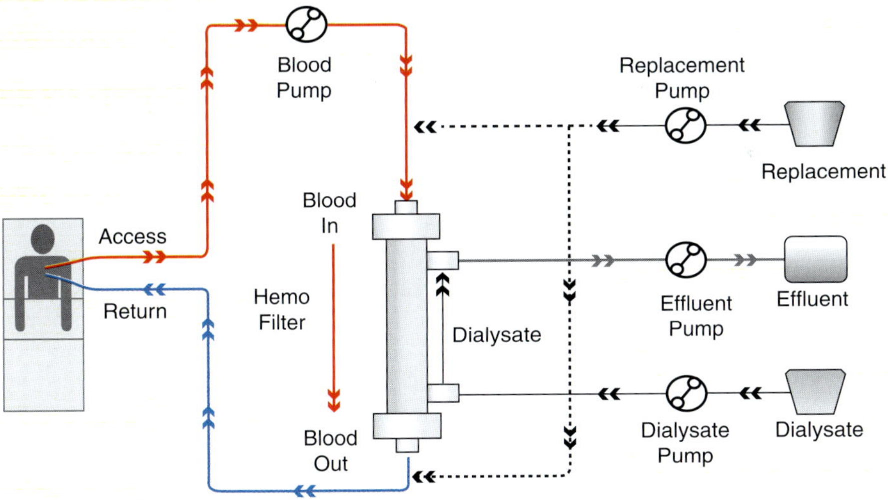

Fig. 8.4 Continuous veno-venous hemodiafiltration (CVVHDF). Simultaneous removal of fluid (filtration) and solutes. Replacement solution is needed to maintain fluid balance. Solutes are cleared by convection and diffusion

8.8.3 Disadvantages of CRRT

- Prolonged anticoagulation – Protocols using regional citrate as an anticoagulant are a reasonable alternative to systemic heparin administration.
- Hypothermia – use blood warmer, especially in infants.
- Dyselectrolytemia – Potassium and phosphate losses can be excessive.
- Solute clearance – CRRT is inferior to HD.
- Depletion of trace elements, essential peptides and (beneficial) cytokines.
- Requires thorough training of nurses, technicians and physicians and is personnel-intensive.
- Expensive equipment and supplies burden health care system, especially where resources are limited.
- Requires a vascular access (in contrast to acute PD).
- Drug elimination differs from conventional HD; pharmacokinetic data are scarce and vary between CRRT modalities.

8.8.4 Vascular Access for CRRT

- Usually via hemodialysis catheter.
- Internal jugular, femoral, and subclavian veins are common sites for acute catheter placement. Try to avoid subclavian vein access (risk of subclavian vein stenosis).
- Choose the shortest and largest caliber catheter that can be placed (highest flows with least resistance) (Table 8.6).
- Neonates: Umbilical lines can be used, but are suboptimal (5 French gauge (Fr) for umbilical artery, 8 Fr for umbilical vein).

8.8.5 CRRT Filter and Machines

- PAES (polyarylethersulfone): HF 1000 (set volume 128 ml).
- AN69 (acrylonitrite): M100 (set volume 107 ml) or M60 (set volume 84 ml), bradykinin release syndrome (BRS) may occur.
  - Risk of "Bradykinin release syndrome" (BRS).
  - Presents clinically as mucosal congestion, hypotension, bronchospasm, and anaphylaxis.

Table 8.6 Choice of vascular catheter sizes

Patient weight	Catheter size (Fr)[a]
3–6 kg (neonate)	5–7
6–15 kg	8
15–30 kg	9
>30 kg	10–12.5

[a] French gauge (Fr divided by 3 = external diameter in mm. Example: 9 Fr = 3 mm external diameter)

  - Thought to arise from bradykinin release when patient's blood comes in contact with the hemofilter. It is most commonly seen with AN69 filters. Clotting factor XII (Hageman factor) in the patient's blood becomes activated when in contact with the filter, and once activated, it stimulates the prekallikrein pathway leading to the production of bradykinin.
  - The syndrome is accentuated if the patient is receiving ACE inhibitors which inhibit the degradation of bradykinin.
- CRRT machines: Prisma, BM 25, BM 11, Hygeia Plus, and Equasmart.

8.8.6 Replacement Fluid

- In many CRRT setups, the replacement fluid is identical to the dialysate fluid
- Various fluids are commercially available (Table 8.7). They can be manufactured by a local (hospital) pharmacy, but the risk of errors is high
- The "ideal" solution is physiological, stable during storage and use, inexpensive, easy to prepare, widely available, fully compatible with added electrolyte
- Replacement fluid can be added before the filter ("pre-dilution") or after the filter ("post-dilution"). In most instances, "pre-dilution" replacement is preferred to increased the clotting-free survival of the filter

8.8.7 Anticoagulation

- If patient has increased bleeding risk, attempt CRRT without anticoagulation (and use calcium containing replacement solutions to avoid hypocalcemia)
- Originally, unfractionated heparin was widely used for systemic anticoagulation (recently also "fragmented" or low-molecular weight heparin). Potential risks of systemic heparinization are bleeding and (rare) heparin-induced thrombocytopenia
- Heparin is increasingly replaced by regional anticoagulation with citrate
- Regional anticoagulation with citrate: use calcium-free replacement and dialysate solutions (see Table 8.7). Patient hypocalcemia is prevented by the infusion of calcium chloride post-filter
- Infuse citrate (ACD-A) via arterial port at a rate of 0.025 (or 1/40) of the blood flow rate (or: 1.5 ml/h for each 1 ml/min blood flow).
  - Hypocalcemia is prevented by infusing calcium chloride post-filter at 0.4× the citrate infusion rate in ml/hour (8 g calcium chloride in 1 L isotonic saline).
  - Beware of hypocalcemia and metabolic alkalosis, and "citrate lock" (patient's total calcium level rises while ionized calcium level remains normal).

8.8.8 CRRT Prescription

- Detailed protocols should be devised considering local needs and adjusted to available equipment and solutions
- Table 8.8 shows the basic outline of a pediatric protocol

Table 8.7 Commercially available CRRT solutions (examples)

Concentration[a] (mmol/l)	Baxter HF (5 l bag)	Hemosol (Hospal) (5 l bag)		Normocarb (240 ml)	Prismasate/PrismaSol (5 l bag)[a]		Prism0Cal (5 l bag)[a]
		L0/LG2/LG4	B0		BK0/3.5	BGK2/0	
Na^+	140	140–142	140	140	140	140	140
Ca^{2+}	1.75[b]	1.75	1.75	0	1.75	0	0
Mg^+	0.75[b]	0.75	0.5	0.75	0.5	0.5	0.5
K^+	2	0/2/4	0	0	0	2	0
Cl^-	117	105–109.5	109.5	107	109.5	108	106
Lac	30	40	3	0	3	3	3
HCO_3^-	–	0	32	35	32	32	32
Glucose (g/dl)	5.5 (100)	0/6/6 (0/110/110)	0	0	0	6 (110)	0

[a]Concentrations are for the final (reconstituted) solution
[b]For conversion from mmol/l into mEq/l, multiply by 2

Table 8.8 CRRT prescription

Description	Fluid flow rates	Comments
Blood prime		Always blood prime if circuit (extracorporeal) volume >10 % of blood volume[a] For extracorporeal volume <10 %, blood prime if hemodynamically instable or requiring PRBC transfusion
Blood flow rate	2–10 ml/kg/min	Try at least 50 ml/min to reduce clotting risk (minimum 25 ml/min). Access is important! Rules of thumb: Neonates 8–12 ml/kg/min Children 4–8 ml/kg/min Older (>50 kg) 2–4 ml/kg/min
Replacement fluid/dialysate rate	1200 ml/1.73 m^2/h	For composition of CRRT solutions, see Table 8.7
Potassium (KCl)	Max. 6 mmol/l	Additives to replacement/dialysate solution
Sodium phosphates (PO_4)	Max. 1.7 mmol/l	
Patient fluid removal (PFR) rate (or "ultrafiltrate" rate, UFR)		PFR (or UFR) is the removal rate of all "non-CRRT" fluids = (citrate + $CaCl_2$ + medication fluids + nutrition) minus (urine output + drains etc.) Note: Current CRRT machines calculate replacement and dialysis fluid rates directly once the non-CRRT fluids are dialed in
Target net hourly fluid deficit (daily target deficit/24)	0.5–2 ml/kg/h	Depending on fluid removal goals: decide how much net fluid to remove over the next 24 h, divide by 24
Citrate[b] (e.g., ACD-A [Anticoagulant Citrate Dextrose, solution A])	0.025 × blood flow rate (= 1/40 blood flow)	Regional anticoagulation Citrate infusion is connected to arterial stopcock access port (pre-filter) Order is often confusingly written as "1.5 × blood flow rate" (blood flow is conventionally given as ml/min)
Calcium chloride ($CaCl_2$) 10 %	0.4 × citrate infusion rate (ml/h)	$CaCl_2$ infusion is connected to Return Port of dialysis catheter or other central venous line port
Clearance (dialysis and pre-filter replacement fluid rates)		Dialysis and (pre-filter) replacement fluid rates (total of 2.4 l/1.73 m^2/h of small solute clearance (1.2 l dialysis + 1.2 l convective)

[a]Extracorporeal circuit volume should not exceed 10 % of child's blood volume. Approximate blood volumes are 85 ml/kg (8.5 % of body weight) in infants (<1 years old), 80 ml (8 %) in children (<20 kg), 75 ml (7.5 %) in older children, and 70 ml/kg (7 %) at 15 years and older

[b]If heparin is used (systemic anticoagulation), dose 10–30 units/kg/h to keep ACT 180–220 or PTT 1.5–2 × normal

8.8.9 Complications of CRRT

- Bleeding
- Hypotension – excessive ultrafiltration
- Hypothermia – use blood warmer, especially in infants
- Membrane reactions – Bradykinin Release Syndrome (BRS), which may be perpetuated by acidic blood (PRBC). Administration of $NaHCO_3$ prior to CRRT (e.g. if serum HCO_3^- <26 mmol/l) may reduce risk of bradykinin release
- Metabolic alkalosis and "citrate lock" (patient's total calcium level rises while ionized calcium level remains normal) – suggests that citrate administration exceeds citrate clearance
- Clotting in the circuit
- Infection
- Electrolyte imbalance (hypokalemia, hypomagnesemia, hypophosphatemia)
- Loss of nutrients

8.9 Long-term Follow Up of Children with AKI

- After an episode of AKI, patients should be followed periodically with urinalysis, renal function and BP measurements
- If there is no recovery of kidney function within three months, the patient is considered to have developed chronic kidney disease (CKD)

Suggested Reading

Akcan-Arikan A, Zappitelli M, Loftis LL, Washburn KK, Jefferson LS, Goldstein SL (2007) Modified RIFLE criteria in critically ill children with acute kidney injury. Kidney Int 71:1028–1035

Askenazi DJ, Goldstein SL, Koralkar R, Fortenberry J, Baum M, Hackbarth R, Blowey D, Bunchman TE, Brophy PD, Symons J, Chua A, Flores F, Somers MJ (2013) Continuous renal replacement therapy for children ≤ 10 kg: a report from the prospective pediatric continuous renal replacement therapy registry. J Pediatr 162:587–592.e3

Bellomo R, Ronco C, Kellum JA, Mehta RL, Palevsky P, Acute Dialysis Quality Initiative workgroup (2004) Acute renal failure – definition, outcome measures, animal models, fluid therapy and information technology needs: the Second International Consensus Conference of the Acute Dialysis Quality Initiative (ADQI) Group. Crit Care 8:R204–R212

Bunchman TE, Brophy PD, Goldstein SL (2008) Technical considerations for renal replacement therapy in children. Semin Nephrol 28:488–492

Cerdá J, Bagga A, Kher V, Chakravarthi RM (2008) The contrasting characteristics of acute kidney injury in developed and developing countries. Nat Clin Pract Nephrol 4:138–153

CRRT Protocols: http://www.pcrrt.com/Protocols%20PCRRT%20Zurich.pdf

de Pont AC (2007) Extracorporeal treatment of intoxications. Curr Opin Crit Care 13:668–673

Fleming GM, Walters S, Goldstein SL, Alexander SR, Baum MA, Blowey DL, Bunchman TE, Chua AN, Fletcher SA, Flores FX, Fortenberry JD, Hackbarth R, McBryde K, Somers MJ, Symons JM, Brophy PD, Prospective Pediatric Continuous Renal Replacement Therapy Registry Group (2012) Nonrenal indications for continuous renal replacement therapy: a report from the Prospective Pediatric Continuous Renal Replacement Therapy Registry Group. Pediatr Crit Care Med 13:e299–e304

Palevsky PM, Liu KD, Brophy PD, Chawla LS, Parikh CR, Thakar CV, Tolwani AJ, Waikar SS, Weisbord SD (2013) KDOQI US commentary on the 2012 KDIGO clinical practice guideline for acute kidney injury. Am J Kidney Dis 61:649–672

Slater MB, Anand V, Uleryk EM, Parshuram CS (2012) A systematic review of RIFLE criteria in children, and its application and association with measures of mortality and morbidity. Kidney Int 81:791–798

Chronic Kidney Disease (CKD) 9

Arpana A. Iyengar and Bethany J. Foster

9.1 Definition of CKD

Chronic kidney disease (CKD) is defined as an abnormality of kidney function, as determined by laboratory tests, urinalysis, or imaging tests, which have been present for at least 3 months. CKD has replaced "chronic renal failure" and "chronic renal insufficiency" as the globally accepted terminology for persistent renal dysfunction. This term, along with the CKD staging system, highlights the fact that there is a wide range in the magnitude of renal dysfunction, which occurs on a continuum.

CKD is underdiagnosed and underreported worldwide, partly due to the asymptomatic nature of the disease. As a result, its prevalence may be underestimated. There exist geographical variations in the epidemiology of CKD, but no region of the world is untouched. The data from various national registries are limited. The epidemiological data from the "ItalKid Project," a prospective population-based registry, reported an incidence of CKD of 12.1 cases per million and a prevalence of 74.7 cases per million age-related population. Based on data from the North American Pediatric Renal Transplant Cooperative Study (NAPRTCS) chronic renal insufficiency (CRI) database, 7,000 patients aged 2–17 years with an estimated GFR (eGFR) of less than 75 ml/min per 1.73 m^2 (1994–2008) have been entered into this voluntary registry.

A.A. Iyengar (✉)
Department of Pediatric Nephrology,
St John's Medical College Hospital,
Bangalore, Karnataka 560034, India
e-mail: arpanaiyengar@gmail.com

B.J. Foster
Division of Pediatric Nephrology,
Department of Pediatrics,
Montreal Children's Hospital,
Montreal, QC, Canada
e-mail: beth.foster@muhc.mcgill.ca

K. Phadke et al. (eds.), *Manual of Pediatric Nephrology*,
DOI 10.1007/978-3-642-12483-9_9,

Table 9.1 Stages of CKD

CKD stage	Description	GFR (ml/min/1.73 m^2)
1	Kidney damage with normal or increased GFR	≥90
2	Kidney damage with mild decrease in GFR	60–89
3	Moderate decrease in GFR	30–59
4	Severe decrease in GFR	15–29
5	Kidney failure	<15 (or dialysis)

9.2 Staging of CKD

The American National Kidney Foundation's Kidney Disease Outcomes Quality Initiative (KDOQI) in their important publication from 2002 (see "Suggested Reading" at the end of the chapter) highlighted the importance of improved and standardized treatment of patients with chronic, often progressive, renal insufficiency prior to reaching dialysis. It popularized the term CKD and laid out a framework of reference (staging) based on GFR (see Table 9.1).

In 2009, the commonly used, pediatric bedside equation for GFR estimation, the "Schwartz formula" was adapted to the IDMS standardized serum creatinine; the new Schwartz (or CKiD) formula uses a $k=36.5$ (for SI units of creatinine, expressed as μmol/l) or $k=0.413$ (for traditional units of creatinine, expressed as mg/dl), for boys and girls of all ages. More precise estimates can be obtained using formulae that include serum cystatin C in addition to serum creatinine.

9.3 Etiology of CKD

In younger children, congenital malformations of the kidneys and urinary tract and metabolic/genetic disorders are the most common causes of CKD, whereas in older children, glomerular and tubular diseases prevail. Common causes of CKD are listed below.

In <5 years of age

- Congenital malformations:
  - Hypoplastic/dysplastic kidneys
  - Reflux nephropathy
  - Obstructive uropathy
  - Posterior urethral valves

- Metabolic/genetic disorders:
  - Oxalosis
  - Polycystic kidney disease
  - Congenital nephrotic syndrome
  - Wilms' tumor

In >5 years of age
- Glomerular disease:
  - Focal segmental glomerulosclerosis
  - Hemolytic uremic syndrome
  - Chronic glomerulonephritis
  - Alport's syndrome
- Tubulointerstitial disease:
  - Chronic tubulointerstitial nephritis
  - Cystinosis
  - Nephronophthisis
  - Nephrotoxic drugs

9.4 Clinical Presentations

Early recognition of CKD is crucial, and therefore, one should have a high index of clinical suspicion especially in the following situations (see Box 9.1).

Chronic kidney disease is often asymptomatic – especially in the early stages. The manifestations are subtle and nonspecific, posing a challenge to the clinician.

The pertinent points in evaluating CKD are given below.

9.4.1 History

Family history:
- Consanguinity
- Abortions
- Renal disease

Box 9.1 High Index of Suspicion for CKD

Abnormal renal imaging
Unexplained anemia
Failure to thrive, not explained by undernutrition or gastrointestinal disorders
Bony deformities
Recurrent urinary infection
Polyuria
Systemic disease with known renal involvement
Hypertension
Persistent proteinuria and abnormal urine analysis
Positive family history of kidney disease
Exposure to nephrotoxic drugs

Antenatal events:

Hydronephrosis – *seen with obstruction*
Oligohydramnios – *secondary to renal dysfunction/obstruction*
Polyhydramnios – *secondary to polyuria*
Large placenta – *seen with congenital (Finnish-type) nephrotic syndrome*

At birth:

Intrauterine growth restriction
Respiratory distress – *associated with lung hypoplasia*
Perinatal asphyxia

Infancy/childhood:

Failure to thrive
Easy fatigability
Developmental delay
Polyuria/polydipsia
Edema
Recurrent fever – *suggesting urinary tract infections*
Recurrent seizures – *secondary to hypocalcemia, hypertension, and uremia*
Refractory anemia
Recurrent vomiting – *seen with metabolic acidosis and uremia*
Bony deformities
Poor urinary stream
Incontinence

9.4.2 Physical Examination

At birth:

Single umbilical artery
Palpable bladder
Spinal defects
Ambiguous genitalia
Dysmorphic features

General:

Short stature
Malnutrition and obesity
Pallor
Edema
Flapping tremors
Hypertension
Rickets/bony deformities
Spinal defects
External genital defects

Systemic:

Lung: tachypnea and pulmonary edema
Heart: cardiomegaly
Abdomen: hepatomegaly, ascites, and abdominal mass
Brain: altered sensorium and neurological deficits

Special areas of focus:

Eye:

Hypertensive retinopathy
Cystine crystals
Chorioretinitis (congenital infections causing nephrotic syndrome)
Aniridia (Denys–Drash syndrome)
Optic atrophy
Retinitis pigmentosa (nephronophthisis)

Ear

Sensory neural deafness (Alport's syndrome, renal tubular acidosis)

Dentition

Dentin/enamel defects (hypophosphatemic rickets)

Skin

Uremic frost

9.4.2.1 Physical Manifestations of a Child with CKD

The spectrum of clinical manifestations of CKD is summarized in Table 9.2.

9.5 Evaluation and Management of CKD

9.5.1 General Aspects

Assessment of renal function:

- *Serial measurements of creatinine*: Serial measurement of serum creatinine is important. An abnormal serum creatinine value persisting for more than 3 months confirms CKD.
- *Creatinine clearance*: As per KDOQI guidelines, measurement of creatinine clearance using 24-h urine collections does not improve the estimate of GFR over that provided by predictive equations like Schwartz's equation but may provide useful information in infants and malnourished children.

Proteinuria:

- Persistent proteinuria is a marker of ongoing renal disease. Reduction of proteinuria may slow progression of CKD. Hence, early detection and intervention are important.

Table 9.2 Clinical manifestations of CKD

Clinical entities	Mechanism
Growth failure	Inadequate caloric intake
	Metabolic acidosis
	Growth hormone resistance
	Renal osteodystrophy
	Anemia
	Chronic volume depletion
Anemia	Decreased erythropoietin production
	Decreased erythrocyte survival
	Iron deficiency
Renal osteodystrophy	Impaired production of active vitamin D: 1,25-$(OH)_2D3$
	Hyperphosphatemia
	Hypocalcemia
	Secondary hyperparathyroidism
Hypertension	Volume overload
	Hyperreninism
Hyperlipidemia	Decreased plasma lipoprotein lipase activity
Cardiovascular problems	
Cardiomyopathy	Uremic toxins
Pericarditis	Hypertension
Arrhythmia	Fluid overload
	Vascular calcification (abnormal Ca/phosphate metabolism)
	Electrolyte disturbances
Neurological problems	
Headache	Uremic toxins
Seizures	Hypertension
Peripheral neuropathy	
Bleeding tendency	Defective platelet function
Hyperkalemia	Decreased GFR
	Metabolic acidosis
	Hyporeninemic hypoaldosteronism
Hyponatremia	Dilutional, solute diuresis, tubular dysfunction
Hyperventilation	Decreased GFR
	Decreased net acid excretion, ammonia synthesis
	Decreased bicarbonate reabsorption
Renal concentration defect	Tubular dysfunction

- Although several novel urinary markers (such as tubular or low molecular weight proteins) show promise of future utility, they should not be used for clinical decision making at present.
- Screening for microalbuminuria: In some specific types of chronic kidney diseases (diabetic nephropathy, hypertension), one should evaluate for microalbuminuria as an early marker of hyperfiltration.

Imaging studies:

- Renal ultrasound:
  - Renal growth monitoring is feasible with serial ultrasonographic measurements of kidney length and volume. These measurements can be plotted against age or body height on reference graphs (nomograms). The reader is referred to the Chap. 17 for further details.
  - Ultrasonography in children with CKD may reveal normal sized/small or large kidneys; hydronephrosis; loss of corticomedullary differentiation.
  - Conditions that may present with normal-sized or enlarged kidneys in CKD are:

    Nephronophthisis
    Focal segmental glomerulosclerosis
    Congenital nephrotic syndrome
    Polycystic kidney disease
    Obstructive uropathy
- Renal Histopathology

  In advanced stages of CKD, renal histopathology may be nonspecific showing widespread glomerulosclerosis, tubular atrophy, and interstitial fibrosis.

Aims of therapy:

- Regular monitoring of associated conditions as per KDOQI guidelines
- Initiation of conservative/supportive therapy for comorbid disorders
- Retarding progression of CKD
- Preparation for renal replacement therapy
- Psychosocial evaluation and support

Clinical action pyramid: The clinical approach and management depends on the stage of chronic kidney disease, as illustrated in Fig. 9.1.

9.5.2 Nutrition and Growth in CKD

Growth and nutrition are strongly interrelated in infants and children with CKD. Infants and young children with CKD are particularly vulnerable to growth failure since nutrition is the primary factor influencing growth in this age group. In contrast, growth hormone is a more important player in growth in older children.

9.5.2.1 Assessment of Nutritional Status and Growth

Height or recumbent length, weight, body mass index (BMI), and head circumference should be measured and plotted on the appropriate growth charts at regular intervals. Growth charts are available from the US National Center for Health Statistics and from the World Health Organization websites.

The US National Center for Health Statistics 2000 Growth Charts LMS tables are available on-line at www.cdc.gov/growthcharts/

The WHO Growth Standards LMS tables are available in downloadable documents online at www.who.int/childgrowth/standards/technical_report/en/index.html

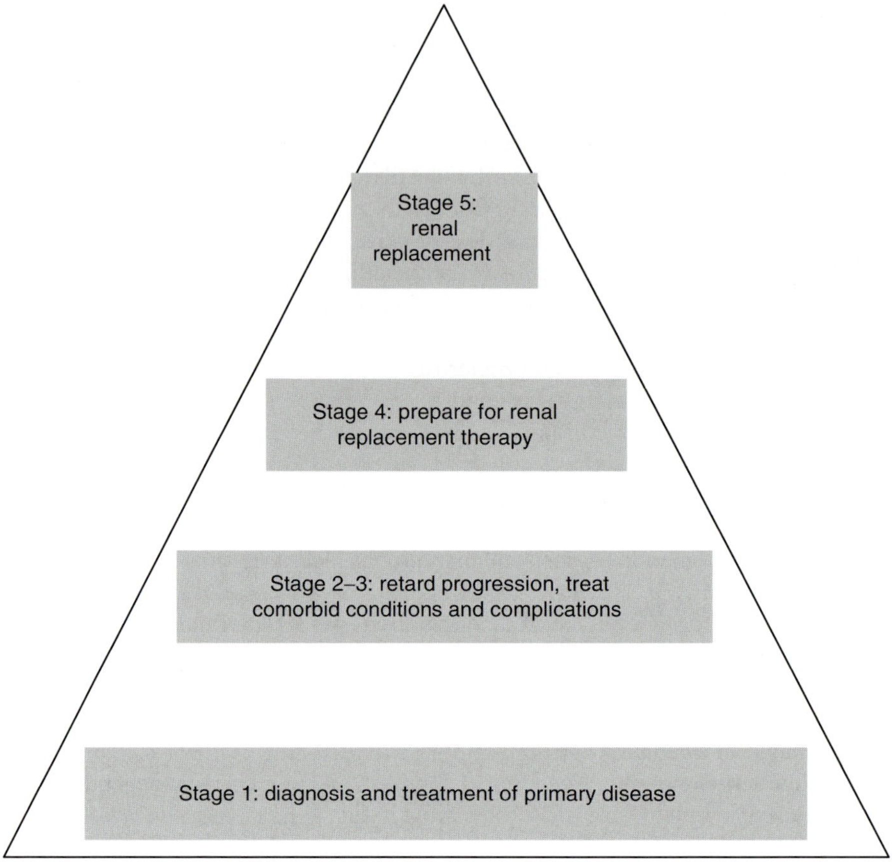

Fig. 9.1 Clinical action pyramid for CKD

Both websites also provide tables of L, M, and S values for each measure to allow the calculation of exact standard deviation score (SDS) using the following equation:

$$\text{SDS} = [(\text{observed measure} \div \text{M})^{\text{L}} - 1] \div (\text{L} \times \text{S}).$$

It is recommended that the following growth and nutritional parameters be evaluated every 1–3 months in children under 3 years of age with CKD stages 2–5 and every 3–6 months in older children:

Dietary intake (3-day diet record or three 24-h dietary recalls)
Length- or height-for-age percentile or standard deviation score (SDS)
Length or height velocity-for-age percentile or SDS
Estimated dry weight and weight-for-age percentile or SDS
Body mass index (BMI)-for-height–age percentile or SDS

Head circumference-for-age percentile or SDS (<3 years old only)

Besides the above-mentioned nutritional parameters, other measures have not been proven to be clinically useful markers of nutrition. These are mentioned below.

- Normalized protein catabolic rate: This has been studied as an objective measure of daily protein intake (DPI) in stable patients receiving maintenance dialysis.
- Serum albumin level was previously considered an index of nutritional status. However, important limitations have been identified with respect to the ability of serum albumin level to function as a reliable marker of malnutrition in the setting of CKD. Hypoalbuminemia may be a better marker of volume overload and/or of systemic inflammation than of inadequate nutrition.
- Dual-energy X-ray absorptiometry (DXA): A whole-body DXA scan provides excellent estimates of fat mass and lean mass. The main limitation of DXA in patients with CKD is that it is unable to distinguish normally hydrated from over-hydrated lean tissue; thus, it may overestimate lean mass in volume-overloaded subjects.
- Bioelectrical impedance analysis (BIA): BIA allows estimation of body fluid compartment volumes, which may then be used to make inferences about body composition. However, despite extensive BIA studies, investigators have been unsuccessful at developing broadly applicable BIA methods that function well at the individual level.
- Subjective Global Assessment (SGA): This method of nutritional assessment using clinical judgment rather than objective measures has been widely used to assess nutritional status of adults with CKD but is not yet recommended in children.

9.5.2.2 Management of Nutrition

Energy intake:

- Both infants and older children should be prescribed a calorie intake according to the estimated energy intake for age, sex, and body size; the formulae required to calculate estimated energy intake are available online at http://www.hc-sc.gc.ca/fn-an/nutrition/reference/table/index-eng.php
- If the recommended daily dietary intake is not achieved by the child and there is suboptimal growth for the age, supplemental nutritional support should be considered.
- Oral intake of an energy-dense diet is preferred especially in resource-poor countries before commercial nutritional supplements are prescribed in children with CKD stages 2–5 and children on dialysis (CKD stage 5D).
- When energy requirements cannot be met with oral supplementation, tube feeding should be considered.

Protein intake:

- Recommendations suggest relative restriction of protein intake as a means of reducing phosphorus intake. Spontaneous protein intake for children on "western diets" generally provides 150–200 % of the dietary reference intake.

- Protein intake is prescribed according to severity of CKD, with intakes between 100 % and 140 % of the dietary reference intake suggested for children with CKD stage 3 and intakes between 100 % and 120 % for children with CKD stages 4–5.

Sodium and fluid:

- Restriction of sodium and fluid is only absolutely necessary in children with oliguric or anuric renal failure (CKD stage 5). In lower stages of CKD, restriction is generally unnecessary. In contrast, children with polyuric renal failure often require sodium and water supplementation.
- Sodium supplementation in the range of an additional 2–4 mmol/kg/100 ml of formula has been shown to be useful in improving growth in infants with polyuric CKD. Sodium supplementation must be accompanied by a high fluid intake. In addition to the volume of formula required to meet caloric needs, these children should receive supplemental water, to take total fluid intake of as high as 180–240 ml/kg/day. Doses of sodium and water should be adjusted according to growth response and serum biochemistry.

Potassium:

- Potassium restriction is usually required only for children with CKD stage 5. However, in some conditions, restriction may be necessary at lower CKD stages. Monitoring of serum potassium levels is essential to determine the need for potassium restriction.

9.5.2.3 The Use of Nutritional Supplements

Table 9.3 summarizes some of the nutritional products available to augment inadequate oral and/or enteral calorie intake when children with CKD are unable to meet their requirements through food and fluids alone.

When nutritional targets are not met through oral intake, enteral tube feeding should be considered. This is rarely necessary outside infancy and very early childhood.

Suggested rates (KDOQI guidelines) for initiating and advancing tube feedings are as follows (Box 9.2):

9.5.2.4 Management of Growth

Early nutritional intervention, along with prevention and treatment of metabolic derangements, is a key component in the preservation of growth in a child with CKD. In children who demonstrate poor growth despite these measures, the addition of growth hormone therapy can be beneficial. Adequate nutritional intake is the most important prerequisite for growth in CKD especially in infancy. The following two algorithms summarize an approach to growth failure in very young and older children (Figs. 9.2 and 9.3).

9.5.2.5 Growth Hormone Therapy

- Initiation of growth hormone therapy:
  - Therapy with (recombinant) growth hormone (rhGH) is indicated in patients with GFR <75 ml/min/1.73 m^2 who have potential for growth, when height SDS is <1.88 (3rd percentile) or height velocity-for-age SDS is <1.88 (3rd percentile) despite adequate nutrition.

Table 9.3 Enteral nutritional supplements for CKD

	Product	Manufacturer	Kcal	Protein (g)	CHO (g)	Fat (g)	Na (mmol)	K (mmol)	Ca (mg)	Po_4 (mg)	Osmolality (mOsm/kg/H_2O)
Infant feeds	Good start	Nestle	67	1.4	7.5	3.4	0.8	1.8	72	25	265
Pediatric feeds	Resource just for kids	Novartis, Nestle	100	3	11	5	2.6	2.9	116	80	390
Adolescent feeds	Ensure	Abbott	106	3.8	17	2.5	3.7	4	128	106	590
Specific feeds in CKD	Novasource renal, Renalcal	Nestle Nestle	200 200	7.4 3.4	20 29	10 8.2	3.9 0	2.1 0	84 0	65 0	700 600

Box 9.2 Tube feeding advancements

Age (years)	Initial hourly infusion	Daily increases	Goal
Continuous feedings			
0–1	1–2 ml/kg/h	1 ml/kg/h	6 ml/kg/h
1–6	2–3 ml/kg/h	1 ml/kg/h	4–5 ml/kg/h
6–14	1 ml/kg/h	0.5 ml/kg/h	3–4 ml/kg/h
14	0.5–1 ml/kg/h	0.4–0.5 ml/kg/h	125 ml/h
Bolus feedings			
0–1	10–15 ml/kg/feed	20–40 ml q 4 h	20–30 ml/kg/feed
1–6	5–10 ml/kg/feed	40–60 ml q 4 h	15–20 ml/kg/feed
1–6			
6–14	3–5 ml/kg/feed	60–80 ml q 4 h	10–20 ml/kg/feed
>14	3 ml/kg/feed	100 ml q 4 h	10 ml/kg/feed

American Journal of Kidney Diseases, Vol 53, No 3, Suppl 2 (March), 2009: p S91–S91

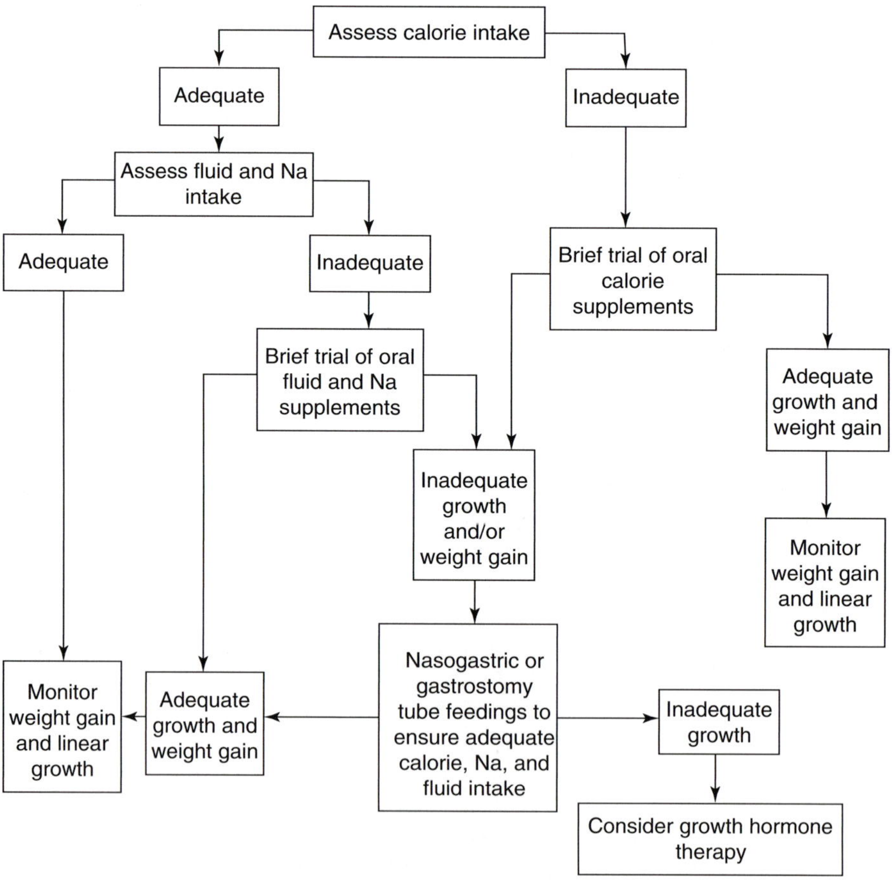

Fig. 9.2 Approach to growth failure in a young child/infant (<2 years) with height SDS –1.88 or worse or height velocity-for-age SDS –1.88 or worse

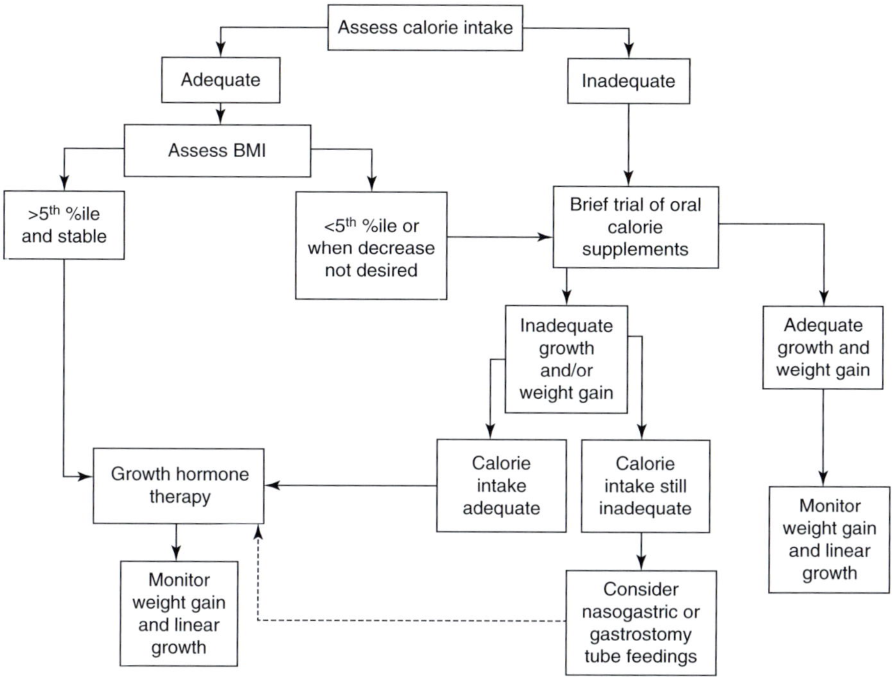

Fig. 9.3 Approach to growth failure in an older child with height SDS –1.88 or worse or height velocity-for-age SDS –1.88 or worse

  - Dose: The initial dose of GH is 0.05 mg/kg/day SC or 30 IU/m^2/week (0.35 mg/kg/week).
- Baseline investigations before starting GH therapy:
  - Hip X-rays and wrist (left-hand wrist) bone age. Problems such as active rickets or a slipped capital femoral epiphysis should be resolved before starting growth hormone therapy.
  - Growth hormone therapy should not be initiated until the PTH level is no greater than twice the target upper limit for CKD stages 2–4 or one-and-a-half times the target upper limit in CKD stage 5.
  - Growth hormone therapy should not be initiated until the phosphorus is no greater than one-and-a-half times the upper limit for age.
- Monitoring of growth hormone therapy:
  - Children receiving GH therapy in stages 2–4 CKD should have calcium, phosphorus, PTH, and alkaline phosphatase monitored at least every 3 months during the first year of therapy and every month during the first 6 months in stage 5.
  - Wrist bone age performed yearly. Height, weight, head circumference (until 3 years of age), pubertal stage, nutritional evaluation, fundoscopic exam at least every 3 months.
  - The target height deficit at the initiation of therapy and duration of treatment are the most important predictors of cumulative height gain. Long-term rhGH therapy in children with CKD has been shown to result in catch-up growth, and many achieve a final height within the normal range.

- With lack of expected response to GH therapy, the following conditions should be ruled out:
  Acidosis
  Malnutrition
  Salt wasting
  Osteodystrophy
  Hypothyroidism
- Indications to stop growth hormone therapy:
  - CKD stages 2–4: PTH level >400 pg/ml; GH should not be restarted until the PTH level is <200 pg/ml.
  - CKD stage 5: PTH level >900 pg/ml; GH should not be restarted until the PTH level is <450 pg/ml.
  - In all stages of CKD, if the patient develops a slipped capital femoral epiphysis or symptomatic high turnover renal osteodystrophy.
  - Epiphyseal closure.
  - Other complications of growth hormone, including pseudotumor cerebri.

9.5.3 Anemia of CKD

Anemia in children in CKD is defined as hemoglobin (Hb) less than the 5th percentile relative to age and sex. Table 9.4 is a guide to diagnose anemia based on hemoglobin values in CKD.

9.5.3.1 Assessment of Anemia

The following investigations are carried out at diagnosis and once in every 3–6 months on follow-up (Box 9.3):

Erythropoietin (EPO) deficiency and iron deficiency are the most important causes for anemia in CKD. Other causes include inflammation, infection, dietary deficiencies, hyperparathyroidism, and aluminum toxicity. Serum iron and the % TSAT reflect the amount of iron immediately available for hemoglobin synthesis. The serum ferritin reflects total body iron stores. A low level of either of these indices may indicate the need for supplemental iron to support erythropoiesis.

The TIBC represents the amount of iron, if added to transferrin that is needed to saturate Tf plus the iron that was already bound to the Tf.

Table 9.4 Diagnosis of anemia in CKD

Age (years)	5th percentile Hb level for boys (g/l)	5th percentile Hb level for girls (g/l)
1–2	107	108
3–5	112	111
6–8	115	115
9–11	12	119
12–14	124	117
15–19	135	115

Box 9.3 Assessment of anemia in CKD

Complete blood count
Mean corpuscular volume (MCV)
Peripheral smear
Reticulocyte count
Serum ferritin
Serum Iron
Total iron binding capacity (TIBC)
Transferrin saturation (TSAT)

Diagnosis of iron deficiency in CKD:

- Low MCV with a high red cell distribution width (RDW)
- Serum ferritin of <20 ng/ml (target 100 ng/ml during iron or erythropoetin therapy)
- Transferrin saturation (serum iron/transferrin or total iron binding capacity ×100 %) of <20 % (0.2; not applicable when the TIBC<200 μcg/dl (<36 mcmol/l))

Iron-replete state: TSAT>20 % and serum ferritin >100 ng/ml (adults on HD: >200 ng/ml)

Iron-deplete state: TSAT<20 % and serum ferritin <100 ng/ml

9.5.3.2 Management of Anemia

Erythrocyte-stimulating agents (ESA) are indicated in CKD when the iron status is adequate and hemoglobin level is below recommended standards mentioned in Table 9.4. Iron deficiency needs to be treated before administrating ESA.

- *Iron therapy*:
  - Oral iron therapy is indicated in doses ranging from 2 to 3 mg/kg up to 6 mg/kg of elemental iron per day in two to three divided doses per day. Oral iron should be taken 2 h before or 1 h after all calcium-based phophate binders and food in order to maximize gastrointestinal absorption.
  - Intravenous (IV) iron therapy is indicated if children do not have a satisfactory response with oral iron therapy. The IV iron formulations currently available include iron dextran, iron sucrose, and sodium ferric gluconate. Sodium ferric gluconate complex in sucrose and iron sucrose appear to be safer than iron dextran.
  - Maintenance IV therapy aims to provide 1–2 mg/kg (maximum of 5 mg/kg/week or 100 mg/dose) of elemental iron per week for 8–10 weeks to achieve a TSAT between 20 % and 50 % and serum ferritin levels of 100–800 ng/ml. Higher doses of intermittent IV iron are usually given less frequently to non-dialysis CKD patients.
  - Resuscitative medication and personnel trained to evaluate and manage anaphylaxis should be available whenever a dose of iron dextran is administered.

  - Frequency of monitoring iron status is once a month during initial ESA treatment and at least every 3 months during stable ESA treatment.
- *Erythropoietin-Stimulating Agents (ESA)*
  - Advantages of ESA:
    - Minimization of blood transfusions
    - Reduced sensitization to histocompatibility antigens
    - Reduced risk of infections and iron overload
  - Erythropoietin Dosage (per kg/week): <1 years: 350 IU, 1–5 years: 275 IU, 5–12 years: 250 IU, >12 years: 200 IU.
  - *Darbepoetin*: Darbepoetin (starting dose of 0.5 μg/kg per week) is equally efficacious for treating anemia associated with CKD. The extended half-life of darbepoetin does provide an advantage by allowing less frequent dosing at 1 μg /kg every 2 weeks.

These apparent differences in the dosing of ESA in children of different ages may be related to an increased presence of non-hematopoietic binding sites of ESA in younger children that may lead to increased clearance of ESA.

- Route: Convenience favors subcutaneous administration in nondialysis patients and IV administration in dialysis patients.
- Monitoring: The frequency of hemoglobin (Hb) monitoring in patients treated with erythropoietin should be at least once a month. Scheduled doses that have been missed should be replaced at the earliest possible opportunity.
- Target hemoglobin: Hb target should be in the range of 11.0–12.0 g/dl (110–120 g/l). A dose increase or decrease of approximately 20 % may be instituted in an attempt to maintain the hemoglobin at the target recommendations.
- ESA resistance: Chronic blood loss, iron deficiency, inflammation/infection, hyperparathyroidism, and autoantibodies are some factors responsible for ESA resistance.
- Complications: Hypertension, vascular access occlusion, and seizures are potential complications of ESA therapy; however, they are not contraindications for its use.

Blood transfusions: Repeated blood transfusions are best avoided in order to reduce the risk of sensitization in potential transplant recipients, iron overload, and transmission of infectious agents. Symptomatic severe anemia may sometimes need blood transfusions. Leukocyte filters should be used while giving these blood transfusions.

9.6 Bone Disease in CKD

The term renal osteodystrophy (ROD) is exclusively used to define alterations in bone morphology associated with chronic kidney disease. The terminology bone mineral disease includes renal osteodystrophy and vascular calcification.

The three main abnormalities seen in renal osteodystrophy or bone mineral disease of CKD are (a) phosphate retention, (b) decreased free calcium level, and (c) decreased 1, 25 hydroxyvitamin D

Phosphate retention and hyperphosphatemia: Phosphate retention begins early in the disease as the glomerular filtration rate (GFR) decreases. Hyperphosphatemia plays a central role in the development of secondary hyperparathyroidism.

Table 9.5 Follow-up investigations in bone disease of CKD

Stage	GFR (ml/min/1.73 m^2)	Calcium, phosphate, total CO_2	PTH and alkaline phosphatase
2	60–89	At least yearly	At least yearly
3	30–59	At least every 6 months	At least every 6 months
4	15–29	At least every 3 months	At least every 3 months
5	<15 or dialysis	At least every month	At least every 3 months

Hypocalcemia: Total serum calcium usually decreases during the course of CKD due to phosphate retention, decreased calcitriol level, and resistance to the calcemic actions of PTH on bone. With compensatory hyperparathyroidism, PTH secretion varies inversely with serum calcium.

Decreased calcitriol activity: Plasma calcitriol levels fall below normal when the GFR is less than 30 ml/min. Low calcitriol levels have also been found in earlier stages of CKD.

Assessment:

1. Clinical symptoms
   Children manifest with renal osteodystrophy in early stages of CKD, and it is recommended to begin screening for bone disease in stage 2 CKD. Symptoms may be subtle with bone pains, abnormal gait, hairline fractures, and bony deformities. Associated clinical entities such as slipped epiphysis, muscle weakness, and extra skeletal calcification may be encountered.
2. Investigations
   - Serum levels of calcium, phosphate, alkaline phosphatase, total CO_2, and parathyroid hormone should be measured in all patients with CKD stages 2 through 5 at regular intervals (see Table 9.5).

The frequencies of measurement of PTH, calcium, phosphorus (phosphate), total CO_2 (bicarbonate), and alkaline phosphatase in stages of CKD are mentioned in Table 9.5.

These measurements should be made more frequently if the patient is receiving concomitant therapy for the abnormalities in the serum levels of calcium, phosphorus, or PTH in a transplant recipient or is a patient being treated with growth hormone therapy (rhGH).

The target range of serum PTH in the various stages of CKD:

Stages 2 and 3: 35–70 pg/ml (or ng/l in SI units)
Stage 4: 70–110 pg/ml
Stage 5: 200–300 pg/ml

Other Aspects of Renal Osteodystrophy

- Newer markers of renal osteodystrophy:
  Markers of bone formation: bone-specific alkaline phosphatase and osteocalcin.
  Markers of bone resorption: tartrate-resistant acid phosphatase and pyridinoline.
  They are not recommended in the routine evaluation of CKD ROD.
- Vitamin D deficiency: If serum PTH is above the target range for the stage of CKD and serum 25-hydroxyvitamin D (25-hydroxy cholecalciferol) should be measured. Vitamin D stores are categorized as vitamin D insufficiency (levels of 25 OH vitamin D of 10–30 ng/ml [25–75 nmol/l]) and deficiency (levels <10 ng/ml [<25 nmol/l]).

- Dual-energy X-ray absorptiometry (DXA) should not be used to monitor bone mineral density (BMD) in children with CKD. X-ray radiography is only indicated in stage 5 CKD and in high turnover bone disease.
- Bone biopsy
  The gold standard diagnostic test for determining the type of bone disease associated with CKD is iliac crest bone biopsy with double tetracycline labeling and bone histomorphometric analysis.
  It is not necessary to perform bone biopsy for most situations in clinical practice.
  High bone turnover is seen secondary to hyperparathyroidism and is seen in untreated children manifesting with skeletal deformities and bone pains. Low bone turnover is due to calcium overload, vitamin D metabolites, and malnutrition and can predispose to extraosseous calcification.
  Indications for bone biopsy:
  (a) Fractures with minimal or no trauma (pathological fractures)
  (b) Suspected aluminum bone disease based upon clinical symptoms or history of aluminum exposure
  (c) Persistent hypercalcemia with PTH levels between 400 and 600 pg/ml.
- Bone radiographs are not routinely indicated but are indicated in patients with clinical manifestations suggestive of avascular necrosis (AVN) and symptomatic proximal femoral slipped epiphyses (SCFE) or for the assessment of skeletal maturation.

9.7 Management of Renal Osteodystrophy

- Principles of management:
  - Control of hyperphosphatemia
  - Control of serum calcium
    - (a) Calcium supplementation
    - (b) Vitamin D therapy
  - Correction of 25 OH vitamin D stores
  - Control of PTH

9.7.1 Phosphate Control

- If serum phosphorus levels exceed upper limits of normal (see Chap. 17.1) despite dietary phosphorus restriction, phosphate binders should be prescribed.
- Calcium-based phosphate binders are used as the initial therapy. Calcium carbonate, calcium acetate, and calcium gluconate are the preferred binders that need to be administered with meals (1 g of calcium carbonate binds 39 mg of phosphate and 1 g of calcium acetate binds 45 mg of phosphate). It is important to continue restriction of dietary phosphate during this therapy. Aluminum- and citrate-based phosphate binders should be avoided in children.

- Sevelamer: Corrected serum calcium of >10.2 mg/dl (2.54 mmol/l) or serum PTH levels <150 pg/ml (150 ng/l) on two consecutive measurements are indications for the use of a non-calcium-, nonaluminum-containing phosphate binder, such as sevelamer. The dose recommended is 120–160 mg/kg/day in three divided doses along with meals. It can be used alone or in conjunction with the calcium-based phosphate binder.

9.7.2 Correction of Serum Calcium

9.7.2.1 Calcium Supplementation

- Patients whose serum levels of corrected total calcium are below the lower limit (<8.8 mg/dl [2.20 mmol/l]) should receive calcium supplements. Therapy for hypocalcemia should include calcium salts such as calcium carbonate or calcium acetate orally, or calcium gluconate or calcium chloride parenterally, and/or oral vitamin D.
- Monitoring:
  If corrected total serum calcium level exceeds 10.2 mg/dl (2.54 mmol/l), therapies that increase serum calcium should be adjusted as follows:
  (a) Calcium-based phosphate binders to be discontinued and the use of non-calcium, nonmetal-based phosphate binders should be considered.
  (b) Active vitamin D sterols should be discontinued until the serum levels of corrected total calcium return to the target range (8.8–9.5 mg/dl [2.20–2.37 mmol/l]).
  (c) If hypercalcemia (serum levels of corrected total calcium >10.2 mg/dl [2.54 mmol/l]) persists despite the discontinuation of therapy with vitamin and/or the modification of calcium-based phosphate binders, dialysis using lower dialysate calcium may be used for 3–4 weeks.
- The serum Ca X P should be maintained at <55 mg^2/dl^2 (<4.4 $mmol^2/l^2$) in adolescents >12 years and <65 mg^2/dl^2 (<5.2 $mmol^2/l^2$) in younger children. This is best achieved by controlling serum levels of phosphorus within the target range.

Dietary Considerations

Calcium and phosphorus

- Calcium intake should be limited to 100–120 % of the dietary reference intake for age, taking into account all sources of calcium, including phosphate binders.
- In CKD stages 3–5 and dialysis, dietary phosphorus intake should be limited to 100 % of the DRI for age when the serum parathyroid hormone (PTH) concentration is above the target range for CKD stage and the serum phosphorus concentration is within the normal reference range for age.
- In CKD stages 3–5 and dialysis, dietary phosphorus intake should be limited to 80 % of the dietary reference intake for age when the serum PTH level is above the target range for CKD stage and the phosphorus concentration exceeds the normal reference range for age.
  Serum phosphate concentration should be monitored at least every 3 months in children with CKD stages 3–4 and monthly in children with CKD stage 5.

Table 9.6 Vitamin D therapy to correct vitamin D status

Vitamin D status	Treatment with ergocalciferol
Vitamin D insufficiency (16–30 ng/ml)	50,000 IU every 4 weeks for 3 months
Vitamin D deficiency (5–15 ng/ml)	50,000 IU every alternate week for 3 months
Severe vitamin D deficiency (<5 ng/ml)	50,000 IU every week for 3 months

9.7.2.2 Vitamin D Therapy

- In CKD stages 2–4: Measure PTH. If serum PTH is above the target range for the stage of CKD, serum 25-hydroxyvitamin D should be measured.
- If the serum level of 25-hydroxyvitamin D is <30 ng/ml (75 nmol/l), supplementation with vitamin D2 (ergocalciferol) should be initiated as mentioned below (Table 9.6).
- The serum levels of corrected total calcium and phosphate should be measured after 1 month and then at least every 3 months.
- If the serum levels of corrected total calcium exceed 10.2 mg/dl (2.54 mmol/l), discontinue ergocalciferol therapy and all forms of vitamin D therapy.
- If 25(OH) vitamin D is normal, discontinue vitamin D therapy.
- Once patients are replete with vitamin D, continued supplementation with a vitamin D-containing multivitamin preparation should be used with annual reassessment of serum levels of 25(OH) vitamin D.

Active Vitamin D Therapy

- In CKD stages 2–4: Active oral vitamin D (calcitriol) should be initiated when:
    1. Serum levels of 25(OH) D are >30 ng/ml (75 nmol/l).
    2. Serum levels of PTH are above the target range for the CKD stage.
    3. Serum levels of corrected total calcium <10 mg/dl (2.37 mmol/l).
    4. Serum levels of phosphorus less than age-appropriate upper limits.
- Dosage adjustments:
    1. If serum levels of PTH decrease to values below the target range for the CKD stage, active vitamin D sterol therapy should be held until serum levels of PTH increase to above the target range; treatment should then be resumed at half the previous dose of active vitamin D sterols.
    2. If serum levels of corrected total calcium exceed 10.2 mg/dl (2.37 mmol/l), active vitamin D sterol therapy should be held until serum calcium decreases to <9.8 mg/dl (2.37 mmol/l); treatment should then be resumed at half the previous dose. If the lowest daily dose of the active vitamin D sterol is being given, alternate-day dosing should be used.
    3. The dosage of active vitamin D sterols should be adjusted downward as follows: If serum levels of phosphorus increase to greater than age-appropriate upper limits, active vitamin D therapy should be held; the dose of phosphate binders should be increased or initiated until the levels of serum phosphorus decrease to age-appropriate levels; then, treatment at half the prior dose of active vitamin D sterol should be resumed.

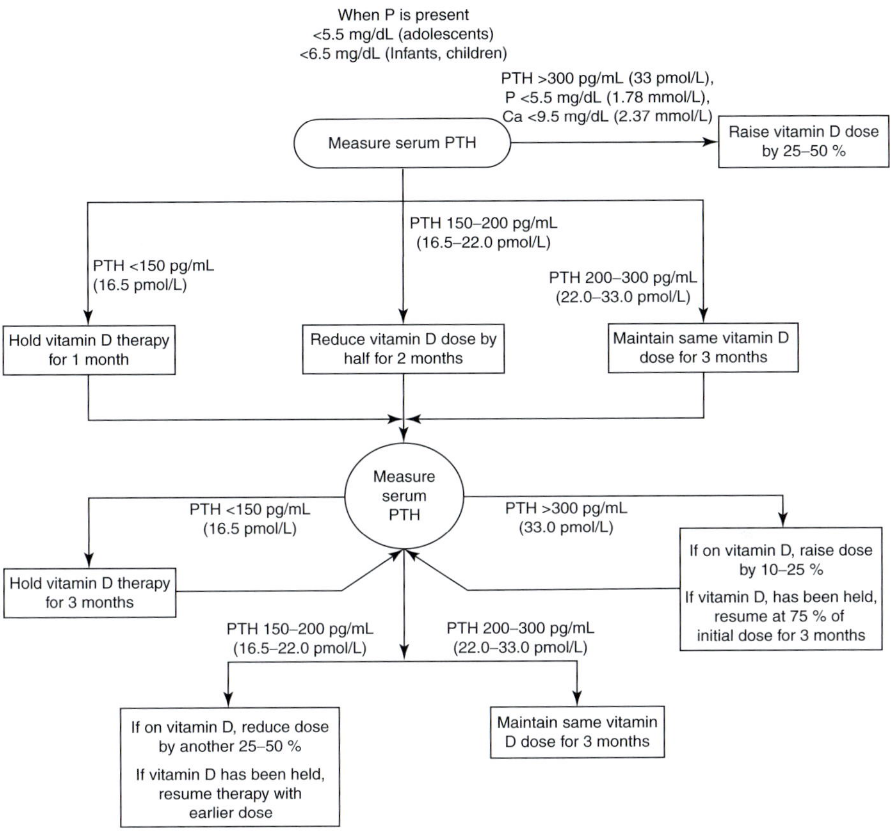

Fig. 9.4 Evaluation and treatment of renal osteodystrophy

Monitoring

Serum levels of calcium and phosphorus should be measured at least monthly for the first 3 months and at least every 3 months thereafter. Serum PTH levels should be measured at least every 3 months.

The approach to evaluating and treating biochemical abnormalities of renal osteodystrophy are summarized in the below algorithm taken from the KDOQI guidelines (Fig. 9.4 and Box 9.4 at the end of this chapter).

1. *Control of PTH*: Calcium and vitamin D supplements and phosphate binders are sufficient in most cases.

Parathyroidectomy

- Following adequate efforts to restrict phosphorus and supplement calcium and vitamin D if intact PTH is persistently high, parathyroidectomy may have a role to play.

  Parathyroidectomy should be considered in patients with severe hyperparathyroidism (persistent serum levels of PTH >1,000 pg/ml [1,000 ng/l]) and disabling

Box 9.4 Summary of KDOQI Recommendations

Serum phosphate: CKD stage 5: >12 years: 3.5–5.5 mg/dl (1.15–1.80 mmol/l), 1–12 years: 4–6 mg/dl (1.30–1.95 mmol/l)
Ca × PO_4: <55 mg^2/dl^2 (<4.4 $mmol^2/l^2$) >12 years and <65 mg^2/dl^2 (<5.2 $mmol^2/l^2$) in younger children
25 OH vitamin D: insufficiency: <30 ng/ml (75 nmol/l), deficiency: <15 ng/ml (<37.5 nmol/l)
Calcium: maintain within normal limits in all stages
PTH (pg/ml): CKD stages 2, 3: 35–70, CKD stage 4: 70–110, CKD stage 5: 200–300
Energy: 100 % of estimated energy requirement
Protein: CKD stage 3:100–140 % of DRI, CKD stages 4–5:100–120 % of DRI
Hemoglobin: 11–12 g/dl (110–120 g/l)

bone deformities associated with hypercalcemia and/or hyperphosphatemia that are refractory to medical therapy.

- Surgical Technique
  Effective surgical therapy of severe hyperparathyroidism can be accomplished by subtotal parathyroidectomy or total parathyroidectomy with parathyroid tissue autotransplantation. Total parathyroidectomy probably is not the procedure of choice in patients who may subsequently receive a kidney transplant, since subsequent control of serum calcium levels may be problematic.

Indications for Orthopedic Surgery

Lower extremity angular deformity should be surgically corrected if the deformity is progressive or severe as defined by interference with gait or by the presence of a mechanical axis deviation of more than 10° between the femur and tibia. Control of secondary HPT is recommended prior to surgical correction.

Symptomatic proximal femoral slipped epiphyses (SCFE) should be surgically stabilized if K/DOQI target values for PTH are not achieved within 3 months of the diagnosis of SCFE.

Metabolic Acidosis

In children, overt acidosis is present when the estimated GFR is less than 30 ml/min per 1.73 m^2. Acidosis may also be present in less severe CKD with conditions associated with renal tubular acidosis. Acidosis is associated with growth impairment because the body utilizes bone buffering to bind some of the excess hydrogen ions.

In CKD stages 1–5, the serum level of total CO_2 should be measured.

In patients >2 years of age, serum levels of total CO_2 should be maintained at >22 mEq/l (22 mmol/l); in neonates and young infants below age 2, serum levels of total CO_2 should be maintained at >20 mEq/l (20 mmol/l).

If necessary, supplemental alkali salts should be given to achieve this goal.

Aluminum Bone Disease

Though aluminum bone disease is seen in patients on dialysis, it can occur in stage 4 or 5 prior to dialysis therapy secondary to intake of medications containing aluminum salts.

Prevention: To prevent aluminum toxicity, the regular administration of aluminum should be avoided and the dialysate concentration of aluminum should be maintained at <10 μg/L.

Monitoring: In children with CKD lower than stage 5, serum levels of aluminum should be measured yearly if children have been exposed to aluminum for 3 months or more in the prior year. Baseline levels of serum aluminum should be <20 μg/l. A deferoxamine (DFO) test should be performed if there are elevated serum aluminum levels (60–200 μg/l) or clinical signs and symptoms of aluminum toxicity or prior to parathyroidectomy if the patient has had aluminum exposure for at least 4 months or more.

Diagnosis: The presence of aluminum bone disease can be predicted by a rise in serum aluminum of >50 μg/l following DFO challenge combined with serum PTH levels of <150 pg/ml (150 ng/l). However, the gold standard for the diagnosis of aluminum bone disease is a bone biopsy showing increased aluminum staining of the bone surface (>15–25 %) using an aluminum-specific stain and often the presence of adynamic bone disease or osteomalacia.

Therapy: In symptomatic patients with serum aluminum levels >60 μg/l but <200 μg/l or increase in aluminum after DFO >50 g/l, DFO should be given to treat the aluminum overload.

9.7.3 Hypertension

Measurement of blood pressure in children should be performed with age- and size-appropriate equipment, and blood pressure values should be interpreted according to normal values adjusted for age, gender, and height percentile, as recommended by the Task Force Report on High Blood Pressure in Children and Adolescents (see also Chap. 7). Target blood pressure in children should be lower than the 90th percentile for normal values adjusted for age, gender, and height or 120/80 mmHg, whichever is lower. More recent randomized trial evidence suggests that maintaining BP below the 50th percentile may be effective in delaying progression of CKD. Intensified blood pressure control with target 24-h blood pressure levels in the low range of normal confers a substantial benefit with respect to renal function among children with chronic kidney disease. The approach to using antihypertensive drugs and drug dose adjustments in CKD is mentioned below.

9.7.3.1 Antihypertensive Drugs in CKD

When the GFR is >50 ml/min/1.73 m^2, thiazides are indicated. When GFR <50 ml/min/1.73 m^2, loop diuretics can be tried. If blood pressure readings are >75th percentile, treatment with angiotensin-converting-enzyme inhibitors/angiotensin receptor blockers is initiated. One may add calcium channel blockers or beta adrenergic blockers, and thereafter, if blood pressure readings are >75th percentile, clonidine, minoxidil, or prazosin may be added.

9.7.4 Cardiovascular Morbidity

Cardiovascular abnormalities such as left ventricular (LV) hypertrophy, LV dysfunction, increased arterial stiffness, increased carotid intima–medial thickness (IMT), and coronary calcification are common in CKD, even in children and young adults. Individuals who are under dialysis are at particularly high risk for CV abnormalities. Hypertension, anemia, fluid overload, hyperphosphatemia, and carnitine deficiency are risk factors contributing to cardiovascular morbidity.

KDOQI recommends the evaluation of dyslipidemia in adolescents upon presentation with CKD stage 5 (GFR <15 ml/min/1.73 m^2 or on dialysis), at 2–3 months after a change in treatment or other conditions known to cause dyslipidemia and at least annually thereafter. The assessment of dyslipidemia should include a complete fasting lipid profile with total cholesterol, LDL, HDL, and triglycerides. Hyperlipidemia in children is defined as lipid levels greater than the 95th percentile for age and gender. The normative data for lipids in children and adolescents currently used are from the Lipid Research Clinics Program from the NIH published in 1980 and can be found in the 2003 KDOQI guidelines for the management of dyslipidemia in chronic kidney disease.

For adolescents with stage 5 CKD and a level of LDL ≥130 mg/dl (3.36 mmol/l), KDOQI recommends treatment to reduce LDL to <130 mg/dl. If LDL is <130 mg/dl, fasting triglycerides ≥200 mg/dl (5.18 mmol/l), and non-HDL cholesterol (total cholesterol minus HDL) ≥160 mg/dl (4.14 mmol/l), treatment should be considered with gemfibrozil (1,200 mg/day) or fenofibrate (48 mg/day). All children with dyslipidemia should follow the recommendations for therapeutic lifestyle changes (TLC), which include diet modification with a reduction in saturated fat intake and increase in fiber intake and moderate physical activity. If LDL cholesterol is ≥160 mg/dl (4.14 mmol/l) and non-HDL cholesterol ≥190 mg/dl, statin therapy (atorvastatin 5–10 mg/day, simvastatin 20 mg/day) is recommended in children older than 10 years.

9.7.5 Infection

The CDC recommendations (2006) of the Advisory Committee on Immunization Practices (ACIP) on the "guidelines for vaccinating kidney dialysis patients and patients with chronic kidney disease" are presented below.

Vaccination is recommended against hepatitis B, influenza (trivalent inactivated influenza vaccine, TIV), and pneumococcal infection (see below).

As per national immunization guidelines, expected exposure/travel or lack of protection, patients may be vaccinated against diphtheria/tetanus (DTap/Tdap/Td), *H. influenza*, hepatitis A, MMR (see below), polio (inactivated/parenteral), rabies, typhoid fever, varicella, and yellow fever.

Hepatitis B vaccine schedule (for <20 years):
Recombivax hepatitis B: 5 μg, 0.5 ml IM, 3 doses at 0.1 and 6 months.
Engerix B: 10 μg, 0.5 ml IM, 3 doses at 0, 1 and 6 months.
The Advisory Committee on Immunization Practices (ACIP): recommends double standard doses to achieve a measurable antibody response.
Serological testing for anti-hepatitis B antibody (anti-HBs) 1–2 months after the third dose. Anti-HBs levels <10 mIU/ml are an indication for revaccination.

Live vaccines such as BCG, oral polio, and measles–mumps–rubella (MMR) are contraindicated while on immunosuppressive therapy or within 6 weeks of their discontinuation.

9.7.6 Pneumococcal Vaccine

Children who have completed the pneumococcal vaccine (13-valent [PCV13] – if available – or 7-valent [PCV7] conjugate vaccine) series before 2 years of age and who have CKD should receive one dose of 23-valent pneumococcal polysaccharide vaccine (PPV23), (≥2 months after the last dose of PCV).

Children ages 24–59 months with CKD should receive two doses of PCV13 (or PCV7, if PCV13 is unavailable) administered 2 months apart followed by one dose of PPV23 administered ≥2 months after the second dose of PCV.

Children aged 24–59 months who have received PPV23 vaccine should receive two doses of PCV7 or 13 administered 2 months apart, 2 months of the last dose of PPV23.

9.7.7 Hematological Issues

Besides anemia, children with advanced CKD demonstrate altered platelet function and abnormal coagulation which may result in bleeding or thrombotic tendency.

- Uremic bleeding is characterized by abnormal prolongation of bleeding time and hemorrhagic symptoms, like skin bleeds, epistaxis, and prolonged bleed from needle puncture sites, hemorrhagic pericarditis, and intracranial and retroperitoneal bleed.
  - The factors responsible for platelet dysfunction are platelet abnormalities, uremic toxins, von Willebrand factor abnormalities, blood vessel abnormalities, and anemia.
  - Correction of uremic bleed: Correct anemia, maintain adequate dialysis, and withdraw antiplatelet agents.

  Desmopressin (DDAVP) is indicated 1 h before surgery at a dose of 0.3 μg/kg subcutaneously (or IV 30 min before surgery), or 2–3 μg/kg intranasally.

  Cryoprecipitate can be administered as infusion of 10 units (bags) in adults in case of active bleed and prior to surgery. If unavailable, frozen plasma (10 ml/kg) may be tried.
- Thrombotic events: Children on hemodialysis are at risk to develop thrombosis at the site of vascular access as well as coronary, cerebral, and retinal arteries.

- Factors responsible for thrombosis are enhanced platelet aggregability, diminished protein C anticoagulant activity, and elevated levels of antiphospholipid, antiprotein C, and antiprotein S antibodies.
- Warfarin should be used only in case of thrombotic events and not prophylactically in CKD.

9.7.8 Fluid Electrolyte and Acid–Base Issues

Despite advanced CKD, children with underlying tubulointerstitial diseases may produce normal or large quantities of urine. On the contrary, children with glomerular diseases may present with oliguria. The fluid management therefore depends on the residual renal function and need not be universally restricted in all cases. Children with underlying tubular disorders in CKD may have hypokalemia as compared to hyperkalemia seen commonly in CKD of a glomerular etiology. Metabolic acidosis may be an early and long-standing feature of tubular diseases.

9.7.9 Psychosocial Issues

It is crucial to have ongoing involvement of child psychologists, medical social workers, and counselors in dealing with the multifaceted problems of CKD in children. Appropriate measures need to be taken to address issues concerning family dynamics, coping skills, decision making, and adherence to therapy. A coordinated team approach works best. Patient education focuses on health monitoring, home care, adherence to medications, schooling, growth, and maturational issues. Financial issues play an important part in decision making and disease management in developing countries where medical care is not supported by health insurance. Transition of care from pediatric to adult care providers also requires attention. One approach is to offer combined pediatric/adult clinics attended by both pediatric and adult nephrologists.

9.8 Retarding Progression of CKD

The modifiable factors contributing to CKD progression are:

- Hypertension
- Proteinuria
- Dyslipidemia
- Nephrotoxic drugs
- Urinary obstruction
- Hyperfiltration

  Interventions to retard progression:

(a) Lowering blood pressures to target systolic and diastolic blood pressures <90th percentile for age, height, and gender. In a pediatric study from Europe, 29.9 % of patients who received intensified blood pressure control reached the end point of 50 % decline of renal function compared to 41.7 % of patients receiving conventional blood pressure control.

(b) Reduction of proteinuria: Angiotensin-converting-enzyme inhibitors (ACEI) and angiotensin receptor blockers (ARB) have potential reno-protective effect by reducing proteinuria, lowering intra-glomerular pressure, and exerting antifibrotic effects. In children with CKD, ACEI have been beneficial in the presence of hypertension and proteinuria. The combination therapy of ACEI and ARB is not yet recommended as a part of standard care.

(c) Phosphorus control: Studies in adults reveal that phosphorus restriction may help retard progression of CKD.

(d) Dietary protein restriction: Children are in a dynamic phase of growth and cannot afford to have restriction in calorie or protein intake.

(e) Prophylactic antibiotics in children with recurrent UTIs; consider urological interventions (clean intermittent catheterization, surgery) when indicated.

(f) Ensure adequate volume status (an issue in children with polyuric CKD).

9.9 Indications for Renal Replacement Therapy

- Laboratory criteria: GFR <15 ml/min/m^2, refractory hyperkalemia, hyperphosphatemia, and metabolic acidosis.
- Clinical criteria: Children with symptoms of nausea, vomiting, malnutrition, growth retardation, fluid overload, hypertension, and uremia, despite optimal medical management.
- Renal transplantation is the renal replacement therapy of choice in children, offering a near normal life to a child with end-stage renal disease (for details refer to Chaps. 10 and 11 on dialysis and transplantation). For children requiring dialysis while awaiting transplantation or for children unable to receive a transplant, peritoneal dialysis is generally the preferred choice as it is child friendly, potentially less costly than in-center hemodialysis, can be offered at home, preserves vascular access, and is more feasible in small infants than hemodialysis.

Conclusion

CKD in children often presents with vague and subtle clinical manifestations. It is crucial to recognize children in early stages of CKD for optimal evaluation and care. Monitoring a child in CKD regularly provides an opportunity to control factors that can aggravate progression of CKD. Management of children with CKD calls for a multidisciplinary team approach. Children who reach end-stage renal disease should promptly be offered suitable renal replacement therapy.

Suggested Reading

KDOQI (2002) Clinical practice guidelines for chronic kidney disease: evaluation, classification, and stratification. Am J Kidney Dis 39:S1–S266

KDOQI (2005) Clinical practice guidelines for bone metabolism and disease in children with chronic kidney disease. Am J Kidney Dis 46(4 Suppl 1):S1–S122

KDOQI (2009) Clinical practice guideline for nutrition in children. Am J Kidney Dis 53(3 Suppl 2):S1–S124

KDOQI, National Kidney Foundation (2006) Clinical practice recommendations for anemia in chronic kidney disease in children. Am J Kidney Dis 47(Suppl 3):S86–S108

KDOQI, National Kidney Foundation (2003) Clinical practice guidelines for managing dyslipidemias in chronic kidney disease. Am J Kidney Dis 41(Suppl 3):S22–S38

Chronic Dialysis

10

Kishore Phadke, Martin Bitzan, and Sudarshan Shetty

10.1 PD

10.1.1 Introduction

Peritoneal dialysis (PD) is a versatile renal replacement therapy (RRT) modality for acute kidney injury (AKI) as well as long-term dialysis.

PD works on the principle of equilibration of blood in the peritoneal capillaries and dialysis fluid in the peritoneal cavity. The dialysis takes place by diffusion and convection.

Peritoneal dialysis in AKI has been described in Chap. 8. This chapter deals with PD in endstage renal disease (ESRD).

Milestones that led to the wide acceptance of PD as a modality for chronic RRT were the development of appropriate peritoneal catheters, the introduction of plastic bags containing stable, standardized dialysis solutions, improved connection technology that helped reducing the infection risk, the invention of automated PD (cyclers) and, more recently, the propagation of light, portable cyclers.

K. Phadke (✉)
Department of Pediatric Nephrology,
Children's Kidney Care Center, St. John's Medical College Hospital,
Koramangala, Bangalore, Karnataka 560034, India
e-mail: kishorephadke@yahoo.co.in

M. Bitzan
Division of Pediatric Nephrology, Montreal Children's Hospital, McGill University,
2300, rue Tupper, Montreal, QC H3H 1P3, Canada
e-mail: martin.bitzan@mcgill.ca

S. Shetty
Department of Pediatrics, K.S. Hegde Medical Academy,
Mangalore, Karnataka 575018, India
e-mail: sudarshan_july4@rediffmail.com

K. Phadke et al. (eds.), *Manual of Pediatric Nephrology*,
DOI 10.1007/978-3-642-12483-9_10, © Springer-Verlag Berlin Heidelberg 2014

Determining the indication for PD, dialysis prescription, and treatment of PD-associated peritonitis are medical acts performed by the nephrologist. However, many aspects of PD can be managed by qualified nurses in conjunction with a nephrologist or trained pediatrician.

The PD team should further include a social worker and a surgeon/urologist.

This chapter can only give the framework for this dialysis modality. Delegation of the preparation and education of the family and the patient by the PD nurse, and day-to-day technical instructions and recognition of potential problems, requires the creation of a set of clearly outlined protocols for all PD-related procedures and for trouble shooting.

A center offering PD should have a knowledgeable member of the medical team that can be reached 7 days a week and 24 hours a day. The major providers of PD equipment have a help-line and personnel to trouble shoot when technical problems arise, and provide hands-on training and useful educational material.

10.1.2 Definitions

10.1.2.1 Principles of PD

- Physical and physiological principles underlying PD is the exchange of solutes and water between the blood (peritoneal capillaries) and the surrounding tissue, and the dialysis solution across the peritoneal membrane.
- The major mechanisms are *diffusive transport* of solutes (based on the concentration gradient between dialysate and blood), *ultrafiltration* (UF; removal of plasma water) and *convective mass transfer* (when solutes and proteins are "dragged" along with the UF). The UF driving force in PD is determined by the osmotic pressure exerted by the dialysate glucose concentration.
- The permeability of the peritoneal membrane (the tissue between the capillary lumen and the peritoneal space) can be increased by inflammation (peritonitis) and impaired by progressive peritoneal fibrosis.
- The surface area of the peritoneal membrane correlates with the body surface area (BSA): this relationship remains constant across patient age groups. Dialysate volume prescription is therefore scaled to BSA, specifically when determining dialysis adequacy and peritoneal transport properties (see Sect. 10.1.4.9).

10.1.2.2 Types of PD

- Chronic PD can be performed manually or with an automated device (cycler).
- CAPD (chronic ambulatory peritoneal dialysis) is typically performed with four exchanges during the day and a long night-time dwell
- CCPD (continuous cycling peritoneal dialysis), consisting of 5–10 nightly exchanges, is possible using a cycling machine and a long daytime dwell (also termed automated PD, or APD).
- Chronic PD depends on the presence of a surgically placed catheter. To avoid pericatheter leakage and minimize infection (PD peritonitis), the catheter is tunneled

and usually has two subcutaneously buried cuffs. Dialysate, additives, and all catheter manipulations and connections have to be done under aseptic conditions.

- Complications to CAPD/CCPD in children include abdominal hernia, back pain, hydrothorax, obesity, and hyperlipidemia.
- Long-term dialysis modifies the peritoneal membrane characteristics, e.g., due to unphysiological, high glucose concentrations, and may decrease dialysis efficiency.
- Commonly used PD terms and abbreviations are found in Box 10.1.
- The principal differences between various types of PD are depicted in Fig. 10.1.

Box 10.1 Types of PD (the PD Alphabet)

APD	Automated peritoneal dialysis (PD; see also "APD-C")
	PD using a "cycler" to effect dialysate infusion and drainage (conveniently performed over night. Can be combined with manual drain or fill cycle during the day if needed)
APD-A	Adapted peritoneal dialysis (also termed APD)
	Sequential use of short dwell times (and small fill volume) to promote ultrafiltration and longer dwell times (with larger fill volume) to promote removal of uremic toxins (e.g., phosphate)
APD-C	"Conventional" automated peritoneal dialysis
	Automated PD using uniform dialysate volumes and dwell times during a given dialysis period
CAPD	Continuous ambulatory peritoneal dialysis
	"Classical" form of PD; advantages are its simplicity, low-cost, and similar efficiency in most patients
CCPD	Continuous cycling peritoneal dialysis
	Long daytime dwell and several cycles overnight. A minority of patients undergoing CCPD does not have daytime dwell (NIPD) and some patients must also do a midday exchange to meet adequacy or ultrafiltration (UF) targets
CFPD	Continuous flow peritoneal dialysis
	Continuous dialysis technique using two separate catheters or a double lumen PD catheter and high dialysate flow rates. Spent dialysate can be regenerated with hemodialysis technology. Theoretical advantages of CFPD are its very high clearances and improved UF. Impractical in most settings
CPD	Continuous peritoneal dialysis
	No "dry" periods; CPD may also denote "chronic PD" (to distinguish from "acute PD")
IPD	Intermittent peritoneal dialysis
	Alternating periods of "wet" and "dry" peritoneum (e.g., cycler changes during the night followed by complete drainage of the peritoneum in the morning; see NIPD)
IPP	(Hydrostatic) Intraperitoneal pressure
IPV	Intraperitoneal volume
NIPD	Nocturnal (nightly) intermittent peritoneal dialysis
	"Dry" abdomen during daytime

(continued)

Box 10.1 (continued)

PD	Peritoneal dialysis
PET	Peritoneal equilibration test
TPD	Tidal peritoneal dialysis
	Exchanges where the peritoneum always contains at least some dialysate (usually at least one-half full). It is used to improve comfort and drainage. TPD may or may not include a daytime dwell
UF	Ultrafiltrate
	Net UF = Total effluent volume – Total fill volume (usually overnight or a 24-h period)

10.1.3 When to Use PD and HD?

10.1.3.1 Advantages of Peritoneal Dialysis

- Ease of procedure (expertise).
- Can be performed with simple equipment and infrastructure.
- Suitable in challenging circumstances: newborns and small infants, hemodynamically unstable patients, peripheral centers where expertise may not be available.
- No systemic anticoagulation
- Compared with conventional hemodialysis (HD), PD is more physiological with lower risk of disequilibrium syndrome.
- Better control of hypertension and anemia with reduced or no need for blood transfusions.
- Residual renal functions may be preserved better than with chronic hemodialysis.
- PD allows a more liberal diet than HD.

10.1.3.2 Challenges of PD

- Abdominal adhesions following previous abdominal surgeries
- Recent abdominal surgery or inflammation
- Occasionally inferior to blood borne dialysis techniques when large ultrafiltration is required within a short time, as in pulmonary edema
- Limitations in hypercatabolic states such as sepsis, burns, heat stroke, or crush injuries
- Risk of peritonitis if strict asepsis is not followed

10.1.3.3 Contraindications to PD

Absolute contraindications

- Omphalocele
- Gastroschisis
- Bladder exstrophy
- Diaphragmatic hernia
- Severe adhesions
- Peritoneal membrane failure

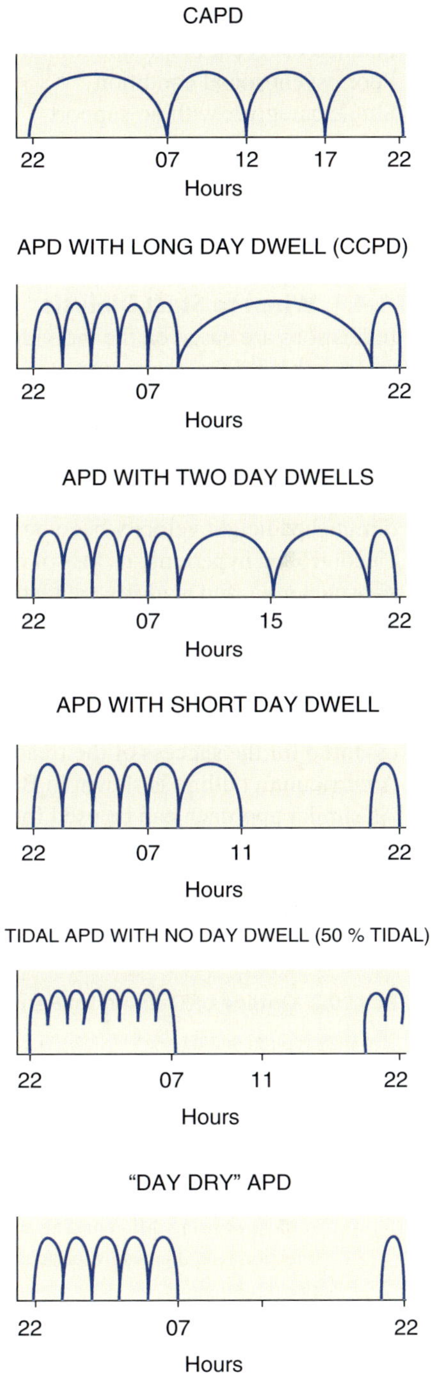

Fig. 10.1 Peritoneal dialysis treatment modalities. For abbreviation see Box 10.1 (From Brenner & Rector's The Kidney, 9th edition; with permission)

Relative contraindications

- Planned or recent major abdominal surgery
- Poor psychosocial condition
- Single caregiver with no support
- Unhygienic home conditions

10.1.4 Initiation of PD

10.1.4.1 When to Start Dialysis

- Indications are based on the individualized combination of clinical, biochemical, and psychosocial assessments
- When the glomerular filtration rate (GFR) reaches 15–10 ml/min/1.73 m^2 and the child is unwell, despite optimal conservative measures, or when the GFR is <10 ml/min per 1.73 m^2
- When signs such as nausea, vomiting, lethargy, restricted daily activities, and diminished height velocity become apparent in a child with advanced CKD
- Uncontrolled hypertension, loss of residual renal functions, hyperkalemia, hyperphosphatemia, and acidosis are factors to be considered in the decision to initiate dialysis

10.1.4.2 Education

- Diligent training of the patient (if applicable) and at least two family members is essential for the success of the treatment and for the PD program.
- A curriculum outline is shown in Box 10.2.
- As similar approach can be used for training new nurses (with adjustments).
- The training is best conducted by a dedicated (PD/dialysis) nurse.

Box 10.2 Outline of Training for Peritoneal Dialysis (Training Curriculum)

1. Background and theory
   - (a) Renal functions
   - (b) Principles of peritoneal membrane transport and dialysis (PD)
   - (c) Effects of fluid and water balance on weight, blood pressure, and survival
   - (d) Composition of dialysis solutions: glucose, electrolytes, lactate, and bicarbonate
   - (e) Purpose of using different dialysis solutions
   - (f) Infection risk, organisms, principles of asepsis/techniques
2. Practical training
   - (a) Training in aseptic techniques
     - (i) Handwashing
     - (ii) Connections
     - (iii) Exit site infections and exit site care
     - (iv) What to do in case of (possible) breaks of sterility (contamination)

Box 10.2 (continued)

(b) Set-up for dialysis: manual PD and cycler (if applicable)
  (i) Step-by-step procedure guide (preferably with visual material)
  (ii) Documentation (charting)
(c) Problem-solving
  (i) Manual PD (CAPD)
  (ii) Cycler alarms and malfunction
(d) Daily measurements
  (i) Body weight
  (ii) Blood pressure and heart rate
  (iii) Recoding and understanding implications
(e) Others: Obtaining a dialysate specimen; administering of intraperitoneal (IP) medications

3. Complications of PD
  (a) Peritonitis
    (i) Signs, symptoms, laboratory diagnostic
    (ii) Steps to follow when peritonitis is suspected
    (iii) Treatment of peritonitis and long-term risks
    (iv) IP antibiotics and their administration
  (b) Exit site and tunnel infection
  (c) Dialysate drain problems
    (i) Constipation
    (ii) Fibrin
    (iii) PD catheter position
  (d) Hyper- and hypotension
  (e) Changes in the amount of ultrafiltrate (UF)
  (f) Dialysate leaks
  (g) Pain related to dialysis
  (h) Bloody or cloudy dialysate effluent
4. Life with PD
  (a) Ordering and managing PD supply
  (b) Record keeping, important phone numbers
  (c) How and when to contact hospital/dialysis center/dialysis team
  (d) Medications and prescriptions
  (e) Clinic appointments
  (f) Home visits
  (g) School, sports, vacation, and travel

The training curriculum has to be adjusted to the needs of the caregiver and patient (family) and nurses in training, respectively. Concrete material is available from the major suppliers (manufacturers) of dialysis equipment, textbooks, and the Internet

- PD training is started before the initiation of therapy or during the healing phase after PD catheter placement.
- "Refresher" sessions and review of caregiver's (patient) performance should be planned and are advisable after each episode of peritonitis or after a prolonged break of PD.

10.1.4.3 PD Catheter Placement and Choice of Catheter

- While trained nephrologists place chronic PD catheters in many (adult) centers, it is usually a dedicated (pediatric) surgeon, who inserts pediatric catheters, generally laparoscopically.
- PD catheters come in a variety of flavors, but all models may not be available in a given center.
- All but neonatal catheters should have 2 cuffs to anchor the catheter in the abdominal wall and reduce the peritonitis risk due to microbial infections.
- The catheter should have a downward or lateral subcutaneous tunnel configuration.
- Perioperative antibiotic prophylaxis to be given within 1 h before the incision for PD catheter placement to reduce the risk of early-onset peritonitis.
- The catheter can be used immediately; however, delayed PD initiation is preferred to allow the catheter to heal in and reduce the risk of pericatheter leaks.

10.1.4.4 Post Catheter Insertion Break-In Protocol

Management immediately after PD catheter insertion

Details see Table 10.1

Management during the healing phase (break-in period)

Table 10.1 Break-in protocol: immediate post-insertion period

Step	Procedure	Instructions
1	X-Ray (plain film)	In operating or recovery room Initiate catheter/peritoneal flushes as soon as patient is back in the ward
2a	Rapid in-out exchanges until clear (about three exchanges)	Peritoneal infusion volume 10 ml/kg Heparin 1,000 units/l in dialysate bag (for the first week) Cefazolin 250 mg/l for the first 12–16 h. Stop the morning after catheter insertion. Alternative antibiotic, if patient allergic
2b	When dialysate is clear, begin hourly exchanges	50 min dwell (including filling time) 10 min drain (depending on fill volume)
2c	Repeat cycles hourly for 12–16 h or less	Individualize according to patient's status
2d	Repeat steps 2a–c for eight more hours	After 16 h if dialysate (effluent) *un*clear or color*ed* and/or *in*appropriate draining Reassess
2e	Proceed to the maintenance phase	After 16 h dialysate clear and colorless, with appropriate draining
3	Prescribe antiemetic PRN for nausea/vomiting and for pain	Antiemetics are used to avoid high intra-abdominal pressures Dimenhydrinate: 5 mg/kg/day q 6 h (IV, IM, PO)
4	Pain management	Morphine: 0.05–0.1 mg/kg/dose PRN q 2–4 h (IV, IM, PO) Antidote: naloxone (IV, IM, PO) <20 kg 0.01–0.1 mg/ml/kg per dose q 3–5 min >20 kg 2 mg per dose q 3–5 min
5	Use stool softeners	Locally available preparations (example, docusate-Na 5 mg/kg/day divided twice daily)

- The break-in period refers to the time immediately following catheter insertion Routinely, dialysis is initiated 2–4 weeks post catheter insertion to allow adequate healing.
- Some centers report no difference in post-insertion complications (esp. pericatheter leak) when the catheter is used earlier. However, there are no prospective, controlled studies comparing different break-in protocols for CAPD and for CCPD/NIPD.
- Risks for PD catheter complications depend on catheter placement technique, (early) initiation of daytime fill, resumption of physical activity, and age.
- The purpose of the break-in procedure is to clear intra-peritoneal blood and fibrin from the catheter, minimize immediate omental adhesion, and reduce the incidence of pericatheter leak by maintaining low intra-abdominal pressure.
  - Pericatheter leakage delays the in-growth of fibrous tissue into the catheter cuff which provides a medium for bacterial growth which may lead to peritonitis or an exit site infection.
  - Intra-abdominal pressure is minimized by the restriction of dialysate volume and of patient activity.
- Dialysis can be initiated in the immediate post-insertion period if there is urgent need for dialysis.
  Starting exchange volumes are 10–20 ml/kg. For details, see Table 10.2.
- Ambulation and sitting position are not permitted when the abdomen is filled with increased volume for the first 6 weeks. Mobilization is permitted if the patient is filled with a small volume as "last fill."
- Heparin: during the first week of dialysis, add 1,000 units/l to the dialysis solution. Decrease to 500 units/l during the second week, if no fibrin or blood clots are seen in the effluent. Then stop heparin.

10.1.4.5 Healing of the PD Exit Site

- Healing of the exit site may take 6–12 weeks.
- Exit site is cleaned and dressed weekly by experienced PD nurse or physician.
- More frequent dressing changes are not warranted (and should be avoided), unless drainage is excessive or dressing becomes soiled or wet.
- Continue 1-weekly dressing changes until exit site is well healed.
- No shower or bath tub during the healing phase.
- Aseptic techniques for dressing changes and cleaning of exit site using sterile gloves and face mask.

Table 10.2 Maintenance phase for patients in need of immediate dialysis

Procedure	Instructions	
Infuse dextrose dialysate containing 1,000 units/l of heparin as follows:	*Time period*	*Volume (ml/kg)*
	1st 24 h	10 ml/kg
	2nd 24 h	15 ml/kg
	3rd 24 h	20 ml/kg for 4 weeks, then 25 ml/kg for 1 week, and then, 30 ml/kg for 4–8 weeks
	To be reassessed after 8 weeks	

- For detailed guidelines of exit site care, see "Consensus Guidelines for the Prevention and Treatment of Catheter-Related Infections and Peritonitis in Pediatric Patients Receiving Peritoneal Dialysis: 2012 Update."

10.1.4.6 Maintenance Dialysis Prescription

- Typical CAPD consists of four daily exchanges with low-strength dextrose concentrations.
- In contrast to typical adult PD prescriptions, pediatric fill volumes have to be adjusted to body size (1,100–1,200 ml/m^2 surface area or 30–40 ml/kg body weight).
- Measurement of hydrostatic intraperitoneal pressure (IPP) helps to evaluate fill volume tolerance in the individual patients. Fill volume exceeding a pressure of 18 cm H_2O in supine position is associated with abdominal pain and decreased respiratory vital capacity.
- Slightly higher fill volume may be tolerated in supine position (NIPD or CCPD).
- The pricing of appropriate sized bags of dialysis solutions and pediatric tubing may be limiting in some countries or settings.
- Protocols for the use of cycler technology are easily available from the major manufactures or suppliers.

10.1.4.7 Choice of PD Solutions

- The choice of dialysate fluid is tailored to the individual patient's clinical needs considering fluid balance, blood pressure, and peritoneal membrane characteristics (see Sect. 10.1.4.9).
- If a cycler is used, solutions of different dextrose concentrations can be mixed to optimize ultrafiltration and solute removal.
- Traditional PD solutions are lactate-based (which is metabolized to bicarbonate, once absorbed, but confers a relatively acidic pH of 5.5) and have a high (ionized) calcium concentration (1.75 mmol/l; see Table 10.3).

Table 10.3 Composition of commonly used Dianeal peritoneal dialysis solution

			PD1[a]			PD4[b]		
	Dextrose ⇒	0.5 %	1.5 %	2.5 %	4.25 %	1.5 %	2.5 %	4.25 %
	Glucose ⇒		1.36 %	2.27 %	3.86 %	1.36 %	2.27 %	3.86 %
			Iso	Medium	Hyper	Iso	Medium	Hyper
Dextrose anhydrate	g/l	5.0	13.6	22.7	38.6	13.6	22.7	38.6
Glucose	mmol/l		75.6	126.1	214.4	75.6	126.1	214.4
Sodium [Na^+]	mmol/l	132	132	132	132	132	132	132
Calcium [Ca^{++}]	mmol/l	1.62	1.75	1.75	1.75	1.25	1.25	1.25
Magnesium [Mg^{++}]	mmol/l	0.75	0.75	0.75	0.75	0.25	0.25	0.25
Chloride [Cl^-]	mmol/l	101	102	102	102	95	95	95
Lactate	mmol/l	35	35	35	35	40	40	40
Osmolality	mOsm/kg	295	340	390	480	340	390	480
pH		5.2	5.5	5.5	5.5	5.5	5.5	5.5

[a]PD1 normal calcium solution
[b]PD4 low calcium solution

Table 10.4 Composition of "second generation" peritoneal dialysis solutions

		Bicarbonate-based ("physiological") solutions			Amino acid-based solution	Icodextrin-based solution
	Glucose ⇒	1.36 %	2.27 %	3.86 %	1.10 %	7.50 %
Dextrose anhydrate	G/l	13.6	22.7	38.6	–	–
Glucose in mmol/l	mmol/l	75.6	126.1	214.4	–	–
Sodium [Na^+]	mmol/l	133	133	133	132	133
Calcium [Ca^{++}]	mmol/l	1.25	1.25	1.25	1.25	1.75
Magnesium [Mg^{++}]	mmol/l	0.25	0.25	0.25	0.25	0.25
Chloride [Cl^-]	mmol/l	96	96	96	96	96
Lactate	mmol/l	15	15	15	40	40
Bicarbonate	mmol/l	25	25	25	–	–
Osmolarity (approx)	mOsm/kg	340	390	480	340	282
pH		7.4	7.4	7.4	6.7	5.5

- Relatively low pH (5.5) and high glucose concentration (exceeding physiological blood sugar concentration by about 15 [1.35 % glucose] to 40-fold [3.86 % glucose]) are believed to be toxic to (peritoneal) mesothelial cells.
- "Second generation" PD solutions have physiological calcium concentrations (1.25 mmol/l) to avoid hypercalcemia and elevated Ca x P product, and a close to physiological pH (e.g., physioneal; see Table 10.4 and a recent overview by García-López E et al. *Nat Rev Nephrol* 2012).
- Supra-physiological glucose concentrations, low pH, and glucose degradation products in PD solution can contribute to peritoneal fibrosis by epithelial-mesenchymal transition or increased fibroblast proliferation leading eventually to peritoneal (UF) failure. Glucose degradation products are also thought to inhibit cell proliferation, retard wound healing, induce apoptosis, downregulate cytokines, and stimulate growth factors (TGF-beta, VEGF).
- Icodextrin-based solutions (e.g., extraneal) can be used to circumvent the rapid dissipation of the osmotic pressure of the dialysis solution needed to achieve the water removal (ultrafiltration) and effective solute clearance.
- Icodextrin is a starch-derived, branched, water-soluble glucose polymer with an average molecular weight between 13,000 and 19,000 that acts as a colloid-osmotic agent. It is slowly absorbed into the blood stream (40 % over 12 h) and metabolized to maltose and other oligosaccharides.
- Problems may arise when blood glucose measuring devices are used that do not differentiate glucose from maltose.
- Icodextrin solutions prolong UF to up to 16 h with improved solute and water clearance compared to glucose-based solutions. Use for long day (CCPD) or overnight dwells (CAPD).
- Use of icodextrin reduces unwarranted weight gain that can be seen with glucose-based solution.
- Some patients may develop eczematous skin reactions.

- Amino acid-based dialysate solutions (Table 10.4) can be used in patients with malnutrition (1 or 2 cycles per day).

10.1.4.8 Adequacy of Dialysis

- Adequate control of body fluid volume and management of hypertension are essential goals in PD.
- Preservation of residual renal function (RRF) as *renal* clearance is as important as *peritoneal* clearance.
- RRF provides a better clearance of middle and large molecules and helps maintenance of euvolemia.
- Creatinine clearance: It is calculated from a 24 h collection of dialysate and urine and normalized to 1.73 m^2 body surface area. A plasma sample is obtained for measurement of creatinine at the midpoint of the timed dialysate and urine collection. The target value is >60 l/week per 1.73 m^2.
- Determination of Kt/V tells us how much dialysis is delivered, but not whether it is adequate.
- Total KT/V should be at least 1.7. Lower values have been linked to poorer outcomes.
- Optimal PD dosing includes small solute and middle molecule clearance, and UF.
  - Small solute clearance is determined by frequency of cycles and volume of fluid per cycle.
  - Middle molecule clearance is determined by duration of contact of dialysate to peritoneum (dwell time).
  - UF is influenced by osmotic pressure (glucose concentration) and peritoneal membrane transport characteristics (see below).
- UF can be increased by higher-strength glucose and shorter dwell times. Some patients will do better with icodextrin than with glucose-containing solutions for longest cycle.
- Dialysis targets do not differ across age groups and body size, or for patients with diabetes.
- Residual renal function should be measured every 3 months.
- Urine volume and ultrafiltration volume should be closely monitored and reviewed by the Nephrology team at each clinic visit, usually once a month.

10.1.4.9 Peritoneal Equilibration Test (PET) Protocol

- The PET enables clinician to individualize the dialysis prescription according to the patient's specific requirements.
- The PET is performed 4-8 weeks post PD initiation and may be repeated yearly. It is also indicated following an episode of peritonitis or when clinical findings suggest altered membrane transport characteristics (e.g., poorly explained fluid overload, worsening hypertension, or rising serum creatinine and urea concentrations and/or uremic symptoms).

Test Procedure

- Under aseptic precautions, prepare two dialysis setups – one to drain the patient, the second to fill the peritoneum and obtain the test samples.

- To improve test reproducibility, the pediatric PET uses a standardized fill volume of 1,100 ml/m^2 of 2.5 % dextrose or 2.27 % anhydrous glucose-containing PD solution.
- On the evening before the test date, infuse 1,100 ml/m^2 of dialysis 2.5 % (2.27 %) solution for single, overnight dwell of 8–12 h.
- Connect and drain abdomen over 20 min. Record volume and send samples for cell count, culture, and protein.
- Prime and connect the second dialysis system and infuse 1,100 ml/m^2 of fresh 2.5 % dialysate over 10 min. Ask the patient to roll intermittently from side to side.
- "Zero dwell time" is the time the infusion is complete.
- Send dialysate samples at 0 and 2 h for glucose and creatinine.
- Draw a single blood sample at midpoint of the test period (+2 h) for sodium, glucose, creatinine, urea, and protein.
- After 4 h, drain the patient completely over 20 min, record the volume and send a third dialysate sample from the drained volume (4 h sample) and resume regular PD.
- Dialysate to plasma (D/P) ratio of creatinine and urea, and dialysate glucose concentrations at the measured points to time 0 (D/D_0) are calculated and plotted as shown in Fig. 10.2.
- Based on the statistical distribution of a representative group of pediatric PD patients (Warady et al. 1996), the peritoneal membrane is characterized as "low," "low average," "high average," or "high" transporter.
- The lines represent the maximal, mean +1 SD, mean, mean −1 SD, and minimal values.
- "High transporters" produce a low ultrafiltrate (due to the rapid transport of glucose from the dialysate) with adequate clearance. Increasing the number of cycles of PD with or without volume adjustments overcomes the problem.
- "Low transporters" demonstrate satisfactory ultrafiltration, but poor clearances. Increased dwell times with minor volume adjustments can rectify the deficit.
- No dietary restrictions are required for the test.
- An abbreviated version over 2 h ("Short PET") appears to vie identical results to the conventional 4-h PET (Warady et al. 2007).

Phosphate removal

- Dialytic phosphate clearance contributes to serum phosphate control. It depends on total dialysate turnover and the prescribed number of cycles, and is more adequately predicted by phosphate than by creatinine equilibration characteristics.
- Given its importance as cardiovascular risk factor in uremia, dialytic phosphate removal should be monitored routinely (Schmitt et al. 2009).
- Future modifications of the PET should include phosphate serum and dialysate measurements.

10.1.4.10 Chronic Exit Site Care

- The goal is to maintain a clean catheter exit site and minimize risk of tunnel infection and/or peritonitis during the dressing change.
- The dressing should be changed at least three times per week, and when the dressing is moist, soiled, or after taking a shower.

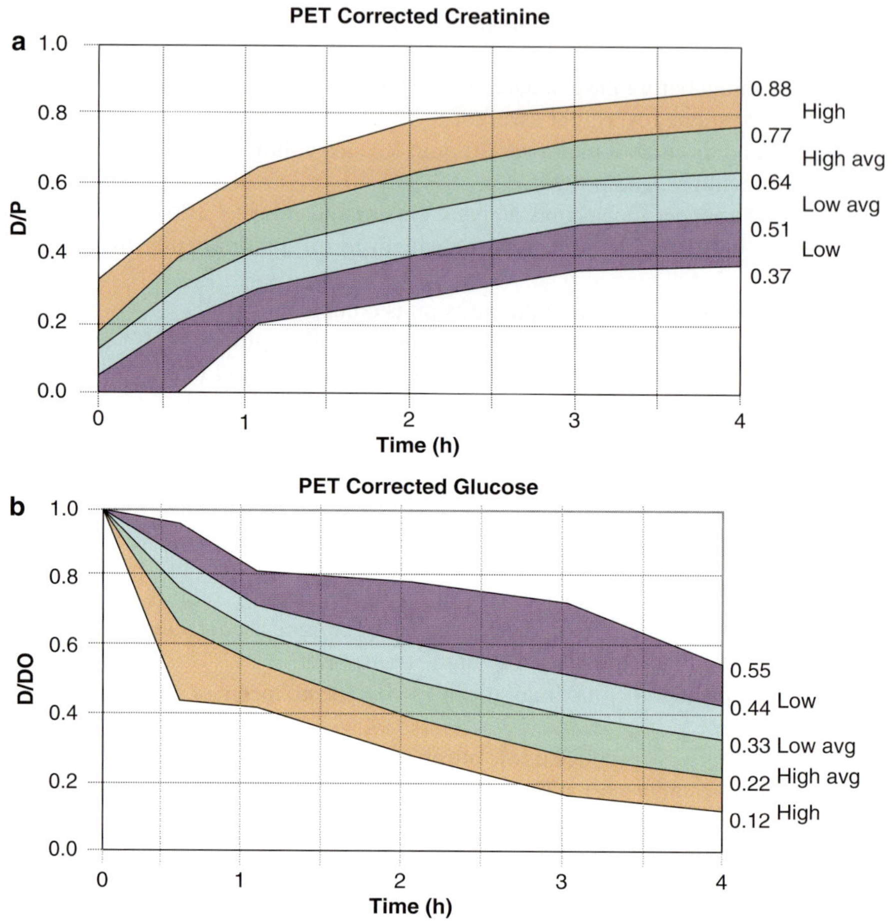

Fig. 10.2 Pediatric PET curves for creatinine (**a**) and glucose (**b**). The original study by Warady et al. 1996 comprised 95 pediatric patients; dialysate test samples were drawn at 0, 0.5,1, 2, 3, and 4 h dwell time, and blood samples at 0 and 4 h

- The exit site is cleaned with sterile antiseptic solution (chlorhexidine, sodium hypochlorite, or octenidine) and sterile gauze.
- A topical antibiotic is applied to the exit site (e.g., gentamicin, mupirocin).
- Excellent hand hygiene before examination of the exit site by patient, caregivers, and health care professionals. This includes handwashing and thorough drying.
- Prophylactic use of mupirocin intranasally or at the exit site reduces the incidence of exit site infection and peritonitis by *S. aureus*.
- A multicenter randomized trial is underway to determine whether daily honey (Medihoney antibacterial wound gel) in nasal staphylococcal carriers reduces the risk of catheter-associated infections in PD patients.

10.1.4.11 Practical Advice (Rules)

Shower and bath

- Shower is allowed with PD exit site exposed to air when the site is well healed (usually after 6 weeks), intact, and after being assessed by PD nurse.
- It is preferred that the PD exit site be covered during the shower.
- When the PD exit site is not intact (erythema, trauma), it should be covered with a medical dressing (e.g., Tegaderm) when showering or bathing.
- A bath is allowed, but PD exit site has to be covered with a gauze and a medical dressing at all times.
- Water must be shallow and not cover the PD exit site.

Activities and Sports

- Avoid contact sports, weight lifting, gymnastics, parachuting, and bungee jumping.
- Swimming is permitted in the ocean or a private swimming pool (after approval by treating nephrologist). PD catheter and exit site must be covered with waterproof dressing (e.g., colostomy bag, Tegaderm).
- Amusement rides are permitted only when exit site is healed.

10.1.5 Complications of PD

10.1.5.1 Mechanical Complications

- Pericatheter leaks (see Table 10.5)
- Positional blockage
- Catheter dislocation

10.1.5.2 Accidental Disconnection Protocol

- Close windows, doors, and ventilation.
- Wash working surface area with alcohol-based disinfectant and wash hands with chlorhexidine 4 % for 2 min, dry hands well.

Table 10.5 Protocol for management of peri-catheter leak

Signs and symptoms	Confirm diagnosis	Corrective measures
Overt fluid leakage at the skin exit site	Confirm leak with glucose dipstick	Discontinue dialysis for 7–10 days
Subcutaneous swelling, local or generalized edema and/or local pallor Weight gain Diminished outflow volume or outflow failure	Nuclear scan or CT scan for suspected peritoneal injury	If discontinuation is not possible due to the patient's condition, return to the break-in schedule (15–20 ml\kg) for 2–3 weeks Perform dialysis only in the supine position, to minimize intra-abdominal pressure If leakage persists, stop PD and switch to hemodialysis for 3–6 weeks If the leakage remains refractory, the PD catheter must be replaced Surgical repair needs to be considered in some situations

- Clamp the PD catheter with a gauze and yellow clamp.
- With aseptic precautions, clean the junction of catheter with chlorhexidine 2 % for 2 min and air dry.
- Repeat the step with alcohol 70 %.
- Replace the old PD transfer set with the new transfer set.
- Unclamp the yellow clamp and drain the patient to flush the bacterial contamination.
- Dialysate culture if contamination is suspected.
- Initiate antibiotic treatment with cefazolin 250 mg/l for 3 days. If cell count shows WBC <100/mm^3, treat for 3 days and stop treatment. If WBC >100/mm^3, continue treatment and change transfer set again when WBC <100/mm^3.

10.1.5.3 Infectious Complication: PD Associated Peritonitis (PDAP)

Diagnosis

- Peritonitis in PD patients is heralded by acute clouding of the dialysate effluent with abdominal pain, vomiting, abdominal distension, UF change, and (rarely) fever, chills and rigor, or (late) shock.
- Conversely, peritonitis should be considered whenever the peritoneal effluent is cloudy.
- Bacterial culture is often positive for coagulase-negative Staphylococci, *S. aureus*, Gram negative organisms (*Escherichia coli*, *Klebsiella* spp., *Pseudomonas aeruginosa*), and *Streptococcus viridans.*

Treatment

- Empiric diagnosis of peritonitis in the presence of effluent WBC count >100/mm^3 with at least 50 % polymorphonuclear leukocytes.
- (Cloudy) dialysate is sent for cell count, differential count, and culture to confirm the diagnosis of peritonitis.
- The differential diagnosis of cloudy effluent is shown in Box 10.3.

10.1.5.4 Empiric Antibiotic Therapy

- In most instances of PD-associated peritonitis, intraperitoneal (IP) treatment is the preferred form of antibiotic administration.

Box 10.3 Differential Diagnosis of Cloudy Effluent

- Infectious peritonitis
- Infectious peritonitis with sterile culture
- Chemical peritonitis
- Eosinophilic effluent
- Hemoperitoneum
- When effluent is taken from a "dry" abdomen
- Malignancy (rare)
- Chylous effluent (rare)

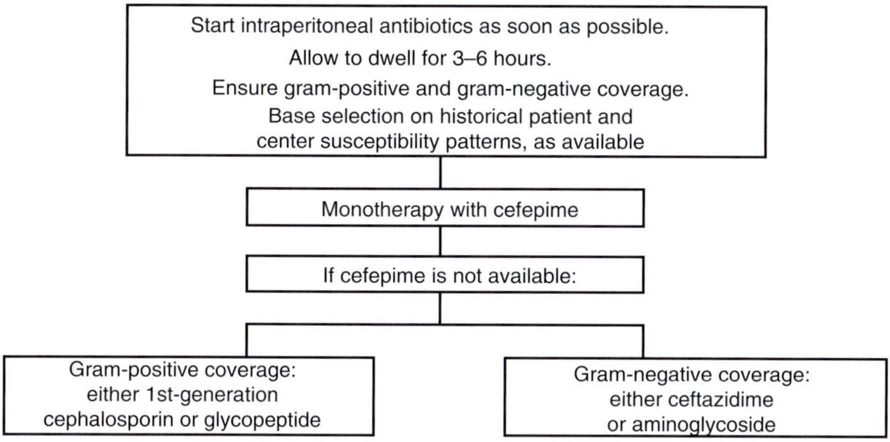

Fig. 10.3 Empiric intraperitoneal antibiotic therapy for PD associated peritonitis (From Warady BA et al. Perit Dial Int 2012; 32:S29–S86)

- Traditionally, treatment is initiated with a first-generation cephalosporin (cefazolin) combined with an aminoglycoside (gentamicin or tobramycin) or ceftazidime.
- Where available and affordable, the International Society for Peritoneal Dialysis (ISPD) Guidelines from 2012 now suggests a fourth-generation cephalosporin (cefepime) as IP monotherapy for empiric treatment.
- Where the center-specific resistance rate of *S. aureus* isolates to methicillin or oxacillin exceeds 10 %, or if the patient has a history of methicillin-resistant *S. aureus* (MRSA) infection or carriage, a combination of a glycopeptide (e.g., vancomycin) with cefepime is suggested (or with a less expensive antibiotic with activity against Gram negative rods, including *P. aeruginosa*) (Fig. 10.3).
- Continuation of antibiotic therapy is directed by the microbiological findings.
- When a Gram positive bacterium is isolated, stop the antibiotics targeting Gram negative organisms (and vice versa). Treatment duration is usually 2 weeks.
- Isolation of *Pseudomonas* spp. calls for treatment with cefepime (or another *Pseudomonas*-active antibiotic, such as piperacilin or ceftazidime) with an aminoglycoside or fluoroquinolone for 3 weeks (Warady et al. 2012).
- For IP antibiotic dosing refer to Table 10.6.

10.1.5.5 Relapsing Peritonitis

- Diagnose "relapsing peritonitis" if peritonitis recurs with the identical organism as in the preceding episode within 4 weeks of completion of antibiotic therapy, based on antibiotic susceptibility and molecular techniques, if available (for the terminology of PD-associated peritonitis see Table 10.7).
- Empiric therapy is reinitiated with relapsing peritonitis. Include susceptibilities of the original organism.
- Directed therapy should be based on in vitro susceptibility of the isolated organism; cefazolin should be avoided.

Table 10.6 Antibiotic dosing for IP therapy

Antibiotics	Dose	
	Loading	Maintenance
Cefazolin/cephalothin	250–500 mg/l	125 mg/l
Cefepime	500 mg/l	125 mg/l
Ceftazidime	250–500 mg/l	125 mg/l
Penicillin G	–	50,000 units/l
Ampicillin	–	125 mg/l
Cloxacillin	–	100–200 mg/l
Vancomycin	500 mg/l	25–30 mg/l
Teicoplanin	200 mg/l	20 mg/l
Tobramycin/gentamicin	8 mg/l	4 mg/l
Cefuroxime	250 mg/l	125 mg/l
Cefotaxime	500 mg/l	250 mg/l
Gentamicin	–	8–10 mg/l
Netilmicin	70 mg/l	4–6 mg/l
Amikacin	150–250 mg/l	6–8 mg/l
Amphotericin B	–	5 mg/l

Table 10.7 Terminology of peritonitis

Recurrent	Episode occurring within 4 weeks of completion of therapy of a preceding peritonitis, but caused by a different organism
Relapsing	Episode occurring within 4 weeks of completion of therapy of preceding peritonitis by the same organism (or a sterile peritonitis)
Repeat	Episode occurring more than 4 weeks after completion of therapy for preceding peritonitis, but caused by the same organism
Refractory	Failure of effluent to clear after 5 days of appropriate antibiotic therapy
Catheter-related	Episode occurring together with an exit site or tunnel infection caused by the same organism (lack of growth from one of the sites)

From: Warady BA et al. Perit Dial Int 2012;32:S29–S86

- Instillation of fibrinolytic agent is suggested.
- PD catheter removal is recommended once peritonitis is controlled.

10.1.5.6 PD Catheter-Related Infections

- Catheter *exit site infection* is diagnosed in the presence of pericatheter swelling, erythema, and tenderness.
- *Tunnel infection* is defined by the presence of erythema, edema, and tenderness along the subcutaneous portion of the catheter, with or without purulent drainage from the exit site (Warady BA et al. Perit Dial Int 2012;32:S29–86).
- A scoring system has been developed to describe changes to the exit site (Table 10.8).
- Oral antibiotic therapy is suggested for the treatment of uncomplicated catheter exit site infections (exit site score^{3}4, or at least 2 with a pathogenic isolate) for a minimum of 2–3 weeks (1 week after resolution of the infection) (see Table 10.9).
- Tunnel infection is treated by oral, IP, or IV route (IP or IV glycopeptides e.g., vancomycin in case of MRSA tunnel infection) (see Table 10.10).

Table 10.8 Exit site infection and exit site scoring system

	Score[a]		
Indication	0	1	2
Swelling	No	Exit only (<0.5 cm)	Including part of or the entire tunnel
Crust	No	<0.5 cm	>0.5 cm
Redness	No	<0.5 cm	>0.5 cm
Pain on pressure	No	Slight	Severe
Secretion	No	Serous	Purulent

[a]Infection should be assumed with a cumulative exit site score of 4 or greater regardless of culture results or in the presence of pericatheter swelling, redness, and tenderness (exit site score of 2 or greater in the presence of a pathogenic organism). From Schaefer F et al. *J Am Soc Nephrol* 1999

Table 10.9 Exit-site infection and corrective measures

Signs and symptoms	Confirm diagnosis	Corrective measures
Redness, tenderness, and/or discharge at the exit site	Patient should be examined by a PD nurse and/or a nephrologist Do a gram stain and culture of the catheter insertion site (if discharge). If exit site is dry, inject sterile saline into exit site and then culture	If the infection is very mild, begin local therapy – mupirocin ointment for 14 days If there is no significant improvement after 24–48 h, begin systemic oral or intraperitoneal antibiotic therapy If the infection is severe, proceed directly to systemic antibiotic therapy. Antimicrobial therapy should be continued for a minimum of 2 weeks resulting in a normal exit site for 1 week. If the infection does not resolve, catheter removal will be necessary

Table 10.10 Tunnel infection and corrective measures

Signs and symptoms	Confirm diagnosis	Corrective measures
Extension of a skin exit-site infection with pain, swelling, nodularity, and redness over the subcutaneous portion of the catheter	Patient should be examined by PD nurse and/or nephrologist	Antibiotics IV or PO are begun as soon as the diagnosis is made
Systemic signs such as fever or malaise "Relapsing" peritonitis due to the same organism	Do a gram stain and culture of the catheter insertion site (if discharge). If exit site dry, inject sterile saline into exit site and then culture	If there is no response after 2 weeks, the catheter must be removed Antimicrobial treatment is then continued for 2–3 weeks

10.1.5.7 Indications for PD Catheter Removal

- Refractory peritonitis
- Relapsing peritonitis
- Repeat (refractory) exit site or tunnel infection
- Fungal peritonitis

- Simultaneous PD catheter removal and replacement after cleaning of the peritoneal effluent (WBC < 100/mm³) in repeated, relapsing peritonitis
- Minimum period of 2–3 weeks between catheter removal and replacement for fungal, enteric, and refractory bacterial peritonitis

10.1.5.8 Non-infectious Complications

- Non-infectious complications of PD, their differential diagnoses, and corrective measures are summarized in Table 10.11.

Table 10.11 Noninfectious complications of PD

PD complication	Confirm diagnosis	Corrective measures
PD catheter exit site leak	Confirm leak with glucose dipstick	Discontinue dialysis for 7–10 days
	CT or nuclear scan with peritoneal infusion	Lower dialysate volume
Outflow failure	Abdominal X-ray (plain and lateral)	Improve bowel motility
		Heparinize dialysis fluid or instill streptokinase or tissue plasminogen activator (TPA) in PD catheter
		Reposition PD catheter under fluoroscopy
Dehydration	Excessive UF	Notify nephrologist. Reassess dry weight
	Twice daily weight	↑ BP: hold PD exchange/dwell, ↑ fluid/salt intake
	Decreased fluid intake	
	Nausea/vomiting (rule out peritonitis and pancreatitis)	↓ PD dextrose concentration
		Bed rest with legs elevated, restrict activity
Fluid overload	Inadequate UF	Notify nephrologist. Reassess dry weight
	Increased fluid intake	↓ fluid/salt intake
	Hypotonic PD solution	↑ PD dextrose concentration
	Excessive dwell time	Reassess fluid intake and output
Muscle cramps	Excessive UF	Notify nephrologist
	Too rapid UF (e.g., dextrose 3.86% solution)	Check serum electrolytes and calcium
	Electrolyte imbalance (↓Ca^{++}, ↓K^{+})	Relief measures: apply heat to area, rub cramp
Air in peritoneal cavity	Infusion of air with the dialysate	Shoulder pain usually resolves in a few days
	Misplacement of the catheter	Notify physician if pain persists
	Bowel perforation	Lie on back, pillow under hips, and drain the fluid
Blood in effluent	Menstruation/ovulation	Pink: clears up in two to three exchanges without specific treatment
	Rupture of tiny peritoneal capillaries	Bloody fluid: check BP and HR. Observe.
		Adjust heparin → prevent clotting of PD catheter
	Possible serious abdominal injury	Call nephrologist

Table 10.11 (continued)

PD complication	Confirm diagnosis	Corrective measures
Protein loss	Average protein losses in effluent: 9 g/day	Check serum albumin and total proteins
	Peritonitis can ↑ protein losses	Call nephrologist and dietician to modify protein intake
Accidental disconnection		Refer to *Accidental Disconnection Protocol*
Pain during dialysate inflow	"Jet" effect	Slower infusion rate
	Abnormally low tidal volume	Have incomplete drainage
	Omentum attachment to PD catheter	Reposition PD catheter
Ultrafiltration failure	Increasing edema, dyspnea, worsening of hypertension	Short dwell times, tidal PD, use of icodextrin
Metabolic complications	Hyponatremia, hypernatremia, hypokalemia, hyperglycemia, metabolic alkalosis, hypoalbuminemia	Take appropriate corrective measures
Intestinal perforation (rare)	Presence of fecal material in the dialysate effluent, new onset of watery diarrhea	Surgical intervention may be necessary
Respiratory distress	When large volumes are used, common in newborns	Reduce dialysate volume, rule out underlying pneumonia, pleural effusion, or atelectasis

10.1.5.9 Rare Complications

Eosinophilic Peritonitis

- Defined by the presence of >100 eosinophils/mm^3 of peritoneal dialysis fluid, eosinophils >10 % of the total WBC count of PD fluid.
- There may be a peripheral blood eosinophilia.
- May occur after catheter insertion or during the treatment phase of peritonitis.
- Peritoneal dialysis fluid cultures are negative, may occur in association with fungal and parasitic infections.
- It is benign and usually resolves spontaneously over 2–6 weeks; intraperitoneal hydrocortisone may be helpful.

Chronic Sclerosing Peritonitis

- Defined by the presence of thickened, fibrosed peritoneal membrane (Inflammation?)
- Presenting clinically with abdominal pain, fever, hemorrhagic PD effluent, deteriorating UF capability.
- Peritoneal calcification, thickened bowel loops may be seen on ultrasound; peritoneal biopsy confirms the clinical diagnosis.
- Associated with a history of prolonged peritoneal dialysis, use of high glucose content of PD solution, recurrent peritonitis.
- May lead to gut obstruction and malnutrition.

- Surgical intervention may be required. Immunosuppression has been tried with no or limited success.
- The patient may have to be transferred to hemodialysis.
- High mortality.

10.1.6 General Antibiotic Prophylaxis for PD Patients

- Procedure prophylaxis recommendations are summarized in Table 10.12.

Table 10.12 Antimicrobial prophylaxis for PD patients

Situation	Indication	Antimicrobial
Presence of risk factors for fungal peritonitis	High baseline rate of fungal peritonitis in the PD unitPEG/GT placement	Nystatin PO 10 000 U/kg daily Fluconazole 3–6 mg/kg IV or PO q 24–48 h (max 200 mg)
Touch contamination	Instillation of PD fluid after disconnection during PD	Cefepime 250 mg/l IP for 3 days Cefazolin 125 or 250 mg/l IP, or Vancomycin 25 mg/l IP (if known colonization with MRSA) ⇒ Positive culture result directs subsequent therapy
Invasive dental procedures		Amoxicillin 50 mg/kg PO (max 2 g) *If allergic to penicillin:* Clindamycin 20 mg/kg PO (max 600 mg) *Alternatives:* Ampicillin 50 mg/kg IV or IM (max 2 g) Cefazolin 25 mg/kg IV (max 1 g) Ceftriaxone 50 mg/kg IV or IM (max 1 g) Clarithromycin or azithromycin 15 mg/kg PO (max 500 mg)
Gastrointestinal procedures	High-risk procedures (esophageal stricture dilation, treatment of varices, ERCP, PEG/GT)	Cefazolin 25 mg/kg IV (max 2 g) *Alternatives:* Clindamycin 10 mg/kg IV (maxi 600 mg) Vancomycin 10 mg/kg IV (max 1 g), if high risk for MRSA infection
	Other gastrointestinal or genitourinary procedure	Cefoxitin/cefotetan 30–40 mg/kg IV (max 2 g) *Alternatives:* Cefazolin 25/kg IV (max 2 g) *plus* metronidazole 10 mg/kg IV (max 1 g), or Clindamycin 10 mg/kg IV (max 600 mg) *plus* aztreonam 30 mg/kg IV (max 2 g)

Based on the "Consensus Guidelines for the Prevention and Treatment of Catheter-Related Infection 2012" (Warady et al. 2012)

Abbreviations: *ERCP* endoscopic retrograde cholangiopancreatography, *GT* gastrostomy tube, *IV* intravenously, *IP* intraperitoneally, *MRSA* methicillin-resistant *Staphylococcus aureus*, *PEG* percutaneous endoscopic gastrostomy, *PO* orally

10.2 Hemodialysis

- Hemodialysis (HD) is an extracorporeal, intermittent form of renal replacement therapy (RRT).
- Technical advances have substantially improved the safety of the procedure. HD is now technical possible in a child of any age, even in infants.
- Acute dialysis serves to prevent death or severe morbidity due to acute kidney injury (AKI) or intoxication with water-soluble (and dialyzable) substances.
- HD is a lifesaving therapy for children with AKI and end-stage renal disease (ESRD). However, any chronic dialysis is inferior to kidney transplantation with respect to normal development and growth, and survival.
- Some aspects of hemodialysis in the setting of AKI are discussed in Chap. 8. The current section describes aspects of chronic HD.

10.2.1 Principles of HD

The goal of HD is to remove accumulated solutes (clearance) and water (ultrafiltration). This is accomplished using a dialysis filter with a semipermeable membrane.

10.2.1.1 Solute Clearance

This occurs by diffusion and convection. Major factors affecting solute clearance are dialyzer size (surface area), blood flow rate, dialysis flow rate (normally 500–800 ml/min; 200 ml/min in SLED – slow low-efficiency dialysis, see Chap. 8) and dialyzer membrane characteristics. Most dialyzers clear solutes up to a molecular weight 5,000–10,000 KD.

1. Diffusion refers to migration of solutes across the semipermeable membrane down a concentration gradient. Small solutes such as urea nitrogen and potassium diffuse rapidly.
2. Convection refers to the passive movement of solutes across the semipermeable membrane along with solvent (solvent drag) in response to a transmembrane pressure. Middle size and larger molecules do not diffuse to a great extent, but may pass through the dialyzer membrane by convection.

Too rapid removal of solutes during dialysis will result in a rapid decrease in serum osmolality and an imbalance between serum and brain cell osmolality causing movement of water into (higher osmolar) brain tissue and cerebral edema. This phenomenon is known as "disequilibrium syndrome" (DES) presents with headache, nausea, and vomiting in mild cases and altered sensorium and seizures in severe cases. High predialysis blood urea concentration increases the disequilibrium risk. To prevent DES, urea clearance should be limited during the first few dialysis sessions, aiming at a blood urea reduction of not more than 30 %.

10.2.1.2 Ultrafiltration

The goal is to finish the dialysis session with the patient at the target weight, often referred to as "dry weight". It is defined as the weight beyond which no further fluid removal is tolerated. Excess fluid removal will result in hypotension, cramps, abdominal pain, headache, nausea, and vomiting. Insufficient fluid removal will result in persistent fluid overload, contributing to hypertension and congestive cardiac failure. Since the fluid is removed from intravascular space and the redistribution of fluid from extravascular to intravascular space is not immediate, aggressive fluid removal rates can lead to hypovolemic symptoms even if correct dry weight is targeted. The child's dry weight adjusted periodically, to balance true body mass increase (and growth) against weight loss due to poor nutrition or chronic inflammation.

Measures to achieve fluid removal without causing symptomatic hypotension are "sodium modeling", where the sodium concentration of the dialysate is set higher during early dialysis, and gradually reduced during the course of the dialysis session, and "noninvasive volume monitoring" (acute change in hematocrit depicts acute change in blood volume).

10.2.2 Differences between "Pediatric Dialysis" and HD in Adults

1. Vascular access problems are common in small children.
2. Low blood flow increase the risk of clotting events.
3. Extracorporeal circuit volume needs be scaled to body size and blood volume using special neonatal or pediatric blood lines. The circuit (tubings and dialyzer) has to be primed with blood or albumin, when it exceeds 8–10 % of the child's total blood volume to prevent hypotension.
4. Cardiac dysfunction is less common in children, compared to adults.
5. Dialysis treatment (frequency and duration), fluid allowance and nutrition have to be optimized to facilitate near normal growth and development.
6. Seizures/CNS manifestations are more commonly encountered in uremic children, in comparison to adults.
7. Support and attention for children and their families needs be individualized. Trained social workers, dieticians, play therapists, school teachers become a part of the dialysis team.

10.2.3 Vascular Access

- Stable, large-bore vascular access is essential for effective dialysis and can pose a challenge, particularly in small children.
- Uncuffed (percutaneous) double lumen catheters are reserved for temporary HD over no more than 1–2 weeks. Different sizes are available for different age groups – newborns (two separate 5 F single lumen or 6.5 F), 3–15 kg (7 F, 12–15 cm), 16–30 kg (9 F, 20 cm), >30 kg (11.5 F, 24 cm).
- Cuffed, tunneled permanent ("perm") catheters are used for long-term use.

- Site of catheter insertion – femoral (restricts mobility and increases infection risk), subclavian (risk of stenosis), internal jugular (preferred). In newborns, umbilical artery (5 F) and vein (8 F) can be considered.
- Arteriovenous shunts (brought out externally) are not recommended. They have a high risk of infection and discconnection with dangerous blood loss; vessels cannot be used later for a permanent vascular access.
- Arteriovenous fistula: the best option for long-term HD, but may be challenging to create in small children; takes 2–3 months to mature.
- Synthetic grafts are usually made from teflon or polytetrafluoroethylene.

10.2.4 Dialysis Prescription

- Dialyzer surface area/body surface area ratio = 0.8–1.0
- Examples of dialyzers and their specifications are listed in Table 10.13 and the following paragraph

Other dialyzers: Cobe – 100HG (prime volume 18 ml, surface area 0.22 m^2, for <10 kg), F_6 (surface area 1.3 m^2, prime volume 82 ml, for 30–40 kg), F_8 (surface area 1.8 m^2, prime volume 110 ml, for >40 kg), Polyflux 140 (surface area 1.4 m^2, prime volume 94 ml, for >30 kg)

- Adult blood lines, pediatric lines, and infant/neonatal lines are available. Choice can be made depending on the size of the child. The prime volumes are 140, 75, 20 ml, respectively.
- Blood flow rate 5–8 ml/kg/min.
- Dialysate flow rates should be at least 1.5–2 times the blood flow rates. Higher dialysate flow rates achieve little additional clearance benefits.
- Dialysate sodium should be equal to or more than serum sodium. Dialysate K concentration is adjusted according to predialysis serum K levels. Standard dialysate Ca concentration is 2.5 mEq/l (1.25 mmol/l); it can be adjusted if there is hypo- or hypercalcemia.
- Fluid removal is adjusted to target body weight; fluid removal should be less than 5 % body weight or not more than 0.2 ml/kg/min.

Table 10.13 Examples of pediatric dialyzers and their characteristics

	F_3	F_4	F_5
Surface area – met^2	0.4	0.7	1.0
UFR ml/h/mm TMP	1.7	2.8	4.0
Urea clearance (25 ml/min)	25	25	25
Urea clearance (200 ml/min)	145	185	205
Prime volume in ml	28	42	72
Weight of child	<12 kg	12–20 kg	20–30 kg

- Dialysis duration: first dialysis should not reduce blood urea by more than 30 %; may give mannitol 0.5–1.0 g/kg/dose during dialysis to prevent disequilibrium syndrome. If the predialysis blood urea levels are high, HD session should not last more than 1–2 h.
- The standard duration of HD sessions is 4 h, three times a week. Hypercatabolic and very young children may require more frequent dialysis.
- Dialyzer material may be cellulose based (can cause complement activation, activation of coagulation cascade) or synthetic (more biocompatible) – Polysulphone, polyamix, polycarbonate, polyamide, or polyacryl-polyamide acrylate.
- Conventional HD uses a low-flux (small pore size) membrane. High-flux dialyzers are more efficient in removing solutes that are larger than urea but may not be more efficient than conventional hemodialysis in removing small solutes. These membranes are more biocompatible and cause less complement activation when blood comes in contact with the dialyzer membrane.
- Blood prime with WBC reduced packed RBCs diluted to a hematocrit of 35 % or 5 % albumin if circuit volume is >10 % of the patient's estimated volume. Isotonic saline or no prime in stable patients if circuit volume is <10 % of blood volume.
- Anticoagulation: Standard is the use (conventional, unfractionated) heparin. Loading dose of heparin 10–30 units/kg followed by 10 units/kg/h, adjusted to keep activated clotting time around 150 % of baseline. Heparin is stopped 30 min before closure of HD. Heparin-induced thrombocytopenia (HIT) is a rare complication.
- Under special circumstances (bleeding disorder, thrombocytopenia, post-operatively), dialysis can be performed with "tight" or no heparinization. Clotting-free dialysis time may be limited; flush dialyzer with 100–200 ml of isotonic saline every 15–30 min, increase ultrafiltration rate to remove this additional fluid, and carefully monitor venous pressure, drip chamber and dialyzer for signs of clotting.

10.2.5 Complications of HD

- Intradialytic hypotension is a common complication in HD. Causes are overzealous or (too) rapid fluid removal (UF), pre-dialysis antihypertensive medication, or bradykinin release. Treat with cessation of ultrafiltration, reduce blood flow, head low position, bolus of saline 5–10 ml/kg. Discontinue dialysis if hypotension is severe. Dry weight of the patient should be reassessed; avoid antihypertensives before dialysis session. Another possible cause is the use of hypotonic (low sodium) dialysate relative to the plasma. Sodium remodeling, online blood volume monitoring, sequential ultrafiltration, and use of intradialytic dobutamine (in patients with poor cardiac reserve) may be beneficial.
- Nausea, vomiting, cramps – treat the cause.

- Disequilibrium – secondary to cerebral edema, gradual reduction of blood urea is recommended. Mannitol may be used as a prophylaxis.
- Air embolism due to technical problem, e.g., at the negative pressure part of the circuit. Air detectors should clamp the return lines. Treatment is to clamp the lines, stop the pump and put the patient head down in left lateral position, give 100 % oxygen, aspirate air from right ventricle if required, and other resuscitative measures.
- Hemolysis – presents with nausea, pains, and dark venous blood. It may be due to contamination, overheating, hypotonicity of dialysate, defective pump, or kinked blood lines. Dialysis should be stopped. Hyperkalemia should be looked for.
- Blood leak – This is due to entry of blood into the dialysate circuit.
- Dialyzer reactions/bioincompatibility – anaphylaxis or first use syndrome, back pain, chest pain, pruritus.
- Fever – pyrogens, presence of contaminants, infection.
- Bleeding – check anticoagulation.
- Related to the access – thrombosis, stenosis, recirculation, infection.

10.2.6 Dialysis Adequacy

- Urea reduction rate (URR) = (1 – urea post HD/urea pre HD) × 100. Adequate dialysis should yield a URR >65 %.
- Formal urea kinetic modeling, single pool – Kt/*V* (Target Kt/*V* >1.2).
- The most commonly used formula:

$$\mathrm{Kt}/V = -\mathrm{In}\,(R - 0.008 \times t) + (4 - 3.5 \times R) \times \left(\mathrm{UF}/W\right)$$

where R = urea post HD/urea pre HD, t = time of dialysis in minutes, UF = ultrafiltration in liters, and W = post dialysis weight in kg.

- "Single pool" refers to assuming that total body water is all in one compartment and that the immediate postdialysis blood urea concentration is representative of total body urea concentration. However, "urea rebound" occurs at a logarithmic rate in the first hour after a dialysis session reflecting diffusion of urea from the intracellular to extracellular space or a "double pool" compartment. Measuring urea 1 h postdialysis would hence truly reflect the delivered Kt/*V*, referred to as "equilibrated Kt/*V*."
- Calculation of *n*PCR (normalized protein catabolic rate) – This is representative of urea generation between dialysis sessions and protein catabolism and is a valuable indicator of recent protein intake. It is equal to $5.43 \times G/\mathrm{Vd} + 0.17$, where G = urea generation rate mg/minute and Vd = post HD total body water = 0.58 × post HD weight in kg. Target it to >1 g/kg/day. The value <1 g/kg/day is predictive of weight and BMI decrease.
- Other indicators – adequacy of ultrafiltration, good control of blood pressure, anemia, acidosis, bone disease, and patient well-being.

10.2.7 Causes of Inadequate Dialysis

- Improper dialysis prescription
- Inadequate blood flow
- Reduction in treatment time
- Dialyzer clotting, leaks
- Recirculation, calculated as (systemic urea-arterial urea) divided by (systemic urea-venous urea); if lines are reversed during dialysis, 15–20 % increase in recirculation is expected to occur.

Suggested Reading

Duagirdas JT, Blake PG, Inq TS (eds) (2006) Handbook of dialysis, 4th edn. Lippincott Williams & Wilkins, Philadelphia

Fischbach M, Issad B, Dubois V, Taamma R (2011) The beneficial influence on the effectiveness of automated peritoneal dialysis of varying the dwell time (short/long) and fill volume (small/large): a randomized controlled trial. Perit Dial Int 31:450–458

Fischbach M, Zaloszyc A, Schaefer B, Schmitt CP (2013) Optimizing peritoneal dialysis prescription for volume control: the importance of varying dwell time and dwell volume. Pediatr Nephrol (in press)

García-López E, Lindholm B, Davies S (2012) An update on peritoneal dialysis solutions. Nat Rev Nephrol 8:224–233

Guest S (ed) (2011) Handbook of peritoneal dialysis, 1st edn. CreateSpace Independent Publishing Platform, Lexington

Schmitt CP, Borzych D, Nau B, Wühl E, Zurowska A, Schaefer F (2009) Dialytic phosphate removal: a modifiable measure of dialysis efficacy in automated peritoneal dialysis. Perit Dial Int 29:465–471

Schmitt CP, Zaloszyc A, Schaefer B, Fischbach M (2011) Peritoneal dialysis tailored to pediatric needs. Int J Nephrol 2011:940267

Warady BA, Alexander SR, Hossli S, Vonesh E, Geary D, Watkins S, Salusky IB, Kohaut EC (1996) Peritoneal membrane transport function in children receiving long-term dialysis. J Am Soc Nephrol 7:2385–2391

Warady BA, Bakkaloglu S, Newland J, Cantwell M, Verrina E, Neu A, Chadha V, Yap HK, Schaefer F (2012a) Consensus guidelines for the prevention and treatment of catheter-related infections and peritonitis in pediatric patients receiving peritoneal dialysis: 2012 update. Perit Dial Int 32(Suppl 2):S32–S86

Warady BA, Schaefer FS, Alexander SR (eds) (2012b) Pediatric dialysis, 2nd edn. Springer, New York

Renal Transplantation

11

Kishore Phadke, Paul Goodyer, and Arpana A. Iyengar

11.1 Introduction

- All children with end-stage renal disease (ESRD), barring any contraindications, should be considered for renal transplantation. It offers (in comparison with the dialysis option) better renal functions, a decrease in morbidity and mortality, improved quality of life, and improved growth, nutrition, and school performance. Children are excellent candidates for renal transplantation since, unlike in adults, comorbidities such as diabetes and advanced cardiac disease are often absent.
- Performing renal transplantation is a team effort. Transplant centers need to develop a network of specialists, e.g., a psychologist, psychiatrist, urologist, gastroenterologist, cardiologist, infectious diseases, and other specialists who become familiar with the transplant evaluation process.
- The donor source could be a living related (LRD; parents, grandparents, siblings above 18 years of age, first degree relatives) or an unrelated (altruistic) individual

The authors acknowledge the contribution of Dr. Lorraine E. Bell to this chapter.

K. Phadke (✉)
Department of Pediatric Nephrology, Children's Kidney Care Center,
St. John's Medical College Hospital, Koramangala, Bangalore, Karnataka 560034, India
e-mail: kishorephadke@yahoo.co.in

P. Goodyer
Division of Pediatric Nephrology, Montreal Children's Hospital,
McGill University, Montreal, QC H3H 1P3, Canada
e-mail: paul.goodyer@mcgill.ca

A.A. Iyengar
Department of Pediatric Nephrology, St John's Medical College Hospital,
Bangalore, Karnataka 560034, India
e-mail: arpanaiyengar@gmail.com

K. Phadke et al. (eds.), *Manual of Pediatric Nephrology*,
DOI 10.1007/978-3-642-12483-9_11, © Springer-Verlag Berlin Heidelberg 2014

(LURDD) or a deceased donor (DD). Living donor allografts have a longer half-life compared to those obtained from deceased donors. This is because of relatively healthy organs and minimization of cold ischemia time in the case of living donors. Increase in cold ischemia time increases the likelihood of acute tubular necrosis (ATN). It also increases the risk of acute rejection due to enhanced expression of HLA antigens and adhesion molecules on the surface of endothelial cells and renal tubular cells.

11.2 Contraindications to Transplantation

Absolute contraindications include active infection, recent malignancy, and progressive neurological diseases of the recipient candidate. Children with recent malignancy should wait for 2 years after achieving remission before undergoing transplantation. Children with advanced mental and functional impairment pose an ethical dilemma. Some children with advanced liver disease may need a combined liver and kidney transplant. Patients with primary hyperoxaluria also benefit from a combined liver and kidney transplant once they have reached ESRD. Most centers transplant children once they weigh at least 10 kg. Few centers perform transplants in children weighing 5–10 kg. Transplantation of patients with vasculitis (e.g., ANCA-associated vasculitis or circulating anti-GBM antibodies) is usually delayed to a year after active disease is controlled.

Desired requirements for a transplant are a compatible blood group and a negative cross match. HLA identical grafts have a longer half-life compared to those that are less matched. Children with HIV infection have been successfully transplanted using strict selection criteria with comparable outcomes. Children with chronic hepatitis B and C infection should undergo liver biopsy and treatment with antiviral drugs prior to transplantation. It is debated, if nonadherence to medical therapy predicts post-transplant nonadherence and graft loss and constitutes a (relative) contraindication for transplantation.

11.3 Pre-transplant Evaluation

11.3.1 Donor

11.3.1.1 Exclusion Criteria for Living Donors

Absolute contraindications:

- Age <18 years
- Hypertension (blood pressure >140/90 mmHg, more than one drug required for control of blood pressure)
- Diabetes (abnormal glucose tolerance test or HbA_1c)
- Proteinuria >300 mg/day
- Abnormal glomerular filtration rate (creatinine clearance <75 ml/min/1.73 m^2)

- History of thrombosis or thromboembolism
- Medically significant illness such as chronic lung disease, recent malignancy, or heart disease
- History of bilateral kidney stones

Relative contraindications:

- Abnormalities of donor kidney (urological, vascular)
- Obesity (>30 % or more above ideal weight)
- Psychiatric disorders

11.3.1.2 Donor Investigations

Mandatory tests:

- Blood group, complete blood counts, prothrombin time, partial thromboplastin time
- Renal function tests, liver enzymes and function tests, fasting blood sugar, lipid profile, thyroid function tests, serum calcium, phosphorous, and uric acid
- Routine urine analysis and urine culture
- Timed urine collection to measure creatinine clearance
- 24 h urine collection to measure urine protein
- Antibicrobial antibodies: HIV, hepatitis B and C, CMV, EBV and T. pallidum (VDRL)
- Renal imaging with pelvic ultrasound in females
- Chest X-ray and electrocardiogram
- Pap smear in females
- Conventional renal angiogram or CT/MRI angiogram

Additional tests:

- Echocardiography
- Cardiac stress test/angiography
- Oral glucose tolerance test
- Mammogram in females
- Cystoscopy
- Renal biopsy

11.3.1.3 Blood Group, Tissue Typing, and Cross Match

- Attempts have been made to overcome blood group barriers by removing blood isoagglutinins by pheresis or immunoadsorption often in conjunction with splenectomy.
- Genes involved in the immune response are clustered in the major histocompatibility complex (MHC) on chromosome 6 which includes human leukocyte antigen (HLA) encoding genes.
- There are two classes of HLA antigens – Class I (HLA A, B, C) and Class II (DP, DQ, and DR). Class I antigens are expressed on nearly all nucleated cells. Class II are expressed only on antigen-presenting cells (APCs) and activated endothelial cells.
- Tissue typing is performed by serologic methods, microlymphocytotoxicity assay (MLC), or by DNA-based methods (PCR).

- Cross match is the process of identifying preformed antibodies in the recipient's serum against donor tissue (lymphocytes).
- Panel reactive antibody (PRA) is a screening test to identify the presence of antibodies to HLA antigens by adding the patient's serum to a panel of cells from multiple donors (ideally drawn from the region where the recipient resides). The percentage of panel cells that are lysed by the serum is then calculated. A 50 % score means that half of the (regional) donor pool or population is expected to give a positive cross match. A score of more than 20 % indicates that the recipient is sensitized. The higher the degree of sensitization (PRA), the more difficult it is to find a compatible donor within the population and the higher the risk of antibody mediated rejection.
- In order to detect specific antibodies, complement dependent cytotoxic assays (CDC), flow cytometry, and microarrays are used.
- The recipient serum should be a fresh sample or not later than 1 month old. A gap of 2 weeks after a blood transfusion or an infection episode should be allowed before performing a tissue cross match. Since heparin may interfere with tissue typing and cross match, heparin-free dialysis should be done for 48–72 h prior to tissue typing and cross match. Pre-transplant cross match is performed within a week prior to living donor transplant.

11.3.2 Recipient

11.3.2.1 Investigations

- Blood group, complete blood counts, prothrombin time, and partial thromboplastin time
- Renal function tests, liver enzymes and function, fasting blood sugar, lipid profile, thyroid function tests, serum calcium, phosphorous, and uric acid
- Urine analysis and culture
- Timed urine collection to measure creatinine clearance and urine protein
- Antimircobial antibodies: HIV, hepatitis B and C, CMV, EBV and T. pallidum (e.g., VDRL)
- Renal imaging with residual urine volume estimation
- Chest X-ray, X-ray for bone age, electrocardiogram, and echocardiography
- Serum complement C3 and C4 and anti-DsDNA if required
- Clotting tests and APLA, anti-cardiolipin antibodies in children with SLE thrombotic disorders or other hypercoagulable states

11.3.2.2 Determining the Cause of ESRD

- In children with congenital and structural urological problems, a thorough evaluation of the lower urinary tract and advance planning is crucial to ensure adequate compliance, storage, and emptying of the bladder. The bladder and urethra should be evaluated by post-void ultrasonography, voiding cystourethrogram, and urodynamic studies, if indicated. Prerequisites for a "ready urinary tract" are residual urine <30 ml, urine flow rate >15 ml/s, normal voiding pattern, distensible bladder of good capacity and compliance, and end filling pressure <30 cm of water.

- There is a potential for recurrence of some pathologic lesions such as focal segmental glomerulosclerosis (FSGS), atypical uremic syndrome (HUS), and membranoproliferative glomerulonephritis (MPGN). Strategies to monitor for disease recurrence and treatment should be in place in advance of the transplantation.

11.3.2.3 Immunization Status

Children should receive all age-appropriate immunizations including hepatitis A and B, varicella, pneumococcal, meningococcal, influenza, and human papillomavirus. Children with a positive Mantoux test should be treated with isoniazid to prevent reactivation of tuberculosis after transplantation.

11.4 Preoperative Management

- Preoperative investigations:
- Complete blood count; PT; aPTT; renal function tests; liver function enzymes and tests; calcium and phosphate; urine routine, microscopy, and culture; chest X-ray; EKG; blood culture; nasal and throat swab; and group and cross match for packed red blood cells (leukocyte-free).
- Transfusions: Transfuse with leukocyte-free packed RBC if Hb <6 g/dl (60 g/l).
- Dialysis orders: The child should be adequately dialyzed. Serum potassium should be <5.5 mmol/l. Keep the patient slightly above his dry weight to favor posttransplant diuresis; saline dialysis (without heparin) should be performed no more than 48 h prior to transplant.
- Indications for pre-transplant nephrectomy:
- Some children will need bilateral nephrectomy either in advance or at the time of transplant. Indications for nephrectomy include (active) nephrotic syndrome with large proteinuria, large polycystic kidneys, intractable hypertension, chronic infections of the kidneys, and nephrolithiasis or excessive polyuria.

11.5 Intra- and Postoperative Management

11.5.1 Surgery

- Infants and children <15 kg may receive an intraperitoneal graft with the renal artery and vein anastomosed to aorta and inferior vena cava, respectively.
- Using the conventional extra peritoneal approach, the vessels are anastomosed to external iliac or common iliac vessels. Right side is preferred as it is easier to expose common iliac vessels.
- The graft ureter is inserted into the bladder using anti-reflux technique.
- Prolonged cold and warm ischemia times are associated with increased risk of early graft dysfunction.

- The circulating blood volume should be expanded immediately prior to unclamping, particularly in small recipients, to accommodate the perfusion demands of the relatively large-sized adult kidney.
- Perioperative antibiotic prophylaxis (e.g. first or third generation cephalosporine).

11.5.2 Fluids and Electrolytes

- *Intraoperative period*: The amount of fluid to be given is guided by the central venous pressure (CVP). Maintain CVP 12–15 cm of water.
- *Postoperative period*: The general guidelines for fluid management are: replacement of insensible losses as 5 % dextrose (D5 %) (400 ml/m^2/day or 35 ml/100 cal), hourly urine replacement as 0.45 % (half-isotonic) saline with 10 mmol/l KCl (and initially 20 mmol/l $NaHCO_3$), nasogastric tube aspirate replacement as D5 % / 0.45 % saline. Maintain CVP between 8 and 10 cm of H_2O. After 48 h, change to fixed rate (orally + intravenous), e.g., 1.5 times the usual maintenance rates. Isotonic saline boluses may be given if urine output <2 ml/kg/h or CVP <3 cm of water.

11.5.3 Monitoring

- Hourly pulse rate, blood pressure, temperature, and oxygen saturation
- Hourly input and output
- Daily body weight
- Laboratory investigations: Serum urea, creatinine, electrolytes, calcium, phosphate, magnesium and capillary or arterial blood gas (if required) every 4–6 h till renal function stabilizes and daily thereafter, complete blood count every 12 h till patient stabilizes and daily thereafter, serum magnesium daily, liver enzymes and function tests every week, cyclosporine or tacrolimus blood levels initially daily, then as required
- Urine analysis, microscopy, and culture at 72 h, at the time of removal of urinary catheter and when clinically indicated
- Baseline renal Doppler ultrasound immediately post surgery and on the third or fourth day
- Dynamic renal scan (99mTC MAG3 or DPTA) within 24 h and then as needed (see below)

11.6 Induction and Maintenance Immunosuppression Protocol

11.6.1 Induction Regime

Induction therapies include use of either polyclonal (equine ATGAM or rabbit Thymoglobulin [rATG]) or monoclonal (anti IL-2R such as daclizumab or basiliximab) antibodies with high dose of IV methylprednisolone. For low-risk transplants (first transplant, unsensitized recipients), most centers use one of the monoclonal antibodies or no induction therapy (there are cost considerations in developing countries). For high-risk transplants (patients with high PRA, re-transplants, and in whom delayed graft function is anticipated), Thymoglobulin is the most commonly used agent.

Many centers employ glucocorticoid sparing or steroid withdrawal protocols. With newer anti-CD52 antibody (alemtuzumab, also known as Campath-1H) and belatacept (CTLA4-Ig), steroid-free protocols with low rejection rates or even calcineurin inhibitor-free protocols may develop.

11.6.1.1 Day 0

Daclizumab (*Zenapax*) – 1 mg/kg/dose (max 50 mg); the calculated volume should be mixed with 50 ml of sterile 0.9 % sodium chloride solution and given via central/peripheral vein over a 15-min period before surgery.

OR

Basiliximab (*Simulect*) – 10 mg for recipients <40 kg and 20 mg for those >40 kg, infused over 20–30 min via central/peripheral vein within 2 h prior to surgery.

OR

Anti-thymocyte globulin (*Thymoglobulin/Atgam*) via central line – rabbit Thymoglobulin (1.5 mg/kg for 4–10 days) or equine Atgam (15 mg/kg for 10–14 days); test dose – intradermal Thymoglobulin (1 μg) or Atgam (5 μg) in 0.1 ml of 1:1,000 dilution and contralateral 0.1 ml sodium chloride injection control. Positive reaction: wheal and/or erythema >10 mm. Observe every 15–20 mm for 1 h; pre-treat all doses with 1 mg/kg (max 50 mg) of diphenhydramine and paracetamol 10 mg/kg/dose; continue MMF/azathioprine at half the dose till ATG is stopped; also halve the dose if platelets $<100 \times 10^9$/l (<100,00/microliter) (ANC $<2 \times 10^9$/l or <2,000/microliter), and hold the dose if platelets $<50 \times 10^9$/l (ANC $<1 \times 10^9$/l);

AND

Intravenous methylprednisolone – 10 mg/kg (max 500 mg) at induction of anesthesia.

11.6.2 Postoperative Immunosuppression

11.6.2.1 Days 0–7

- Cyclosporine: Calcineurin inhibitor, oral, 12–15 mg/kg/day divided in two doses; in children <6 years, 500 mg/m^2/day in two or three divided doses; intravenous (IV) if orally not possible. IV dose is about 1/3 of total oral dose, ~3.5 mg/kg as continuous infusion or in two/three divided doses; in children <6 years, the IV dose is 150–165 mg/m^2. Intravenous cyclosporine should be given for 48–72 h and then switched to oral therapy. The drug is diluted 1:20 to 1:100 with 5 % glucose or normal saline, maintain 12-h trough level between 150 and 250 ng/ml, and withhold if serum creatinine is persistently above 3.0 mg/dl (>27 micromol/l). Monitoring of CSA drug levels is critical due to substantial interindividual variation in absorption and multiple drug and food interactions. Target levels must be adjusted according to assay methods and patient age. Peak levels (C2) may correlate better with drug exposure and toxicity than 12-hour trough levels.

- Tacrolimus: Calcineurin inhibitor, oral, 0.2–0.3 mg/kg/day in two divided doses and intravenous, 0.05–0.10 mg/kg/day as continuous infusion; maintain a 12-h trough level between 10–15 ng/ml; reduce or withhold if serum creatinine persistently above 3.0 mg/l (27 umol/l), i.e., DGF.
- *Prednisolone*/methylprednisolone (MPS): Day 1, 10 mg/kg IV MPS, and day 2–7, 2 mg/kg IV MPS or prednisolone 2 mg/kg; prednisolone 1.5 mg/kg if MMF is used.
- Azathioprine – oral, 2 mg/kg; reduce the dose by 50 % if total white count is $<4 \times 10^9$/l (<4,000/microliter); and withhold if absolute neutrophil count $<1.5 \times 10^9$/l (<1,500/microliter) or total white count $<3 \times 10^9$/l (<3,000/mm^3).
- Mycophenolate mofetil (MMF)/sodium (1,000 mg MMF equivalent to 720 mg of mycophenolate sodium) – oral, 600 mg/m^2/dose 12 hourly (max: 1 g); reduce the dose by 50 % if tacrolimus is used concomitantly; and omit if absolute neutrophil count $<1.5 \times 10^9$/l (<1,500/microliter).

11.6.3 Maintenance Immunosuppression

- Cyclosporine – After 1 month, reduce every month by 1 mg/kg till 6 mg/kg/day, maintaining the target trough level; after 6 months, reduce cyclosporine dose to 4–5 mg/kg/day. The recommended blood 12-h trough levels are 150–250 ng/ml within 3 months and 100–200 ng/ml after 3 months by RIA method.
- Tacrolimus – The dose of tacrolimus is reduced to 0.1–0.2 mg/kg/day after 3 months. The recommended blood 12-h trough levels are 10–15 ng/ml in first 2 weeks, 8–10 ng/ml in first month, 6–8 ng/ml for 2 months, and 5–7 ng/ml after 2 months.
- Prednisolone – The tapering schedule is as follows: 0.6 mg/kg/day by 2 weeks, 0.3 mg/kg/day by 1 month, 0.15 mg/kg/day by 2 months, and thereafter as a maintenance dose of 0.15 mg/kg/day; after 1 year, prednisolone may be given on alternate days.
- Azathioprine – Long-term maintenance dose: 1.5–2.0 mg/kg/day.
- Mycophenolate mofetil – Oral: 600 mg/m^2/dose 12 hourly, reduce dose by 50 % if tacrolimus is used as a concomitant immunosuppression.

11.6.4 Alternative Drugs for Calcineurin Inhibitor Toxicity or Avoidance (Inhibitors of Mammalian Target of Rapamycin [mTOR])

- Sirolimus: Loading dose 3 mg/m^2 in patients ≥13 years who weigh less than 40 kg. The maintenance dose is 1 mg/m^2/day (1/3 of loading dose); for >40 kg, a loading dose of 6 mg should be given, followed by a maintenance dose of 2 mg/day. Sirolimus dose should be adjusted to obtain whole blood trough concentrations of 16–24 ng/ml (chromatographic method) for the first year following transplantation. Thereafter, the target sirolimus concentrations should be 12–20 ng/ml. It is recommended that sirolimus be taken 4 h after cyclosporine dose. However, some authors advise against the combination of calcineurin and mTOR inhibitors.

- *Everolimus* – The recommended dose is 0.8 mg/m^2 (maximum 1.5 mg) bid. In the absence of recommendations for drug levels in children, a trough level of 3–8 ng/ml is suggested.

11.7 Posttransplant Complications

11.7.1 Delayed Graft Function (DGF)

- Delayed graft function is much more common in organs transplanted from deceased compared to live donors, especially with prolonged cold ischemia time.
- It is defined by the lack of reaching normal kidney function 3 days after transplantation. A more stringent definition includes the need for dialysis within the first week post transplant.
- The most frequent cause of DGF is acute tubular necrosis (ATN), which can be precipitated by prolonged warm or cold ischemia time, hypotension, or use of vasoconstrictors in the donor and recipient.
- The differential diagnoses of DGF include hyperacute or accelerated allograft rejection which can mimic ATN or be present concomitantly, vascular thrombosis, FSGS (focal segmental glomerulosclerosis) recurrence, and rarely hemolytic uremic syndrome.
- When urine output dwindles, always exclude Foley's catheter obstruction, urinary obstruction due to blood clots, and urine leakage e.g., due to dehiscent ureter anastomosis.
- After ruling out urinary obstruction, ultrasound with Doppler and dynamic nuclear renal scan is performed using MAG3 or DPTA (see above). Adequate renal blood flow with impaired excretion is consistent with ATN.
- Dynamic nuclear renal scan also allows the detection of urine leakage and graft thrombosis (lack of uptake/perfusion by the graft).
- Graft biopsy indicated if rejection or disease recurrence are suspected. Surgical exploration may be warranted in case of vascular thrombosis. Calcineurin inhibitors may be withheld till the issues are resolved.

11.7.2 Acute Rejection (AR)

- Acute rejection is usually indicated by an asymptomatic rise in serum creatinine level.
- It often occurs in the first 3 months. Delayed rejections are frequently due to nonadherence with therapy and much less amenable to treatment.

- Dehydration, calcineurin inhibitor toxicity, urinary tract infection, urinary tract obstruction, and BK virus nephropathy should be excluded.
- The diagnosis of AR is made by examining a core biopsy of the transplanted kidney. Banff classification (see Box 11.1) is widely used to define the type of rejection in transplant biopsies.
- Histologically, AR can be T-cell-mediated (TCMR) or antibody-mediated (AMR). AMR is more common in highly sensitized, re-transplants and in transplants across blood group and positive cross match barriers. Immunofluorescence (IF) or immunoperoxidase staining show deposition of C4d in peritubular capillaries and/or antibodies to donor HLA class I and class II antigens (DSA).
- Standard treatment of acute cellular (T-cell mediated) rejection consists of giving intravenous methylprednisolone in daily doses of 10 mg/kg (max: 500–1,000 mg) for 3 consecutive days.
- Treatment of steroid resistant rejection – Monoclonal OKT3 antibodies at a dose of 2.5 mg for children weighing <30 kg and 5 mg for children >30 kg for 10–14 days.

  OR

  Anti-thymocyte globulin (Atgam): It is given in a dose of 15 mg/kg through a central venous line for 10–14 days.

Box 11.1 Transplant biopsy: Banff criteria

1. Normal
2. Antibody-mediated rejection (deposition of C4d in peritubular capillaries and/or circulating donor-specific antibodies) (a) Acute antibody-mediated rejection (i) ATN-like (ii) Capillary – glomerulitis, neutrophils, and/or mononuclear cells in peritubular capillaries (iii) Arterial – transmural inflammation/transmural change (b) Chronic antibody-mediated rejection
3. Borderline changes
4. T-cell-mediated rejection (TCMR) (a) Acute TCMR 1. (I) – significant interstitial infiltration, foci of tubulitis (divided into IA and IB) 2. (II) – intimal arteritis (divided into IIA and IIB) 3. (III) – transmural arteritis and/or arterial fibrinoid changes (b) Chronic active TCMR (c) Chronic allograft arteriopathy
5. Interstitial fibrosis and tubular atrophy Grades I, II, and III: <25 %, 26–50 %, and >50 % cortical area, respectively
6. Others: Changes not due to rejection

Source: KDIGO clinical practice guidelines for the care of kidney transplant recipients: Am J Transplant 9 (suppl 3): S 1–155

OR
Rabbit anti-thymocyte globulin (Thymoglobulin): 1.5–2.0 mg/kg for a total of 10–14 days. CD3+ cell count >20 cells/mm^3 should be maintained.
- Treatment of antibody-mediated acute rejection: Usually difficult to treat and associated with poor prognosis. High-dose immunoglobulins and rituximab may be used. Some have used plasmapheresis with variable results.

11.7.3 Infections

- Transplant recipients are at risk of opportunistic infections due to chronic immunosuppression.
- The spectrum of infections and infectious organism varies with time from transplantation (see Box 11.2) and the intensity or type of immunosuppression (e.g., due to rejection treatment).

11.7.3.1 CMV Infection

- Infection can be transmitted by the graft (mainly to CNV negative recipients) or occur de novo, or due to reactivation.
- It can be asymptomatic or clinically severe affecting multiple organ systems, including bone marrow (leukocytopenia, thrombocytopenia, anemia), colitis, pneumonia, hepatitis, or allograft dysfunction.
- Treatment: IV ganciclovir 5 mg/kg/dose 12 hourly for 14–21 days, reduction in immunosuppression may be required if disease is severe; oral valganciclovir for treatment of mild to moderate CMV disease – 15 mg/kg/day (max 900 mg); in refractory CMV disease, CMV hyperimmune globulin, in addition to ganciclovir, may improve clinical response. The dose is 400 mg/kg/dose on days 1, 2 and 7, followed by 200 mg/kg weekly × 2; alternatively, 500 mg/kg may be administered weekly ×2 doses and then alternate weeks for 5 more doses.

Box 11.2 Infections after organ Transplantation

Infection in the first month posttransplant
Infection conveyed with a contaminated allograft
Infections related to invasive procedures: wound, urinary, respiratory, and catheter infections
Infections 1–6 months posttransplant
Cytomegalovirus, Epstein-Barr virus, hepatitis B and C, varicella-zoster, HSV, parvovirus B19, and fungal infections such as Aspergillus and Pneumocystis jirovecii (PJP, formerly known as PCP)
Infection >6 months posttransplant
Community acquired infections, urinary tract infections, hepatitis B and C, and Cryptococcus neoformans, Molluscum contagiosum, common warts

11.7.3.2 Varicella

- In immunosuppressed patients, varicella my case severe disease, including encephalitis and pneumonia, or death.
- Treatment: IV acyclovir 500 mg/m^2/dose (<12 years old) or 10 mg/kg/dose (12 years and older) every 8 h as slow infusion till lesions are crusted (max 1,500 mg/m^2/day). This is followed by oral acyclovir 20 mg/kg/dose (500–600 mg/m^2/dose) 4–5 times/day for a total of 14 days.
- Good hydration should be ensured to minimize acyclovir nephrotoxicity.
- MMF may increase acyclovir (and valacyclovir) serum levels.

11.7.3.3 Polyoma BK Virus Infection

- Polyoma BK virus has been recognized to cause clinical and histological features mimicking acute rejection.
- Bimodal distribution: 1–6 weeks or 5–18 months after transplantation.
- Tubulointerstitial nephritis, hemorrhagic cystitis, ureteral stenosis, and graft dysfunction.
- Serum and urine PCR for BK virus, decoy cells in urine, and immunoperoxidase staining for SV40 (Simian virus 40) large T antigen in a graft biopsy.
- Managed with reduced immunosuppression, IVIG, leflunomide, cidofovir, or quinolone antibiotics.

11.7.3.4 Prophylaxis

- Perioperative antibiotic prophylaxis: Intravenous cefotaxime/cefazolin.
- Cytomegalovirus (CMV) prophylaxis:
  1. Duration of prophylaxis is 3 months except if positive donor to negative recipient, when the duration of prophylaxis is 6 months.
  2. Ganciclovir : The dosage depends on creatinine clearance (CrCl), 5 mg/kg/dose intravenously 12 hourly (CrCl >70 ml/min/1.73 m^2); reduce the dose by 50 % if CrCl between 70 and 25 ml/min/1.73 m^2; reduce the dose by 75 % if CrCl <25 ml/min/1.73 m^2; given for up to 2 weeks followed by oral ganciclovir 30 mg/kg/dose three times a day.
  3. Valganciclovir: 15 mg/kg/dose (max 450 mg); 15/mg/kg alternate days if GFR <40 ml/min/1.73 m^2; and 15 mg/kg twice weekly if GFR less than 25 ml/min/1.73 m^2.
  4. In high-risk recipient (positive donor to negative recipient) CMV, immunoglobulin may be considered as adjunctive prophylaxis 200 mg/kg on day 0, followed by 150 mg/kg at weeks 2, 4, 6, 8, and 10 and 100 mg/kg/day at weeks 12–16.
- Antibiotic prophylaxis for UTI/stent: Nitrofurantoin, 1 mg/kg/day.
- Pneumocystis jirovecii prophylaxis: Co-trimoxazole 3–5 mg/kg/dose of trimethoprim alternate days or three consecutive days per week for 3–6 months. Note that co-trimoxazale can increase the creatinine level (reversible).
- Varicella: Varicella-zoster immunoglobulin – 0.4–1.2 ml/kg IM or 125–625 iu/dose IM within 72 h of exposure.

11.7.4 Chronic Allograft Dysfunction (CAD)

- Chronic allograft dysfunction, previously known as chronic allograft nephropathy, is defined as gradual and irreversible decline in graft function.
- Contributory factors leading to CAD include immunological factors (episodes of acute rejection, chronic rejection, and presence of donor-specific antibodies) and nonimmunological factors (chronic cyclosporine/tacrolimus toxicity, recurrence of native kidney disease, de novo glomerulonephritis, hypertension, hyperglycemia, hyperlipidemia, donor and recipient size mismatch, and donor age)
- Rescue therapy with sirolimus or everolimus, instead of cyclosporine/tacrolimus and mycophenolate instead of azathioprine are common strategies employed to retard the progression of chronic graft dysfunction.
- Managing other complications like hypertension, proteinuria, and hyperlipidemia may slow down deterioration of graft function.

11.7.5 Surgical Complications

The common surgical complications include wound infection, bleeding, graft thrombosis, urinary leak, renal artery stenosis, and lymphocele.

11.7.6 Metabolic Complications

- Hypomagnesemia may occur due to renal tubular wasting of magnesium as a result of tacrolimus, cyclosporine, or diuretic use.
- Hyperkalemia may be due to tacrolimus or cyclosporine toxicity, acute rejection, and urinary obstruction or due to ACE inhibitors or co-trimoxazole therapy.
- Hypophosphatemia may occur due to persistent secondary hyperparathyroidism of ESRD. Sometimes it may take about 12 months for it to resolve.
- Dyslipidemia may occur due to steroids, tacrolimus, cyclosporine, or sirolimus.

11.7.7 Recurrence of Disease in Allograft (Table 11.1)

- Patients with recurrent glomerular diseases have a poorer allograft survival compared to those with no recurrence.
- Recurrences of FSGS occur in about 40 % of transplanted grafts. Age 6–12 years at disease onset, rapid progression to ESRD, mesangial hypercellularity on native biopsy, and recurrence in previous transplant markedly increase the risk of recurrence. The efficacy of plasma exchange and immunoadsorption in treatment of recurrent FSGS has been addressed in small studies with variable results.

Table 11.1 Recurrent glomerulonephritis in renal allograft

Type of glomerulonephritis	Rate of recurrence (%)
FSGS	20–40
IgA nephropathy	50
Membranoproliferative GN	20
Hemolytic uremic syndrome	10–50
Henoch-Schonlein purpura	30–80
Lupus nephritis	5–10

- The other glomerular diseases which recur in transplanted kidney are IgA nephropathy, membranoproliferative glomerulonephritis, atypical hemolytic uremic syndrome, and lupus nephritis. Therapeutic decisions to manage disease recurrence in the graft are based on anecdotal data and information extrapolated from treatment of the primary diseases in native kidneys.
- In view of high risk of recurrence, patients with primary hyperoxaluria are advised to undergo combined liver and kidney transplantation.

11.7.8 Lymphoproliferative Disease (PTLD)

- Associated with Epstein-Barr virus (EBV) infection. Serial measurements of EBV DNA, best in form of quantitative PCR, define patients at risk. High viral copy numbers do not "prove" the presence of PTLD, but may indicate "over immunosuppression".
- Its PTLD incidence varies from 1 to 10 % of pediatric renal transplant recipients.
- EBV seronegative recipient of a kidney from an EBV seropositive donor (EBV mismatch), CMV infection, and induction therapy with ATG and anti-rejection therapy with the combination of calcineurin inhibitor and sirolimus are considered risk factors for the development of PTLD.
- The clinical manifestation of PTLD is variable: nonspecific viral syndrome, weight loss, sore throat, abdominal pain, lymphadenopathy, tonsillar enlargement, focal neurological signs, and severe infectious mononucleosis-like illness with lymphoproliferative tumor masses in multiple organs and allograft dysfunction. Mortality is substantial.
- Therapeutic management includes reduction or discontinuation of immunosuppression, IV gammaglobulin, chemotherapy, and rituximab.

11.7.9 Hypertension

- Side effect of steroids, cyclosporine A, tacrolimus; acute and chronic rejection; and transplant renal artery stenosis.
- Uncontrolled hypertension contributes to deterioration of graft function and increases cardiovascular risk.

11.7.10 Growth

- Height velocity improves after transplantation but may remain suboptimal.
- Growth is assessed by height deficit Z score.
- Growth is better in those who receive transplant at an early age, have good allograft function, and are on minimal (<6 mg/m^2/day) or alternate day steroids. Some children may benefit from human recombinant growth hormone (GH) therapy. High cost of GH therapy may be a prohibitive factor in developing countries.
- Obesity or excessive weight gain may be a problem in some children. Less than 5 % children develop IDDM (insulin-dependent diabetes mellitus) after transplantation. The risk of IDDM is higher with use of tacrolimus as compared to cyclosporine.

11.8 Renal Transplantation in Countries/Regions with Limited Resources

Renal transplantation is the treatment modality of choice in management of children with end-stage renal disease (ESRD). Technical advances in recent years have made renal transplantation a safe and reliable therapy. This option is offered to almost all children with ESRD from the developed world. However, children from countries or regions with limited resources face many hurdles to benefit from this option. These hurdles are outlined below.

Many children with ESRD in developing countries reach the hospitals late in a sick moribund state. This is due to late detection of chronic renal diseases and poor access to medical care. It is not uncommon that they receive medical attention for the first time when they present with life-threatening emergencies like pulmonary edema or encephalopathy. In the absences of affordable medical insurance, payments for treatment may drain the financial resources of families and leave them unable to meet the costs of renal transplantation.

The children may receive suboptimal dialysis and supportive therapy due to financial constraints resulting in malnutrition, stunted growth and severe renal dystrophy. Due to lack of affordability, they may not receive erythropoietin and risk sensitization due to blood transfusions instead. Families my resort to unproven indigenous therapies giving false hopes for miraculous cure.

Many countries do not have nationwide registries. Hence, it is not possible to ascertain the exact burden of chronic kidney disease. Pediatric renal care is unevenly distributed. These services are concentrated in metropolitan cities with scarcity of infrastructure and expertise in peripheral areas.

Renal replacement therapy is an expensive treatment. Many countries do not have governmental support or insurance to cover costs of renal care. Treatment of chronic diseases in children is accorded low priority in the public health domain compared with malnutrition and acute infectious diseases. The patients have to pay for dialysis, transplantation surgery, and immunosuppressive medications out of their pockets, thus making renal transplantation a distant dream.

There are issues regarding kidney donations. Misconceptions exist about consequences of organ donation, its ill effects on health, productivity, and life span. Cultural beliefs and superstitions may come in the way. Working members of the family may not volunteer for organ donation for fear of losing their capacity to earn. A sustained active deceased donor program may not exist, eliminating a source of organs. Living unrelated donors are admissibile in some countries. However, this avenue is generally limited to the rich minority. While a (supervised) "paid organ donation program" may alleviate some of the access problems, the practice is controversial due to remaining nontransparencies, and ethical concerns.

For the above-mentioned reasons, the outcomes of chronic kidney disease are generally poor for the majority. This perpetuates passive attitudes and apathy among the society about kidney diseases in children, making them believe that having end-stage renal disease is an "end of the road" situation!

Early detection and timely referral of children with kidney disease to tertiary centers, sensitizing the medical fraternity and the society as a whole to chronic kidney diseases and transplantation, seeking financial help from philanthropists, and developing a sustained deceased donor program will go a long way in fulfilling the gap between the needs and the reality.

Suggested Reading

Cochat P, Fargue S, Mestrallet G, Jungraithmayr T, Koch-Nogueira P, Ranchin B, Zimmerhackl LB (2009) Disease recurrence in paediatric renal transplantation. Pediatr Nephrol 24:2097–2108

Comoli P, Ginevri F (2012) Monitoring and managing viral infections in pediatric renal transplant recipients. Pediatr Nephrol 27:705–717

Danovitch GM (2009) Handbook of kidney transplantation, 5th edn. Lippincott Williams & Wilkins, Philadelphia/London

Dharnidharka VR, Abdulnour HA, Araya CE (2011) The BK virus in renal transplant recipients-review of pathogenesis, diagnosis, and treatment. Pediatr Nephrol 26:1763–1774

Fine RN, Weber SA, Harmon SE, Kelly DA, Olthoff KM (2007) Pediatric solid organ transplantation, 2nd edn. Wiley-Blackwell, Malden/Oxford

Morris P, Knechtle SJ (2001) Kidney transplantation: principles and practice, 5th edn. Saunders, Philadelphia

Rizvi SA, Zafar MN, Lanewala AA, Naqvi SA (2009) Challenges in pediatric renal transplantation in developing countries. Curr Opin Organ Transplant 14:533–539

Shapiro R, Sarwal MM (2010) Pediatric kidney transplantation. Pediatr Clin North Am 57: 393–400

Vinai M, Waber P, Seikaly MG (2010) Recurrence of focal segmental glomerulosclerosis in renal allograft: an in-depth review. Pediatr Transplant 14:314–325

Oncology and Kidney

12

Anand Prakash and David Mitchell

12.1 Renal Tumors

12.1.1 Wilms' Tumor

12.1.1.1 Incidence

- Most common primary renal tumor of childhood
- Constitutes 6 % of all pediatric malignancies
- Common age at diagnosis: 1–5 years (75 %)
- Usually sporadic; 1 % are familial
- Bilateral disease occurs in 5 %
- Occurs as part of a syndrome in 2–4 % cases (see Table 12.1)

12.1.1.2 Presentation

- Incidental detection of a painless abdominal mass in the flank – most common presentation
- Hypertension – seen in 25 % cases
- Hematuria – seen in 15 % cases – most often microscopic hematuria
- Rarely – polycythemia, urinary infection, abdominal pain, pleural effusion, cardiac failure, diarrhea
- Associated anomalies may be seen – hypospadias, cryptorchidism, hemihypertrophy, and aniridia

A. Prakash (✉)
Department of Pediatrics,
St. John's Medical College Hospital,
Sarjapur Road, Bangalore, KA 560034, India
e-mail: anandprakash94@gmail.com

D. Mitchell
Division of Pediatric Oncology,
Montreal Children's Hospital, McGill University,
2300 rue Tupper, Montreal, QC H3H 1P3, Canada
e-mail: david.mitchell@muhc.mcgill.ca

K. Phadke et al. (eds.), *Manual of Pediatric Nephrology*,
DOI 10.1007/978-3-642-12483-9_12,

Table 12.1 Congenital syndromes associated with Wilms' tumor

Syndrome	Features	Risk of developing Wilms	Gene locus
WAGR	*W*ilms *A*niridia *G*enitourinary malformation Mental *r*etardation	30 % Bilateral:15 %	Deletion of WT1 gene on chromosome 11p13
Denys-Drash syndrome	Pseudohermaphroditism Nephrotic syndrome	90 %	11p13
Frasier syndrome	Male hermaphroditism Primary amenorrhea Chronic kidney disease	8 %	11p13
Beckwith-Wiedemann syndrome	Macrosomia Neonatal hypoglycemia Macroglossia Omphalocele Visceromegaly Renal anomalies Hemihypertrophy	5 %	Loss of imprinting of heterozygosity of WT2 on chromosome 11p15
Perlman syndrome	Fetal gigantism Bilateral renal hamartomas Visceromegaly Unusual facies	33 %	Not known
Simpson-Golabi-Behmel syndrome	Course facies Macrosomia Macrocephaly Renal and skeletal anomalies	10 %	Xq26
Blooms	Short stature Photosensitivity	3 %	15q26
Trisomy 13, 18	Multiple congenital anomalies	Low	Not known

12.1.1.3 Evaluation

1. Abdominal ultrasound:
   - Confirm origin and extent of renal mass
   - Assess extent into renal vein and inferior vena cava
   - Assess opposite kidney for involvement
2. CT abdomen
   - Confirm above findings and rule out liver metastasis
3. Chest X ray and CT chest
   - To rule out pulmonary metastasis
4. Complete blood count
5. Renal functions
6. Urinalysis
7. Coagulation profile (possibility of acquired von Willebrand disease)

Table 12.2 Staging system for Wilms' tumor

Stage	NWTS	SIOP
I	Tumor is limited to kidney Totally excised There is no tumoral involvement in surgical margin The vessels of renal sinus are not involved There is no tumoral rupture before or during removal	Tumor is limited to kidney No tumor cells at the surgical margin The vessels of renal sinus are not involved Intrarenal vessels may be involved
II	Tumor is outside the kidney Totally removed Local spillage and intrarenal vessels could be involved	Tumor extends outside of the kidney Totally resected but capsule, adjacent tissues, renal sinus and renal vessels can be involved
III	Intra-abdominal tumor Renal hilus, abdominal lymph nodes are involved Diffuse spillage Peritoneal involvement Thrombus in vena cava	Incomplete resection Intra-abdominal lymph node involvement but renal hilus lymph node positivity makes it stage II Ureteral, peritoneal, and caval involvement Preoperative or perioperative biopsy or rupture Peritoneal metastases
IV	Hematogeneous or distant lymph node metastases	Hematogeneous and extra-abdominal lymph node metastases
V	Bilateral renal tumors	Bilateral renal tumors

With permission from Nephron Clin Practice 2008: 108: c83–c90

12.1.1.4 Staging

There are two types of staging based on the NWTS (North American) and the SIOP (European) approach to the therapy (Table 12.2).

12.1.1.5 Histopathology

Wilms' tumors characteristically have triphasic histology (blastemal, epithelial, stromal components). Features of anaplasia (bizarre nuclear enlargement, hyperpolyploidy, atypical mitotic figures) are looked for. Anaplasia is defined as focal of diffuse. Based on above features, the tumors are stratified as with favorable and unfavorable histologies.

12.1.1.6 Therapy

Treatment of Wilms' tumor is based on:

1. Staging
2. Histology (favorable vs. unfavorable)
3. Molecular features: loss of heterozygosity of chromosome 1p and 16q

The modalities of surgery, chemotherapy, and radiotherapy are used. The timing and sequence of these vary based on the protocol followed for treatment.

NWTS (North American) approach: Surgery upfront (if possible) → chemotherapy +/– radiotherapy

SIOP (European) approach: Neoadjuvant chemotherapy → surgery → adjuvant chemotherapy +/– radiotherapy

Both protocols have overall similar outcomes.

12.1.1.7 Surgery

Tumor mass is resected completely. Partial nephrectomy is done only for bilateral Wilms, solitary, or horseshoe kidney.

Care should be taken to avoid tumor spill or incomplete removal during surgery. This reduces incidence of tumor recurrence. The tumor spill makes radiotherapy an essential part of treatment.

12.1.1.8 Chemotherapy

The duration and number of chemotherapeutic agents administered depends on the staging and histology of the resected tumor. The common agents used are vincristine, actinomycin D, and doxorubicin for favorable histology. The above agents with cyclophosphamide and etoposide are used for unfavorable histology.

Chemotherapy upfront is used in the following situations:

1. Bilateral Wilms
2. Tumor thrombus extending into the IVC
3. Extremely large and "difficult to resect" tumors

The SIOP protocols use chemotherapy upfront in an attempt to make surgery safer and to decrease the risk of tumor spill.

12.1.1.9 Radiation Therapy

- Local flank radiation is recommended for patients with anaplasia and stage III (residual tumor post surgery/spill) or stage IV (metastatic) tumors.
- Whole abdomen radiation is required in diffuse tumor spills.
- Whole lung irradiation is given for pulmonary metastasis.

12.1.1.10 Bilateral Wilms' Tumor

- Occurs in 5 % of Wilms' tumor patients.
- Have poorer outcome than unilateral disease of comparable histology, age of patient, and stage of tumor.
- Aim of treatment is to eradicate the tumor with maximum preservation of renal tissue.
- Preoperative chemotherapy is given to decrease tumor size.
- Bilateral partial nephrectomies are then performed.

12.1.1.11 Prognosis

Overall prognosis of Wilms' tumor is favorable. The 5-year overall survival is more than 90 %. A higher stage and anaplastic histology are associated with poorer prognosis.

Relapse-free survival based on stage of disease:

Stage I	89.7 %
Stage II	87.1 %
Stage III	75.1 %
Stage IV	62.5 %

12.1.1.12 Long-Term Concerns Post-therapy for Wilms' Tumor

- Renal impairment
  - The potential late effects after nephrectomy are proteinuria, hypertension, hyperfiltration, and renal insufficiency.
  - Renal insufficiency is also due to radiation therapy if given.
  - Patients with bilateral Wilms' and syndromes associated with Wilms are at increased risk of renal toxicity.
  - Renal dysfunction may occur many years after nephrectomy. Patients with WAGR syndrome are particularly at risk for late onset renal failure.

    Blood pressure and urine analysis checks are to be done yearly post treatment.
- Other complications
  - Cardiac toxicity secondary to anthracyclines
  - Second neoplasms
- Recurrence of tumor
  - Abdominal ultrasonograms (USG) are recommended to look for recurrence or tumor developing in other kidney (metachronous Wilms' tumor):
    - USG every 3 months for 2 years, then yearly for 3 years
    - If presence of nephrogenic rests in the resected kidney
      - Age <48 months at diagnosis: every 3 months for 6 years
      - Age >48 months at diagnosis: every 3 months for 4 years
    - USG every 3 months till age of 8 years for children with syndromes prone for Wilms' tumor

12.1.2 Other Renal Tumors

12.1.2.1 Clear Cell Sarcoma of Kidney

- Constitutes 3 % of renal tumors.
- Occurs often with bone metastasis.
- Following resection and radiation therapy, intensive chemotherapy with cyclophosphamide, etoposide, vincristine, and doxorubicin is given.
- Higher rate of relapse and death than Wilms' tumor.

12.1.2.2 Malignant Rhabdoid Tumor

- Constitutes 1.8 % of renal tumors
- Highly malignant
- Often metastatic to liver, lung, or brain at presentation
- Prognosis poor – mortality 80 % for all stages

12.1.2.3 Congenital Mesoblastic Nephroma

- Low-grade spindle cell tumor from renal medulla
- Usually presents in the first 3 months of life
- Complete nephrectomy is usually adequate

12.1.2.4 Renal Cell Carcinoma

- Constitutes 5 % of renal tumors.
- Pediatric subtypes are distinct from adult.
- Surgery is mainstay of therapy.

12.1.3 Tumor Lysis Syndrome

Tumor lysis syndrome (TLS) constitutes a group of metabolic abnormalities that result from the rapid release of intracellular metabolites from lysed tumor cells. This may lead to hyperuricemia, hyperkalemia, hyperphosphatemia, and hypocalcemia. The degree and rapidity of the process determines if a patient will develop acute kidney injury and/or other complications which may even be life threatening in some instances.

TLS usually occurs spontaneously or within 12–72 h of initiation of chemotherapy. Rapidly proliferating tumors, high tumor load, and the degree of sensitivity of the tumor cells to chemotherapy determine the incidence and severity of TLS.

12.1.3.1 Definition

TLS can be defined in laboratory terms or in clinical terms:

Laboratory TLS is defined by the occurrence of two or more of the following serum values before or after anticancer treatment (given 3 days before to 7 days after the start of anticancer treatment):

(i) Uric acid: Increase by more than 25 % from baseline (if a recent baseline value is available), or values ≥476 μmol/L (8 mg/dL)
(ii) Potassium: Increase by more than 25 % from baseline (if a recent baseline value is available), or values ≥6.0 mmol/L (6 mg/L)
(iii) Phosphorus: Increase by more than 25 % from baseline (if a recent baseline value is available), or values ≥1.45 mmol/L (4.5 mg/dL) in adults and ≥2.1 mmol/L (6.5 mg/dL) in children
(iv) Calcium: Decrease by more than 25 % from baseline (if a recent baseline value is available), or values ≤1.75 mmol/L (7 mg/dL)

Though other biomarkers (NGAL, KIM, IL-18) of acute kidney injury have been evaluated in TLS, none are of routine clinical use at present.

Clinical TLS is defined by the presence of laboratory TLS and at least one of the following clinical alterations:

1. Acute kidney injury (estimated glomerular filtration rate ≤60 mL/min/1.73 m^2)
2. Cardiac arrhythmia
3. Seizures

12.1.3.2 Clinical Manifestations of TLS

Nausea, vomiting, diarrhea, anorexia, lethargy, edema, fluid overload, hematuria, congestive heart failure, cardiac arrhythmias, seizures, muscle cramps, tetany, syncope, and sudden death

Common malignancies where TLS is common are Burkitt's lymphoma, T cell lymphoblastic lymphoma, acute myeloid leukemia, and acute lymphoblastic leukemia. TLS is rare in solid tumors but can occasionally occur with neuroblastoma and germ cell tumors.

12.1.3.3 Risk Factors for TLS

- Type of malignancy
- Tumor burden (stage/serum LDH levels)
- White blood cell (WBC) counts (>50,000/mm^3)
- Altered renal functions at presentation

The risk stratification system provides for early recognition of clinical settings where TLS is likely and allows for preventive steps in management.

Low-risk disease – less than 1 % chances of developing TLS

Intermediate risk – a risk of 1–5 % of developing TLS

High-risk disease – a risk of greater than 5 % of developing TLS

Some risk stratification systems have been developed by regional entities. Each system, however, addresses different diseases, uses different criteria, and establishes different thresholds for risk.

12.1.3.4 Mechanisms of AKI in TLS

In the initial stages, elevated uric acid levels may cause a drop in GFR due to formation of uric acid crystals causing tubular obstruction. This along with cell lysis leads to elevation of serum potassium. The decrease in GFR also contributes to elevation of phosphate and a consequent decrease in serum calcium. The altered calcium and phosphate levels contribute to deposition of calcium phosphate crystals in the tubules and a further worsening of renal function. The vicious cycle of a decreased GFR contributing to electrolyte disturbances which in turn lead to a further drop in GFR manifests with laboratory and, later, clinical features of TLS. Preexisting renal dysfunction, dehydration, acidic urine, oliguria, and rarely primary involvement of the kidneys by the malignancy contribute to severity of TLS.

12.1.3.5 General Principles of Management

The early recognition of risk of TLS may allow for prevention of major metabolic changes, obviating the need for renal replacement therapy.

1. Ensure adequate hydration, i.e., 3 L/m^2/day and a urine output of 80–100 mL/m^2/h
2. Potassium-free fluids are chosen as hyperkalemia may occur suddenly.
3. Furosemide 0.5–1 mg/kg/day in two divided doses may be given to ensure a good urine output.
4. Allopurinol at 100 mg/m^2/dose q8 hourly is started to combat hyperuricemia. It can be given orally or IV. It is started for 1–2 days before starting chemotherapy and continued till features of TLS resolve. It acts as a competitive inhibitor of xanthine oxidase and prevents formation of new uric acid. It is therefore not useful in severe hyperuricemia where rasburicase (see below) is more effective.
5. Regular hourly monitoring of urine output and 6–12 hourly monitoring of BUN, serum creatinine, uric acid, serum calcium, phosphate, and electrolytes, depending on the risk and the severity of ongoing TLS.

6. Rasburicase (0.1–0.2 mg/kg) one dose in 50 cc normal saline as infusion over 30 min and is repeated if clinically indicated. (It is avoided in patients with G6PD deficiency.) Early use of rasburicase especially in high-risk cases is the standard of care and may help in preventing dialysis and delays in initiating chemotherapy.
7. Mild asymptomatic hypocalcemia does not require aggressive treatment. Calcium gluconate administration may lead to worsening of precipitation of calcium phosphate in the tubules. For symptomatic hypocalcemia, cautious use of single dose of calcium gluconate may be considered.
8. Urinary alkalinization is not routinely practiced. It may play a role when serum uric acid is elevated but may be counterproductive when there is hypercalcemia and hyperphosphatemia as alkalinization leads to calcium phosphate precipitation in the kidney.

12.1.3.6 Indications of Renal Replacement Therapy

Indications for the initiation of renal replacement therapy in TLS include persistent hyperkalemia, severe metabolic acidosis, volume overload unresponsive to diuretic therapy, and overt uremic symptoms, including pericarditis and severe encephalopathy. Dialysis may be initiated "prophylactically" before the development of overt uremic symptoms in response to severe, progressive hyperphosphatemia (>6 mg/dL or >1.94 mmol/L) or severe symptomatic hypocalcemia. The appropriate timing for this criterion remains unresolved. Frequent (daily) dialyses are recommended considering the continuous release into the bloodstream of purine products, potassium, and other metabolites resulting from lysed tumor cells. The timing of dialysis and the dialysis dose should be linked to the severity of TLS.

12.1.3.7 Management of Electrolyte Abnormalities in TLS

Abnormality	Therapy
Hypocalcemia	
Asymptomatic	No therapy
Symptomatic	Calcium gluconate 10 % 1 mL/kg slow IV with cardiac monitoring
Hyperkalemia	
Moderate (>6.0 mmol/L)	Potassium-free fluids Cardiac monitoring
Severe (>7 mmol/L)/ symptomatic	Potassium-binding resins – sodium polystyrene 1 g/kg orally IV calcium gluconate 10 % 1 mL/kg Sodium bicarbonate 1–2 mEq/kg IV (Do NOT give calcium and bicarbonate in the same line) Insulin with dextrose (0.1 U/kg +25 %D 2 mL/kg) Dialysis
Hyperphosphatemia	Administer phosphate binder Dialysis
Renal dysfunction	Fluid management Correction of drug doses as required Dialysis

12.2 Chemotherapy-Induced Renal Dysfunction

Chemotherapeutic agents used in pediatric oncology have various renal toxic effects. Drug nephrotoxicity is a complication which may limit and hamper lifesaving therapy.

This section describes some of the common chemotherapy drugs and the renal dysfunction they produce. The chapter on nephrotoxicity (Chap. 16) and Appendix (Chap. 17) may also be referred.

12.2.1 Risk Factors for Chemotherapy-Induced Renal Dysfunction

Disease related:

- Renal infiltration (lymphoma/leukemia)
- Urinary obstruction
- Volume depletion (vomiting, diarrhea)
- Metabolic derangements (hyperuricemia, hypercalcemia)

Drug related:

- High drug doses and prolonged course of therapy
- Crystal formation in tubular lumens
- Insoluble drugs
- Direct nephrotoxicity
- Pharmacogenetics (polymorphisms of P450 enzyme systems)

12.2.2 Sites of Renal Injury

Renal vasculature:

Bevacizumab (VGEF inhibitor)
Tyrosine kinase inhibitors
Mitomycin C
Cisplatinum
Gemcitabine

Glomeruli:

Interferon
Pamidronate

Tubulointerstitial:

- ATN: Carboplatin/cisplatin, ifosfamide
- Tubulopathies
  - Fanconi syndrome: cisplatin, ifosfamide, and azacitidine
  - Salt wasting: cisplatin and azacitidine
  - Magnesium wasting: cisplatin, cetuximab
  - Nephrogenic diabetes insipidus: cisplatin, ifosfamide
  - Syndrome of inappropriate antidiuresis: cyclophosphamide and vincristine
  - Crystal nephropathy: methotrexate

12.2.3 Renal Toxicity of Selected Chemotherapeutic Drugs

Cisplatin:

- Causes both AKI and CKD.
- Toxicity is dose related (>200 mg/m^2 cumulative dose).
- Affects most commonly the tubules, also the renal vasculature and glomeruli.
- Tubular injury manifests as AKI.
- Renal toxicity in usually reversible but can be permanent.
- Mechanism of toxicity is tubular cell apoptosis and necrosis due to intracellular activation of caspase and kinase pathways.
- Tubulopathy can also manifest as proteinuria, phosphaturia, Fanconi syndrome or sodium wasting, hypomagnesemia, and nephrogenic DI.
- Treatment of renal manifestations is mainly supportive.
- Prevention of kidney injury – forced diuresis with normal or hypertonic saline.
- Prophylactic use of magnesium supplementation also helps reduce the risk of nephrotoxicity.
- In the presence of renal dysfunction, cisplatin may need to be withheld, dose reduced, or substituted by another drug if possible.
- Sodium thiosulfate, amifostine, N acetyl cysteine, and liposomal formulations have been tried to reduce nephrotoxicity.
- Carboplatin and oxaliplatin may be less nephrotoxic and are used in patients at high risk of renal dysfunction.

Carboplatin:

- Less nephrotoxic than cisplatin; degree of nephrotoxicity depends on the creatinine clearance as 60–70 % of drug excretion is through the kidneys.

Ifosfamide:

- Main toxicity are tubulopathies, proximal tubular damage, Fanconi syndrome, and nephrogenic diabetes insipidus.
- Chloroacetaldehyde is the toxic metabolite of ifosfamide.
- Dose (>60 g/m^2) and underlying CKD contribute to degree of toxicity.
- Rarely a permanent tubulopathy causing phosphaturia leads to osteomalacia and growth problems in children.
- Renal toxicity is prevented by adequate hydration.
- Mesna does not have a role in protecting against the tubular dysfunction of ifosfamide.

Cyclophosphamide:

- Though not directly nephrotoxic, it is associated with hemorrhagic cystitis because of the toxic metabolite acrolein.
- Adequate hydration and the concomitant use of mesna prevent this complication.

Methotrexate:

- Nephrotoxicity occurs with high-dose therapy (1–12 g/m^2).
- AKI occurs because of precipitation of methotrexate and its metabolites in the distal tubular lumen.
- Risk factors for AKI include dehydration, sluggish urinary flow, acidic urine, and underlying kidney disease.
- Toxicity is prevented by adequate hydration, alkalinization of urine, and ensuring adequate urine output.

- Leucovorin is given to reduce renal and hematological toxicity of methotrexate after 24–48 h of methotrexate infusion.
- Glucarpidase, a compound which cleaves methotrexate into nontoxic metabolites, is used when methotrexate levels are very high.
- High-flux hemodialysis is useful but associated with post-dialysis plasma rebound in levels.

Mitomycin C:

- Associated with renal dysfunction with microangiopathic hemolytic anemia
- Occurs in 20 % of patients with cumulative dose of 100 mg

12.2.4 Drugs Which Do Not Require Dose Modifications Based on Renal Dysfunction

- Actinomycin D
- Busulfan
- Daunorubicin
- Doxorubicin
- 5-Flurouracil
- Idarubicin
- 6 Mercaptopurine
- Mitoxantrone
- Procarbazine
- 6-Thioguanine
- Thiotepa
- Vinblastine
- Vincristine

12.3 Secondary Hypertension in the Oncology Setting

12.3.1 Tumors Associated with Hypertension

- Wilms' tumor
- Neuroblastoma
- Ganglioneuroblastoma
- Abdominal lymphoma
- Pheochromocytoma
- Teratoma

12.3.2 Mechanism of Hypertension

- Increased renin secretion:
  - Renal artery compression
  - Renal parenchymal compression
  - Ectopic renin secretion by tumor

- Renal vein thrombosis
- Increased intracranial pressure due to intracranial tumors/CNS leukemia
- Secondary to steroids, cyclosporine, and amphotericin B
- Pain

12.3.3 Evaluation of Hypertension

- Document systolic/diastolic BP >95th percentile for age and gender
- Fever, pain may temporarily elevate BP
- Abdominal CT scan
- Urine and plasma catecholamine levels
- Renin levels
- CT head if indicated
- Renal Doppler US if indicated

12.3.4 Management

- Hypertensive emergencies to be managed as per guidelines given in the chapter on hypertension.
- Long-acting ACE inhibitors or calcium channel blockers may be used for long-term control.
- During as well as immediate postsurgery for neuroblastoma, hypertensive crisis may occur and should be monitored.
- Hypertension of raised intracranial pressure due to tumors is treated with dexamethasone or mannitol.
- Definitive treatment of hypertension is by cytotoxic therapy of primary tumor.

12.4 Oligoanuria in the Oncology Setting

Prerenal, renal, and postrenal causes of decreased renal function can all occur in a child with a newly diagnosed malignancy or on treatment for the same.

12.4.1 Prerenal Causes

- Septic shock
- Emesis, poor oral intake
- Profuse infectious diarrhea

12.4.2 Renal Causes

- Tumor lysis syndrome
- Chemotherapy-induced AKI (cisplatin, methotrexate, ifosfamide)
- Antibiotic and antifungal (amphotericin) use

12.4.3 Postrenal Causes

- Bulky abdominal/pelvic tumors – obstruct ureters and bladder
  - Lymphomas, germ cell tumors, neuroblastoma, sarcomas
- Intravesicular blood clots – ureter and bladder obstruction
- Urinary retention due to sacral nerves affected by opioids or vinca alkaloids

12.4.4 Therapy

- Ensure adequate hydration
- Bladder catheterization or ureter stents
- Surgery for abdominal mass
- Stop or replace nephrotoxic agents by less toxic agents
- Management of AKI – non-dialytic and dialytic therapies, as required

12.5 Renal Dysfunction and Stem Cell Transplantation

Stem cell transplants (SCT) are now performed for a wide range of oncological, hematological, and metabolic diseases in children. This chapter gives an overview of stem cell transplantation and focuses on various causes for renal dysfunction in this setting.

12.5.1 Overview of Stem Cell Transplantation (SCT)

The SCT procedure involves infusion of hematopoietic stem cells (precursor blood cells which have the ability to differentiate into all the major cell lines of blood). The stem cells may be sourced from a human donor (allogeneic SCT) or may be harvested from the patient, stored, and given back to the patient (autologous SCT).

- Allogeneic transplants are done when the goal is to replace the diseased hematopoietic system with a new one, e.g., acute myeloid leukemia, relapsed acute lymphoblastic leukemia, aplastic anemia, and severe combined immunodeficiency. The source of stem cells from the donor for an allogeneic transplant needs to be HLA matched to the recipient. The source may be a sibling or an unrelated donor from a donor registry. The stem cells from the donor may be sourced from the bone marrow or peripheral blood. Cord blood units stored in public cord blood banks are also a source which is being used increasingly.
- Autologous transplants are done when the goal is to give high doses of chemotherapy to cure malignancy. However, the doses of chemotherapy involved are too toxic for the bone marrow to regenerate without stem cell support, e.g., metastatic neuroblastoma and relapsed Hodgkin's lymphoma. The stem cells for autologous SCT are harvested from the patient prior to giving high-dose chemotherapy.

12.5.2 The Steps of SCT

The steps for SCT include conditioning, infusion of stem cells, and marrow recovery.

12.5.2.1 Conditioning

It includes the chemotherapy +/– radiotherapy given to the patient prior to the infusion of stem cells. The purpose of conditioning is to clear the marrow of native cells, kill any residual malignant cells, and cause adequate immunosuppression such that when the new stem cells are transplanted, they are taken up and not rejected by the recipient. The conditioning regimens vary based on the disease and age of the patient. Based on the degree of myelotoxicity, regimens are termed myeloablative or non-myeloablative transplants. The toxicity of chemotherapy, time for recovery of the marrow, and chances of complications vary based the type of conditioning given. Common drugs used for condition include busulfan, cyclophosphamide, melphalan, and fludarabine. Radiotherapy given as total body irradiation (TBI) is done as a part of conditioning, particularly for leukemia.

12.5.2.2 Stem Cell Infusion

Following conditioning, stem cells are infused, usually through a central venous access.

12.5.2.3 Marrow Recovery

The process of marrow recovery follows infusion of the stem cells. Recovery of blood counts is termed engraftment. It is during this stage that various complications can occur causing both morbidity and mortality. The time taken for engraftment varies based on the source of stem cells. Peripheral blood stem cells take about 2 weeks; bone marrow harvests take about 3 weeks and cord blood transplants, about 4 weeks for engraftment.

The common complications that occur at this stage include:

1. Sepsis: Bacterial, fungal infections are common particularly before engraftment. Viral infections can occur even after engraftment due to the lymphotoxic immunosuppression which needs to be continued following SCT.
2. Sinusoidal obstruction syndrome (SOS): This is characterized by edema, tender hepatomegaly, jaundice, and ascites soon after conditioning. It occurs secondary to chemotherapy like busulfan and cyclophosphamide which cause endothelial damage and thrombosis of hepatic veins (formerly called veno-occlusive disease)
3. Graft rejection: Failure to engraft can cause prolonged bone marrow failure and recurrence of native bone marrow disease.
4. Graft versus host disease (GVHD): In this complication, the lymphocytes from the donor attack the immunosuppressed recipient. It is characterized by skin, liver, and gut manifestations. All SCT recipients are given immunosuppressants as GVHD prophylaxis. Severe grades of GVHD need higher doses of immunosuppression making the patient prone to both infections and drug toxicity.

12.5.3 Renal Complications Following SCT

12.5.3.1 Acute Kidney Injury (AKI)

AKI is not uncommon and the etiology is often multifactorial.

Risk factors for AKI:

- Sepsis
- Sinusoidal obstruction syndrome
- Thrombotic thrombocytopenic purpura
- GVHD
- Hypertension
- Use of nephrotoxic medications – cyclosporine, amphotericin B, ganciclovir

Salient observations from retrospective reviews:

- Mortality is two to three times higher in patients with AKI.
- Median time for occurrence of AKI is 40 days posttransplant.
- AKI without other causes is most often due to nephrotoxic drugs.
- Up to 45–50 % of patients have a doubling of creatinine and dialysis is required in about 1 % cases.

12.5.3.2 Chronic Kidney Disease

CKD can occur as a long-term complication of SCT

Risk factors:

- AKI at the time of SCT
- Total body irradiation at the time of transplant
- GVHD
- Long-term usage of calcineurin inhibitors

Salient features of CKD:

- Hypertension and proteinuria cause progressive worsening of CKD.
- Drugs for prevention of GVHD may play an important role. Cyclosporine and other calcineurin inhibitors have been recognized as important factors contributing to renal dysfunction.
- The most reproducible and reliable diagnostic features are tubular atrophy, interstitial fibrosis, and calcineurin inhibitor arteriolopathy.
- Radiation-induced renal damage is a consequent to degeneration and sclerosis of the arterioles and capillaries, with secondary destruction of the glomeruli and tubules, associated with interstitial fibrosis.

12.5.3.3 Nephrotic Syndrome

It is a rare complication after allogeneic SCT. It may be a complication of chronic GVHD and may be seen after abrupt discontinuation of cyclosporine.

12.5.3.4 Renal Complications Associated with Sinusoidal Obstruction Syndrome (SOS)

Most cases of SOS are mild and self-limiting and resolve within a few days. Careful fluid and electrolyte balance monitoring is adequate therapy for mild cases. Severe cases can be life threatening and lead to serious derangements in fluid balance and hepatorenal function.

Principles of management are:

- Early recognition of severe SOS (rapid and early rise of bilirubin and weight) needs therapy with defibrotide that attempts to reverse the ongoing damage within the hepatic sinusoids.
- Extravascular fluid accumulates as free water and sodium are retained in the setting of low albumin. Loop diuretics and spironolactone are to be used judiciously since they may worsen intravascular volume depletion.
- In the setting of renal compromise, monitoring of blood levels of cyclosporine, tacrolimus, aminoglycosides, vancomycin, and other potentially nephrotoxic drugs is important.

12.5.4 Pretransplant Screening and Post-SCT Monitoring of Renal Status

Pretransplant renal evaluation can identify patients at risk of CKD. Renal functions, GFR, and urine protein analysis should be performed at yearly intervals in all patients after SCT. Renal biopsy should be considered in patients with unclear chronic kidney disease after transplantation.

Suggested Reading

Ali Varan (2008) Wilms' tumor in children: an Overview. Nephron Clin Pract 108:c83–c90. doi:10-1159/000113012

Cairo MS, Coiffier B, Reiter A, Younes A, TLS Expert Panel (2010) Recommendations for the evaluation of risk and prophylaxis of tumor lysis syndrome (TLS) in adults and children with malignant diseases: an expert TLS panel consensus. Br J Haematol 149(4):578–586

Coiffier B, Altman A, Pui CH, Younes A, Cairo MS (2008) Guidelines for the management of pediatric and adult tumor lysis syndrome: an evidence-based review. J Clin Oncol 26(16): 2767–2778

Ellis MJ, Parikh CR, Inrig JK, Kanbay M, Patel UD (2008) Chronic kidney disease after hematopoietic cell transplantation: a systematic review. Am J Transplant 8(11):2378–2390

Kersting S, Koomans HA, Hené RJ, Verdonck LF (2007) Acute renal failure after allogeneic myeloablative stem cell transplantation: retrospective analysis of incidence, risk factors and survival. Bone Marrow Transplant 39(6):359–365

Lam AQ, Humphreys BD (2012) Onco-nephrology: AKI in the cancer patient. Clin J Am Soc Nephrol 7(10):1692–1700

Perazella MA (2012) Onco-nephrology: renal toxicities of chemotherapeutic agents. Clin J Am Soc Nephrol 7(10):1713–1721

Pizzo PA, Poplack DG (eds) Ch 29. In: Renal tumors: principles and practice of pediatric oncology. Lippincott Williams

The Kidney and the Tropics 13

Anita Shet

13.1 Introduction

Tropical renal diseases are infectious or toxin-mediated diseases that affect the kidney and occur predominantly in tropical and subtropical regions. The pathogenesis of renal complications in tropical conditions is multifactorial. Factors which are unique to the tropics and which may play a role in specific renal outcomes include the distinct type of prevalent pathogens, vegetation and disease vectors, the increased population density, high prevalence of malnutrition, and the use of local alternative medications. With increasing global travel, tropical diseases are no longer confined only to the tropics but are increasingly seen in nontropical areas as well.

13.2 Classification

1. **Infections**
   (a) ***Parasitic infections***
   Malaria
   Schistosomiasis
   Filariasis
   Visceral leishmaniasis
   (b) ***Bacterial infections***
   Leptospirosis
   Rickettsial infections

A. Shet, MD
Department of Paediatrics,
St John's National Academy of Health Sciences,
Bangalore, KA 560034, India
e-mail: anitashet@gmail.com

K. Phadke et al. (eds.), *Manual of Pediatric Nephrology*,
DOI 10.1007/978-3-642-12483-9_13, © Springer-Verlag Berlin Heidelberg 2014

Enteric pathogens
Renal and genitourinary tuberculosis

(c) ***Viral pathogens***
Viral hemorrhagic fever (dengue, hantavirus, yellow fever virus)

2. **Toxic injuries**
Snakebite nephropathy
Scorpion bites
Natural medicines

13.3 Malaria

Introduction: Malaria is caused by the protozoan *Plasmodium* and is a huge public health burden globally, particularly in children. The overall incidence of malarial nephropathy is low at 2–5 % among those living in endemic areas; however, up to 30 % of nonimmune visitors with malaria develop renal complications (Fig. 13.1).

Transmission: The parasite is transmitted by the Anopheles mosquito. Of the 4 plasmodium species, nephropathy is seen most frequently with *P. falciparum* and rarely with *P. vivax* and *P. ovale*. "Quartan malarial nephropathy" associated with *P. malariae* infections in children causing nephrotic syndrome and chronic renal failure observed in the 1970s in Africa has become extremely rare with no recent reports in the literature (Fig. 13.2).

Clinical Features: The classic features of malaria are spiking fevers with rigors. Other features are malaise, headache, nausea, and hypotension. Chronic anemia and splenomegaly are observed in endemic areas. Severe infection may include acute kidney injury, coma and seizures, pulmonary edema, acute respiratory distress syndrome (ARDS), jaundice, shock, and disseminated intravascular coagulation.

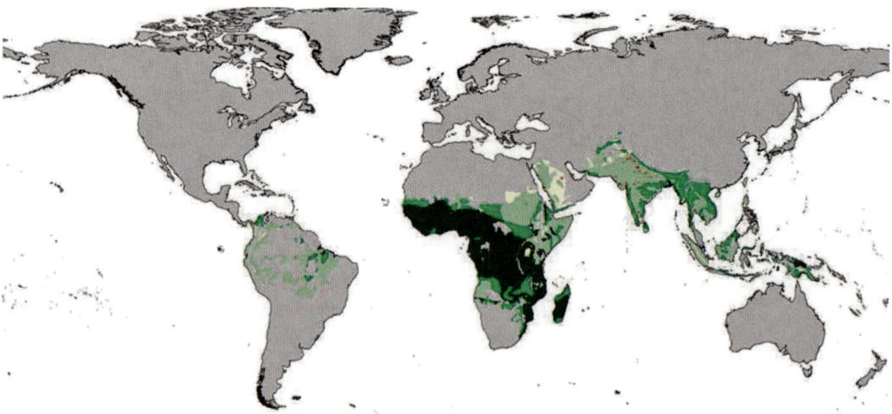

Fig. 13.1 Global distribution of *Plasmodium falciparum*. *Light green*, childhood infection prevalence is <10 %; *medium green*, prevalence 11–50 %; *dark green*, prevalence >50 % (Source: WHO)

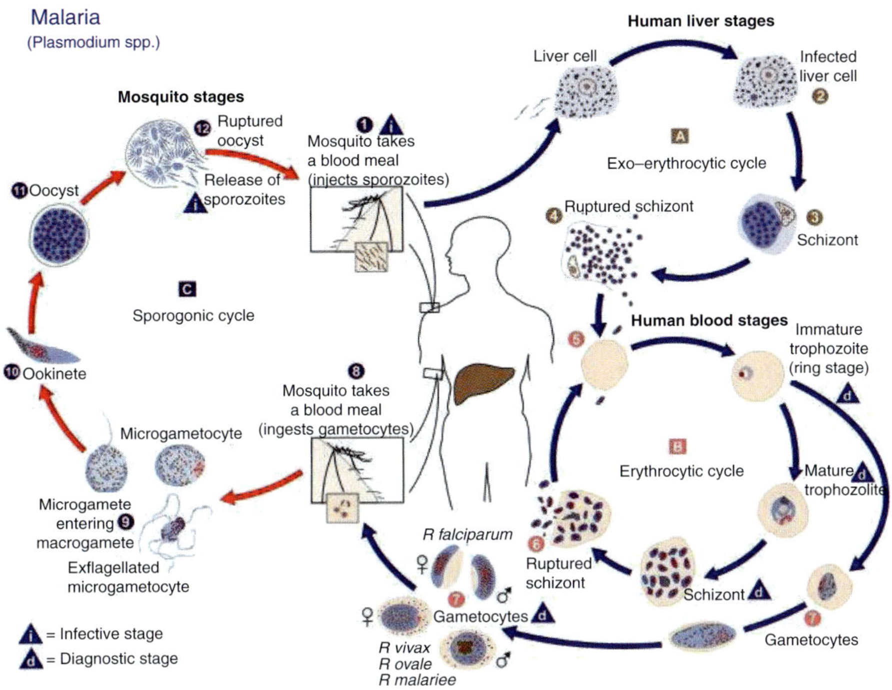

Fig. 13.2 Life cycle of *Plasmodium species* (Source: Public Health Image Library, # 3405)

Renal Involvement: Transient proteinuria in uncomplicated malaria lasts usually less than 1 week after initiation of antimalarial therapy and can be observed in 30 %.

Malarial acute kidney injury (MAKI) is defined as an abrupt reduction (<48 h) in renal function or serum creatinine >3 mg/dl in a child with falciparum malaria (WHO criteria). It is seen in about a third of those with cerebral malaria, and is usually oliguric, and accompanied by hyperkalemia and acidosis.

The causes of MAKI in malaria may be multifactorial:

1. Shock leading to hypotension and reduced renal perfusion.
2. Intravascular hemolysis and hemoglobinuria (black water fever) often associated with use of antimalarial drugs such as quinine, halofantrine, or mefloquine.
3. Disseminated intravascular coagulation (DIC) and rhabdomyolysis are rare causes.
4. Antimalarial drugs may precipitate hemolysis in glucose-6-phosphate dehydrogenase (G6PD)-deficient individuals resulting in hemoglobinuria and AKI.

Renal Pathophysiology: The predominant lesions are acute tubular necrosis, mild proliferative glomerulopathy, and varying degrees of interstitial nephritis. *P. falciparum* is associated with alteration in red cell surface structure resulting in increased cytoadherence to vascular endothelial cells and red cell sequestration, which in turn interferes with microcirculatory flow with subsequent multiorgan involvement. In severe hemolysis, vacuolization of proximal tubular cells and hemoglobin deposition in tubules are seen. Immunofluorescence shows mesangial C3 and IgM deposition. EM shows subendothelial and mesangial electron-dense deposits with granular, fibrillar, and amorphous material. Immune complexes of malarial antigen can be present in the glomerular basement membrane.

Diagnosis: Blood smear examination using thick and thin smears stained with Giemsa stain revealing the presence of asexual forms of *P. falciparum* is diagnostic. Staining with the fluorescent dye acridine orange increases sensitivity. Rapid diagnostic tests (RDTs) that detect the presence of *P. falciparum*-specific antigens are also in use.

Treatment: The main principles of treatment are (1) prompt use of combination antimalarial drugs (quinine or artemisinin derivatives; no dosage adjustment is required in the presence of renal dysfunction unless quinine needs to be given as a parenteral dose beyond 48 h; in this situation, two-thirds dose can be administered), (2) maintenance of fluid and electrolyte balance, (3) renal replacement therapy at the earliest indication, (4) treatment of associations and infections, and (5) careful use of concomitant drugs (avoid nephrotoxic drugs such as aminoglycosides, NSAIDS, and ACE inhibitors). The use of diuretics should be avoided. In severe disease, partial exchange transfusion has been used when the parasite index is >20 % in order to remove infected red blood cells from circulation and reduce parasite burden and also alleviate microcirculatory obstruction, although a clear consensus on indications has not yet been achieved.

Prognosis: Malarial AKI may resolve completely and is not usually associated with chronic renal disease or hypertension. The overall mortality from malarial AKI varies between 15 and 50 %. Survival rates are better when hemodialysis rather than peritoneal dialysis was instituted early.

13.4 Schistosomiasis

Introduction: Schistosomiasis is a highly prevalent helminthic infection, and human pathogenic species include *Schistosoma haematobium* (African subcontinent) and *Schistosoma mansoni* (Latin America) which are associated with renal and bladder involvement.

Transmission: Infection is acquired by contact with freshwater snails, which are the intermediate hosts. The infective agent is the cercaria which penetrates the skin and gains access to the bloodstream and reaches the portal and perivesical venous plexus via lymphatics where it rapidly grows to its adult bisexual form.

13.4.1 *Schistosoma haematobium*

Natural History: For *S. haematobium*, the female lays eggs into the submucosa of the bladder from where they are shed by the urine. The ova cause hypersensitivity reaction in the bladder leading to pseudotubercle formation, fibrosis, bladder outlet obstruction, and cystitis and predispose to squamous cell carcinoma of the bladder.

Renal Involvement: Renal clinical symptoms of *S. haematobium* infections are painful, terminal hematuria; increased frequency; and dysuria.

Renal Pathophysiology: Urine analysis shows RBCs, parasite eggs, and occasionally eosinophiluria (refer to Fig. 13.3). Pyuria and bacteriuria are seen with secondary

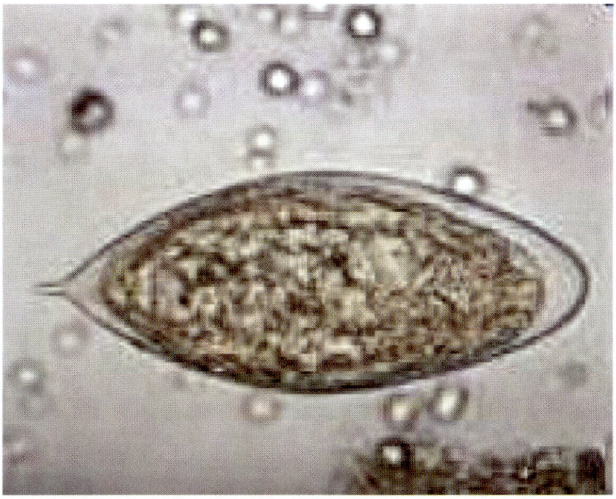

Fig. 13.3 Urine microscopy shows schistosoma ova with terminal spines (Source: CDC, Atlanta, USA)

bacterial infection. Functional consequences depend on extent of fibrosis and include partial obstruction at the lower ureteral ends, bladder neck obstruction, impaired detrusor contractility, vesicoureteral reflux, and hydronephrosis. Chronic infection can predispose towards developing squamous cell carcinoma of the bladder.

13.4.2 *Schistosoma mansoni*

Natural History: *S. mansoni* infects the portal venous plexus and causes colorectal disease and hepatic fibrosis.

Renal Involvement: Nephrotic edema and hypertension are seen in typical hepatosplenic schistosomiasis. Glomerulonephritis may be due to immune-mediated glomerular injury and may present with immune complex deposits in the kidney. Clinical manifestations may include proteinuria, sometimes nephrotic range, edema, and hypertension. Biopsy may show (i) exudative glomerulonephritis, (ii) mesangiocapillary glomerulonephritis, (iii) focal segmental sclerosis, and (iv) renal amyloidosis. IF may show IgG and IgA deposits.

Diagnosis: The gold standard of diagnosis is the demonstration of ova in urinary sediment (*S. haematobium*) or stool (*S. mansoni* and *S. japonicum*).

Treatment: Treatment is praziquantel 40 mg/kg/day in two divided doses for 1 day.

13.5 Filariasis

Introduction: Lymphatic filariasis is caused by the three different types of nematodes: *Wuchereria bancrofti*, *Brugia malayi*, and *Brugia timori*. For global distribution of filariasis, refer to Fig. 13.4.

Transmission: The disease is transmitted by different types of mosquitoes. The female mosquito releases microfilaria into the bloodstream. Infective larvae migrate

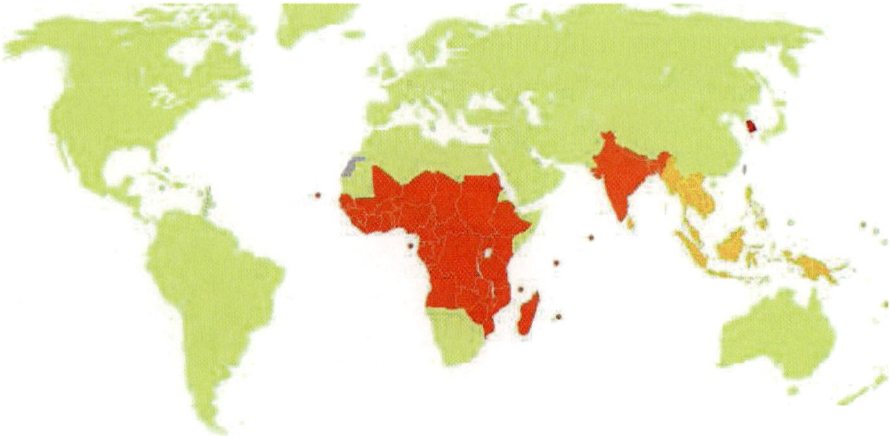

Fig. 13.4 Global distribution of filariasis (Source: World Health Organization 2002)

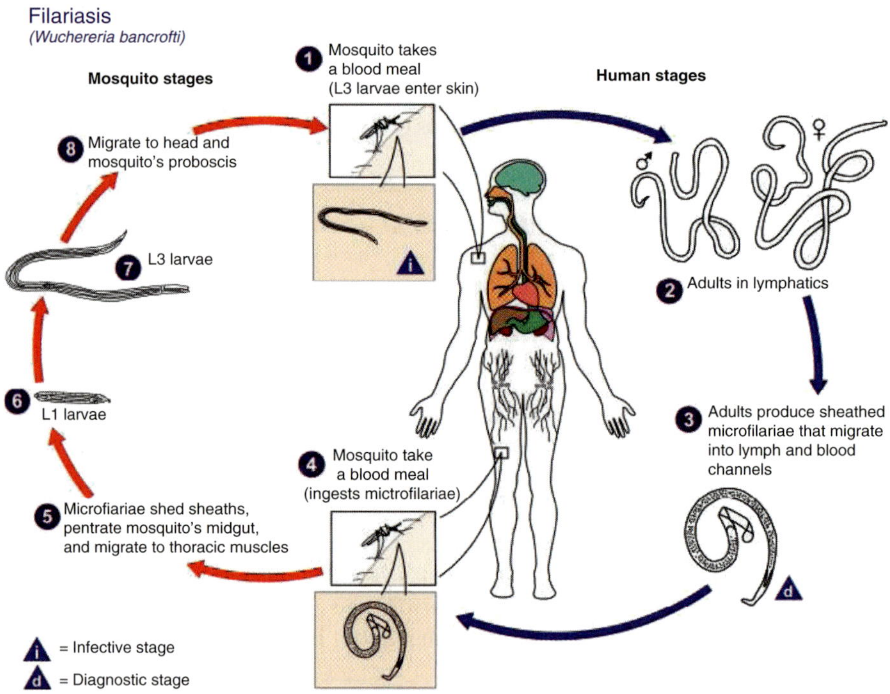

Fig. 13.5 Life cycle of *Wuchereria bancrofti* (Source: Public Health Image Library, #3425)

into the lymphatics where they slowly mature to adult worms, mate, and may reside for decades. Refer to Fig. 13.5 for life cycle of *Wuchereria bancrofti*.

Clinical Features: The disease ranges from asymptomatic subclinical infection to acute manifestations such as adenolymphangitis, filarial fever, and tropical pulmonary eosinophilia and chronic manifestations such as lymphedema (elephantiasis), secondary infections, and renal involvement. Eosinophilia is typically found in all cases.

Renal Involvement: Microscopic hematuria and proteinuria, possibly immune complex glomerulonephritis. Chyluria occurs in bancroftian filariasis when the intestinal lymphatics drain into the renal pelvis, leading fat and protein losses through the urine and causing secondary nutritional deficiencies.

Renal Pathophysiology: Histology shows diffuse mesangial proliferative glomerulonephritis with C3 depositions. Eosinophils and microfilaria may be seen in glomerular capillaries.

Diagnosis: The standard for diagnosis is microscopic detection of microfilariae on a thick blood film. Filarial antigen assays are also available.

Treatment: Diethylcarbamazine (DEC) is the drug of choice and is effective against both microfilaria and adult filarial worms. The earlier recommended dose of this drug was 6 mg/kg given daily for 12 days. Recent studies have shown that a single dose of DEC 6 mg/kg is as effective as the above standard regimen. Other treatment options are ivermectin and albendazole. Annual treatment in endemic areas has been shown to decrease prevalence. Management of chyluria may require special low-fat, high-protein diet with supplementation of middle-chain fatty acids.

13.6 Onchocerciasis

General: Also known as river blindness, this parasitic disease is found in sub-Saharan Africa and sometimes in Central and South America and is caused by the roundworm, *Onchocerca volvulus*. Humans acquire onchocerciasis through the bite of *Simulium* black flies. Skin involvement is common and consists of intense pruritus and inflammation resulting in papules, plaques, hyperpigmentation, and widespread lichenified onchodermatitis. Ocular involvement is also common, often leading to blindness.

Renal Involvement: Onchocerca volvulus is associated with higher incidence of proteinuria and nephrotic syndrome in hyperendemic regions in Africa. Histology can show different types of glomerulonephritis (minimal change, mesangioproliferative, chronic sclerosing GN). Onchocercal antigens as well as IgM, IgG, and C3 can be detected on IF. Treatment with diethylcarbamazine may help to resolve early glomerular lesions but usually fails to treat renal lesions once nephrotic syndrome is manifested.

13.7 Visceral Leishmaniasis (Kala-azar)

Introduction: This zoonosis is caused by Leishmania species, obligate intracellular parasites of mononuclear phagocytes. Three species, *L. donovani* (Asia and East Africa), *L. chagasi* (South America), and *L. infantum* (Mediterranean region), are responsible for the “visceral” manifestations.

Transmission: The vector is the female phlebotomine sand fly, and there are several mammalian hosts including canines, rodents, and man. The incubation period ranges from 2 to 6 months.

Clinical Features: A cutaneous ulcer may develop at the site of the primary bite. Typical manifestations are fever, anorexia, weight loss, massive splenomegaly, and hepatomegaly. Hematological abnormalities such as anemia, leukopenia, and thrombocytopenia are also seen.

Renal Involvement: May occur in 50 % of those with visceral leishmaniasis and manifests as proteinuria, microscopic hematuria, or pyuria. AKI and acute interstitial nephritis have also been reported. In addition, the common modality of treatment, antimony compounds, may be associated with renal dysfunction.

Renal Pathophysiology: Mesangial proliferative GN or a focal proliferative GN, or a generalized interstitial nephritis with interstitial edema, and focal tubular degeneration. Immunofluorescence may show deposition of IgG, IgM, and C3 within the glomeruli. Electron-dense deposits in the basement membrane and mesangium may be seen through EM.

Diagnosis: Direct visualization of amastigote forms of the parasite in Giemsa- or Wright-stained tissue specimens leads to definitive diagnosis. Serological tests are not widely available.

Treatment: Amphotericin B is the main treatment. Pentavalent antimonial agents such as sodium stibogluconate were used earlier but are associated with severe toxicity, as well as high drug resistance in India.

Prognosis: Untreated visceral leishmaniasis is nearly always fatal. Renal disease is mild and typically resolves after treatment.

13.8 Leptospirosis

Introduction: Leptospirosis is a zoonosis with a high prevalence in tropical areas and is caused by a filamentous spirochaete belonging to the genus *Leptospira. Leptospira interrogans* is the only human pathogenic strain. Disease occurs throughout the year, with an increase in incidence seen during the monsoon season, or after natural disasters such as floods or hurricanes.

Transmission: The common vectors for this infection are wild and domesticated mammals such as rodents, dogs, pigs, cattle, horses, and others. The pathogen can survive for long periods in renal tubules of infected asymptomatic animals and up to months in untreated water. Human infection occurs incidently through contact with water or soil contaminated by urine of infected animals. The usual portals of entry are abraded skin and exposed mucosae.

Natural History: Disease manifestation varies from subclinical infection to self-limited anicteric febrile illness to severe, potentially fatal disease. After an incubation period of 2–26 days, the majority of those infected present with a mild anicteric illness. Only 10 % become severely ill with jaundice and multiorgan involvement in Weil's disease which is associated with a mortality of 50 %.

Clinical Features: The usual illness follows a biphasic course. The leptospiremic phase is characterized by high fever with chills, headache, myalgias, skin rashes, nausea, vomiting, and conjunctival effusion for 3–9 days, followed by 2 days of defervescence. Subsequently, the immune phase sets in, featuring recurrence of fever, aseptic meningitis, and uveitis. The severe form or Weil's disease is constituted by renal insufficiency, hepatic dysfunction, thrombocytopenia, hemorrhagic manifestations, myocarditis, and high mortality.

Renal Involvement: Renal involvement is almost universal in leptospirosis and includes proteinuria, pyuria, hematuria, and hyaline and granular casts even in absence of renal dysfunction. The incidence of leptospirosis-induced acute kidney injury varies from 10 to 60 % of infected patients and is typically associated with polyuria and hypokalemia with increased fractional excretion of potassium. Hypomagnesemia and hypophosphatemia may also be present. Hypotension is also found in several cases and is often unresponsive to volume expansion and inotropic support.

Renal Pathophysiology: Leptospiral nephropathy is characterized by interstitial nephritis and tubular damage with relative glomerular sparing. Histopathological features include tubular necrosis and tubulointerstitial inflammation with infiltration by lymphocytes, plasma cells, macrophages, and polymorphonuclear leukocytes. In addition, glomerular mesangial hyperplasia with C3 and IgM deposition and, occasionally, glomerular infiltration of inflammatory cells can be found.

Diagnosis: Diagnosis can be made by serologic testing using IgM-specific dot enzyme-linked immunosorbent assay or microscopic agglutination test (MAT). Direct smear of lesions using dark field microscopy to demonstrate the organisms can be used in some cases. Culture of organisms from blood or urine is less frequently done.

Treatment: Treatment should be instituted as soon as the diagnosis is suspected as it shortens the clinical course and severity of infection. Penicillin G (200,000–250,000 U/kg/day in divided doses every 4–6 h) is recommended for serious infection. Less serious infections can be treated with doxycycline (2 mg/kg/day divided into two doses for children >8 years of age) or amoxicillin (50 g/kg/day in three divided doses). Duration of treatment is 7–14 days. Supportive management includes correction of hypotension and fluid and electrolyte imbalance. Dialysis may be necessary in severe AKI.

Prognosis: Poor prognostic factors include older age, hypotension, pulmonary complications, hyperbilirubinemia, and hyperkalemia. Children have better outcomes compared to adults. Survivors may have a residual defect in tubular concentrating ability.

13.9 Rickettsial Infections

Introduction: Rickettsioses are important emerging infections caused by infection with a family of microorganisms that have both viral and bacterial features.

Transmission: Arthropods such as ticks, lice, and mites are the common vectors, and infection occurs when humans get bitten by these infected vectors.

Clinical Features: Infected individuals present with an acute febrile illness, erythematous rashes, and widespread vasculitis.

Renal Involvement: Subclinical renal involvement secondary to vasculitis probably occurs in many of the rickettsial diseases. In certain rickettsiosis, Rocky Mountain spotted fever (*Rickettsia rickettsii*), tick typhus (*Rickettsia conorii*), and Q fever (*Coxiella burnetii*), clinical renal involvement may be more common and may manifest as elevated creatinine and urea along with metabolic acidosis.

Renal Pathophysiology: Rickettsia multiply in endothelial cells causing focal areas of endothelial cell proliferation, perivascular mononuclear cell infiltration, and thrombosis. Renal biopsy shows interstitial vasculitis and acute tubular necrosis.

Diagnosis: Serology is the mainstay of diagnosis and is based on detection of IgM antibodies to species-specific rickettsial antigens. Previously, the Weil-Felix assay, a nonspecific test that detected the presence of cross-reacting antibodies, was used but is no longer recommended due to its low sensitivity and specificity.

Treatment: Doxycycline (2.2 mg/kg every 12 h) for 1–2 weeks is indicated for children of any age along with intensive support of shock and multiorgan failure as necessary. Acute dialysis may be required until renal function returns to normal.

13.10 Enteric Pathogens

Enteric infections can cause hypovolemia and acute kidney injury of prerenal etiology. In addition, *Escherichia coli*, Yersinia, Campylobacter, and Salmonella have been associated with different forms of glomerulonephritis. Shigella dysenteriae and E. coli 0157:H7 can cause diarrhea-associated HUS (refer to Chap. 3.7.4).

13.10.1 Salmonellosis

Typhoid fever caused by *Salmonella typhi* is characterized by fever, malaise, and hepatosplenomegaly. Renal involvement is rarely severe, but >50 % show asymptomatic glomerular involvement with abnormal urine analysis (hematuria, proteinuria, usually <1 g/24 h) during the febrile phase. Acute tubular necrosis might occur in most severe cases. Significant renal disease occurs in <6 % with mesangial proliferation and IgM, IgG, and C3 deposition on IF. Salmonella Vi antigens have been demonstrated within the glomeruli. Recovery is usually complete and occurs in 2–3 weeks.

13.10.2 Yersinia Infections

Infections caused by *Yersinia enterocolitica* and *Y. pseudotuberculosis* are characterized by fever, abdominal pain, and diarrhea. Transient proteinuria is found in

25 % of acute infections and elevated creatinine in 10 % of cases. Renal biopsy shows mild mesangial glomerulonephritis or IgA nephropathy. *Y. pseudotuberculosis* is also known to cause tubulointerstitial nephritis causing acute kidney injury, especially in children. Mild degrees of proteinuria, glycosuria, and sterile pyuria are also found. AKI develops 1–3 weeks after onset of fever and follows a benign course with complete recovery.

13.10.3 Cholera

Epidemic diarrheal illness caused by *Vibrio cholerae* may sometimes be associated with acute kidney injury and rhabdomyolysis. Rapid intervention with fluid replacement is essential to prevent hypovolemic shock and circulatory collapse in most cases. Doxycycline is useful in some cases for shortening the duration of symptoms.

13.11 Renal and Genitourinary Tuberculosis

Renal tuberculosis (TB) is rarely reported in children, and most cases are reported in adults. In recent years, there appears to be a reemergence of renal tuberculosis due to HIV infection. Following hematogenous spread, several renal cortical foci are formed, although these foci have little tendency to progress. Renal involvement usually occurs years to decades after the primary infection, although several cases of short incubation period in children are reported. Among very young children, renal tuberculosis is seen along with military TB.

Clinical Features: The onset may be insidious and may manifest when the bladder is involved. Urinary frequency, dysuria, hematuria, and flank pain may be seen, along with fever, loin pain, and hypertension. Lab evaluation can reveal sterile acid pyuria and hematuria. AKI due to tuberculosis is very rare. Tuberculosis of the epididymis presents as a scrotal swelling with later development of a hard, craggy epididymis. Caseation necrosis leads to the development of sinuses.

Diagnosis: The definitive diagnosis is the isolation of *Mycobacterium tuberculosis* from the urine or directly from the renal or genitourinary lesion. Newer modalities like PCR are useful, although limited by availability factors and false-positive rates. Needle aspiration or renal biopsy may demonstrate granulomas or acid-fast bacteria. Tuberculous skin test (TST) may be used as an adjunct diagnostic aid. Imaging studies such as ultrasound and CT scan may be helpful in identifying kidney lesions. The most common findings of renal parenchymal masses, scarring, calcification, cavitation, and hydronephrosis due to stricture may be seen in imaging studies.

Renal Pathophysiology: In classical TB of the kidney, renal damage is caused by obstruction or massive caseous destruction. Mesangial proliferation, which is not usually seen with other forms of interstitial nephritis, is also common. TB granulomatous interstitial nephritis has been well described and is thought to be secondary to the immune response against TB.

Treatment: Treatment includes combination antituberculosis therapy for 12 months. Either daily or intermittent therapy has been recommended. Reconstructive surgery is useful in the case of ureteral stricture or contracted bladder. Radical surgery in the form of a nephrectomy may be done for a nonfunctioning kidney especially if hypertension is present.

13.12 Viral Hemorrhagic Fevers

Viral hemorrhagic fevers are diseases caused by different families of RNA viruses that are transmitted through the bite of an infected arthropod or by inhalation of particles of rodent excreta.

13.12.1 Dengue

Introduction: Dengue virus is a *flavivirus* transmitted by the mosquito *Aedes aegypti* and other *Aedes* species. There are four dengue serotypes that are closely related antigenically; infection with one serotype produces lifelong immunity to that serotype but poorly protects against the remaining serotypes. The global dengue belt is depicted in Fig. 13.6.

Clinical Features: After an incubation period of 3–14 days, the infection is characterized by biphasic fever, malaise, rash, and lymphadenopathy. The classic features of dengue hemorrhagic fever (DHF) are fever, minor or major hemorrhagic manifestations, thrombocytopenia, and evidence of increased capillary permeability which can result in serositis, hypoalbuminemia, and raised hematocrit. In 20–30 % of cases, DHF is complicated by shock (dengue shock syndrome) as well as hypotension.

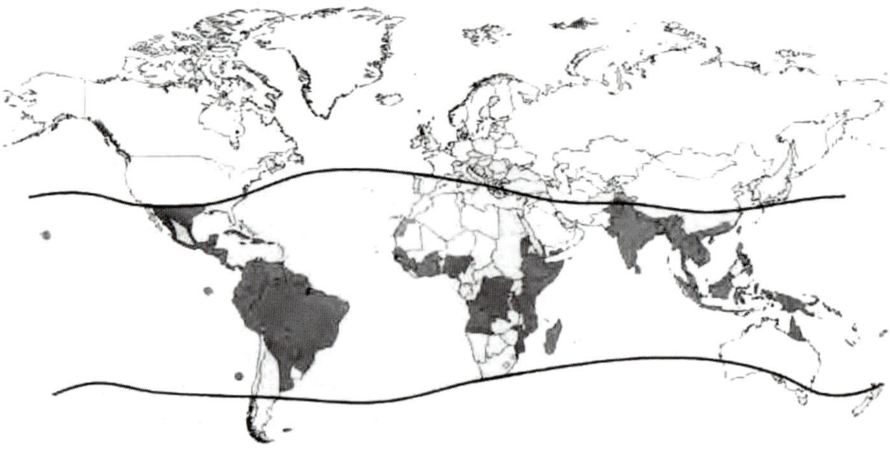

Fig. 13.6 The global dengue belt (Source: WHO 2008)

Renal Involvement: Renal involvement is not common. Severe dengue infections can give rise to shock and multiorgan dysfunction, leading to prerenal AKI and acute tubular necrosis. Other renal manifestations include azotemia, proteinuria, glomerulonephritis, and hemolytic-uremic syndrome.

Renal Pathophysiology: Histopathology shows mesangioproliferative glomerulonephritis, endothelial swelling, interstitial edema, perivascular infiltration by mononuclear cells, and tubular degeneration. IF shows deposits of IgM, IgG, and C3.

Diagnosis: Clinical criteria are used in making a diagnosis of dengue fever and may be confirmed by lab parameters. In early infection, viral antigen detection in serum or cerebrospinal fluid using immunofluorescence or ELISA may be helpful. PCR may also be used for virus detection. Serological diagnosis may be performed once the fever has subsided and the second week has begun.

Treatment: Management of dengue is supportive and includes fever control, fluid management, and control of bleeding. Fluid management that is guided by clinical response and serial hematocrit levels is currently practised. Full management guidelines may be found in the WHO 2009 dengue management document. Renal replacement therapy is rarely indicated unless there is fluid overload or severe multiorgan failure.

Prognosis: Complete recovery is the norm with adequate supportive management.

Dengue-Like Viruses: ***These*** are distributed globally and can have similar clinical manifestations. Some examples are as follows:

- Chikungunya (Togavirus)—Africa, India, and Southeast Asia
- O'nyong-nyong (Togavirus)—East Africa
- West Nile fever (Flavivirus)—Europe, Africa, Middle East, India, and North America

13.12.2 Hantavirus

Introduction: Hantavirus infection is a rare tropical disease of hemorrhagic fever with renal syndrome caused by an RNA virus in the Bunyaviridae family. Previously, hantaviruses have been recognized to cause two separate syndromes: hemorrhagic fever with renal syndrome (HFRS) in Eurasia and hantavirus pulmonary syndrome (HPS) in the Americas, although this dichotomy is increasingly becoming indistinct as the disease has overlapping features and is found in other parts of the world.

Transmission: Rodents are the reservoir; infection to humans occurs via inhalation of rodent excreta or direct inoculation through skin cuts or abrasions.

Clinical Features: After incubation period of 2–5 weeks, the disease presents with flu-like symptoms. In hantavirus pulmonary syndrome, severe respiratory distress may occur. In severe cases, thrombocytopenia and disseminated intravascular coagulation (DIC) occur.

Renal Involvement: Renal involvement is common with proteinuria, hematuria, pyuria, and decreased GFR. In severe cases, increased vascular permeability and vascular endothelial injury result in hypovolemia, decreased renal perfusion, and acute kidney injury.

Renal Pathophysiology: Histopathology shows acute tubular necrosis, interstitial edema and hemorrhages, and later interstitial monocyte infiltration. Glomerular changes are less remarkable, showing mild hypercellularity and IgM, IgG, and C3 deposits.

Diagnosis: Serological tests are used for diagnosis.

Treatment: There is no specific treatment for the virus; dialysis and supportive measures for renal failure may be required.

Prognosis: Recovery is generally complete; chronic renal failure and hypertension are rare.

13.12.3 Yellow Fever

Introduction: Yellow fever is endemic in the African subcontinent and is caused by the yellow fever virus, belonging to family Flaviviridae and transmitted by Aedes aegypti mosquito. Despite the presence of the vector, this disease is not seen in Asia.

Clinical Features: The spectrum of clinical manifestations is variable, ranging from mild febrile illness to severe hemorrhagic fever.

Renal Involvement: Acute kidney injury with oliguria may occur within 5 days of the severe form of the disease with hemorrhagic manifestations, jaundice, and DIC.

Renal Pathophysiology: Histology may show features of acute tubular necrosis in severe cases.

Diagnosis: Serology with detection of specific IgM is the main method of diagnosis, although sometimes PCR may also be used.

Treatment: Management is mainly supportive and involves treatment of AKI; renal replacement may be necessary in severe cases.

13.13 Snakebite Nephropathy

Introduction: Snakebites are common in the tropics and are caused by either hemotoxic or myotoxic snakes. Most bites are attributed to snakes belonging to Colubridae, Elapidae, Viperidae, and Hydrophidae families. *Bothrops* and *Crotalus* snakes are common in Latin America. For differentiation between poisonous and nonpoisonous snakes, refer to Figs. 13.7.

Clinical Features: Clinical symptoms can vary from local pain and swelling to systemic involvement with hypotension, hemorrhage, disseminated intravascular coagulation, abdominal pain, central nervous system symptoms, and paralysis.

Renal Involvement: Proteinuria, hematuria, pigmenturia, and acute renal failure are common renal manifestations. Proteinuria is usually transient and mild (<500 mg/day), except after Russell's viper bites where nephrotic range proteinuria may be seen. Hematuria (either microscopic or macroscopic) is often seen after hemotoxic snakebites, the incidence as high as 35 %. Pigmenturia (hemoglobinuria or myoglobinuria) is associated in occurrence with intravascular hemolysis or rhabdomyolysis, respectively.

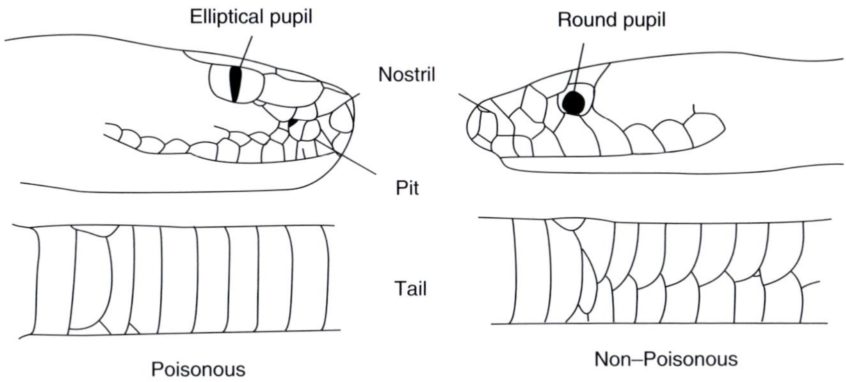

Figs. 13.7 Distinguishing a poisonous from a nonpoisonous snake. (1) Pupil shape: poisonous snakes have elliptical pupils as opposed to round pupils in nonpoisonous snakes. (2) A distinctive nostril or "pit" is seen in poisonous snakes. (3) Scale arrangement: the underside scales are arranged in a single row in poisonous snakes (Source: WHO)

Acute kidney injury (AKI) manifests as oliguria, hyperkalemia, and hyperuricemia, with high CPK and LDH levels, and may be due to several reasons:

1. Shock leading to prerenal AKI.
2. Hemoglobinuria due to hemolysis and myoglobinuria due to rhabdomyolysis.
3. DIC with fibrin thrombi in the glomeruli leading to microangiopathic hemolytic anemia and thrombocytopenia, with a hemolytic-uremic syndrome-like picture.
4. Direct nephrotoxicity of the venom.
5. Sepsis and hypersensitivity to antivenom are rare causes.

Renal Pathophysiology: Snake venoms can cause cellular injury through enzymes and cytokines and initiate a sepsis-like process. AKI can occur due to shock or due to intravascular hemolysis (hemotoxic snake) or rhabdomyolysis (myotoxic snake).

Renal Histopathology: Renal biopsy and histology can show a varied picture:

1. Tubulointerstitial: most common; degeneration of tubular cells, necrosis, interstitial infiltrates, and edema.
2. Glomerular: focal segmental mesangial proliferation, areas of necrosis, thrombosis, and mesangiolysis. IF may show IgM and C3 deposits occasionally.
3. Cortical necrosis: necrosis of all elements with thrombi in the vessels.
4. Vascular: segmental necrotizing vasculitis.

Treatment: Management includes specific antivenom treatment; monovalent antivenoms are preferred over polyvalent. In situations where antivenom is not available, plasmapheresis or blood exchange has been used. Early and frequent peritoneal dialysis or hemodialysis is important for survival. Urine alkalinization has a role if there is pigmenturia or if the snake is known to be myotoxic/hemotoxic and renal failure is not yet established. Caution is necessitated as administration of sodium bicarbonate in the setting of acute renal failure can be dangerous, leading to further fluid overload and hyperosmolality.

Prognosis: With adequate treatment, renal recovery is generally complete and takes 2–4 weeks. Residual renal dysfunction and cortical calcification may be sequelae of cortical necrosis.

13.14 Scorpion Bite Nephropathy

Certain scorpions present in tropical countries may be responsible for causing acute kidney injury following a sting. The onset of disease is characterized by the occurrence of hemoglobinuria within 24 h of the sting. Other manifestations include oliguria, edema, hemolytic anemia, and hemolytic jaundice. Renal pathophysiology includes acute tubular necrosis and disseminated intravascular coagulation. AKI can develop within a few days after the sting. Renal biopsies often show mesangial proliferation, variable degrees of tubular changes, and mild interstitial infiltration.

13.15 Natural Medicines Causing Nephropathies

The use of alternative medicines derived from plants and animals is widespread globally, particularly in the tropics. In India and Africa, up to 60–80 % of the population depend on traditional healers and untested herbal medications. These medications are not tested for safety, and since the kidney plays an important role in their metabolism and excretion, acute kidney injury is a common manifestation of their toxicity. In addition, there is easy availability of over-the-counter medications, which may be either allopathic approved medications which are used without a valid prescription or indigenous medications which can cause renal injury. The usual renal lesions include acute tubular necrosis, cortical necrosis, and interstitial nephritis. A high index of suspicion is required to prevent missed diagnosis and to reduce mortality.

Natural medicine	Indications for use	Mechanism of kidney injury
St John's wort, derived from *hypericum perforatum*	Depression and anxiety	Induces cytochrome P450 activity. Can precipitate AKI in kidney transplant patients due to allograft rejection
Alfalfa juice, noni juice	Nutritional supplement	Hyperkalemia
Saw palmetto/ chlorophyll	Benign prostatic hyperplasia	Hyperkalemia
Ginkgo biloba	Memory stimulant	Hemorrhagic complications
Cape aloe (aloin or aloe extract)	Hypertension, eczema, constipation	Hemorrhagic gastroenteritis and acute tubular necrosis
Propolis	Anti-inflammatory, antibiotic, and dietary supplement	Acute kidney injury

Natural medicine	Indications for use	Mechanism of kidney injury
Hydrazine sulfate	Cancer cure	Acute kidney injury
Cat's claw	Cirrhosis, gastritis, gonorrhea, and rheumatism	Acute kidney injury
Aristolochia pistolochia	Weight loss supplement	Acute kidney injury
White willow bark	Back pain, fever, osteoarthritis, headache, and dysmenorrhea	Acute kidney injury
Raw carp bile	Fever, cough, hypertension, stress	Acute kidney injury

Conclusions

Tropical diseases are a well-known cause of acute kidney injury. However, the majority are preventable with early diagnosis and treatment. In almost all cases, treatment of underlying disease and providing supportive care are critical in alleviating the renal damage. Appropriate referral and judicious use of fluids, electrolytes, and renal replacement therapy are major contributory factors towards an uneventful recovery in most cases.

Suggested Reading

Andrade L, de Francesco DE, Seguro AC (2008) Leptospiral nephropathy. Semin Nephrol 28(4):383–394

Avner ED (ed) (2009) Pediatric nephrology. Springer, Berlin

Burdmann EA (2008) Acute kidney injury in the tropics. Semin Nephrol 28(4):319

Das BS (2008) Renal failure in malaria. J Vector Borne Dis 45(2):83–97

Geary DF, Franz S (eds) (2008) Comprehensive pediatric nephrology. Elsevier Health Sciences, Philadelphia

Guerrant RL (ed) (2006) Tropical infectious diseases. Elsevier, Inc, Philadelphia

Jha V, Rathi M (2008) Natural medicines causing acute kidney injury. Semin Nephrol 28(4):416–428

Lima EQ, Nogueira ML (2008) Viral hemorrhagic fever-induced acute kidney injury. Semin Nephrol 28(4):409–415

Nguansangiam S, Day NP, Hien TT, Mai NT, Chaisri U, Riganti M et al (2007) A quantitative ultrastructural study of renal pathology in fatal Plasmodium falciparum malaria. Trop Med Int Health 12(9):1037–1050

Sarah L, Larry P, Charles P (eds) (2008) Principles and practice of pediatric infectious diseases, 3rd edn. Elsevier, Philadelphia

Schrier RW (ed) (2007) Diseases of the kidney and urinary tract. Lippincott Williams & Wilkins, Philadelphia

Sitprija V (2006) Snakebite nephropathy. Nephrology (Carlton) 11(5):442–448

World Health Organization (2009) Dengue guidelines for diagnosis, treatment, prevention and control. World Health Organization, Geneva, Available at: www.searo.who.int/LinkFiles/Dengue_Guideline-dengue.pdf

HIV and the Kidney

14

Anita Shet

14.1 Introduction

Renal disease is an increasingly important complication of HIV infection in children. In the era before highly active antiretroviral therapy (HAART) was widely available, HIV-associated nephropathy was common in perinatally infected children, and up to 40 % of children were found to have clinical evidence of renal disease. With the availability of HAART, there is increased survival, and HIV has been transformed into a chronic disease. HIV-associated renal disease is being identified in more children at later ages and continues to be a significant reason for morbidity and mortality.

Tests for HIV

Tests for HIV
Diagnostic
HIV rapid antibody test
HIV ELISA
HIV western blot
DNA PCR (for infants only)
Monitoring tests
CD4 T cell count
HIV viral load (RNA copies/ml)

A. Shet, MD
Department of Pediatrics,
St John's National Academy of Health Sciences,
Bangalore, KA 560034, India
e-mail: anitashet@gmail.com

K. Phadke et al. (eds.), *Manual of Pediatric Nephrology*,
DOI 10.1007/978-3-642-12483-9_14, © Springer-Verlag Berlin Heidelberg 2014

14.2 Spectrum of HIV-Associated Renal Disease

Children with HIV infection can present with a wide spectrum of renal abnormalities, which may be due to direct HIV-specific viral activity in renal tissues, due to complications of drugs used in the setting of HIV disease or renal disease specifically associated with HIV co-infections and comorbidities. The age of onset of renal disease is variable and may be found in children as young as 2 years of age.

14.2.1 HIV-Associated Nephropathy (HIVAN)

14.2.1.1 Introduction

HIVAN is the most frequent renal manifestation of HIV infection and consists of glomerular and tubulointerstitial disease. It can occur at any stage of HIV disease, although it is most commonly seen in advanced stages with CD4 T cell counts <200 cells/mm^3.

14.2.1.2 Timeline

Children may present with renal manifestations at any stage of HIV disease. Typically, proteinuria or azotemia develops 2–5 years after the onset of HIV infection. Mean duration from the onset of proteinuria to development of ESRD ranges from 8 months to 3 years.

14.2.1.3 Pathogenesis

HIVAN is established as a result of direct HIV infection of the renal epithelium.

14.2.1.4 Genetic Aspects

HIVAN is found more often in certain races, such as African Americans, and among those with a family history of ESRD, suggesting a genetic predisposition to HIVAN development.

14.2.1.5 Clinical Features

HIV-infected children may present with classic features of nephrotic syndrome, including heavy proteinuria, oedema and hypoalbuminemia. Proteinuria is the earliest and most consistent clinical finding in HIVAN and is a useful screening tool. Other presenting features include haematuria, hypertension or manifestations of renal tubular acidosis and acute kidney injury. The presence of "urine microcysts", which are tubular epithelial cells grouped together in the urine sediment, indicates HIVAN with renal tubular injury.

14.2.1.6 Ultrasonography

Renal ultrasound classically shows enlarged, echogenic kidneys.

14.2.1.7 Unique Histological Findings

A characteristic finding is "collapsing" focal and segmental glomerulosclerosis with podocyte hypertrophy and hyperplasia. Marked podocyte hyperplasia may sometimes cause obliteration of the urinary space, forming "pseudocrescents".

Other spectra of glomerular changes include minimal change disease, mesangial hyperplasia and lupus-like nephritis. Tubular changes include microcystic tubular dilation with interstitial cellular infiltrates. The presence of numerous tubuloreticular inclusions within the cytoplasm of glomerular and peritubular capillary endothelial cells is characteristic of HIVAN.

14.2.1.8 Treatment

The primary treatment strategy for childhood HIV-related renal disease includes direct control of HIV infection using antiretroviral therapy. Without HAART, HIVAN can progress to ESRD within weeks to months.

Steps in Specific Management of HIVAN

1. Highly active antiretroviral therapy (HAART)	Standard combination treatment for HIV infection. Observational studies have indicated resolution of HIVAN after starting HAART. HAART can also slow down the rate of progression of HIVAN to ESRD.
2. Angiotensin-converting enzyme inhibitors (ACE inhibitors)	Can be used when HAART alone is not enough to resolve proteinuria. In children, improvement of proteinuria and hypertension has been observed.
3. Steroids	Good response seen in children with HIV-associated minimal change disease. No observed sustained benefit in HIVAN.
4. Cyclosporine	Observational studies reveal remission of proteinuria among children with steroid-resistant renal disease that is not responsive to HAART.

Clinical Vignette

A 4-year-old girl presented with fever, facial swelling and abdominal distension during the previous month. She had 2 episodes of lower respiratory tract infection in the past 6 months. On examination, she had facial oedema and generalized lymphadenopathy. She was moderately underweight and mildly stunted. Her blood pressure was normal. Systemic examination revealed hepatosplenomegaly with ascites. Other examination findings were normal.

Her laboratory tests revealed haemoglobin of 92 g/l and white cell count of 17.4×10^9/l with 46 % neutrophils and 52 % lymphocytes. Her serum albumin was 29 g/l, with normal liver transaminases (ALT = 25 U/l, AST = 32 U/l) and normal cholesterol, blood urea nitrogen, serum creatinine and electrolytes. Her urine albumin was 3+ on three occasions and her urine protein/creatinine ratio was 1.4. Further testing revealed a positive HIV rapid antibody test. Her mother was also tested and found to be HIV infected. Her father has passed away 2 years ago due to a “lung infection”, but no records were available. The child's CD4 T cell count was 346 cells/mm^3 and CD4 percent was 14.2 %. A renal ultrasound showed bilateral enlarged echogenic kidneys, and a renal biopsy showed mesangial hyperplasia and microcystic tubular dilatation.

A diagnosis of perinatally acquired HIV infection and HIV-associated nephropathy (HIVAN) was made, and she was started on a three-drug antiretroviral therapy (ART) regimen consisting of zidovudine, lamivudine and nevirapine. A month after starting this treatment, proteinuria had disappeared and ascites had resolved. On follow-up at 3 months, she was asymptomatic, her weight had improved by 4 kg, and her CD4 count had increased to 502 cells/mm^3 (CD4 percentage: 18 %), and physical and laboratory evaluation revealed complete resolution of HIVAN.

14.2.2 Other HIV-Related Intrinsic Diseases of the Kidney

14.2.2.1 HIV-Associated Haemolytic Uremic Syndrome (HUS) and Thrombotic Microangiopathy

This is an atypical, fatal form of HUS characterized by an insidious onset, preserved urine output and the absence of preceding diarrhoea. There are features of renal insufficiency, microangiopathic haemolytic anaemia and thrombocytopenia. Children often present before 2 years of age and may progress rapidly to ESRD or to death from infectious or bleeding complications. Renal pathology consists of thrombotic microangiopathic glomerular lesions with accumulation of fibrin and accompanying microcystic tubular changes.

14.2.2.2 HIV-Associated Glomerulonephritis (GN)

1. IgA nephropathy with immune complexes containing HIV proteins
2. Membranous GN similar to lupus nephritis
3. Membranoproliferative GN associated with mixed cryoglobulinemia

14.2.2.3 Tubulopathy

Common renal tubular disorders in HIV-infected children include hypercalciuria, nephrocalcinosis, crystalluria, hyperchloremia and metabolic acidosis, resulting in sodium-, potassium- and phosphate-wasting states. These metabolic complications may be in part responsible for the growth impairment frequently seen in HIV-infected children.

14.2.3 Renal Manifestations of HIV Disease

HIV-Associated Proteinuria

Early finding in HIV-associated nephropathy is a manifestation seen in many conditions.

Glomerulopathy	Post-infectious glomerulonephritis IgA nephropathy Haemolytic uremic syndrome HIV-associated glomerulopathy
Tubulopathy	HIV-associated renal tubular diseases
Others	Co-infections (hepatitis C virus) Renal tuberculosis

HIV-Associated Pyuria

(centrifuged urinary sediment of >4 leukocytes per high-power field)

Infections	Opportunistic infections with renal involvement (e.g. *Mycobacterium tuberculosis*) Pyelonephritis and cystitis by gram-negative bacteria, *neisseria gonorrhoea*
Interstitial nephritis	Cytomegalovirus, adenovirus and BK virus Drug-induced interstitial nephritis
Renal calculi and crystalluria	Associated with some antiretroviral drugs (e.g. indinavir) Other drugs used in the setting of HIV (e.g. acyclovir)

Haematuria in HIV-Infected Children

Origin	Urinalysis picture	Causes
Renal causes	Dysmorphic erythrocytes	Glomerulonephritis Nephrotic syndrome
Post-renal causes	Non-dysmorphic erythrocytes	Renal calculus Crystal aggregates Renal or bladder carcinoma Infection in urogenital system
Other	Erythrocytes absent from urinalysis	Haemoglobinuria Myoglobinuria

Acute Kidney Injury (AKI) in HIV-Infected Children

There is a wide range of HIV-related conditions that can have the final common pathway of acute kidney injury.

Classification of AKI	Pathogenesis and aetiology
Pre-renal	Intravascular volume depletion (vomiting, diarrhoea, dehydration)
	Sepsis, infections that result in capillary leakage
	Hypotension
	Decreased renal blood flow
Renal	Acute tubular necrosis
	Interstitial nephritis (antibiotics, CMV infection)
	Immune complex glomerulonephritis
	Thrombotic thrombocytopenic purpura
Post-renal	Tubular obstruction (acyclovir)
	Intrinsic ureteral obstruction (calculus, indinavir crystals)
	Extrinsic ureteral obstruction (lymphoma, massive lymphadenopathy)

14.2.4 Secondary Renal Effects

14.2.4.1 HIV-Associated Opportunistic Infections

Specific opportunistic infections affecting the kidney may be seen in the setting of HIV infection:

1. BK virus-associated haemorrhagic cystitis and nephropathy.
2. Hepatitis C virus-associated membranoproliferative GN.
3. Fungal infections such as cryptococcosis, renal candidiasis is a possibility.

14.2.4.2 Immune Reconstitution Inflammatory Syndrome (IRIS)

Immune reconstitution syndrome following HAART in HIV-infected patients is characterized by paradoxical inflammatory worsening of symptoms and organ functions despite improvement in surrogate markers of HIV infection such as CD4 cells and viral load. Although these are very rare in children, some common examples reported among adults include disseminated tuberculosis with renal involvement leading to acute kidney injury, renal cryptococcosis, inflammatory interstitial nephritis and even immune reconstitution sarcoidosis presenting with hypercalcemia and acute kidney injury.

Treatment in most cases involves continuation of HAART and additional use of steroids or in milder cases, nonsteroidal anti-inflammatory agents. If a previously untreated quiescent infection has manifested, then treatment of the specific infection is also warranted.

14.2.4.3 Drug-Induced Nephropathy

Mechanisms of drug-induced nephropathy seen in HIV-related conditions include:

1. Crystallization: indinavir, saquinavir and nelfinavir have been implicated in nephrolithiasis, causing dysuria, renal colic, urinary obstruction and interstitial nephritis.
2. Drug interactions: ritonavir, when combined with tenofovir and indinavir, can cause acute kidney injury.
3. Tubular cytotoxicity: tenofovir and other NRTIs such as stavudine and zidovudine can exert mitochondrial toxicity and tubular dysfunction, resulting in Fanconi syndrome, lactic acidosis and metabolic disturbances.
4. Chronic kidney disease: protease inhibitors and nucleoside reverse-transcriptase inhibitors (NRTIs) are associated with diabetes, insulin resistance, dyslipidemia and lipodystrophy with resulting chronic kidney injury.
5. Acute tubular necrosis: caused by drugs commonly used in the setting of HIV such as amphotericin B, pentamidine, foscarnet and cidofovir. (Table 14.1)

Table 14.1 Renal complications of antiretroviral agents used in HIV-infected children

Antiretroviral agent	Renal toxicity	Special consideration
Nucleotide reverse-transcriptase inhibitor (NRTI)		
Tenofovir	Proximal tubular toxicity and features of Fanconi syndrome. (Toxicity is higher when combined with ritonavir-containing regimens)	Annual monitoring of renal function, serum phosphorus and urinalysis for proteinuria and glycosuria
	Nephrogenic diabetes insipidus	Reduced dosage required for impaired renal function
Nucleoside reverse-transcriptase inhibitors (NRTI)		
Didanosine	Hypokalemia, hyperuricemia, Fanconi syndrome, lactic acidosis	Monitor for lactic acidosis Reduced dosage required for impaired renal function Dose to be administered after dialysis
Zidovudine	Rhabdomyolysis, lactic acidosis	
Stavudine	Fanconi syndrome, lactic acidosis	Permanent discontinuation of drug is recommended in case of proven lactic acidosis
Non-nucleoside reverse-transcriptase inhibitors (NNRTI)		
Nevirapine	No described renal toxicity	An extra dose to be given after dialysis
Protease inhibitors (PI)		
Indinavir	Nephrolithiasis, urinary tract obstruction, interstitial nephritis	Maintain urine output >1.5 ml/kg/day. Regular monitoring of urinalysis and serum creatinine
Ritonavir	Acute kidney injury	May potentiate nephrotoxicity of other agents (indinavir, tenofovir)

(continued)

Table 14.1 (continued)

Antiretroviral agent	Renal toxicity	Special consideration
HIV-1 fusion inhibitor		
Enfurvirtide	Membranoproliferative GN	
Other antiviral drugs		
Acyclovir	Crystal-induced obstructive nephropathy	Dosage adjustment is recommended in those with renal impairment
Foscarnet	Acute kidney injury, nephrogenic diabetes insipidus	
Antifungal drugs		
Amphotericin B	Acute kidney injury, distal renal tubular acidosis, nephrocalcinosis	Monitoring of blood urea nitrogen and serum creatinine required. Renal impairment is usually reversible after discontinuing drug
Antibacterial drugs		
Aminoglycosides	Acute kidney injury	Monitoring of peak and trough drug levels recommended
Ciprofloxacin	Allergic interstitial nephritis	
Sulphonamides	Azotemia, obstructive nephropathy, allergic interstitial nephritis	

14.3 Approach to a Child with HIV and Suspected Renal Disease

Many HIV-infected children with renal disease may be asymptomatic in the early stages, and screening strategies aim at early identification of renal involvement in these children (Fig. 14.1).

14.4 Dosing Adjustments for Antiretroviral Drugs in Chronic Kidney Disease

Nucleoside and nucleotide reverse-transcriptase inhibitors (NRTIs) are primarily excreted by the kidneys; thus, reduced dosage is required in those with impaired renal function. NRTIs are also easily removed by dialysis and should be administered *after* dialysis. On the other hand, the non-nucleoside reverse-transcriptase inhibitors (NNRTIs) and protease inhibitors (PIs) are tightly plasma bound and are primarily metabolized by the liver; hence, dose adjustment is not required. (Table 14.2)

14.5 Renal Replacement Therapies in HIV-Infected Patients

14.5.1 Dialysis

- Good infection control practices in the dialysis unit need to be established.
- Haemodialysis and peritoneal dialysis are well-established therapeutic modalities among HIV-infected children with ESRD and are known to prolong survival times.

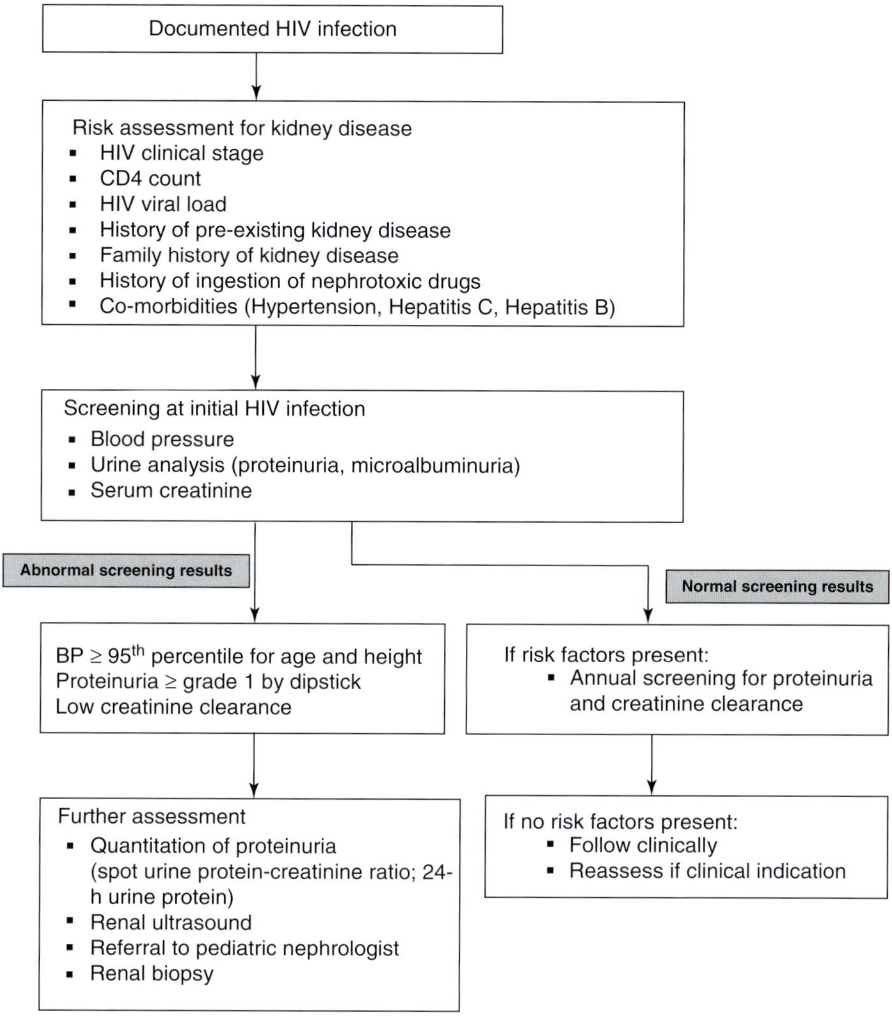

Fig. 14.1 Approach to a child with HIV infection: screening algorithm for HIV-associated kidney disease

- Children who are younger at initiation and those with higher CD4 T cell count have better prognosis.
- Peritoneal dialysis: more convenient, however higher risk of infection, particularly peritonitis caused by *Pseudomonas* species, atypical mycobacterium and fungal pathogens.
- Haemodialysis may also be used but is associated with risk of bloodstream infections and thrombosis. A dedicated haemodialysis machine is not necessary for use in HIV-infected patients; however, good infection control practice is mandatory.
- Dialysate fluid should be handled as a contaminated body fluid as HIV may be recovered from peritoneal dialysis effluent for up to 7 days after the procedure.

Table 14.2 Drug dosing in renal impairment

Antiretroviral agent	Creatinine clearance (ml/min)	Paediatric dose	Adult dose
NRTI			
Abacavir No dose adjustment necessary	Normal	8 mg/kg BD	300 mg BD
Didanosine (enteric-coated capsules)		*20–25 kg*	*25–60 kg*
	Normal	200 mg QD	250 mg QD
	10–59	100 mg QD	125 mg QD
	<10 or HD	60 mg QD	75 mg QD
Emtricitabine Give dosage after dialysis		*3 m–17years*	*>18 years*
	Normal	6 mg/kg OD	200 mg QD
	30–49	6 mg/kg Q48H	200 mg Q48H
	15–29	6 mg/kg Q72H	200 mg Q72H
	<15, HD	6 mg/kg Q96H	200 mg Q96H
Lamivudine		*<50 kg*	*≥50 kg*
	Normal	4 mg/kg BD	150 mg BD
Give dosage after dialysis	30–49	4 m/kg QD	150 mg QD
	15–29	4 mg/kg first dose, then 2.6 mg/kg QD	150 mg first dose, then 100 mg QD
	5–14	4 mg/kg first dose, then 1.3 mg/kg QD	150 mg first dose, then 50 mg QD
	<5 or HD	Unknown	50 mg first dose, then 25 mg QD
Stavudine Give dosage after dialysis		*≤30 kg*	*>30 kg*
	Normal	1 mg/kg BD	30 mg BD
	26–50	0.5 mg/kg BD	15 mg BD
	10–25 or HD	0.5 mg/kg QD	15 mg QD
Tenofovir	Normal	*<12 years (investigational)*	*≥12 years and >35 kg*
		8 mg/kg QD	300 mg QD
	30–49	Not recommended	300 mg Q48H
	10–29	Not recommended	300 mg twice weekly
	HD		300 mg QWeekly
Zidovudine		*4–9 kg 9–30 kg*	
	Normal	12 mg/kg, 9 mg/kg	300 mg BD
	<15 or HD	4 TID 3 TID	100 mg TID
NNRTI			
Nevirapine No dose adjustment necessary	Normal	<8 years: 200 mg/m^2 ≥ 8 years: 120–150 mg/m^2	*Adult* 200 mg BD
	HD	An additional 200 mg dose of nevirapine following each dialysis treatment is recommended	

(continued)

Table 14.2 (continued)

Antiretroviral agent	Creatinine clearance (ml/min)	Paediatric dose	Adult dose
Efavirenz No dose adjustment necessary	Normal	*Dose (mg HS)* 10–14 kg: 200 15–19 kg: 250 20–24 kg: 300 25–32 kg: 350 33–39 kg: 400	*≥40 kg* 600 mg HS
Protease inhibitors	No dose adjustment necessary		
Atazanavir	Unboosted atazanavir should not be used		
Lopinavir/ritonavir	For patients receiving haemodialysis, once-daily dosing should not be used		

Modified from (1) Guidelines for use of ART in HIV-infected adults and adolescents, December 2009, and (2) Guidelines for use of ART in pediatric HIV infection (Both are accessible at http://www.aidsinfo.nih.gov/)

- All HIV-uninfected patients who undergo routine dialysis should be tested for HIV and other blood-borne infections annually.
- Outcomes in dialysis: No systematic analysis available. A cohort study showed increased mortality among HIV-infected ESRD children on haemodialysis compared to similar HIV-uninfected children, although the incidence of infections in both groups remained similar.

14.5.2 Renal Replacement Therapies in HIV-Associated Renal Disease

Renal Transplantation and HIV Infection

General considerations

An accepted therapeutic modality for those with HIV infection and ESRD.

Transplantation in HIV-infected children has improved survival compared to HIV-infected adults.

The post-transplant immunosuppressant drugs used are similar to those used in non-HIV transplants.

Ethical issues

The appropriateness of transplanting scarce organs for those with HIV infection and its attendant risk factors when there are other non-HIV infected patients also requiring transplantation is debatable.

The consideration of using HIV-infected donors for HIV-infected recipients is not appropriate due to the risk of introducing variant HIV quasi-species into the recipient, resulting in adverse outcomes.

HIV-specific inclusion criteria
CD4 >200 cells/μL for at least 6 months
Undetectable HIV viraemia (>50 copies/ml) for at least 6 months
Demonstrable adherence and a stable HAART regimen for at least 6 months
Absence of AIDS-defining illness following successful immune reconstitution after HAART
Available antiretroviral treatment options in the future
No evidence of cirrhosis on liver biopsy if co-infected with HBV or HCV
HIV-specific exclusion criteria
Poor adherence to HAART
Three-class drug resistance and lack of future HIV treatment options
Documented history of progressive multifocal leukoencephalopathy (PML)
EBV- and HHV 8-related lymphoproliferative disorders (lymphoma and multicentric Castleman's syndrome)
Outcomes
The most recent report on renal transplants in HIV-infected adults (with high CD4 counts and virological suppression on HAART) indicates good patient survival rates at 1 and 3 years (95 and 88 %, respectively) and acceptable graft survival rates (90 and 74 %, respectively).

14.6 Prognosis

With the advent of highly active antiretroviral therapy, the prognosis of children with HIV-related renal disease has improved markedly. The following baseline features may be associated with a worse outcome:

- Advanced HIV clinical stage and higher degree of immunosuppression
- Poor nutritional status
- Presence of severe opportunistic infections
- Poor response to antiretroviral therapy

Certain demographic factors such as African descent ethnicity and older age are associated with worse prognosis. Although survival of patients requiring dialysis remains low, renal transplantation is an increasingly promising treatment modality for HIV-associated end-stage renal disease. Although patients with early initiation of antiretroviral therapy experience a slower progression to ESRD, the presence of kidney disease portends a worse prognosis in HIV-infected patients with respect to both morbidity and mortality. Thus, the screening and identification of early renal involvement in HIV disease is essential.

Conclusion

HIV infection is associated with a diverse range of renal disease. With increasing availability of first-line and second-line antiretroviral therapy in resource-limited settings and other areas globally, survival is likely to be prolonged, and the nature and distribution of HIV-associated kidney disease will likely continue to evolve. Careful diagnosis and management of HIV-associated kidney disease may minimize the adverse effects of renal disease on the growth and development of these children.

Suggested Reading

Bhagani S, Sweny P, Brook G (2006) Guidelines for kidney transplantation in patients with HIV disease. HIV Med 7:133–139

Centers for Disease Control and Prevention (2001) Recommendations for preventing transmission of infections among chronic hemodialysis patients. MMWR Recomm Rep 50(5):1–43

Gordillo R, Kumar J, Del Rio M, Flynn JT, Woroniecki RP (2009) Outcome of dialysis in children with human immunodeficiency virus infection. Pediatr Nephrol 24(1):171–175

Guidelines for use of antiretroviral agents in HIV-1-infected adults and adolescents, January 2011 and (2) Guidelines for use of antiretroviral agents in pediatric HIV infection, Aug 2010. (Accessible at http://www.aidsinfo.nih.gov/

Gupta SK, Eustace JA, Winston JA et al (2005) Guidelines for the management of chronic kidney disease in HIV-infected patients: recommendations of the HIV Medicine Association of the Infectious Diseases Society of America. Clin Infect Dis 40:1559–1585

Ray PE, Xu L, Rakusan T, Liu XH (2004) A 20-year history of childhood HIV-associated nephropathy. Pediatr Nephrol 19:1075–1092

Salliot C, Guichard I, Daugas E et al (2008) Acute kidney disease due to immune reconstitution inflammatory syndrome in an HIV-infected patient with tuberculosis. J Int Assoc Physicians AIDS Care (Chic) 7(4):178–181

Stock PG, Barin B, Murphy B, Hanto D, Diego JM, Light J et al (2010) Outcomes of kidney transplantation in HIV-infected recipients. N Engl J Med 363(21):2004–2014

Newborn and the Kidney

15

P.N. Suman Rao

15.1 Introduction

The advances in neonatal care and improved survival of extremely premature infants have broadened the field of neonatal nephrology significantly. Improved neonatal care has created a new set of complications such as neonatal nephrocalcinosis and catheter-related thromboembolic disease. Managing complex neonatal renal problems is a challenge for the team of neonatologists and nephrologists.

Diseases affecting the newborn kidney may be inherited or congenital or related to certain key events occurring in the perinatal period. Consequently, the practice of neonatal nephrology has some unique features. These are discussed below.

15.2 Nephrogenesis

- Nephrogenesis starts from the fifth week of intrauterine life. It is completed by 35 weeks of gestational age, forming about one million nephrons in one kidney.
- The glomerulus is a third of the size of the adult glomerulus, and the tubules are short and immature even at term.
- The full-term infant is born with as many nephrons as he or she will ever have. In the preterm infant, nephrogenesis continues after birth but is subject to damage by diseases and drugs.

P.N. Suman Rao, MD, DM
Department of Neonatology,
St John's National Academy of Health Sciences,
Bangalore, KA 560034, India
e-mail: raosumanv@rediffmail.com

K. Phadke et al. (eds.), *Manual of Pediatric Nephrology*,
DOI 10.1007/978-3-642-12483-9_15, © Springer-Verlag Berlin Heidelberg 2014

15.3 Foetal Origin of Adult Diseases (Barker's Hypothesis)

- There is a direct relation between birth weight and number of glomeruli at birth. Low birth weight infants (both preterm infants and intrauterine growth-restricted infants) have reduced number of nephrons at birth.
- Number of nephrons formed at birth is a determinant of renal functions later in life. Reduced glomerular number may be associated with hypertension and chronic kidney disease in later life.

15.4 Amniotic Fluid

- The most important function of the prenatal kidney is maintenance of adequate amniotic fluid. The excretory and homeostatic functions of the kidneys begin only in the postnatal period. Alterations in amniotic fluid volume may indicate renal problems.
- Throughout most of the pregnancy, the mean amniotic fluid index (AFI) is approximately 12–14 cm, declining after 33 weeks. The average AFI near term is 12 cm, with the 95th percentile being approximately 20 cm and the 5th percentile being approximately 7 cm (Table 15.1).

Table 15.1 Amniotic fluid volume

Amniotic fluid volume	Maximal vertical pocket	Amniotic fluid index
Normal	>2 – <8 cm	>8 – <25 cm[a]
Polyhydramnios	≥8.0 cm	≥25 cm
Moderate oligohydramnios	≥1 – ≤2 cm	>5 – <8 cm
Severe oligohydramnios	<1 cm	<5 cm

[a]The average AFI near term is 12 cm; AFI >20 cm should be considered high

15.4.1 Oligohydramnios (Table 15.2)

Table 15.2 Causes of oligohydramnios

Renal causes	Non-renal causes
Congenital anomalies: Renal agenesis Polycystic kidneys Multicystic dysplastic kidneys Ureteral or urethral obstruction	Foetal: Chromosomal abnormalities Intrauterine growth restriction Intrauterine foetal demise Rupture of membranes (occult or overt)
Maternal medications: Prostaglandin synthetase inhibitors Angiotensin-converting enzyme inhibitors	Maternal: Uteroplacental insufficiency Placental: Twin-to-twin transfusion Placental infarction

15.4.2 Polyhydramnios (Table 15.3)

Table 15.3 Causes of polyhydramnios

Renal causes	Non-renal causes
Foetal:	Foetal:
Congenital nephrotic syndrome	Chromosomal abnormalities
Bartter syndrome	Congenital anomalies (a) Gastrointestinal – duodenal or oesophageal atresia, tracheo-oesophageal fistula, congenital diaphragmatic hernia (b) Craniofacial – anencephaly (c) Pulmonary – cystic adenomatoid malformation (d) Cardiac – arrhythmias (e) Skeletal dysplasias
	Anaemia
	Foetal hydrops
	Maternal:
	Diabetes – gestational, type II
	Placental:
	Twin-to-twin transfusion
	Chorioangioma

15.5 Perinatal Changes in Kidney Functions

15.5.1 Renal Blood Flow (RBF)

- RBF accounts for only 2–3 % of cardiac output in the foetus.
- At birth, it increases to 15–18 % of cardiac output.
- Increase in RBF results in increased GFR and increased urine output.

15.5.2 Glomerular Filtration Rate (GFR)

- During foetal life, GFR increases progressively from 14 ml/min/1.73 m^2 at 32–34 weeks' gestation to 21 ml/min/1.73 m^2 at term.
- The GFR rises quickly after birth, doubling by 2 weeks of age. It continues to increase postnatally, achieving adult values of 118 ml/min/1.73 m^2 by the age of 2 years (see Table 15.4).
- The rate of GFR maturation is a function related to postconceptional age and not postnatal age. The postnatal rise in GFR in preterm infants is slower than in term neonates. This requires modification of drug dosages and frequency of drug administration.

Table 15.4 Renal functions and gestational age

Age	Glomerular filtration rate (ml/min/1.73 m^2)	Renal blood flow (ml/min/1.73 m^2)	Maximum urine osmolality (mOsm/kg)	Serum creatinine (mg/dl)[a]	Fractional excretion of Na (%)
Newborn					
32–34 weeks of gestation	14±3	40±6	480	1.3	2–5
Term	21±4	88±4	800	1.1	<1
1–2 weeks	50±10	220±40	900	0.4	<1
6 months–1 year	77±14	352±73	1,200	0.2	<1
1–3 years	96±22	540±118	1,400	0.4	<1
Adult	118±18	620±92	1,400	0.8–1.5	<1

[a]Convert serum creatinine values in mg/dl to μmmol/l in SI units by multiplying with 88

15.5.3 Urine Concentrating Capacity

- The newborn infant has a limited ability to concentrate urine. The maximal urine osmolality is 500 mOsm/l in premature infants and 800 mOsm/l in term infants.
- The impaired concentrating capacity is due to short loops of Henle, shallow medullary tonicity gradient and diminished responsiveness of the collecting ducts to ADH.
- Infants fed on high protein diets show a significant improvement in urinary concentrating capacity.
- The inability to concentrate urine makes the newborn more vulnerable to dehydration.

15.5.4 Urine Diluting Capacity

- Though the diluting ability of the term newborn is the same as an adult (50 mOsm/l), the ability to excrete a water load is limited due to the low GFR.
- The excessive administration of water may place the newborn infant at a high risk for dilutional hyponatremia and hypervolemia. In preterm infants, it may result in opening of the ductus arteriosus (PDA).

15.5.5 Urine Output

- Factors that determine urine output include water balance, solute load and renal concentrating ability. Minimum urine volume = Urine solutes to be excreted/maximum urine osmolality.
- A neonate receiving the usual renal solute load of 7–15 mOsm/kg/day with a renal concentrating capacity of 500 mOsm/kg would require a minimal urine output of approximately 1 ml/kg/h. Hence, oliguria is defined as urine flow rate <1 ml/kg/h.

- Normal urine output in a newborn is 1–5 ml/kg/h.
- The first urine: Documentation of the first void is important. Ninety-eight percent of term infants void during the first 30 h of life. A delay in urination for up to 48 h should not be a cause for immediate concern in the absence of a palpable bladder, abdominal mass or other signs or symptoms of renal disease.
- A failure to void for longer than 48 h warrants prompt investigations to rule out impairment of renal functions.

15.5.6 Postnatal Changes in Distribution of Body Water

- Body water is distributed in well-defined compartments that undergo marked developmental changes.
- At birth, the percentage of body weight represented by water is approximately 75 % in term infants and even greater in premature infants. As gestational age increases, total body water and extracellular water decrease and intracellular fluid content increases.
- A reduction in body weight in the first 7–10 days of life is physiologic. This physiologic weight loss is largely the result of a reduction in the extracellular compartment of body water. Term infants lose approximately 7–10 % and preterm infants 10–15 % of the ECF. Perturbations of this normal transitional physiology can lead to imbalances in sodium and water homeostasis.
- Excess loss of body weight (>10 %) postnatally is commonly seen in exclusively breastfeeding babies who feed poorly. This may be associated with hypernatremic dehydration. Monitoring of postnatal weight loss and intensive lactation support are required for prevention of hypernatremic dehydration.
- Insensible water loss also increases with the use of phototherapy and radiant warmer, but decreases with the use of humidified gases during ventilation.
- In preterm infants, high fluid intake may be associated with a higher incidence of symptomatic patent ductus arteriosus and necrotising enterocolitis.

15.5.7 Vasoregulatory Mechanism of the Neonatal Kidney

- Both renin and angiotensin II are high in the foetus and neonate. Plasma renin activity (PRA) is inversely related to gestational age in the foetus and newborn, decreasing from 60 ng/ml/h at 30 weeks to about 10–20 ng/ml/h at term.
- Newborns have high circulating levels of prostaglandins (PG) that counteract the highly activated vasoconstrictor state of the neonatal microcirculation.
- The use of ACE inhibitors in pregnancy results in decreased placental perfusion, foetal hypotension, oligohydramnios and neonatal renal failure.
- PG synthesis inhibitors can have a deleterious renal vasoconstrictor effect in the immature kidney, e.g. maternal indomethacin. Cyclooxygenase type 2 (COX-2) enzyme is necessary for late stages of nephrogenesis, and deficiency of COX-2 activity leads to pathologic changes in cortical architecture and eventually renal

failure. There is potential risk of nephrotoxicity while using drugs like indomethacin for pharmacological closure of patent ductus arteriosus. It can cause reduction in renal perfusion, GFR and urine output. However, these normalise on discontinuation of the treatment.

15.5.8 Sodium

- The fractional excretion of sodium (FENa) decreases progressively from 20 % during early foetal life to 0.2 % in the full-term newborn.
- Premature infants (<34 weeks) have elevated FENa, which may exceed 5 % during the first few days of life. They require higher sodium supplementation (3–5 mmol/kg/day).
- Though preterm breast milk has higher sodium than term breast milk (25 mmol/l vs. 7 mmol/l), preterm infants often have a state of negative sodium balance and loss of body weight during the first 2 weeks of life (i.e. hyponatremia of prematurity). Use of antenatal corticosteroids in pregnant women at risk of preterm delivery reduces FENa.
- Adaptation to the extrauterine environment involves a physiologic natriuresis in the first 4–5 days of life. Soon after the immediate postnatal period, term infants are in a state of positive sodium balance, a requisite for somatic growth, particularly of bone. The tendency of the neonatal kidney to retain sodium during this period may become problematic under conditions of salt loading. Full-term newborn infants given a sodium load in excess of 12 mmol/kg/day experience a rise in serum sodium levels, abnormal increase in weight and generalised oedema.

15.5.9 Potassium

- Like sodium, potassium is critical for somatic growth. In contrast to adults, neonates greater than 30 weeks' gestational age must maintain a positive potassium balance.
- Premature newborns tend to have higher plasma potassium concentrations.
- Potassium levels >6.5 mmol/l are observed in 30–50 % of VLBW infants in the first 48–72 h even in the absence of potassium intake. Extreme premature infants <27 weeks may have life-threatening bradycardia due to hyperkalemia in the first few days.
- Antenatal corticosteroids reduce the incidence of hyperkalemia (>6.5 mmol/l) in the preterm infants.

15.5.10 Acid-Base Balance

- Newborn infants have a lower bicarbonate concentration than adults. The low GFR limits the ability of the neonate to adequately handle an acid load.
- Preterm neonates frequently have mild to moderate normal anion gap acidosis, as a consequence of low renal bicarbonate threshold in the premature kidney.

The bicarbonate threshold is 21 mmol/l in the term infant, 18 mmol/l in the preterm infant and 14 mmol/l in the extremely premature infant, and it reaches adult levels of 24–26 mmol/l only after the first year.

- Effective urinary acidification is usually acquired by the age of 1 month even in premature infants, independent of the gestational age at birth. Antenatally, administered glucocorticoids stimulate the maturation of the acid-base homeostatic mechanisms.
- Physiologically, low serum bicarbonate in the newborn may cause misdiagnosis of renal tubular acidosis.
- High protein intake in total parenteral nutrition or high protein formulas may result in metabolic acidosis in the premature infant. However, this is far less common with the current third-generation amino acid and formula preparations.

15.5.11 Calcium and Phosphate

- As higher calcium and phosphorus are required for the growing skeleton, the foetus is hypercalcemic relative to the maternal levels. This suppresses parathormone release. The release of PTH lags behind the postnatal calcium fall, and the physiologic nadir of serum calcium occurs in the first 2 days of life. Although this nadir is still within normal adult range, it represents a significant decrease compared to foetal levels.
- The normal urine calcium/creatinine is higher in infants. The risk of nephrocalcinosis is increased with calciuric drugs such as furosemide and glucocorticoids especially in preterm infants with bronchopulmonary dysplasia. Substituting furosemide with thiazide diuretics reduces this risk.
- Neonates excrete only 60 % of the intestinally absorbed phosphate and have a higher phosphate concentration than adults.

15.5.12 Uric Acid

- Cord blood uric acid is higher than in maternal blood. The urinary uric acid then progressively reduces, slowly in preterm newborns.
- Despite poor renal tubular reabsorption of uric acid, obstruction by uric acid crystals is rare in the neonatal period. Relative alkaline urine prevents its precipitation.
- A high urinary uric acid-to-creatinine ratio is a marker of perinatal asphyxia (>0.95 in term infants). Uric acid nephropathy has been described rarely in neonates with acute kidney injury (AKI) secondary to perinatal asphyxia.

15.5.13 Glucose

Glycosuria is common among neonates. Maximum tubular reabsorption of glucose is lower in preterm infants. Hence, presence of glucose in urine is commonly seen in preterm babies.

15.6 Assessment of Foetal Renal Functions

15.6.1 Foetal Glomerular Filtration Rate (GFR)

- Measurement of foetal serum cystatin C or beta 2 microglobulins assess foetal glomerular function. They also help in prognostication of postnatal renal function.
- Foetal serum cystatin C is independent of gestational age. Mean serum cystatin C level is 1.6 mg/l with 2 mg/l being the upper limit of normal.
- Beta 2 microglobulin decreases with gestational age, and the upper limit can be calculated from 7.19 (mg/l) to 0.052(mg/l) × gestational age (weeks). It has a higher sensitivity (87 %) than cystatin C in predicting postnatal renal dysfunction.

15.6.2 Foetal Urine

The following measurements in foetal urine indicate good prognosis in foetal hydronephrosis (Table 15.5):

Table 15.5 Factors predicting good long-term function in foetal hydronephrosis

Foetal urine	Values
Sodium	<100 mmol/l
Chloride	<90 mmol/l
Osmolality	<210 mOsm/kg
Calcium	<2 mmol/l
Phosphate	<2 mmol/l
Beta 2 microglobulin	<2–4 mg/l
Protein	<20 mg/dl
Urine output	>2 ml/h

15.7 Clinical Practice

15.7.1 History

15.7.1.1 Family History

- Polycystic kidney disease (autosomal dominant or autosomal recessive), congenital nephrotic syndrome, Bartter syndrome.
- Metabolic disorders with renal manifestations such as cystinosis and tyrosinemia (autosomal recessive).
- Vesicoureteric reflux also has a familial predilection.

15.7.1.2 Antenatal History

- Routine anomaly scan – structural renal malformations such as hydronephrosis, agenesis and cystic dysplasia can be diagnosed in utero.

- Oligohydramnios (amniotic fluid index <8) may be an indicator of severe renal dysfunction.
- Elevated alpha-fetoprotein in amniotic fluid occurs in congenital nephrotic syndrome.
- A history of maternal exposure to medications and teratogens (captopril, indomethacin) is critical in investigation of neonatal renal failure.
- Diabetes mellitus in the mother predisposes the infant of diabetic mother to renal vein thrombosis.
- TORCH infections in mother may lead to congenital nephrotic syndrome.

15.7.2 Physical Examination

- Potter's sequence: The best-known physical indicator of bilateral severe renal disease is the Potter's sequence caused by severe oligohydramnios, which in turn causes foetal deformation by compression against the uterine wall. The characteristic facial features include wide-set eyes, a depressed nasal bridge, a beaked nose, a receding chin and posteriorly rotated low-set ears. Other associated anomalies include a small, compressed chest wall, with resulting pulmonary hypoplasia and arthrogryposis.
- Renal anomalies are part of many syndromes such as VACTREL, Jeune syndrome, Zellweger syndrome and various trisomies.
- The commonest cause for an abdominal mass in a newborn is a renal mass.
- Palpable bladder may be a sign of obstructive uropathy.

15.7.3 Extra-Renal Indicators for Newborn Renal Disease (Table 15.6)

Table 15.6 Indicators in the newborn for genitourinary disorders

Findings	Associated renal anomaly
Placental oedema	Congenital nephrotic syndrome
Single umbilical artery	VUR, megaureter, agenesis, dilatation of collecting system
Abnormal external auricles	Agenesis, dysplasia
Aniridia, hemihypertrophy	Wilm's tumour
Abnormal vertebrae	Agenesis, ectopia, dysplasia
Meningomyelocele	VUR, neurogenic bladder, hydronephrosis, double ureter, horseshoe kidney
Imperforate anus	Agenesis, duplication, hypospadias, VUR
Severe hypospadias	PUJ obstruction, ectopic kidney, VUR
Spontaneous pneumothorax	Hypoplasia, agenesis, polycystic kidney disease, dysplasia, urethral valves
Supernumerary nipples	Hydronephrosis, duplication
Ambiguous genitalia	Congenital adrenal hyperplasia, mesangial sclerosis, Wilm's tumour

15.7.4 Laboratory Evaluation

15.7.4.1 Urine Analysis

- Diaper urine specimens are reliable for pH estimation and qualitative determination of glucose, protein and blood.
- Suprapubic bladder aspiration is considered the collection method of choice in newborns and is safe even in infants with very low birth weight. Intra-abdominal pathology or bleeding disorders are contraindications.
- Colour: A common finding is pink or reddish-brown staining of the diaper which is confused with bleeding. This is often due to urate crystals.
- Glycosuria: Glycosuria is common in the most premature infants and is rare after 34 weeks.
- Proteinuria: Protein excretion is higher in premature infants and decreases progressively postnatally (Table 15.7).

Table 15.7 Proteinuria during the first days of life

Gestational age (weeks)	Mean and range (mg/m^2/h)
<28	0.86 (0.2–1.33)
30	2.08 (0–9.4)
32	2.32 (0–5.22)
34	2.48 (0–13.07)
36	1.27 (0–4.60)
40	1.29 (0–6.14)

15.7.5 Assessment of Renal Functions

15.7.5.1 Serum Creatinine

- In term infants, the serum creatinine level gradually decreases from 1.1 mg/dl to a mean value of 0.4 mg/dl within the first 2 weeks of life.
- However, in preterm infants, the plasma creatinine level may rise in the first 48 h before beginning to fall to a mean value that is higher than term infants.
- Practically, a reasonably accurate estimate of GFR can be made from the serum creatinine concentration by using an empirically derived formula that has been applied to normal preterm and term infants (refer Sect. 1.4).

Table 15.8 Normal serum creatinine values in term and preterm infants (mean + SD)

	<28 weeks	28–32 weeks	32–37 weeks	>37 weeks
Age (days)	Serum creatinine mg/dl	Serum creatinine mg/dl	Serum creatinine mg/dl	Serum creatinine mg/dl
3	1.05+0.27	0.88+0.25	0.78+0.22	0.75+0.2
7	0.95+0.36	0.94+0.37	0.77+0.48	0.56+0.4
14	0.81+0.26	0.78+0.36	0.62+0.4	0.43+0.25
28	0.66+0.28	0.59+0.38	0.40+0.28	0.34+0.2

Convert serum creatinine values in mg/dl to µmmol/l in SI units by multiplying with 88

Issues with Serum Creatinine as a Biomarker of Acute Kidney Injury

- At birth and in the first few days, it reflects the maternal creatinine and not the infant's renal function.
- In newborns, GFR is low, particularly in preterm infants. At lower GFR, serum creatinine overestimates renal functions due to tubular secretion.
- Defining acute kidney injury (AKI) based on an increase in serum creatinine concentration may exclude term neonates with serum creatinine <1.5 mg/dl who fail to show the normal decrease in serum creatinine values observed in the first days/weeks of life in healthy neonates. Failure of the serum creatinine to decrease postnatally may be a sign of AKI.
- Bilirubin levels in premature infants are normal at birth, rise in the first several days and return to normal after a few weeks. If the Jaffe method of serum creatinine is used, this may have an impact on the interpretations of values obtained.

15.7.5.2 Other Markers

- Serum cystatin C is a proteinase inhibitor produced by all nucleated cells, freely filtered across the glomerular capillaries, almost completely reabsorbed and catabolised in the renal proximal tubular cells. However, its claim as a superior marker of neonatal GFR has not been proved.
- Various other biomarkers of kidney injury, such as serum and urinary neutrophil gelatinase-associated lipocalin (NGAL), urinary interleukin 18 and kidney injury molecule-1 (KIM-1), are under evaluation.

15.7.6 Radiological Examination

Details are given in Sect. 1.7. Certain considerations in the newborn are as follows:

- In neonates, the ultrasound appearances are distinctive because the renal cortex has echogenicity equal to or greater than that of liver and spleen (in older children the cortex is hypoechoic relative to other organs). This increased echogenicity of the renal cortex is due to relatively high density of glomeruli which persists till 3–4 months. The neonatal kidney also demonstrates prominent, hypoechoic pyramids because of the larger medullary volume present. This finding may persist until 1 year of age and should not be confused with a dilated collecting system. Medullary hyperechogenicity may be normally seen in the first 2 weeks postnatally due to transient tubular stasis of Tamm-Horsfall protein. It may also be seen in nephrocalcinosis.
- The neonatal kidney demonstrates a paucity of sinus fat. Therefore, the central portion will not be echogenic. The anteroposterior diameter of the renal pelvis is measured (<5 mm, normal; 5–9 mm, borderline; >10 mm, abnormal).
- The length of the kidney in millimetres is approximately equal to the gestational age in weeks.

- Common causes of large echogenic kidneys: ARPKD, diffuse cystic dysplasia, renal vein thrombosis, congenital nephrotic syndrome.
- Common causes of small echogenic kidneys: multicystic dysplasia, cortical and medullary necrosis.
- Blood flow through renal vessels can be assessed by Doppler ultrasound. This may be indicated for the evaluation of haematuria, hypertension and acute kidney injury, especially if there is history of umbilical artery catheterisation.
- Radioisotopic renal scan using mercaptoacetyltriglycine (MAG 3) or 99mTc-DTPA is indicated in renovascular hypertension, lack of visualisation of a kidney by ultrasound, preoperative evaluation for assessment of severity of urinary tract obstruction, and for evaluation of differential renal functions. It is usually done about 4 weeks after birth.
- Intravenous urography is of limited value during the first 15 days of life. Because of the hyperosmolality of the contrast agent, it may induce cellular dehydration and aggravate acute kidney injury.
- Computed tomography (CT) and magnetic resonance imaging (MRI): Gadolinium-enhanced magnetic resonance (MR) angiography is the investigation of choice in suspected renovascular hypertension.

15.8 Fluids, Electrolytes and Acid-base Issues in the Newborn

15.8.1 Sodium

15.8.1.1 Hyponatremia

Hyponatremia is more common in preterm babies than term babies.

The common causes unique to neonates are:

- Renal losses:
  - Immaturity of renal tubules – This is commonly seen in extremely premature infants.
  - Renal salt wasting – congenital adrenal hyperplasia, Bartter syndrome.
  - Chronic lung disease treated with long-term diuretic therapy.
- GI losses:
  - Necrotising enterocolitis
  - Congenital surgical conditions requiring stoma
- Following repeated drainage of CSF in posthaemorrhagic hydrocephalus
- Excess intrapartum infusion of sodium-free fluid to the mother
- Syndrome of inappropriate diuresis – due to perinatal asphyxia, intraventricular haemorrhage, pneumonia

Signs and Symptoms of Hyponatremia

Premature infants with late hyponatremia are generally asymptomatic. Some may develop poor weight gain, apnoea and neurological symptoms such as irritability and convulsions.

- Clues: Abnormal change in weight, ambiguous genitalia, palpable kidneys, hypertension, hyperkalemia, failure to thrive.
- Severe hyponatremia may be a risk factor for sensorineural hearing loss. Neonatal hyponatremia may have unfavourable influences on cognitive and mental development in later life.

Management of Hyponatremia

- If the baby has been on IV fluids and is in the first week of life, the most likely diagnosis is iatrogenic fluid overload. The treatment is fluid restriction. Watch out for hypoglycemia which may necessitate an increase in the concentration of IV dextrose infused.
- Measurement of urine sodium will determine if the infant is losing sodium excessively or attempting to conserve sodium.
- If serum sodium is between 120 and 135 mmol/l, restriction of fluids will suffice. Serum sodium must be monitored at least 12 hourly.
- If hyponatremia is associated with symptoms like seizures or if hyponatremia is less than 120 mmol/l, it requires prompt correction with 3 % hypertonic saline in a dose of 5 ml/kg over 4–5 h.
- Hyponatremia unresponsive to above therapy is an indication for dialysis.
- Babies with non-oliguric acute kidney injury may have very large urinary sodium losses of up to 10 mmol/kg/day, and these must be replaced.

15.8.1.2 Hypernatremia

The commonest cause of hypernatremia in the term infant is inadequate milk intake. Mothers need lactation support for "exclusive breastfeeding" (Table 15.9).

Table 15.9 Common causes of hypernatremia specific to neonates

Water deficit	
Inadequate intake	Ineffective breastfeeding Child neglect or abuse
Increased insensible losses	Extreme premature infants Radiant warmers Phototherapy
Renal losses	Diabetes insipidus – central, nephrogenic
Excessive sodium	
Improperly mixed formula, excess sodium bicarbonate, intravenous hypertonic saline, hyperaldosteronism	

Signs and Symptoms of Hypernatremia

- Clues: abnormal change of weight, poor feeding, seizures.
- Daily weight of all newborns must be monitored. If the weight loss exceeds 10 % of the birth weight, serum sodium should be checked for hypernatremic dehydration and intensive lactation support given.

Management of Hypernatremia

- If salt overload: Stop salt intake, maintain normal hydration and allow the kidneys to excrete the excess salt.
- If water deprivation/dehydration:
  - In extremely premature infants, hypernatremia due to increased insensible water loss can be prevented by nursing in humidified incubators rather than open radiant warmers.
  - Restore plasma volume (orally if hypernatremia is due to feeding problems and if the infant is able to tolerate).
  - The plasma sodium should not drop too rapidly (<10 mmol in 24 h). Too rapid reduction in sodium can precipitate intracranial bleeding.

15.8.2 Potassium

Newborns are less likely to have hypokalemia (serum potassium <3.5 mmol/l) than older infants. Hypokalemic conditions like Bartter syndrome may not manifest with hypokalemia at the onset. On the other hand, ELBW (extremely low birth weight) infants may have life-threatening bradycardia, induced by hyperkalemia (serum potassium >6.0 mmol/l) in the first few days. A laboratory report of hyperkalemia in a newborn should not be interpreted as a result of "squeezed/haemolysed sample" until all potential causes of hyperkalemia are excluded. A repeat sample should be ordered. Hyperkalemia is commonly seen in settings of asphyxia, hypothermia, post exchange transfusion or in infants with congenital adrenal hyperplasia. The details of management of hyperkalemia are given in Chap. 2. Oral administration of kayexalate (K-binding resin) is not recommended in preterm infants because of risk for necrotising enterocolitis. Rectal administration is effective. Complications include gastric bezoars, caecal perforation, bowel opacification, hypernatremia, fluid retention and constipation. In sick newborns, insulin-glucose infusion is the most effective measure in reducing potassium levels.

15.8.3 Calcium

Hypocalcemia is defined as serum calcium <7 mg % in preterm infants and <8 mg % in term infants or an ionised calcium <4.4 mg %. The specific conditions causing hypocalcemia in the newborns include prematurity, infant of diabetic mother, perinatal asphyxia, maternal hyperparathyroidism and phototherapy. The infants present with nonspecific features such as jitteriness, apnoea, cyanosis and seizures. The treatment is elaborated in Chap. 2. Oral calcium, being hypertonic, has the potential risk of precipitating necrotising enterocolitis in preterm infants.

Hypercalcemia is defined as serum calcium >11 mg/dl (>2.75 mmol/l) or ionised calcium >5.4 mg/dl (>1.35 mmol/l). The causes unique to the neonatal age include hypophosphatemia of prematurity, maternal hypoparathyroidism and subcutaneous fat necrosis. The clinical features are nonspecific and the treatment is elaborated in Chap. 2.

15.8.3.1 Osteopenia of Prematurity (Rickets)

- Rickets in the newborn period is most frequently caused by nutritional deficiency. It can affect more than 30 % of ELBW (extremely low birth weight) infants.
- The primary cause is calcium and phosphorus deficiency: prolonged low Ca and/ or low phosphorus in parenteral nutrition, prolonged intake of unfortified human milk in preterm infants, chronic use of loop diuretics.
- Vit D deficiency is not a cause for osteopenia of prematurity.
- It usually presents at 2–6 months postnatally after discharge from the neonatal unit. Most cases are diagnosed from incidental radiographic features of generalised bone demineralisation and widening, cupping and fraying of the distal metaphyses. It may also present with respiratory distress, failure to wean from a ventilator or fractures. Dual-energy x-ray absorptiometry allows a more accurate quantification of the degree of bone mineralisation.
- Grading of osteopenia based on x-ray of right forearm: grade 0, normal bone; grade 1, mineral rarefaction only; grade 2, cupping and fraying of metaphyses; grade 3, fractures.
- Prevention is by ensuring optimal Ca and P intake in parenteral nutrition and fortifying preterm breast milk. Preterm infants require 120–180 mg/100 Kcal of calcium and 80–110 mg/100 Kcal of phosphorus. 800 IU of vitamin D is sufficient with adequate mineral intake. If diuretics are required as in chronic lung disease, it is more preferable to use thiazides rather than furosemide. Biochemical monitoring with calcium, phosphorus and alkaline phosphatase is required and hypercalciuria should be prevented by providing calcium and phosphorus in the right ratio of 2:1. Serum phosphorus should be maintained above 6 mg/dl (91.94 mmol/l).
- Urinary calcium and phosphorus should be measured. The simultaneous presence of both calcium and phosphorus in spot urine samples in a ratio of less than 0.5 indicates that both are provided in sufficient amounts. The absence of either indicates a deficiency of one of these minerals.
- Rickets due to osteopenia of prematurity rapidly heals with treatment but may result in long-term poor linear growth in ELBW infants.

15.8.4 Late Metabolic Acidosis

- Premature infants may present with poor weight gain and hyperchloremic metabolic acidosis in the second to third week of life.
- It is the result of the milk formula that contains excessive metabolic acid precursors that overload the immature kidney's ability to excrete them.
- With the newer milk preparations for premature infants, late metabolic acidosis has largely disappeared.

15.9 Acute Kidney Injury (Acute Renal Failure)

Neonatologists continue to use the term "acute renal failure (ARF)" rather than the term "acute kidney injury". Classification and staging systems using various criteria like AKIN or RIFLE (see Chap. 8) are not in routine day-to-day practice, in neonatal nephrology.

Renal failure is suspected if:

- Urine flow <0.5 ml/kg/h and/or
- If serum creatinine is elevated >2 SD for the gestational age (refer Table 15.4) or
- Serum creatinine is rising at the rate of 0.3 mg/dl/day.

15.9.1 Classification of ARF

A. Based on Urine Output

Oliguric renal failure is defined as urine output <1 ml/kg/h unresponsive to fluid challenge accompanied by serum creatinine >1.5 mg/dl.

Non-oliguric renal failure is defined as serum creatinine >1.5 mg/dl for at least 24 h, but urine output is >1 ml/kg/h. Thirty to fifty percent of neonatal renal failures are non-oliguric and have a better prognosis.

B. Based on Aetiology

Prerenal failure, intrinsic renal failure, post-renal or obstructive renal failure

15.9.2 Incidence

The incidence of ARF in critically ill neonates is between 8 and 24 %, and the mortality rates are between 10 and 61 %. AKI is more frequent in premature, low birth weight infants. The occurrence of ARF results in threefold rise in risk of mortality.

15.9.3 Approach to ARF

15.9.3.1 History

- Maternal drug ingestion (captopril, indomethacin)
- Maternal illness (diabetes)
- Abnormal antenatal ultrasound (oligohydramnios, renal anomaly)
- Perinatal asphyxia
- Abnormal urinary stream
- Urinary retention
- Vomiting, diarrhoea
- Rate and type of fluid administration and urine output
- Use of nephrotoxic drugs (aminoglycosides, amphotericin B)

15.9.3.2 Symptoms and Signs

The symptoms are nonspecific like lethargy, poor feeding, vomiting and seizures. The neonate may show excessive weight gain, oedema, anaemia, abdominal mass, ascites and cardiac arrhythmias. There may be indicators for renal disease (Table 15.6).

15.9.4 Causes of ARF in Newborn (Table 15.10)

Table 15.10 Causes of renal failure in newborn

Prerenal	Intrinsic	Obstructive
Systemic hypovolemia	Congenital abnormalities	Congenital malformations
Dehydration	Congenital dysplasias	Ureterocele
Haemorrhage	Renal agenesis	Posterior urethral valves
Septic shock	Polycystic kidney disease	Vesicoureteric reflux
Systemic vasodilators	Maternal drugs	Megacystis-megaureter
Necrotising enterocolitis	ACE inhibitors	PUJ obstruction
Operative fluid loss	Cyclooxygenase inhibitors	Prune belly syndrome
Renal hypoperfusion	Others	Extrinsic compression
Cardiac failure	Haemoglobinuria	Sacrococcygeal tumour
Respiratory failure	Myoglobinuria	Hematocolpos
Asphyxia	Renal vascular thrombosis	Intrinsic obstruction
Indomethacin	Pyelonephritis	Fungal ball
	Nephrotoxins	Neurogenic bladder

15.9.5 Some Neonatal Conditions Associated with Renal Failure

1. Respiratory distress syndrome – severe hypoxemia often seen in severe respiratory distress syndrome or in persistent pulmonary hypertension can affect renal functions and cause vasomotor nephropathy. This is aggravated by positive pressure ventilation which can reduce renal perfusion.
2. Perinatal asphyxia – ARF with asphyxia results usually in non-oliguric renal failure. Hence, serum creatinine should be serially monitored. Oliguric ARF has a worse prognosis. Persistent oliguria (present for at least 36 h after birth) in asphyxiated term and preterm newborn is a poor prognosticator of future neurodevelopmental outcome.
3. Bilateral renal artery thrombosis – is a known complication of umbilical artery catheterisation, particularly if umbilical arterial catheter is in high position.
4. ARF in twin pregnancies could occur due to hypovolemia following twin-to-twin transfusion syndrome (TTTS) or death of a co-twin.
5. Closure of abdominal wall defects – could reduce venous return and cardiac output, causing ARF.

6. Fungal sepsis – ARF in a neonate with systemic candidiasis can occur due to parenchymal involvement and/or due to drug nephrotoxicity (amphotericin B), and/or due to urinary obstruction by fungus balls. Bilateral candida-related obstructive uropathy can induce oligo-anuric ARF. Preterm infants are more prone to this complication.

15.9.6 Diagnosis of ARF

Table 15.11 depicts the differentiation between prerenal and intrinsic renal failure.

Table 15.11 Renal failure indices in the newborn

Test	Prerenal ARF	Intrinsic ARF
BUN/Cr ratio (mg/mg)	>30	<20
FENa (%)[a]	≤2.5	≥3.0
Urinary Na (mmol/l)	≤20	≥50
Urinary osmolality (mOsm/kg)	≥350	≤300
Urinary-specific gravity	>1.012	<1.014
Renal failure index (RFI)	Low (<1)	High (>4)
Ultrasonography	Normal	May be abnormal
Response to volume challenge	UO >2 ml/kg/h	No increase in UO

[a]Fractional excretion of sodium (FENa) varies inversely with both gestational age and postnatal age in neonates. High urinary sodium excretion observed in very premature infants is a great drawback to the use of FENa in this population. FENa indicative of intrinsic renal failure: 31 weeks' gestational age, >3 %, and 29–30 weeks' gestational age, >6 %

15.9.7 Management of ARF

- General principles of management are similar to those for acute kidney injury in older children (Chap. 8).
- Fluids: Restrict fluids to insensible water losses (500 ml/m^2/day or 30 ml/kg/day) plus urine output and other measured losses. In extremely premature infants, the insensible water losses may be as high as 100 ml/kg/day.
- Role of theophylline: Theophylline, by virtue of being an adenosine antagonist, reverses the intrarenal vasoconstrictor state, in vasomotor nephropathy in preterm infants. Prophylactically, it may reduce the renal dysfunction in asphyxiated term neonates. Though it is promising, it is still not a recommendation in neonatal renal failure.
- Indications for dialysis

Renal replacement therapy is indicated when conservative therapy fails to control complications such as fluid overload, hypertension, congestive heart failure, severe hyponatremia, hyperkalemia and metabolic acidosis.

Methods of dialysis: Peritoneal dialysis (PD) is the preferred method in neonates. Hemofiltration or hemodiafiltration (HDF) may be considered when PD is contraindicated or inefficient as in necrotising enterocolitis or shock. Availability of small dialysers and securing a vascular access in small babies pose special problems for the neonates.

The prognosis is extremely poor in renal agenesis or in severe multisystem involvement; aggressive management then may not improve outcomes.

15.10 Neonatal Hypertension (Fig. 15.1)

Blood pressure increases approximately 1–2 mmHg/week for the first 4 weeks of life.

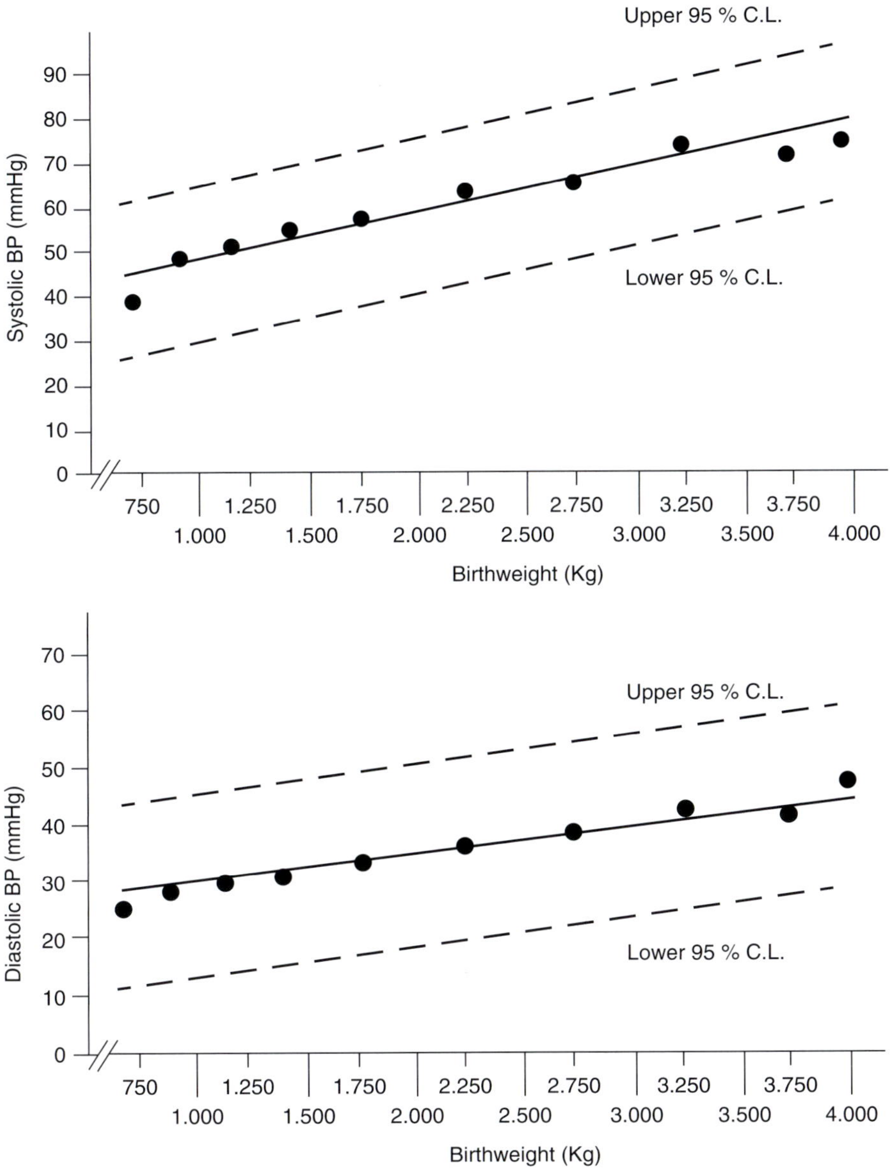

Fig. 15.1 Nomograms for blood pressure in newborn based on birth weight, gestational age and postconceptional age (Zubrow AB et al.: Determinants of blood pressure in infants admitted to neonatal intensive care units: A prospective multicenter study: Neonatal Blood Pressure Study Group. J Perinatol 15:470, 1995)

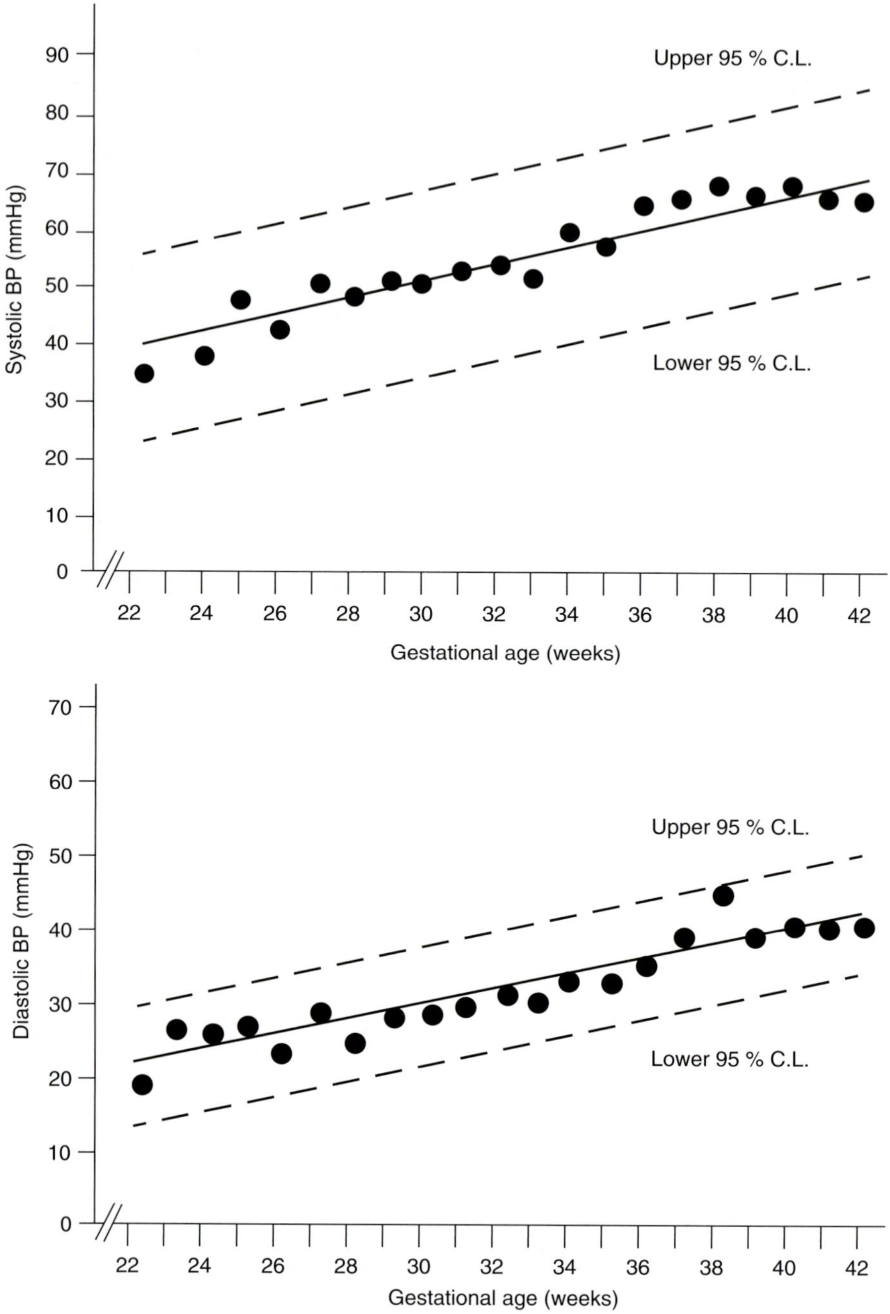

Fig. 15.1 (continued)

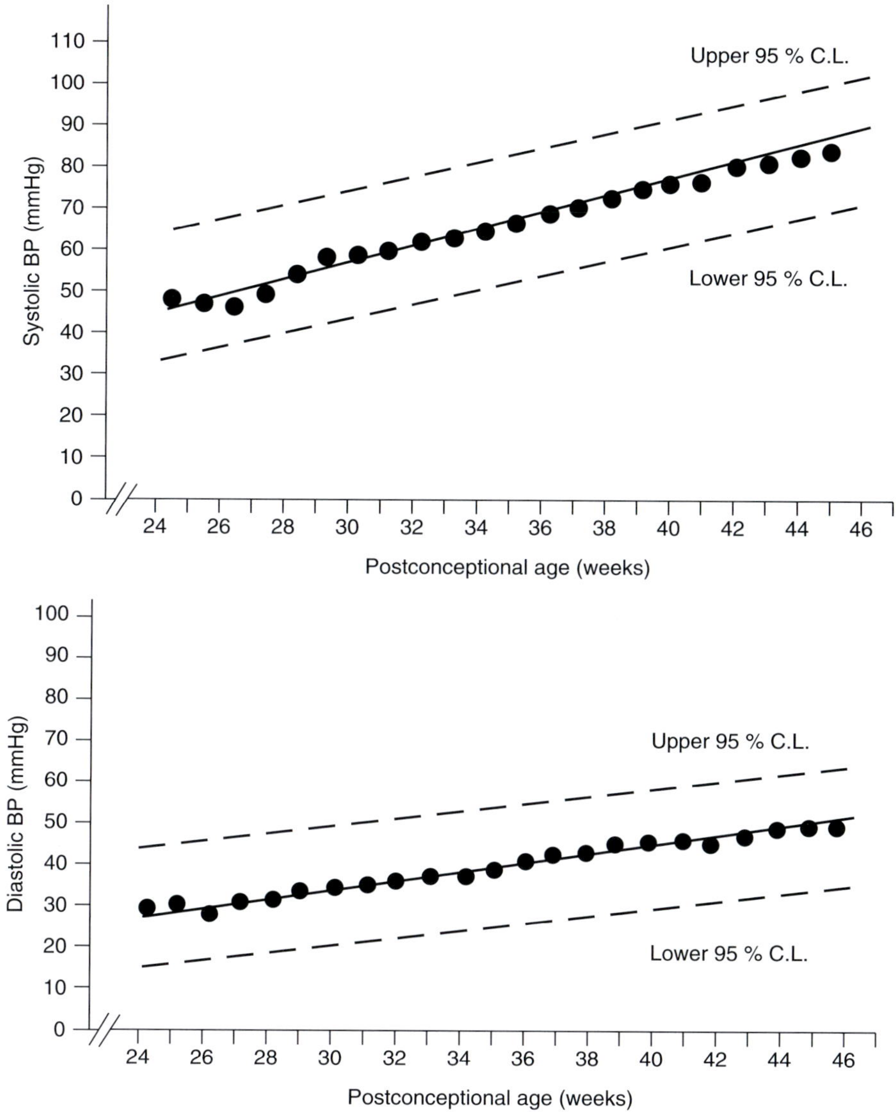

Fig. 15.1 (continued)

Table 15.12 Causes of neonatal hypertension

Renovascular disease (commonest)	Renal arterial thrombosis Renal arterial stenosis Renal venous thrombosis
Renal parenchymal disease	ARPKD
Cardiovascular disorders	Coarctation of the aorta
Neurologic disorders	Seizures Intracranial hypertension Drug withdrawal
Endocrine	CAH – 11-beta-hydroxylase deficiency Thyrotoxicosis
Drugs	Catecholamines Corticosteroids
Miscellaneous	Bronchopulmonary dysplasia Neuroblastoma

15.10.1 Presentation

Neonatal hypertension can have a variable presentation ranging from being asymptomatic to nonspecific symptoms like lethargy and poor feeding; cardiopulmonary symptoms such as tachypnoea, cyanosis, impaired perfusion, vasomotor instability and congestive heart failure; neurologic symptoms like tremors, hypertonicity, hypotonicity, opisthotonus, asymmetric reflexes, hemiparesis, seizures, apnoea or coma; and renal symptoms including acute renal failure.

15.10.2 Measurement of BP

Invasive method – from an in situ arterial line
Noninvasive method – Oscillometry, the cuff bladder should measure two-thirds the length of the extremity.

15.10.3 Investigations

In addition to 4-limb BP (to rule out coarctation of aorta), urinalysis, serum electrolytes, blood urea nitrogen, serum creatinine and serum calcium, special investigations include ultrasonography of the kidneys with a Doppler flow study of the aorta and renal arteries, echocardiography (to exclude aortic coarctation and evaluate the left ventricular mass) and rarely thyroid function studies and urinary studies for catecholamines, 17-hydroxysteroids and 17-ketosteroids.

15.10.4 Management

The treatment of hypertension includes oral or intravenous drug therapy depending on its severity. In severe hypertension, BP should not be lowered more than 25 %

within 6–8 h to prevent cerebral ischemia. Nicardipine, labetalol or nitroprusside are used in severe hypertension; the rate of infusion is adjusted to achieve the desired level of blood pressure. Less severe hypertension is managed with oral antihypertensive medications. ACE inhibitors are used in lower doses, carefully monitoring serum electrolytes and renal functions. Beta blockers are avoided in neonates with chronic lung disease. Nifedipine should be used with caution as it may cause rapid correction of blood pressure.

15.11 Nephrocalcinosis in the Premature Infant

- Nephrocalcinosis is a common complication occurring in 27–65 % of VLBW premature infants. Infants with bronchopulmonary dysplasia (with history of use of loop diuretics, aminophylline and total parental nutrition) are particularly prone to develop nephrocalcinosis.
- Ultrasonographic screening is recommended for all infants on treatment for chronic lung disease.
- Treatment includes restricted use of loop diuretics and corticosteroids and judicious use of calcium supplements, maintaining a high urine flow rate.
- The goal of therapy is to maintain the spot urinary calcium-to-creatinine ratio <0.86 mg/mg for infants <7 months of age.
- In 50 % affected infants, it resolves spontaneously in 5–6 months without adverse consequences.
- The long-term consequences of nephrocalcinosis are unclear; impairment of urine concentrating abilities may be seen.

15.12 Renal Vein Thrombosis (RVT)

- RVT has a definite predilection for the neonatal period.
- Common predisposing conditions include severe dehydration (hemoconcentration), in infants of diabetic mothers, cyanotic congenital heart disease, sickle-cell disease, sepsis and indwelling umbilical venous catheters.
- It presents with a palpable mass, haematuria, albuminuria and thrombocytopenia. If both kidneys are involved, the infant will develop features of renal failure.
- Ultrasound Doppler findings include presence of echogenic filling defects in the main renal vein and absence of renal venous flow surrounding the thrombus. Enlarged echogenic kidneys with loss of corticomedullary differentiation are typically seen.
- Treatment is supportive. Underlying problem should be corrected. Thrombolytics are indicated in bilateral RVT. Thrombectomy may not improve the outcomes.
- Detailed workup for thrombophilia is suggested. This includes a detailed family history and coagulation profile including prothrombin time, activated partial thromboplastin time and levels of protein C, protein S and antithrombin III. The clinical utility of testing for other prothrombotic states such as factor V Leiden

and prothrombin G20210A mutations, hyperlipoproteinemia, hyperhomocysteinemia needs to be individualised.

Suggested Reading

Askenazi DJ, Ambalavanam N, Goldstein SL (2009) Acute kidney injury in critically ill newborns: what do we know? What do we need to learn? Pediatr Nephrol 24:265–274

Gouyon JB, Guignard JP (2000) Management of acute renal failure in newborns. Pediatr Nephrol 14:1037–1044, © IPNA 2000

Oh W, Guignard JP, Baumgart S (2008) Nephrology and fluid electrolyte physiology: neonatology Questions and Controversies. Sauders Elsevier, Philadelphia

Satlin LM (2005) Renal disease. In: MacDonald MG, Mullett MD, Seshia MMK (eds) Avery's neonatology pathophysiology and management of the newborn, 6th edn. Lippincott Williams and Wilkins, Philadelphia

Vogt BA, Dell KM, Davis IR (2005) The kidney and urinary tract. In: Martin RJ, Fanaroff AA, Walsh MC (eds) Neonatal-perinatal medicine – diseases of fetus and infant, 8th edn. Mosby Elsevier, Philadelphia

Nephrotoxicity 16

Anil Vasudevan and Nivedita Kamath

16.1 Introduction

- Nephrotoxins are an important cause of acute kidney injury (AKI) in children. They may also be the cause for chronic kidney disease (CKD).
- There are several factors which increase vulnerability of the kidney to nephrotoxic injury. The kidney is an important site for metabolism of various drugs. The large blood flow through glomeruli and peritubular vessels, the large surface area available for uptake of nephrotoxic compounds, the high concentration of drugs within the tubular lumen which promotes intracellular uptake and precipitation and crystallization within tubules, multiple transport systems which concentrate the drug or its metabolite within tubular cells, and the high metabolic rate of renal tubular cells which makes it susceptible to injury with mild oxygen depletion are some of them.
- Endogenous substances like hemoglobin, myoglobin, and uric acid are toxic to the tubules and cause AKI. Commonly used drugs like NSAIDs and antibiotics can be toxic to the kidney. Often, there may be more than one drug which

A. Vasudevan (✉)
Department of Pediatric Nephrology, Children's Kidney Care Center,
St. John's Medical College Hospital, Koramangala,
Bangalore, KA 560078, India
e-mail: anil.vasudevan@sjri.res.in

N. Kamath
Department of Pediatric Nephrology, Children's Kidney Care Center,
St. John's Medical College Hospital,
Koramangala, Bangalore,
KA 560078, India
e-mail: n_shenoy25@yahoo.com

K. Phadke et al. (eds.), *Manual of Pediatric Nephrology*,
DOI 10.1007/978-3-642-12483-9_16, © Springer-Verlag Berlin Heidelberg 2014

contributes to kidney injury. Renal injury associated with drugs may involve more than one mechanism. Critically ill children, neonates, and children with preexisting renal disease are at maximum risk of nephrotoxicity.

Risk Factors for Nephrotoxicity

Extremes of age
Volume depletion
Concomitant use of several nephrotoxic medications
Compromised renal function
Drug dose, frequency, and duration related

- The spectrum of nephrotoxicity can vary from subtle manifestations to severe kidney injury. Though AKI is the most common renal injury produced by nephrotoxic agents, prolonged exposure to certain drugs may predispose to chronic kidney disease, e.g., NSAIDs.
- The diagnosis of nephrotoxicity is often missed or delayed due to the presence of coexisting risk factors, subtle manifestations, and lack of availability of early markers. A high index of suspicion; use of urinary biomarkers of renal injury, e.g., β-2 microglobulin, retinol-binding protein, and neutrophil gelatinase-associated lipocalin (NGAL) in early stages; and monitoring of drug levels may help in early diagnosis and prompt treatment of nephrotoxicity.
- Pseudonephrotoxicity must be suspected when drugs which inhibit tubular secretion of creatinine (e.g., cimetidine, trimethoprim) or drugs which interfere with the laboratory estimation of creatinine (e.g., cefoxitin, flucytosine) cause a rise in creatinine in the absence of other manifestations of renal injury.

Mechanisms of Nephrotoxicity

Alteration of renal hemodynamics/vasoconstriction resulting in decreased renal perfusion: Nonsteroidal anti-inflammatory drugs (NSAIDs), angiotensin-converting enzyme inhibitors (ACE inhibitors), calcineurin inhibitors, norepinephrine, radiocontrast agents, and diuretics
Acute tubular injury: Aminoglycosides, amphotericin B, vancomycin, NSAIDs, contrast media, acetaminophen, cyclosporin, cisplatin, IV immunoglobulin, mannitol, heavy metals
Acute interstitial nephritis: Ciprofloxacin, methicillin, penicillin G, ampicillin, cephalosporins, rifampicin, sulfonamides, NSAIDs, contrast media, thiazides, furosemide, phenytoin, allopurinol, cimetidine

Tubular obstruction:
Sulfonamides, methotrexate, methoxyflurane, triamterene, acyclovir, ethylene glycol, protease inhibitors, pigments (hemoglobin, myoglobin), statins (rhabdomyolysis)
Hypersensitivity angiitis:
Penicillin G, ampicillin, sulfonamides
Thrombotic microangiopathy:
Mitomycin C, cyclosporine, oral contraceptives
Glomerulopathy: NSAIDs, gold, penicillamine
Papillary necrosis: NSAIDs
Nephrocalcinosis: Furosemide

16.2 Endogenous Nephrotoxins

16.2.1 Hemoglobinuria

A Case Vignette

A 7-year-old boy is brought with history of fever for 3 days and history of passing reddish urine since day one. There is history of oliguria but no edema. On examination, his vitals are stable, and there is no hypertension. He has pallor but no organomegaly. Investigations show hemoglobin of 6 g/dl (3.72 mmol/l), peripheral smear showing anisopoikilocytosis, nucleated RBCs and burr cells, reticulocyte count of 3.5 %, LDH (lactate dehydrogenase) 3,300 units/l (55 μkat/l), and serum haptoglobin levels are undetectable. Urinalysis shows no proteinuria and no RBC but is positive for hemoglobin. Serum creatinine is 1.5 mg/dl (132 μmmol/l).

16.2.1.1 Causes of Hemoglobinuria

- Genetic defects: Glucose-6-phosphate dehydrogenase deficiency, paroxysmal cold hemoglobinuria, march hemoglobinuria
- Infections: Malaria, clostridia
- Transfusion reaction
- Chemical agents: Quinine sulfate, benzene, hydralazine, fava beans
- Venoms: Snakes, spiders
- Traumatic/mechanical destruction: Prosthetic valves, disseminated intravascular coagulation, extracorporeal circulation
- Miscellaneous: Heatstroke

16.2.2 Myoglobinuria

A Case Vignette

A 5-year-old girl was admitted after sustaining multiple fractures and crush injury following a road traffic accident. On the third day in the hospital, she had reddish urine. Her urine routine shows no RBC, but benzidine test is positive. Her hemoglobin is 10 g/dl (6.2 mmol/l) after transfusion, peripheral smear and reticulocyte counts are normal, LDH is 2,550 units/l (42.4 μkat/l), and creatinine phosphokinase (CPK) is 10,500 units/l (167.5 μkat/l).

16.2.2.1 Causes of Myoglobinuria

- Traumatic muscle injury: Crush injury, pressure necrosis, severe burns
- Drugs/toxins: Barbiturates, benzodiazepine, HMG-CoA reductase inhibitors, fibric acid derivatives, salicylates, carbon monoxide, ethylene glycol, snake and insect venoms, succinylcholine, propofol
- Genetic disorders: Phosphorylase deficiency, phosphofructokinase deficiency, α-glucosidase deficiency, carnitine palmitoyl transferase deficiency
- Infections: Influenza, tetanus, gas gangrene, Coxsackie virus, leptospirosis, HIV
- Excessive muscular activity: Vigorous exercise, status epilepticus, tetany
- Ischemia: Arterial occlusion
- Electrolyte and endocrine/metabolic disorders: Hypokalemia, hypophosphatemia hypothyroidism, hypothermia, and hyperthermia
- Immunologic diseases: Polymyositis, dermatomyositis

16.2.3 Clinical Presentation of Hemoglobinuria and Myoglobinuria (Pigment Nephropathy)

The presenting features of pigment-induced nephrotoxicity include oliguria and reddish urine; oliguria lasts for 7–10 days. Urine analysis shows acidic pH, no RBCs in the urine, and positive benzidine test suggesting hemoglobinuria/myoglobinuria. Granular casts/pigment casts may also be seen. Hyperkalemia disproportionate to renal failure is usually seen in case of massive hemolysis/rhabdomyolysis. Fractional excretion of sodium is generally low. In case of hemolysis and hemoglobinuria, pallor is seen. There will be evidence of hemolysis in the form of elevated reticulocyte count, peripheral smear showing features of hemolysis and elevated LDH, and low serum haptoglobin suggesting intravascular hemolysis. In case of myoglobinuria, there may be evidence of muscle injury and history of drug intake along with elevated LDH and CPK levels.

16.2.4 Pathophysiology of Pigment Nephropathy

The cause of pigment-associated acute tubular necrosis (ATN) is not well defined. The proposed mechanisms are (a) hypovolemia and ischemia, (b) direct tubular toxicity, and (c) tubular obstruction with pigment casts.

16.2.5 Treatment of Pigment Nephropathy

- Forced alkaline diuresis: Give fluids intravenously or orally, a one and a half to two times the maintenance rate depending on the condition of the child to target a normal central venous pressure and urine output of >3 ml/kg/h. Sodium bicarbonate (50–100 mmol) can be added to 1 l of 0.45 NS with dextrose, with the aim of maintaining the urine pH >6.5.
- Mannitol: Ensures good diuresis, acts as a free radical scavenger, and increases renal blood flow. It can be given at 3–5 ml/kg/dose every 8 h. Check plasma osmolality and osmolal gap while on mannitol and consider stopping mannitol if signs of fluid overload or if plasma osmolal gap exceeds 55 mOsm/kg.
- Consider renal replacement therapy if there is resistant hyperkalemia, rapidly rising serum potassium, oligoanuria, volume overload, or severe metabolic acidosis (pH <7.1).
- Recovery is usually complete.

16.2.6 Uric Acid Nephropathy

- Acute uric acid nephropathy is seen in patients with leukemias/lymphomas who develop massive cell lysis (tumor lysis syndrome) resulting in release of uric acid. Hyperuricemia causes uricosuria and uric acid crystal deposition and obstruction of renal tubules.
- Risk factors for uric acid nephropathy include urine pH less than 5.0, dehydration, rapid response to chemotherapy, elevated serum uric acid, and preexisting renal dysfunction.
- Lesch-Nyhan syndrome is a genetic disorder of uric acid metabolism which can result in uric acid calculi and nephropathy.
- Uric acid nephropathy is characterized by elevations in blood urea nitrogen, creatinine, potassium, uric acid, and phosphate concentrations and a decrease in the serum calcium levels.
- Acute kidney injury due to acute uric acid nephropathy is oliguric. Elevations in BUN and serum creatinine typically develop 2 days after the initiation of chemotherapy and return to baseline after 7–10 days.
- The urinary uric acid-to-creatinine ratio greater than 1 is consistent with acute uric acid nephropathy.

- Prophylaxis as well as treatment of tumor lysis syndrome includes the use of xanthine oxidase inhibitors, forced diuresis, and urinary alkalinization. Dialysis may be required in some cases.
- Rasburicase, a recombinant form of urate oxidase, is an option for treatment of uric acid nephropathy. It is given in the dose of 0.2 mg/kg/day as an IV infusion over 30 min.
- Prophylaxis:

  Prior to chemotherapy, ensure hydration. Measure uric acid and creatinine levels. If renal function is normal, start with fluids at twice the maintenance rate (3 l/m^2/day). Monitor intake-output strictly and watch for signs of fluid overload. Diuretics may be used to maintain a good urine output. Allopurinol can be added prophylactically in patients with hyperuricemia or if there is high tumor burden.

Urinary pH should be maintained above 7.0, titrating intravenous bicarbonate therapy.

- Fluid overload, refractory hyperkalemia, hyperphosphatemia, and acidosis may be indications to initiate dialysis.
- Recovery is usually complete.

16.3 Exogenous Nephrotoxins

16.3.1 NSAIDs (Nonsteroidal Anti-inflammatory Drugs)

A Case Vignette

A 3-day-old neonate, born at 32 weeks of gestation, weighing 1.4 kg, is started on indomethacin at 2 mg/kg/day for closure of a significant patent ductus arteriosus. The baseline creatinine is 0.4 mg/dl (35.2 μmmol/l). Two days later, the creatinine is found to be 1.1 mg/dl (96.8 μmmol/l).

NSAIDs are the most commonly used "over-the-counter" drugs which have a wide range of toxicity and may manifest as:

1. Acute kidney injury: This may be due to alteration of renal hemodynamics, acute tubulointerstitial nephritis, or papillary necrosis.
2. Chronic kidney disease.
3. Electrolyte abnormalities: Salt retention, hyperkalemia.
4. Fetal/neonatal renal failure: Maternal ingestion of nimesulide in the late trimester causes severe oliguric renal failure in newborns which may be irreversible.

16.3.1.1 Acute Kidney Injury

- NSAIDs precipitate acute kidney injury in conditions with impaired GFR due to inhibition of the compensatory vasodilatation caused by prostaglandins at the efferent arteriole.

- Volume depletion, neonatal period, congestive cardiac failure, and hypoalbuminemia are risk factors.
- The renal toxicity is dose, drug, and duration related. Aspirin is least likely and indomethacin is most likely to cause AKI. Ibuprofen, diclofenac, and naproxen have an intermediate nephrotoxicity.
- COX-2 selective NSAIDs (rofecoxib, celecoxib) also induce renal dysfunction especially in high-risk patients.
- Onset is usually 1–5 days after ingestion and may be oligoanuric or nonoliguric.
- Usually renal failure is reversible upon discontinuation of NSAIDs. If NSAIDs must be used in a child who has poor renal perfusion, a drug with a short half-life should be used (e.g., aspirin, sulindac).
- NSAIDs also cause tubulointerstitial nephritis which may present as acute kidney injury.
- Typically manifests as oliguric or nonoliguric AKI with nephrotic range proteinuria and eosinophiluria or leukocyturia.
- AKI is usually reversible.

16.3.2 Antibiotics

16.3.2.1 Aminoglycosides

- Aminoglycosides are eliminated unchanged almost entirely by the kidneys. They are highly charged cations which bind to tubular epithelial cells of S_1 and S_2 segments of proximal tubules from where they are reabsorbed by pinocytosis via megalin and are translocated into the lysosomes. Accumulation induces an injury cascade, phospholipid hydrolysis, formation of electron dense myeloid bodies, and progression to cell necrosis.
- Risk factors for aminoglycoside toxicity:
  - Patient-related factors: Newborns, preexisting renal disease, intravascular volume depletion, and Mg, K, Ca deficiency
  - Drug-related factors: Recent aminoglycoside therapy, large doses, treatment for more than 15 days
  - Concomitant use: Amphotericin B, cisplatin, cephalosporin, and furosemide
- Nephrotoxicity is drug, dose, and duration related. The order of relative toxicity of aminoglycosides, from the most toxic to the least, is neomycin, gentamicin, tobramycin, and amikacin.
- A variety of tubular dysfunction syndromes, Fanconi syndrome, hypomagnesemia and hypokalemia, and antidiuretic hormone resistance, are observed.
- Clinical manifestations: Usually nonoliguric, starts within 5–10 days following exposure to drug.
- Enzymuria is the first indicator of aminoglycoside toxicity. Tubular proteinuria and glycosuria may be seen. Hypokalemia and hypomagnesemia are common. The other significant toxicity is ototoxicity, to which there may be a genetic predisposition.
- Usually, the acute kidney injury is reversible but may take days to weeks.
- Serum aminoglycoside levels must be checked in all patients who are on therapy for 3–5 half-lives (2–3 doses) of the drug. The trough level is checked 30 min

prior to the dose and peak level is checked after 30 min of intravenous infusion. The peak and trough levels are specific for each drug and also the conditions for which the drug is being administered. Recommended peak and trough levels for amikacin are 20–30 mcg/ml and <10 mcg/ml, respectively.

Prevention of Aminoglycoside Toxicity

Identify risk factor – patient- and drug-related factors
Single daily dose
Administer as an infusion and not as a bolus
Minimum duration of treatment
Avoid other concomitant nephrotoxic drugs
Avoid dehydration
Corrected doses if reduced GFR
Estimate trough blood levels and titrate dose
Use alternative non-nephrotoxic drugs if possible

16.3.2.2 Beta-Lactam Antibiotics

- Penicillins, cephalosporins, and carbapenems are all associated with nephrotoxicity. Cephaloridine and imipenem are most nephrotoxic.
- Cefotaxime, ceftazidime, and meropenem are nephrotoxic and require dose adjustments in renal failure.
- Ceftriaxone and cefoperazone are not nephrotoxic and hence do not require dose adjustments in renal failure.
- Clinical features: Usually an idiosyncratic response. They may present as oliguric or nonoliguric renal failure. Acute tubulointerstitial nephritis presents as nonoliguric renal failure and may be associated with systemic manifestations like fever, rash, and arthralgia. Urinalysis shows tubular proteinuria, pyuria, and eosinophiluria.
- Lipid peroxidation, acylation, inactivation of tubular proteins, and inhibition of mitochondrial respiration are the major mechanisms of nephrotoxicity.
- Acute tubulointerstitial nephritis (TIN) due to hypersensitivity can also cause renal failure, especially with drugs like methicillin.
- Generally resolves spontaneously; steroids may be helpful in acute TIN.
- Administration of probenecid may help to reduce the nephrotoxic effect of beta-lactam antibiotics.

16.3.2.3 Glycopeptide Antibiotics (Vancomycin)

- Usually asymptomatic and manifests only as rise in serum creatinine levels.
- The exact mechanism of action is not known. Accumulation in the lysosomes of the proximal tubule contributes to nephrotoxicity.
- Nephrotoxicity is related to the dose and duration of therapy.

- Risk factors are high baseline serum creatinine, concomitant nephrotoxic drugs, and existing liver disease.
- Nephrotoxicity is usually reversible.
- Therapeutic drug monitoring helps to titrate therapy in high-risk groups. The target trough level is 10 mcg/ml.

16.3.2.4 Others

- Sulfonamides and their acetylated metabolites are poorly soluble in acidic urine and may precipitate leading to intrarenal obstruction. This can be prevented by adequate fluid intake and alkalinization of urine.
- Trimethoprim can cause hyperkalemia by blocking amiloride-sensitive channels. It blocks tubular secretion of creatinine causing pseudonephrotoxicity.

16.3.3 Antifungals

16.3.3.1 Amphotericin B

- The drug interacts with membrane cholesterol at the distal tubule and leads to formation of aqueous pores resulting in increased permeability and back diffusion of H+, Na+, and Cl^- resulting in "backleak" type of distal renal tubular acidosis and vasopressin-resistant polyuria. It also causes reduced GFR secondary to afferent arteriolar vasoconstriction.
- The toxicity is related to the cumulative dose, dosing frequency, duration, and formulation (lipid and liposomal formulations are less nephrotoxic).
- The risk factors for nephrotoxicity are salt depletion, concomitant use of diuretics, cyclosporine or aminoglycoside antibiotics, abnormal renal functions, and young age.
- It clinically manifests as distal renal tubular acidosis, hypokalemia, hypomagnesemia, and decreased GFR secondary to afferent arteriolar vasoconstriction.
- Salt supplementation reduces the incidence and severity of nephrotoxicity. Normal saline infusion (10–15 ml/kg) pre- and post-amphotericin B dose is recommended. Use of lipid-based formulations of amphotericin B may produce less nephrotoxicity, without affecting clinical effectiveness.

16.3.4 Antivirals

16.3.4.1 Acyclovir and Ganciclovir

- The toxicity of these drugs may be due to direct tubular toxicity or due to intrarenal obstruction due to crystal deposits. These drugs are excreted by glomerular filtration and tubular secretion. They form insoluble crystals which precipitate in the distal tubule.
- Risk factors include high doses of intravenous acyclovir, volume depletion, and preexisting renal disease.

- Clinical features: Usually asymptomatic; however, symptoms may develop within 24–48 h after starting therapy. Nausea, vomiting, flank pain, or abdominal pain may occur. Urinary findings include crystalluria (needle shaped crystals), hematuria, pyuria, and proteinuria.
- The renal insufficiency is generally reversible and renal function returns to normal by 1 week.
- Infusing the drug slowly over 1–2 h and hydrating the child adequately to maintain a high urinary flow help lower the risk for renal toxicity. Probenecid coadministration may reduce the tubular secretion of acyclovir.

16.3.4.2 Other Antivirals

- Foscarnet: Drug toxicity profile is similar to acyclovir. It also causes functional renal tubular defects like hypophosphatemia, hypokalemia, and nephrogenic diabetes insipidus.
- Cidofovir: Causes proximal tubular necrosis and renal failure.
- Tenofovir: Presents with proximal tubular dysfunction resulting in Fanconi syndrome.
- Indinavir: Causes crystalluria resulting in obstruction and renal failure. It may also present as renal calculi and chronic renal dysfunction. The crystals appear as flat rectangular plates in fan-shaped or starburst aggregates.

16.3.5 Chemotherapeutic Drugs

16.3.5.1 Cisplatin

- Cisplatin is an inorganic platinum compound that may induce acute and chronic renal toxicity. Carboplatin is less nephrotoxic when compared to cisplatin. Cisplatin decreases the GFR and also acts as a direct tubular toxin.
- The nephrotoxicity is dose related.
- Clinical features: Usually presents with polyuria, tubular proteinuria, and tubular loss of potassium, magnesium, sodium, phosphate, and amino acids.
- Hypomagnesemia is a striking feature of cisplatin toxicity and may take weeks to improve.
- Prevention of nephrotoxicity: Infusion of mannitol and saline has been used to maintain good urine output and reduce nephrotoxicity. Dosage should not exceed 25–33 mg/m^2/week. The administration of cisplatin in hypertonic saline is associated with better tolerability.
- Sodium thiosulphate administration also protects the kidneys. The role of amifostine, a free radical scavenger, has been approved for use with cisplatin. N-Acetylcysteine, free radical scavengers, and liposomal formulations are being tried to reduce the nephrotoxic effects of platinum compounds.

16.3.5.2 Ifosfamide

- Unlike cyclophosphamide, ifosfamide is associated with significant nephrotoxicity. Ifosfamide and its metabolites like chloroacetaldehyde have been found to be toxic to cells.

- The incidence is variable and depends on cumulative dose (>60 g/m^2), rapidity of administration, concomitant nephrotoxic drugs like platinum compounds, and age of patient.
- Clinical features: Presents with features of tubular injury resulting in nonoliguric renal failure, associated with tubular wasting of glucose, phosphate, low molecular weight proteins, and bicarbonate and loss of concentrating ability.
- Though usually reversible, chronic hypophosphatemia, rickets, and chronic kidney disease also have been found as late consequences of ifosfamide toxicity.
- Mesna which is used to prevent hemorrhagic cystitis does not offer any protection against nephrotoxic effects of ifosfamide.

16.3.5.3 Cyclophosphamide

- Though cyclophosphamide is not a nephrotoxic drug, it can cause hemorrhagic cystitis.
- Syndrome of inappropriate antidiuresis (SIAD) may also be seen with cyclophosphamide.

16.3.5.4 Methotrexate

- The nephrotoxicity has been attributed to the precipitation of the drug and its metabolites within the tubular lumen and also due to direct tubular toxicity.
- Clinical presentation: Methotrexate toxicity is associated with decrease in GFR and increase in serum creatinine.
- Usually reversible and may require about 2 weeks for recovery.

16.3.6 Calcineurin Inhibitors (Cyclosporine and Tacrolimus)

- Mechanism of action: The nephrotoxic effects may be acute or chronic.
  - Acute nephrotoxicity: Hemodynamically mediated, dose dependent, reversible reduction in GFR due to afferent arteriolar vasoconstriction. Damage to the vascular endothelium may result in hemolytic uremic syndrome resulting in acute kidney injury. Proximal tubular defect includes impaired secretion of uric acid and urea, hyperkalemia, and hyperchloremic metabolic acidosis. It can also cause hypomagnesemia.
  - Chronic nephrotoxicity: Defined as 20 % or greater irreversible reduction in GFR. It is characterized by morphological changes including tubular atrophy, striped interstitial fibrosis, vascular hyalinosis, and glomerular sclerosis. This may not be dose dependent and not reversible.
- Drugs like ketoconazole, macrolides, and metoclopramide which inhibit the metabolism of calcineurin inhibitors may potentiate toxicity.
- Clinical features: May be asymptomatic and recognized only by monitoring of creatinine levels. May manifest as delayed graft function in the post-transplant period. It may be difficult to distinguish calcineurin toxicity from graft rejection. In children with nephrotic syndrome, calcineurin toxicity may be a differential diagnosis for progression of focal segmental glomerulosclerosis. Monitoring of serum levels may help in titrating the dose of calcineurin inhibitors.
- Acute nephrotoxicity usually resolves spontaneously with cessation of therapy.

16.3.7 Angiotensin-Converting Enzyme (ACE) Inhibitors and Angiotensin Receptor-Blocking Agents (ARB)

- Clinical features: Oliguria and hyperkalemia are common manifestations.
- Usually reversible on reduction of dose or cessation of the drug.
- Fetopathy and severe oliguric renal failure in newborn have been reported with maternal ingestion of ACE inhibitors.
- The main mechanism of acute renal dysfunction is due to inhibition of the afferent arteriolar dilatation and efferent arteriolar constriction which is a compensatory autoregulatory response of angiotensin II in order to maintain the GFR.
- Risk factors for renal dysfunction are dehydration, hypovolemia, congestive cardiac failure, renal artery stenosis, and concomitant use of other nephrotoxic medications like NSAIDs. They must be used with caution in patients with solitary kidney and renal artery stenosis.

16.3.8 Paracetamol

- Usually presents as AKI due to acute tubular necrosis with proteinuria, granular casts in the urine, hematuria, and pyuria.
- Paracetamol/acetaminophen: Though hepatotoxicity is the most common manifestation of paracetamol poisoning, nephrotoxicity is also known.
- Nephrotoxicity is attributed to the depletion of sulfates and glutathione resulting in the accumulation of the toxic metabolite N-acetyl-p-benzoquinone imine (NAPQI).
- The serum creatinine peaks at 7 days and returns to normal within a month.
- N-acetylcysteine may be considered in the management of nephrotoxicity.

16.3.9 Radiocontrast Agents

- Radiocontrast agents are tri-iodinated benzoic acid derivatives which are freely filtered at the glomerulus.
- Clinical features: Nonoliguric renal failure characterized by an elevation in serum creatinine within 24 h of exposure is typical. Rarely, it may be oliguric. The serum creatinine peaks at 3–5 days and returns to baseline within 14 days. Urine analysis may show tubular proteinuria and granular casts. Fractional excretion of sodium remains low (<1 %).
- An absolute rise of serum creatinine of ≥0.5 mg/dl within 48 h of exposure to a contrast or a 25 % increase in serum creatinine from baseline within 48 h of exposure is defined as contrast-induced nephropathy (CIN). Other sensitive markers like cystatin C and NGAL (neutrophil gelatinase-associated lipocalin) are being studied as early indicators of renal dysfunction.
- Mechanism of action: Renal medullary ischemia due to vasoconstriction is the most important pathophysiological mechanism resulting in tubular cell hypoxia and damage. Hyperviscosity of the contrast media and osmolar load also result

in medullary hypoxia. Free radical injury may contribute to worsening of renal failure.

- Risk factors for CIN: Preexisting renal dysfunction, congestive cardiac failure, hypovolemia, younger age, concomitant NSAIDs, and diuretics are known risk factors. Diabetes mellitus and myocardial infarction are important risk factors in adults.
- Pharmacokinetic properties of contrast media which predispose to CIN: High osmolality, high viscosity, and higher volumes of contrast are known risk factors. Low-osmolar agents (iohexol, iodixanol) may have benefit over iso-osmolar agents in reducing the risk of CIN.
- Usually recovery is spontaneous, with <1 % requiring dialysis.
- Prevention:
  (a) Intravenous hydration: Hydration with isotonic saline prior to contrast administration has been found to be useful in reducing the risk of CIN.
  (b) Sodium bicarbonate has been shown to be effective in reducing the risk of CIN.
  (c) N-acetylcysteine: Has shown significant reduction in the risk of CIN.
  (d) Diuretics may be used only in situations of fluid overload. There is no role for use of mannitol.
  (e) The role of theophylline, dopamine, and acetazolamide in preventing CIN is unclear.

Protocol for Prevention of Contrast-Induced Nephropathy
Ensure adequate hydration – isotonic saline started at 1 ml/kg/h at least 2 h prior to contrast administration and continued for 6–12 h following the procedure.
Sodium bicarbonate – 3 ml/kg bolus over 1 h prior to the procedure and 1 ml/kg/h for 6 h after the procedure.
N-acetylcysteine 1,200 mg/1.73 m^2 twice a day, orally on the day before and on the day of the procedure.

16.3.9.1 Nephrogenic Systemic Fibrosis (NSF)

- Nephrogenic systemic fibrosis is the result of systemic toxicity in patients with impaired renal function who have subsequent impaired clearance of gadolinium and related compounds.
- Gadolinium is a non-iodinated contrast agent used for magnetic resonance angiography and digital subtraction angiography. The risk of nephrotoxicity with gadolinium was thought to be minimal, and hence, it was considered to be a substitute for iodinated contrast agents in high-risk groups. Later, it was discovered that NSF could be a complication of using gadolinium in patients with renal insufficiency.
- Nephrogenic systemic fibrosis is a condition seen in patients with renal dysfunction exposed to gadolinium. Gadolinium-based agents are rapidly excreted by normal kidneys. In patients with CKD, the time for these agents in circulation is increased and they dissociate into linear chelates. The free gadolinium chelates are responsible for NSF. This primarily involves the skin resulting in fibrosis and myxedema-like features. The early changes are pain, pruritus, erythema, and

edema which usually begin over the legs and later progress to involve the entire body, sparing the head and neck. Usually seen within 18 months following exposure to gadolinium, this condition may also affect the liver, heart, and skeletal muscle. In late stages, there can be severe contractures resulting in deformities.

- The proposed mechanism of action is release of free gadolinium ions which deposit in the skin resulting in fibrosis.
- It can be fulminant and fatal in <5 % cases.
- Prevention:
  (a) Avoid use of gadolinium-based contrast in children with renal dysfunction.
  (b) Use of low-dose gadolinium.
  (c) Hemodialysis initiated following exposure may be helpful in clearance of gadolinium in patients with GFR <30 ml/1.73 m^2/min. Peritoneal dialysis is not effective.
- Treatment of nephrogenic systemic fibrosis are as follows:

Corticosteroids, sodium thiosulfate, intravenous immunoglobulin, phototherapy, and ultraviolet radiation have been used as modalities for the treatment of nephrogenic systemic fibrosis.

16.3.10 Miscellaneous

16.3.10.1 Herbal Medications

- Chinese herbal medicines use aristolochic acid derived from Aristolochia plant species which is known to cause aristolochic acid nephropathy, endemic Balkan nephropathy, and reversible renal Fanconi syndrome.
- Aristolochic acid nephropathy and endemic Balkan nephropathy present with tubular proteinuria, proximal tubulopathy, sterile pyuria, and anemia. It causes chronic kidney disease and can predispose to urothelial malignancies. The progress to ESRD is rapid in aristolochic acid nephropathy (1–2 years) as compared to endemic Balkan nephropathy (15–20 years).
- Traditional medicinal products contain several plant products and heavy metals which can induce various renal problems like acute tubular necrosis, acute or chronic interstitial nephritis, Fanconi syndrome, dyskalemia, arterial hypertension, papillary necrosis, and urolithiasis and urothelial cancer. Glycyrrhiza (licorice) may induce arterial hypertension and hypokalemia.
- Mushrooms (Cortinarius species) are known to cause acute kidney injury due to the toxic substance orellanine. Acute tubular necrosis and acute interstitial nephritis are seen.

16.3.10.2 Ethylene Glycol and Methanol

- Ethylene glycol (EG) and methanol are components of antifreeze or transmission fluid. The ingestion, usually accidental or suicidal, results in severe high anion gap metabolic acidosis and AKI.
- Untreated, three phases have been described as follows: (1) neurologic stage, with hallucinations, stupor, and coma; (2) cardiovascular toxicity with cardiac failure; and (3) renal failure due to acute tubular necrosis.

- The compounds are not themselves toxic, but their metabolites are. Metabolism is initiated by alcohol dehydrogenase (ADH) and results in oxalate and organic acids for ethylene glycol and formic acid and formaldehyde for methanol.
- Oxalic acid combines with calcium to form calcium oxalate crystals in the renal tubules.
- Other laboratory findings: Calcium oxalate crystalluria, hematuria, and hypocalcemia.
- Ethanol and fomepizole are specific antidotes which inhibit alcohol dehydrogenase and prevent metabolism of ethylene glycol into toxic metabolites.
- Mild cases may require only symptomatic treatment.
- In moderate to severe cases, criteria for antidotal therapy in EG poisoning are the following:
  - EG concentration in serum above 200 mg/l
  - Patient's history of ingestion of a toxic dose of EG and an osmolar gap of more than 10 mOsm/kg
  - Suspicion of EG poisoning by history or clinical symptoms and two of the following criteria: Arterial blood pH <7.3, serum bicarbonate concentration <20 mmol/l, osmolar gap >10 mOsm/kg, and crystals of calcium oxalate in urine sediment
  - Fomepizole is better tolerated in children; loading dose of 15 mg/kg, followed by four bolus doses of 10 mg/kg every 12 h
- Hemodialysis is recommended if the EG serum level is above 500 mg/l.

16.3.10.3 Heavy Metals

- Lead: Lead toxicity may be acute or chronic. It has several systemic manifestations like abdominal pain, cognitive deficits, peripheral neuropathy and arthralgia, a lead line at the junction between tooth and gum, and anemia with basophilic stippling. The nephrotoxic effects may manifest as a Fanconi syndrome with damage to the proximal tubule.

  The acute effects of lead on the kidney are generally reversible. Chronic lead toxicity results in progressive tubular atrophy and interstitial fibrosis resulting in chronic kidney disease. It can also cause nephrotic syndrome, hyperuricemia, and hypertension.
- Cadmium: Chronic exposure to cadmium causes chronic kidney disease and osteoporosis.
- Mercury: Acute mercury poisoning can cause tubular necrosis and AKI. Long-term exposure can cause membranous nephropathy.

16.3.10.4 Animal Toxins

- Snake envenomation (refer to Chap. 13).
- Animal stings: Sting by animals (e.g., spiders, arthropods, scorpions) can induce nephrotoxicity in the form of acute tubular necrosis, acute interstitial nephritis, hemolytic uremic syndrome, nephrotic syndrome, and, rarely, pigment nephropathy. Marine animals (e.g., carp, jellyfish, and sea anemones) can also induce acute tubular necrosis, proteinuria, and nephrotic syndrome.

16.3.10.5 Melamine Poisoning

Melamine formaldehyde is an adulterant in powdered milk formula to increase the nitrogen content of the food. The "outbreak" of renal stones in children following consumption of adulterated milk in China has brought melamine poisoning into light. Cyanuric acid, the metabolite of melamine, is implicated in the nephrotoxicity. The toxic effects can be acute or chronic. It can present with nephrolithiasis and AKI. The usual clinical features are hematuria, flank pain, and dysuria. The symptoms are due to renal stones (melamine, uric acid, and triple ammonium phosphate) and due to urinary tract infections. The symptoms are seen within 3–6 months following consumption of melamine. Hypertension, edema, and acute kidney injury may be seen in severe cases. Melamine stones are radiolucent and are usually multiple and bilateral. Urine analysis shows microscopic hematuria with or without proteinuria. Melamine crystals appear as fan-shaped crystals on microscopy. Long-term exposure to melamine can cause bladder calculi and transitional cell carcinoma. Treatment for renal calculi and AKI is conservative. Rarely, surgical removal of calculi is indicated. Food and Drug Administration (FDA) gives a safety limit of exposure to melamine and its structural analogues as <0.63 mg/kg/day.

Conclusions

Nephrotoxic renal injury is an important and preventable cause of AKI as well as CKD in children. The spectrum of nephrotoxicity is varied and requires a high index of suspicion for early diagnosis. Most common cause for nephrotoxic renal injury is "drug toxicity." A drug may cause nephrotoxicity by several mechanisms and different drugs may share common mechanism of nephrotoxicity. Altered hemodynamics, acute tubular necrosis, or acute interstitial nephritis contributes to acute kidney injury. Nephrotoxic injury can be prevented by appropriate dose reduction in renal failure, avoiding concomitant use of nephrotoxic medications, and monitoring of drug levels, whenever possible. The drug toxicity may also present as chronic kidney disease.

Suggested Reading

Bacchetta J, Dubourg L, Juillard L, Cochat P (2009) Non-drug-induced nephrotoxicity. Pediatr Nephrol 24:2291–2300

Cronin RE (2010) Contrast induced nephropathy: pathogenesis and prevention. Pediatr Nephrol 25:191–204

Hau AK, Kwan TH, Li PK (2009) Melamine toxicity and the kidney. J Am Soc Nephrol 20(2):245–250

Lopez-Novoa JM, Quiros Y, Vicente L, Morales AI, Lopez-Hernandez FJ (2011) New insights into the mechanism of aminoglycoside toxicity: an integrative point of view. Kidney Int 79:33–45

Patzer L (2008) Nephrotoxicity as a cause of acute kidney injury in children. Pediatr Nephrol 23:2159–2173

Penfield J (2008) Nephrogenic systemic fibrosis and the use of gadolinium based contrast agents. Pediatr Nephrol 23:2121–2129

Appendix 17

Jyoti Sharma and Anil Vasudevan

17.1 Normal Reference Values of Blood and Urine Chemistries

Different laboratories may have different reference ranges; different methods of testing may be used. Hence, consult your laboratory for its analytic methods and for its range of normal values. 17.1.1 gives normal reference values of routinely performed blood and urine chemistries while evaluating a child with renal disease.

Serum (S), plasma (P), whole blood (W), heparinised (H), day (d), months (mo), year (y).

17.1.1 Blood Chemistries

Analyte	Specimen	Age	Reference values (conventional)	Reference values (SI)
Amylase	S, P	Any	30–100 U/l	30–100 U/l
Albumin	P	Any	3.9–4.5 g/dl	39–45 U/l
Aldosterone	P	Any	<36 ng/dl	<1,000 pmol/l

(continued)

J. Sharma (✉)
Department of Pediatrics, Bharati Vidyapeeth Deemed University Medical College, Pune, MH 411040, India
e-mail: jyotivsharma@gmail.com

A. Vasudevan
Department of Pediatric Nephrology, Children's Kidney Care Center, St. John's Medical College Hospital, Koramangala, Bangalore, KA 560078, India

Department of Pediatrics, Children's Kidney Care Center, St. John's Medical College Hospital, Koramangala, Bangalore, KA 560078, India
e-mail: anil.vasudevan@sjri.res.in

K. Phadke et al. (eds.), *Manual of Pediatric Nephrology*,
DOI 10.1007/978-3-642-12483-9_17,

Analyte	Specimen	Age	Reference values (conventional)		Reference values (SI)
Alkaline phosphatase	S		U/l		U/l
		Up to 1 y	150–420		150–420
		>1 y	100–320		100–320
Anion gap (Na [Cl+HCO_3^-])	P (H)	Any	7–16 mEq/l		7–16 mmol/l
Anti-deoxyribonuclease B (anti-DNAse B)	S	4–6 y	240–480 U		240–480 U
		7–12 y	480–800 U		480–800 U
Antidiuretic hormone (ADH, vasopressin)	P		Plasma osmolality (mOsm/l)	Plasma ADH (pg/ml)	Plasma ADH (ng/l)
			270–280	<1.5	<1.5
			280–285	<2.5	<2.5
			285–290	1–5	1–5
			290–295	2–7	2–7
			295–300	4–12	4–12
Base excess	W		mmol/l		mmol/l
		Newborn	(−10)–(−2)		(−10)–(−2)
		Infant	(−7)–(−1)		(−7)–(−1)
		Child	(−4)–(+2)		(−4)–(+2)
Bicarbonate	W		mEq/l		mmol/l
		Newborn	17–24		17–24
		2 mo to 2 y	16–24		16–24
		>2 y	22–26		22–26
Calcium, ionized (Ca)	S, P (H)		mg/dl		mmol/l
		24–48 h	4.0–4.7		1. 00–1.17
		>2 d	4.8–4.92		1.12–1. 23
	W	Any	2.24–2.46		1.12–1. 23
Calcium (total)	S		mg/dl		mmol/l
		24–48 h	7.0–12.0		1.75–3.00
		4–7 d	9.0–10.9		2.25–2.73
		Child	8.8–10.8		2.20–2.70
Chloride	S, P		97–110 mmol/l		97–110 mmol/l
Cholesterol	S		120–263 mg/dl		3.1–6.8 mmol/l
C-reactive protein	S		0–0.5 mg/dl		47.6 nmol/l
Creatinine Jaffe, kinetic, or enzymatic	S, P		mg/dl		μmol/l
		Newborn	0.3–1.0		27–88
		1 week to 2 mo	0.1–0.6		10–56
		>2 mo to 1 y	0.2–0.4		18–35
		Child	0.3–0.7		27–62
		Adolescent	0.5–1.0		44–88

Analyte	Specimen	Age	Reference values (conventional)	Reference values (SI)
Cystatin C	S	Preterm neonates	mg/l	mg/l
			1.34–2.57	1.34–2.57
		Full-term infants	1.36–2.23	1.36–2.23
		>8 d to 1 y	0.75–1.87	0.75–1.87
		>1–3 y	0.68–1.90	0.68–1.90
		>3–16 y	0.51–1.31	0.51–1.31
D-dimer levels	P		Positive titers ≥1:8	
Ferritin	S		ng/ml	μg/l
		1 mo	200–600	200–600
		2–5 mo	50–200	50–200
		6 mo–15 y	7–140	7–140
Fibrinogen	P		1.5–4.0 g/l	1.5–4.0 g/l
Haptoglobin	P	Neonate	5–48 mg/dl	50–480 mg/l
		>1 mo	26–185 mg/dl	260–1,850 mg/l
Iron	S		22–184 μg/dl	4–33 μmol/l
Lactate dehydrogenase	S		U/l	U/l
		Up to 9 y	150–500	150–500
		10–19 y	120–330	120–330
Magnesium	P		1.2–2.6 mg/dl	0.48–1.05 mmol/l
Osmolality	S		275–295 mOsmol/l H_2O	275–295 mmol/l H_2O
Parathyroid hormone (intact)	P		1–43 pg/ml	0.6–6.0 pmol/l
Phosphorus	S, P (H)		mg/dl	mmol/l
		0–5 d	4.8–8.2	1.55–2.65
		1–11 d	3.8–6.5	1.25–2.3 0
		12–19 y	2.9–5.4	0.95–1.7 5
Potassium	S, P		mEq/l	mmol/l
		<2 mo	3.0–7.0	3.0–7. 0
		2–12 mo	3.5–6.0	3.5–6. 0
		>12 mo	3.5–4.5	3.5–4.5
Sodium	S	135–145 mEq/l		135–145 mmol/l
Total iron-binding capacity (TIBC)	S	250–400 μg/ml		45–72 μmol/l
Urea	S, P		mg/dl	mmol/l
		<1 y	8.1–28.0	2.9–10.0
		1–2 y	5.0–15.0	1.8–5.4
		>2 y	8.1–19.9	2.9–7.1
Uric acid	S		mg/dl	μmol/l
		1–5 y	1.7–5.8	100–350
		6–11 y	2.2–6.6	130–390
		12–19 y	Males: 3.0–7.7	180–460
			Females: 2.7–5.7	160–340

(continued)

Analyte	Specimen	Age	Reference values (conventional)		Reference values (SI)
Vitamin D 25(OH)D	S		ng/ml		nmol/l
			<5	Severe deficiency	<12.5
			5–15	Moderate deficiency	12.5–37.44
			16–30	Insufficiency	40–75
1, 25-dihydroxyvitamin D	S		16–65 pg/ml		42–169 pmol/l

17.1.2 Urine Chemistries

24-h urine			Random urine		
	Conventional units	SI units		Conventional units	SI units
Albumin	–	–	Albumin/creatinine (microalbuminuria)	mg/g	(mg/mmol)
			Normal	<3	<0.3
			Follow-up	30–300	3–30
			High	>300	>30
Calcium			Calcium/creatinine	mg/mg	(mmol/mmol)
	<4 mg/kg/d	<0.1 mmol/kg/d	<7 mo	0.86	0.53
			7–18 mo	0.60	1.5
			19 mo to 6 y	0.42	1.1
			>6 y	0.22	0.6
Chloride	100–200mEq/d	100–200 mmol/d			
Citrate	>150 mg/1.73 m²/d	0.8 mmol/1.73 m²/d	Citrate/creatinine	g/g	mol/mol
			0–5 y	0.2–0.42	0.12–0.25
			>5 y	0.14–0.25	0.08–0.15
Creatinine	≥15 mg/kg/d				
Cystine			Cystine/creatinine	mg/g	(mol/mmol)
	<10 y: <13 mg/1.73 m²/d	<55 μmol/1.73 m²/d	<1 mo	<180	<85
	>10 y: <48 mg 1.73 m²/d	200 μmol/1.73 m²/d	1–6 mo	<112	<53
			>6 mo	<38	<18
Oxalate			Oxalate/creatinine	mg/g	mmol/mol
	<45 mg/1.73 m²/d	<0.5 mmol/1.73 m²/d	0–6 mo	<288	<360
			7–24 mo	<139	<174
			2–14 y	<80	<100
			>16 y	<32	<40
Phosphate excretion				TmP/GFR = (SP-U Cr)/	Neonate = 6.9 mg/dl >neonate-16 y=3.2–4.5 mg/dl

24-h urine			Random urine		
	Conventional units	SI units		Conventional units	SI units
Protein			Protein/creatinine	mg/mg	mg/mmol
	<4 mg/m^2/h		6–24 mo	<0.5	<50
			>24 mo	<0.2	<20
Uric acid	<815 mg/1.73 m^2/d or <35 mg/kg/d	<4.89 mmol/ 1.73 m^2/d 0.21 mmol/kg/d	(Urine uric acid) × (S creatinine/urine creatinine) (all values in same units mg/dl or mmol/l)	<0.56 mg/dl GFR	<0.03 mmol/l GFR

17.2 Conversion from Conventional Units to International Units (SI)

There is a lack of uniformity across the world in the units used for reporting clinical biochemistry values. Conventional units give values in mg/dl or mg/L, or mm Hg. SI units are used for reporting these values in other parts of the world. 17.2 gives typical values for common biochemical parameters in both units and indicates the "conversion factors".

Laboratory test	Conventional units	SI units	To convert to SI units
ALT (alanine aminotransferase)	units/l	μkat/l	×0.01667
Albumin	g/dl	g/l	×10
Alkaline phosphatase	units/l	μkat/l	×0.01667
Aldosterone	ng/dl	nmol/l	×0.0277
Amylase, serum	units/l	nkat/l	×0.01667
Anion gap	mEq/l	mmol/l	No conversion
AST (aspartate aminotransferase)	units/l	μkat/l μkat/l	×0.01667
Bicarbonate	mEq/l	mmol/l	No conversion
Bilirubin	mg/dl	μmol/l	×17.1
Calcium, serum	mg/dl mEq/l	mmol/l	×0.25 ×0.50
Calcium, urine	mg/24 h	mmol/24 h	×0.025
Calcitonin	pg/ml	ng/l	×1.0
Chloride	mEq/l	mmol/l	No conversion
Cholesterol, total	mg/dl	mmol/l	×0.02586
Cortisol, serum	μg/dl	nmol/l	×27.59
Creatinine	mg/dl	μmol/l	×88

(continued)

Laboratory test	Conventional units	SI units	To convert to SI units
Creatinine clearance	ml/min	ml/s	×0.0167
Creatine kinase	units/l	μkat/l	×0.01667
C3/C4 complement	mg/ml	g/l	×0.01
Glucose, urine	g/dl	mmol/l	×0.05551
Glucose, plasma	mg/dl	mmol/l	×0.05551
GGT (gamma-glutamyl transferase)	U/l	45 U/l	No conversion
Haptoglobin	mg/dl	μmol/l	×0.10
Hemoglobin	g/dl	mmol/l	×0.6206
Iron (total) and total iron-binding capacity	μg/dl	μmol/l	×0.179
LDH (lactate dehydrogenase)	U/l	μkat/l	×0.016667
Lactic acid (lactate)	mg/dl	mmol/l	×0.111
Magnesium	mg/dl	mmol/l	×0.411
Mean corpuscular hemoglobin concentration (MCHC)	g/dl	g/l	×10
MCV (mean corpuscular volume)	μm^3 μm^3	fl fl	No conversion
Parathyroid hormone	pg/ml	ng/l	No conversion
Phosphorus	mg/dl	mmol/l	×0.323
Platelets	$10^3/\mu l$	$10^9/l$	No conversion
Potassium	mEq/l	mmol/l	No conversion
Renin	pg/ml	pmol/l	×0.0237
Sodium	mEq/l	mmol/l	No conversion
Triglycerides (fasting)	mg/dl	mmol/l	×0.01129
Urea, plasma (BUN)	mg/dl	mmol/l	×0.357
Uric acid	mg/dl	μmol/l	×59.48
25-hydroxyvitamin D	ng/ml	nmol/l	2.496
1,25-dihydroxyvitamin D	pg/ml	pmol/l	2.6

Katal (*kat*) a unit of catalytic activity, used especially in the chemistry of enzymes, *μkat* (microkatals), *nkat* (nanokatals) per L, *mmol* (millimoles), *μmol* (micromoles), *nmol* (nanomoles), *pmol* (picomoles)

17.3 Important Drug Dosages

17.3.1 Antihypertensives

Medication	Dosage	Formulations	Remarks
Amlodipine Calcium channel blocker	0.1 mg/kg/dose (max. dose: 5 mg) PO QD to BID; may be gradually increased to a max. dose of 0.6 mg/kg/24 h up to 20 mg/24 h	Tabs: 2.5, 5, 10 mg Oral suspension: 1 mg/ml can be compounded into stable suspension	Ideal in low renin- or volume-dependent hypertension
Atenolol Beta blocker	0.5–1 mg/kg/dose PO QD; max. dose: 2 mg/kg/24 h up to 100 mg/24 h. IV administration rate not to exceed 1 mg/min	Tabs: 25, 50, 100 mg Oral suspension: 2 mg/ml Injection: 0.5 mg/ml (10 ml)	Avoid in asthma, cardiac failure
Captopril Angiotensin-converting enzyme (ACE) inhibitor	Neonate: 0.01–0.05 mg/kg/dose PO Q8–12 h Infant <6 mo: 0.01–0.5 mg/kg/dose PO Q8–12 h Child: 0.3–0.5 mg/kg/dose PO Q8–12 h Should be administered 2 h before or after meals	Tabs: 12.5, 25, 50, 100 mg Oral suspension: 0.75,1 mg/ml	Contraindicated in pregnancy and in suspected renal artery stenosis; monitor serum potassium and creatinine periodically to monitor for hyperkalemia and azotemia. Avoid use with high-flux dialysis membranes since anaphylactoid reactions have been reported
Clonidine Central alpha agonist	5–10 mcg/kg/24 h PO ÷ Q8–12 h, may increase at 5–7 d intervals up to 25 mcg/kg/24 h PO ÷ Q6 h IV: 2–6 mcg/kg, infusion. Onset of action: 10 min. Duration: 15–30 min	Tabs: 0.1, 0.2, 0.3 mg Oral suspension: 0.1 mg/ml Transdermal patch: 0.1, 0.2, 0.3 mg/24 h (7 d patch) Conversion to patch only after establishing effective oral dose	Sudden cessation of therapy can lead to severe rebound hypertension. If patient is receiving both clonidine and a beta blocker and both are to be discontinued, the beta blocker should be withdrawn several days prior to tapering clonidine. If converting from clonidine over to a beta blocker, introduce the beta blocker several days after discontinuing clonidine (following taper)

(continued)

Medication	Dosage	Formulation	Remarks
Enalapril Angiotensin-converting enzyme (ACE) inhibitor Enalaprilat (IV)	Infant and child: 0.1–0.6 mg/kg/24 h PO, increase PRN over 2 week, up to 5 mg/24 h ÷ QD to BID IV: 0.005–0.01 mg/kg/dose QD to TDS, administer over 5 min, up to 5.0 mg Q 6 h may be tolerated for up to 36 h. Onset of action within 15 min	Tabs: 2.5, 5, 10, 20 mg Oral suspension: 0.1, 1.0 mg/ml Injection: 1.25 mg/ml	See remarks for captopril
Fosinopril Angiotensin-converting enzyme (ACE) inhibitor	For children >50 kg 5 mg/d PO QD; may increase to 40 mg/d	Tabs: 10 mg	See remarks for captopril
Esmolol Very short-acting beta blocker	2–6 mcg/kg/min, onset of action within seconds, duration 10–20 min	100 mg/10 ml	–
Hydralazine Vasodilator	Infant and child: 0.75–1 mg/kg/24 h PO ÷ Q6–12 h (max. dose: 25 mg/dose), increase dose over 3–4 week. Adolescent: 0.1–0.5 mg/kg/dose IM or IV Q4–6 h. Max. dose: 20 mg/dose. IV: onset of action (10–30 min), duration (4–12 h)	Tabs: 10, 25, 50, 100 mg Injection: 20 mg/ml (1 ml) Oral liquid: 1.25, 4 mg/ml	Vasodilators act on vascular smooth muscle. Palpitations, dizziness, headaches, gastrointestinal discomfort, and sodium and water retention are common side effects. Used in combination with diuretics or beta blockers. Hydralazine can cause a lupus-like syndrome in slow acetylators. Adjust dose in renal failure
Irbesartan Angiotensin-II receptor blockers (ARBS)	≥ 6 y: 75 mg QOD. Max. 300 mg/24 h	Tabs: 75, 150, 300 mg	Contraindicated in pregnancy. Use with caution in renal artery stenosis
Labetalol Alpha and beta blocker	PO: 4–40 mg/kg/24 h ÷ BID. Max. 1,200 mg/24 h. IV infusion: 0.5–3 mg/kg/h; onset of action within 5–10 min, lasts for 2–3 h with infusion	Tabs: 100, 200, 300 mg Oral suspension: 10, 40 mg/ml Injection: 5 mg/ml (20, 40 ml)	Extremely potent, can be used in hypertensive crisis. Contraindicated in asthma, heart failure, and insulin-dependent diabetics

Lisinopril Angiotensin-converting enzyme (ACE) inhibitor	6–16 y: 0.07 mg/kg/dose PO QD. Max. initial dose: 5 mg/dose, titrate up to 0.6 mg/kg/24 h or 40 mg/24 h Use lower initial dose if using with a diuretic Onset of action: 1 h, maximal effect in 6–8 h	Tabs: 5, 10, 20 mg	See remarks for captopril
Losartan Angiotensin-II receptor blockers (ARBS)	≥6 y: 0.75 mg/kg/dose PO QD up to 50 mg/24 h Max. dose: 1.4 mg/kg/24 h or 100 mg/24 h	Tabs: 25, 50, 100 mg Oral suspension: 2.5 mg/ml; contains 2.12 mg potassium per 25 mg drug	Use with caution in angioedema (current or past), volume depletion, hepatic or renal impairment (contains potassium), hyperkalemia, renal artery stenosis, and congestive cardiac failure. Not recommended in patients <6 y or with GFR <30 ml/min/1.73 m^2. Contraindicated in pregnancy
Metoprolol Beta blocker	Child ≥1 y: 1–2 mg/kg/d PO ÷ BID. Max. dose: 6 mg/kg/24 h up to 200 mg/d	Tabs: 25, 50, 100 mg Oral liquid: 10 mg/ml Injection: 1 mg/ml (5 ml)	Avoid in asthma, cardiac failure
Minoxidil Vasodilator	0.1–0.2 mg/kg/24 h PO QD, dose may be increased in increments of 0.1–0.2 mg/kg/24 h at 3-d intervals	Tabs: 2.5, 10 mg	Palpitations, dizziness, headaches, gastrointestinal discomfort, and sodium and water retention are common side effects. Minoxidil is usually used in patients with resistant hypertension. May cause hirsutism and pericardial effusion
Nicardipine Calcium channel blocker	0.5–3 mcg/kg/min IV	25 mg/10 ml	Onset within 15 min, duration 15–30 min
Nifedipine Calcium channel blocker	Hypertensive urgency: 0.25–0.5 mg/kg/dose Q4–6 h PRN PO/SL. Max. dose: 10 mg/dose or 1–2 mg/kg/24 h. Hypertension: 0.25–0.5 mg/kg/24 h ÷ Q12–24 h. May increase to max. dose: 3 mg/kg/24 h up to 120 mg/24 h	Caps: 5, 10 mg (0.34 ml), 20 mg (0.45 ml). Sustained-release tabs: 30, 60, 90 mg	Ideal for post-renal-transplant hypertension, use with caution in children with acute CNS injury. On sublingual administration, a small amount is absorbed via the sublingual route; most effects are due to swallowing and oral absorption. Extended-release nifedipine tablets must be swallowed whole

(continued)

Medication	Dosage	Formulation	Remarks
Phentolamine	0.05–0.1 mg/kg/dose up to a max. single dose 5 mg IM/IV, 1–2 h prior to surgery, repeat Q2–4 h PRN	Injection: 5 mg vial	Indicated for management of hypertension prior to surgery for pheochromocytoma. Monitor blood pressure and heart rate continuously. Use with caution in arrhythmias and cerebral vascular spasm/occlusion. Contraindicated in renal impairment
Prazosin Peripheral alpha antagonist	0.05–0.1 mg/kg/d, max. 0.4 mg/kg/d	Tabs: 1, 2, 5 mg	May cause hypotension and syncope, especially after first dose
Propranolol Beta blocker	PO: 0.5–1 mg/kg/24 h ÷ Q6–12 h. Increase dose Q3–5 d PRN; max. dose: 8 mg/kg/24 h	Tabs: 10, 20, 40, 60, 80, 90 mg. Extended-release caps: 40, 60, 80, 120, 160 mg. Oral solution: 20, 40 mg/5 ml. Injection: 1 mg/ml (1 ml)	Avoid in asthma, cardiac failure
Ramipril Angiotensin-converting enzyme (ACE) inhibitor	0.05 mg/kg/d PO QD up to 10 mg	Tabs: 2.5, 5.0 mg	See remarks for captopril
Sodium nitroprusside Vasodilator	As IV infusion: 0.5–8.0 mcg/kg/min Onset of action within seconds	50 mg/2 ml	Light sensitive; protect the solution from light, but tubing does not need to be covered. Monitor serum thiocyanate levels when used for >48 h or infusion rate >4 mg/kg/min. or patients with renal failure; keep thiocyanate levels <8 mmol/l
Valsartan Angiotensin-II receptor blockers (ARBS)	0.8–3.0 mg/kg/24 h	Tabs: 80 mg	Contraindicated in pregnancy. Use with caution in renal artery stenosis

17.3.2 Diuretics

Useful in oliguric states and in volume-related hypertension. Electrolytes should be monitored. Side effects are volume depletion and hypokalemia (hyperkalemia with potassium-sparing diuretics).

Hydrochlorothiazide	0.5–1 mg/kg/24 h QD PO; max. dose: 3 mg/kg/24 h up to 50 mg/24 h	Tabs: 12.5, 25, 50, 100 mg. Caps: 12.5 mg	May cause hypercalcemia, hyperuricemia, and hyperlipidemia. May not be effective when creatinine clearance is <50 ml/1.73 m^2/min
Metolazone	0.2–0.4 mg/kg/24 h ÷ QD to BID PO	Tabs: 2.5, 5, 10 mg. Oral suspension: 1 mg/ml	Contraindicated in patients with hepatic coma or hypersensitivity to sulfonamides or thiazides
Loop diuretics			
Furosemide	Neonate: 0.5–1 mg/kg/dose Q8–24 h. Max. dose: 2 mg/kg/dose. Beyond neonatal period: 0.5–2 mg/kg/dose Q6–12 h. As infusion: 0.05 mg/kg/h, titrate to effect, up to 1 mg/kg/h	Tabs: 20, 40, 80 mg. Injection: 10 mg/ml (2, 4,10 ml). Oral solution: 10 mg/ml, 40 mg/5 ml	Use with caution in hepatic disease; ototoxicity may occur, especially when used with aminoglycosides. May cause hyperuricemia and hypercalciuria. Prolonged use in premature infants may result in nephrocalcinosis
Bumetanide	0.015–0.1 mg/kg/dose	Tabs: 0.5, 1, 2 mg	Has greater diuretic activity than furosemide but varies with patient and route
Potassium-sparing diuretics	Use with caution in renal or hepatic dysfunction and when used along with ACE inhibitors or ARBs		
Spironolactone	Neonate: 1–3 mg/kg/24 h ÷ QD to BID PO. Child: 1–3.3 mg/kg/24 h ÷ QD to QID PO	25, 50 mg	Hyperkalemia, agranulocytosis, hirsutism, gynecomastia
Amiloride	0.4–0.625 mg/kg/dose PO QD. Max. 20 mg/d	Tabs: 5 mg	
Triamterene	1–2 mg/kg/d PO BID. Max. 4 mg/kg/d up to 300 mg	Tabs: 50 mg	

17.3.3 Immunosuppressants

Anti-thymoctye globulin (ATG) monomeric IgG from rabbit serum (Thymoglobulin) or equine serum (Atgam)	1.5 mg/kg/d IV for 14 d, then alternate day for 14 d. Additional alternate day therapy up to a total of 21 doses can be given	50 mg of horse gamma globulin/ml. Dilute ATG for IV infusions in an inverted bottle of sterile vehicle so the undiluted ATG does not contact the air inside. Concentration should not be>4 mg ATG/ml	Test dose: intradermal thymoglobulin (1 μg) or Atgam (5 μg) in 0.1 ml of 1:1,000 dilution and contralateral 0.1 ml sodium chloride injection as control. Positive reaction: wheal and/or erythema >10 mm. Observe every 15–20 mm for 1 h. Generalized rash, tachycardia, dyspnea, hypotension, or anaphylaxis precludes any additional administration of ATG. Pretreat all doses with 25–50 mg of diphenhydramine and paracetamol 10 mg/kg/dose. Do not administer to a patient who has had a systemic reaction during prior administration of Atgam or any other equine gamma globulin preparation. ATG should be administered into a vascular shunt, A-V fistula, or a high-flow central vein through an in-line filter with pore size 0.2–1.0 μm. Infuse over at least 4 h. Total time in dilution should not be >24 h. Dilution of ATG in dextrose is not recommended. ATG (diluted or undiluted) should not be shaken because denaturation of the protein may occur. Side effects: fever, chills, leukopenia, thrombocytopenia, dermatologic reactions (e.g. rash, pruritus, urticaria, wheal, and flare), arthralgia, chest or back pain, diarrhea, headache, hypotension, night sweats, pain at the infusion site, and peripheral thrombophlebitis
Azathioprine	Initial: 3–5 mg/kg/d, IV/PO QD. Maintenance: 1–3 mg/kg/d IV/PO QD	Tabs: 50, 75, 100 mg	Toxicity: bone marrow suppression, rash, stomatitis, hepatotoxicity, alopecia, arthralgia, and GI disturbances. Monitor CBC, platelets, total bilirubin, alkaline phosphatase, BUN, and creatinine. Adjust dose in renal failure
Chlorambucil	0.2–0.3 mg/kg/d. Cumulative dose should not exceed 8 mg/kg	Tabs: 2.0 mg	Marrow suppression, seizures, hemorrhagic cystitis

Cyclophosphamide (CTX)	2.5–3.0 mg/kg/d PO QD for 8–12 weeks; 500–750 mg/m²/dose IV monthly for six doses	Tabs: 10, 50 mg. IV solution: 200, 500 mg, 1 g/vial	Adverse effects: leukopenia, cardiomyopathy, hemorrhagic cystitis, emesis, direct ADH effect. Long term: infertility, cardiomyopathy, secondary malignancy, leukoencephalopathy. Cumulative dose to be kept below 168 mg/kg. For IV infusion, patient should be given IV hydration: 2 l/m²/d. Some patients may require antiemetic: should be given an hour before starting the infusion; MESNA IV at 20 % of dose of CTX for 4 doses at 0, 3, 6, and 9 h to protect the bladder. Adjust dose of CTX for renal failure
Cyclosporine	Titrated according to plasma drug levels (refer to Chapters 3.3.1 and 11)	Tabs: 25, 100 mg. Oral solution: 100 mg/ml (50 ml). IV: 50 mg/ml	May cause nephrotoxicity, hepatotoxicity, hypomagnesemia, hyperkalemia, hyperuricemia, hypertension, hirsutism, acne, GI symptoms, leukopenia, sinusitis, gingival hyperplasia, and headache. Encephalopathy and convulsions may occur. Use with caution with other nephrotoxic drugs (e.g., amphotericin B, aminoglycosides, nonsteroidal anti-inflammatory drugs, and tacrolimus). Plasma concentrations increase with use of fluconazole, ketoconazole, itraconazole, erythromycin, clarithromycin, diltiazem, verapamil, nicardipine, carvedilol, and corticosteroids and decrease with use of carbamazepine, nafcillin, rifampin, phenobarbital, octreotide, and phenytoin
Deflazacort	1.5 mg/kg/d	Tabs: 6, 18, 24, 30 mg Oral suspension: 6 mg/ml	In patients with hepatic impairment, blood levels of deflazacort may be increased therefore, the dose should be adjusted to the minimum effective dose. Other side effects similar to prednisolone
[a]Dexamethasone	Anti-inflammatory P0, IV, IM: 0.5–0.9 mg/24 h Q6–12 h	Tabs: 2 5, 0.5, 7.5, 15, 24 mg Injection: 4, 8, 16, 24 mg/ml	–
Everolimus	0.8 mg/m² (maximum 1.5 mg) BID	Tabs: 5, 10 mg	No recommendation for drug levels available in children but safe to maintain a trough level of 3.0–8.0 ng/ml

(continued)

[a]Hydrocortisone	Adrenal insufficiency: 100 mg/m^2/d. Anti-inflammatory: 1.5 mg/kg/d in 3–4 doses. Renal transplantation: 2 mg/kg/dose Q 6 h	Tabs: 5, 10 mg. Hydrocortisone acetate injection: 25, 50 mg/ml. Hydrocortisone sodium succinate injection: 100, 250, 500 mg, 1.0 g vial. Hydrocortisone phosphate injection: 50 mg/ml, 2 ml single-dose vial	–
Intravenous immunoglobulin (IVIG) Derived from human blood and provides immediate antibody levels with a half-life of 21–29 d	Recommended infusion rates for 5–6 % IVIG: 0–15 min: 0.5 ml/kg/h 15–45 min: 1 ml/kg/h 45–75 min: 2 ml/kg/h Remainder: 4 ml/kg/h Half of above infusion rates for 10–12 % concentration		Dosing adjustment is needed with renal impairment; avoid use when CrCl <10 ml/min. Infuse separately from all other products/solutions and at room temperature. The solution should be colorless, particle-free, and non-turbid. Stable for a maximum of up to 4 h from time of dispensing *Adverse reactions*: antigenic reactions that include flushing of face, nausea, chills, fever, dizziness, headache, muscle cramps, myalgias, hypotension, wheezing, urticaria, pruritus, dyspnea, and anaphylaxis (hypotension, sudden dyspnea, respiratory distress, chest pain/tightness, and shock). Serious outcomes such as hemolysis and renal dysfunction have been observed. Anaphylaxis is more likely to occur with initial dose of IVIG; adrenaline should be available for treatment of an anaphylactoid reaction *Contraindications* are selective IgA deficiency, history of anaphylactic episode following previous IVIG infusion, dehydration, diabetes mellitus, preexisting renal insufficiency, and sepsis. Patients receiving large volumes of fluid due to 5 % IVIG concentration and large dosage requirements should be observed for signs of fluid overload. Risk of inflammatory reactions is higher in patients with agammaglobulinemia or severe hypogammaglobulinemia receiving the first dose
Levamisole	2–3 mg/kg/48 h PO	Tabs: 50, 150 mg	Leukopenia, rash, fever, dysgeusia, myalgias

[a]Methylprednisolone	Anti-inflammatory/ immunosuppressive: PO/IM/IV 0.5–1.7 mg/kg/24 h Q6–12 h. Pulse IV dose 30 mg/kg/dose infusion over 1–2 h	Tabs: 2, 4, 8, 16, 24, 32 mg. Na succinate injection: 40, 125, 500, 1,000, 2,000 mg. Acetate injection: 20, 40, 80 mg/ml (IM repository)	Close BP monitoring required during and after the infusion. May increase cyclosporine and tacrolimus levels
Mycophenolate	600 mg/m²/dose PO BID, max. 2,000 mg/24 h	Mycophenolate mofetil (MMF). Tabs: 250, 500 mg	Mycophenolate mofetil (MMF) is a pro-drug for mycophenolic acid (MPA). A 720 mg dose of mycophenolate sodium (MPS) is equivalent to 1,000 mg of MMF (would provide the nearest molar equivalent of MPA).
	400 mg/m²/dose BID, up to a max. of 1,440 mg/24 h	Mycophenolate sodium (MPS): enteric-coated, delayed-release monosodium salt of MPA. Tabs: 180, 360, 720 mg	Delayed-release tablets should not be interchanged with the other oral dosage forms on an equivalent mg-to-mg basis.
		Powder for oral suspension, when reconstituted: 200 mg/ml	Mycophenolate mofetil tablets and capsules or mycophenolate sodium delayed-release tablets should not be crushed, chewed, or cut.
		Injection: 500 mg/20 ml mycophenolate mofetil	Common side effects include headache, hypertension, diarrhea, vomiting, bone marrow suppression, fever, opportunistic infections, and sepsis. May increase risk for malignancies. Periodic blood count monitoring required. Injection: must be reconstituted and diluted to a concentration of 6 mg/ml using 5 % dextrose injection. Incompatible with other intravenous solutions. Must be administered as a slow infusion; begin infusion within 4 h from reconstitution and dilution of the drug
[a]Prednisolone	1–2 mg/kg/d Q 6–8 h PO	Tabs: 5, 10, 20 mg. Oral syrup: 5, 15 mg/5 ml	Side effects: mood changes, seizures, hyperglycemia, GI bleeding, hypertension, sodium and water retention, hypothalamus-pituitary-adrenal axis suppression, osteopenia, growth suppression, cushingoid effects, and cataracts may occur with prolonged use. Concurrent barbiturates, carbamazepine, phenytoin, rifampicin, and isoniazid may reduce effects
[a]Prednisone	2 mg/kg/24 h PO Q6–8 h (max. dose: 80 mg/24 h)	Tabs: 1, 2.5, 5, 10, 20, 50 mg. Oral syrup/ solution: 1 mg/ml, 5 mg/ml	Similar to prednisolone

(continued)

Rituximab (RIT): chimeric monoclonal antibody that acts by inhibiting CD20-mediated B-cell proliferation and differentiation	375 mg/m²/dose. Total number of doses and frequency vary with the underlying condition	Vials: 100/10 and 500 mg/50 ml. Dilute in 0.9 % sodium chloride or 5 % glucose to a concentration of 1–4 mg/ml. Mix gently to avoid foaming; diluted solution may be refrigerated (2–8 °C) for up to 24 h	Infusion rate: 1 mg/kg/h for initial dose (maximum initial rate 50 mg/h), increasing rate by 50 mg/h every 30 min to a maximum of 400 mg/h Subsequent infusions: may be started at 100 mg/h, increased by 100 mg/h, increments at 30-min intervals (to a max. of 400 mg/h). If 100 mg/h is not tolerated, start subsequent infusions at a maximum tolerated rate *Premedication* orally 30–60 min prior to each infusion: paracetamol 15 mg/kg PO (max. 1 g) and an antihistamine, e.g., promethazine 0.125 mg/kg. A corticosteroid (hydrocortisone) may be given if required *Adverse effects*: fever, chills, and rigors. Other infusion-related symptoms include nausea, vomiting, urticaria, headache, bronchospasm, dyspnea, angioedema, and hypotension. Cytokine release syndrome manifests as severe dyspnea and hypoxia. Adverse reactions are more severe with the first infusion; time to onset is 30–120 min and may be fatal. Anaphylaxis can occur at any stage of treatment Emergency treatments (adrenaline, hydrocortisone) should be available. Patients with preexisting pulmonary disease may be at greater risk of respiratory adverse effects. Concomitant nebulized salbutamol may be considered Monitor temperature, pulse, and blood pressure at baseline and every 30 min up to 2 h following completion of infusion to exclude any delayed reactions. If stable, infusion rate is to be increased gradually. Consider withholding antihypertensive medication for 24 h to prevent hypotension. Screen for hepatitis B before starting rituximab as treatment may reactivate infection; continue to monitor for signs of infection during and, for several months, after treatment. Stop rituximab if fulminant hepatitis develops. Cardiac monitoring may be required for patients with cardiac dysfunction as rituximab may exacerbate or induce arrhythmias. Severe gastrointestinal adverse effects including bowel obstruction and perforation have been reported

Sirolimus	Patients ≥13 y who weigh <40 kg: initial loading dose should be 3 mg/m^2. Maintenance dose: 1 mg/m^2/d (1/3 of loading dose) If >40 kg, loading dose: 6 mg. Maintenance dose: 2 mg/d.	Tabs: 1, 2 mg Oral solution: 1 mg/ml	Maintain target trough level (whole blood trough concentrations of 16–24 ng/ml by chromatographic method) for the first year following transplantation. Thereafter, 12–20 ng/ml. Sirolimus should be taken 4 h after cyclosporine
Tacrolimus	0.15 mg/kg/dose PO, BID, maximum dose 10 mg	Caps: 0.5, 1.0, 5.0 mg	Adverse effects are nephrotoxicity, seizures, glucose intolerance, tremor, headache, insomnia, hypertension, renal dysfunction, hypomagnesemia, hyperglycemia, lymphoma, and liver enzyme elevation.
	IV: 0.3–0.15 mg/kg/24 h by continuous infusion Adjust with trough levels: Age – Trough level 0–2 mo – 10–12 ng/ml 3–6 mo – 8–10 ng/ml >6 mo – 5–8 ng/ml	Oral suspension: 0.5 mg/ml IV: 5 mg/ml	Tacrolimus is a substrate of the CYP 450 3A4 drug metabolizing enzyme. Calcium channel blockers, imidazole antifungals (ketoconazole, itraconazole, fluconazole, clotrimazole, posaconazole), macrolide antibiotics (erythromycin, clarithromycin, troleandomycin), cisapride, cimetidine, cyclosporine, danazol, methylprednisolone, and grapefruit juice can increase serum tacrolimus levels; carbamazepine, caspofungin, phenobarbital, phenytoin, rifampicin, rifabutin, and sirolimus may decrease levels
Monoclonal antibodies			Severe acute (within 24 h) hypersensitivity reactions may occur on initial exposure and on reexposure: include anaphylactoid reactions such as urticaria, pruritus, sneezing, hypotension, tachycardia, dyspnea, bronchospasm, and respiratory failure
Basiliximab: immunosuppressant, induction agent, chimeric murine/human monoclonal antibody, selectively directed against interleukin-2 receptor alpha chain expressed on surface of T-lymphocytes in response to antigenic challenge	2-dose regime IV. 10 mg for those <40 kg. 20 mg for those >40 kg. As an infusion over 20–30 min or as bolus via central/peripheral vein, within 2 h prior to shifting for surgery	20 mg sterile lyophilized powder	Asthenia, fatigue, edema, nausea, vomiting. Cases of suspected cytokine release syndrome (CRS) have been reported

(continued)

Daclizumab Humanized IgG1 monoclonal antibody that binds specifically to alpha subunit of interleukin-2 receptor expressed on the surface of activated lymphocytes	Pre-transplantation day 0: 1 mg/kg/dose (max. 50 mg). Calculated volume should be mixed with 50 ml of sterile 0.9 % sodium chloride solution; should be given within 4 h of preparation over 15 min, before shifting for surgery. Can be refrigerated at 2–8 ^{0}C for maximum of 24 h	25 mg/5 ml vial	Safe and effective from 11 months to 17 y of age. The standard course of therapy is 5 doses; first dose should be given no more than 24 h before transplantation, and 4 remaining doses at intervals of 14 d
Muromonab-CD3 [Orthoclone (OKT3)] Murine monoclonal antibody	Initial dose: 0.1–0.3 mg/kg IV bolus over 5 min. Max. dose: 2.5 mg (<30 kg) or 5 mg (>30 kg) IV. Further doses to be adjusted by total lymphocyte (<100/mm^3) or CD3 (<20/mm^3) counts	Sterile solution contains 1 mg/ml (5 ml ampoule)	Risk of anaphylaxis: premedicate patient 30 min before with diphenhydramine, methylprednisolone and acetaminophen. Filter each dose with 0.22 μm filter before administering. Give IV bolus over 1 min at a final concentration of 1 mg/ml. Keep refrigerated

[a]For relative potencies of corticosteroids, see table below

Relative potencies of corticosteroids

Drug	Anti-inflammatory effect (mg)	Sodium-retaining effect (mg)
Hydrocortisone	100	100
Cortisone	80	80
Prednisolone	20	100
Prednisone	20	100
Methylprednisolone	16	0
Dexamethasone	2	0

17.3.4 Electrolyte Supplements

Drugs	Dosage	Formulations	Remarks
Bicitra	2–3 mEq/kg/24 h PO ÷ Q6–8 h	100 g sodium citrate 60 g citric acid per ml	1 ml = 1 mEq of base equivalent
K-Lyte effervescent tablet	2–3 mEq/kg/24 h PO ÷ Q6–8 h	Tab K citrate 2.5 g	1 tab = 25 mEq of K, 25 mEq base
Polycitra	2–3 mEq/kg/24 h PO ÷ Q6–8 h	110 g potassium citrate, 100 g sodium citrate, 66.8 g citric acid per ml	1 ml = 2 mEq base equivalent, 1 mEq Na, 1 mEq K; sour taste and laxative effect
Polycitra-K	2–3 mEq/kg/24 h PO ÷ Q6–8 h	220 g potassium citrate, 66.8 g citric acid per ml	1 ml = 2 mEq base equivalent, 2 mEq K; K salts should be used with caution in patients with renal functional impairment
Shohl solution	2–3 mEq of bicarbonate/kg/24 h PO ÷ Q6–8 h	140 g citric acid, 90 g sodium citrate per 1,000 ml	1 ml = 1 mEq base equivalent
Sodium bicarbonate	2–3 mEq/kg/d. Higher doses required for patients with proximal RTA	IV 's' Solution (7.5 %) Tabs: 325, 650 mg	1 ml = 0.9 mEq bicarbonate, 325 mg = 4 mEq, 650 = 8 mEq bicarbonate. Watch for hypernatremia, tetany, hypokalemia
Potassium chloride	1–2 mEq/kg/d10 % solution (Potchlor), 15 ml = 20 mEq of potassium	Syrup Kesol: 5 ml = 13 mEq of potassium	Injection potassium chloride (15 %, 10 ml/ampoule), 1 ml = 2 mEq of potassium

17.3.5 Phosphate Supplements

Neutra Phos	Phosphate: 30–90 mg/kg/d (0.25–0.5 mmol/kg/d PO, Q 4–6 h). Hypophosphatemic rickets: 1–5 g/24 h Q 4–6 h	Neutra Phos packet 250 mg or tab 250 mg, 125 mg, 114 mg PO_4. Solution: 250 mg PO_4/75 ml	250 mg PO_4 = 8 mmol PO_4, (7.125 mEq Na, 7.125 mEq K per tab or packet of powder)
Phosphate Sandoz		Effervescent tab: sodium acid phosphate, sodium bicarbonate, potassium bicarbonate	PO_4: 500 mg (16 mmol), 469 mg (20.4 mmol Na^+). Potassium: 123 mg (3.1 mmol K^+). Citric acid (anhydrous): 800 mg
Joulie solution		1,000 ml = 136 g dibasic sodium phosphate, 58.8 g phosphoric acid	1 ml = 30 mgPO_4 (1.6 mmol) Use with caution in patients with renal impairment. Be aware of sodium and/or potassium load when supplementing phosphate. May cause nausea, vomiting, abdominal pain, or diarrhea

17.3.6 Calcium and Vitamin D Supplements

Calcium carbonate	45–65 mg of elemental calcium/ kg/24 h PO ÷ QID	250, 500 mg tablets	1,000 mg = 22.3 mEq base. Side effects: constipation, hypercalcemia, hypophosphatemia, hypomagnesemia, nausea, vomiting, headache, and confusion. Administer with plenty of fluids. As a phosphorus-lowering agent, administer with meals
Calcium chloride	IV: 0.2 ml/kg/dose for hypocalcemia, hyperkalemia, magnesium toxicity. Maximum IV rates: IV push: donot exceed 100mg/min. IV infusion: 45–90 mg/kg/h with a maximum concentration of 20 mg/ml	10 % solution	1 ml = 100 mg calcium chloride = 27 mg or 0.7 mmol elemental Ca. Slow infusion and monitor for bradycardia and hypotension. Extravasation may lead to necrosis. Hyaluronidase may be helpful for extravasation. Central line is the preferred IV route of administration
Calcium gluconate	0.5 ml/kg/dose, slow IV. Max IV infusion rates: IV push: Do not exceed 100mg/min (1ml/min). IV infusion: 120–240 mg/kg/h (1.2–2.4 ml/kg/h)	10 % solution	1 ml = 100 mg calcium gluconate = 9 mg elemental Ca. Slow infusion and monitor for bradycardia and hypotension
Calcidiol (alphacalcidiol): 1 hydroxycholecalciferol	Children < 20 kg: 0.05 µg/kg/d. Children > 20 kg body: 1 µg/d	0.25, 0.5 microg 1 µg	Monitor plasma levels of calcium, phosphorus, alkaline phosphatase, and parathyroid hormone. Side effects: polydipsia, polyuria, constipation, hypotonia, metastatic calcification, headache, vomiting
Calcitriol (1,25-dihydroxycholecalciferol)	Renal failure: 0.01–0.05 µg/ kg/24 h	0.25 µg, 0.5 microg	Active and most potent vitamin D metabolite available. Side effects same as calcidiol

17.3.7 Miscellaneous Drugs

Acyclovir	*Immunocompetent, Zoster*: IV: 30 mg/kg/24 h or 1,500 mg/m²/24 h Q8 h × 7–10 d. PO: 4,000 mg/24 h ÷ 5 times/24 h × 5–7 d for patients ≥12 y *Varicella*: IV: same as Zoster. PO: 80 mg/kg/24 h ÷ QID × 5 d. Max. dose: 3,200 mg/24 h. *Immunocompromised, HSV*: IV: 750–1,500 mg/m²/24 h÷ Q8 h × 7–14 d. *PO*: 1,000 mg/24 h ÷ 3–5 times/24 h × 7–14 d. *HSV prophylaxis*: IV: 750 mg/m²/24 h ÷ Q8 h during risk period. *PO*: 600–1,000 mg/24 h ÷ 3–5 times/24 h during risk period	Caps: 200 mg. Tabs: 400, 800 mg. Oral suspension: 200 mg/5 ml. Ointment: 5 % (15 g). Cream: 5 % (2 g). Powder injection(with sodium): 500,1,000 mg. Injection in solution (with sodium): 50 mg/ml (contains 4.2 mEq Na/1 g drug)	*Use with caution* in patients with preexisting neurologic or renal impairment or dehydration. Adequate hydration and slow (1 h) IV administration are essential to prevent crystallization in renal tubules. Do not use topical product on the eye or for the prevention of recurrent HSV infections. Oral absorption is unpredictable (15–30 %). Use ideal body weight for obese patients when calculating dosages. Resistant strains of HSV and VZV have been reported in immunocompromised patients (e.g., advanced HIV infection) Can cause renal impairment and has been infrequently associated with headache, vertigo, insomnia, encephalopathy, GI tract irritation, elevated liver function tests, rash, urticaria, arthralgia, fever, and adverse hematologic effects. Probenecid decreases acyclovir renal clearance. Acyclovir may increase the concentration of tenofovir and meperidine and its metabolite (normeperidine)
Albumin	0.5–1 g/kg IV as infusion	5 % (50 mg/ml) (50, 250, 500 ml), 25 % (250 mg/ml) (20, 50, 100 ml). Both concentrations contain 130–160 mEq Na/l	Fluid overload, hypertension, cardiac failure
Amphotericin B	0.5–1.5 mg/kg/24 h IV QD as infusion over 2 h	50 mg vials	Common infusion-related reactions include fever, chills, rigors, nausea, vomiting, hypotension, and headache; may premedicate with acetaminophen and diphenhydramine Acute side effects: fever, chills, myalgias, diarrhea, dyspnea, skin rash, low back pain, phlebitis, and severe tissue injury in case of extravasation. Renal, hepatic, electrolyte, and hematologic status need to be monitored for thrombocytopenia, hypokalemia, hypomagnesemia, hypocalcemia, hyperglycemia, and increases in liver enzymes and bilirubin. Some decrease in GFR occurs, hence increases in BUN and creatinine
Amphotericin B lipid complex	5 mg/kg/d	5 mg/ml	Shake the vial gently until there is no yellow sediment at the bottom prior to withdrawing the dose. Use 18 G needle to draw drug. Mix in 5 % dextrose water to a final concentration of 1–2 mg/ml; solution stable for 48 in refrigerator for 8 h at room temperature. Infuse over 24 h; flush line with 5 % dextrose before and after medication if used for any other drug. Fever and chills are common after first dose. Rise in creatinine and hypokalemia may occur

(continued)

Amphotericin B liposomal complex	3–5 mg/kg/d. 6 mg/kg/d for cryptococcal meningitis	Injection: 50 mg powder	Reconstitute with 12 ml water for injection to obtain 4 mg/ml suspension. Withdraw volume of suspension needed from vial; attach 5 μm filter to syringe when injecting dissolved drug to final infusion solution (5, 10, 20, or 25 % DW) of concentration of 0.5–2.5 mg/ml. This solution should be used within 24 h. Do not mix with NS or any other drug. Flush IV line with 5 % D and infuse over 2 h. Infusion protocol: as for conventional amphotericin B
Atorvastatin	Children >6 y: 10–80 mg/l over 24 h	Tabs: 10, 20, 40 mg	Dyspepsia, flatulence, pancreatitis, hepatitis, arthralgia, myalgias
Atropine	0.01–0.02 mg/kg/dose. Max. 5.0 mg ½h before the procedure	0.5 mg/ml	Tachycardia, tremors, ataxia, dry and hot skin, blurring of vision
Calcitonin	4–8 IU/kg/dose IM or SC q6–12 h	Injection: 200 units/ml	
Chloral hydrate	Sedative: 50–75 mg/kg/24 h PO/PR ÷ Q6–8 h. Max. dose: 500 mg/dose. Sedation for procedures: 50–75 mg/kg/dose PO/PR 60 min prior to procedure; may repeat in 30 min if needed, up to a total max. dose of 120 mg/kg or 1 g for infants and 2 g for children	Caps: 500 mg. Syrup: 250, 500 mg/5 ml. Suppository : 325, 500, 650 mg	Contraindicated in patients with hepatic disease. Avoid use in moderate/severe renal failure. Use with caution with IV furosemide or warfarin. May cause GI irritation, excitement, hypotension, and myocardial/respiratory depression. Peak effects occur within 30–60 min
DDAVP	0.1–0.4 mg PO (max. dose: 0.6 mg) or nasal spray at 20–40 μgm at bedtime	Tabs: 0.1, 0.2 mg. Nasal spray:10 μ/puff	Patient is advised not to take fluids 1 h before and 8 h after taking the drug to prevent water intoxication. Side effects: transient headache, nausea, abdominal pain
Erythropoietin (Recombinant human erythropoietin)	Start at 50–300 U/kg/dose thrice per week. For children receiving hemodialysis up to 450 U/kg/dose 2–3 times per week	1,000, 3,000, 5,000, 10,000 IU	Monitor hematocrit, BP, clotting times, platelets, BUN, and serum creatinine. Peak effect in 2–3 week. May cause hypertension, seizure, hypersensitivity reactions, headache, edema, dizziness, hyperviscosity, and clotting of vascular access. SC route provides sustained serum levels compared to IV route
Fentanyl	Injection: 50 mcg/ml	Sedation/analgesia Neonate and infant: 1–4 mcg/kg/dose IV Q2–4 h PRN. Child: 1–2 mcg/kg/dose IV/IM Q30–60 min PRN	
Ferrous sulfate/ gluconate	3–4 mg/kg/24 h Q TID	Numerous over-the-counter preparations. Ferrous sulfate (20 % elemental Fe), ferrous gluconate (12 % elemental Fe), Ferrous fumarate (33% elemental Fe) polysaccharide-iron complex and ferrous bis-glycinate chelate caps with mg elemental Fe). 60, 150 mg (150 mg contains 50 mg vitamin C). Elixir 100 mg/5 ml	Iron preparations are variably absorbed. Less GI irritation when given with or after meals. Vitamin C, 200 mg per 30 mg iron, may enhance absorption. Liquid iron preparations may stain teeth; hence give with dropper or drink through straw. May produce constipation, dark stools, nausea, and epigastric pain. Iron and tetracycline inhibit absorption. Antacids may decrease iron absorption

Fluconazole	Tabs: 50, 100, 150, 200 mg. Injection: 2 mg/ml (100, 200 ml); contains 9 mEq Na/2 mg drug Oral suspension: 10 mg/ml (35 ml), 40 mg/ml (35 ml)	Loading dose: 12 mg/kg IV. Maintenance: 3–6 mg/kg IV or PO QD	Cardiac arrhythmias may occur when used with cisapride; concomitant use is contraindicated. May cause nausea, headache, rash, vomiting, abdominal pain, hepatitis, cholestasis, and diarrhea. Neutropenia, agranulocytosis, and thrombocytopenia have been reported. Inhibits CYP 450, may increase effects, toxicity, or levels of cyclosporine, midazolam, phenytoin, rifabutin, tacrolimus, theophylline, warfarin, oral hypoglycemics, and azathioprine. Rifampin increases fluconazole metabolism
Ganciclovir	Children >3 mo Induction therapy: 10 mg/kg/24 h ÷ Q12 h IV for 14–21 d. IV maintenance therapy: 5 mg/kg/dose QD IV or 6 mg/kg/dose QD IV for 5 d/week. Oral maintenance therapy following induction: 30 mg/kg/dose PO Q8 h with food Prevention of CMV in transplant recipients Induction therapy (7–14 d): 10 mg/kg/24 h ÷ Q12 h IV. IV maintenance therapy: 5 mg/kg/dose QD or 6 mg/kg/dose QD for 5 d/week	Injection: 500 mg (contains 4 mEq Na per 1 g drug). Caps: 250, 500 mg. Oral solution: 25, 100 mg/ml	Limited experience with use in children <12 y old. Contraindicated in severe neutropenia (ANC<500/mm^3) or severe thrombocytopenia (platelets<25,000/mm^3). Reduce dose in renal failure; oral absorption is poor; consider using the pro-drug, valganciclovir, for better bioavailability Common side effects: Neutropenia, thrombocytopenia, retinal detachment, confusion. Drug reactions alleviated with dose reduction or temporary interruption. Ganciclovir may increase didanosine and zidovudine levels, whereas didanosine and zidovudine may decrease ganciclovir levels. Immunosuppressive agents may increase hematologic toxicities. Amphotericin B, cyclosporine, and tacrolimus increase risk for nephrotoxicity. Imipenem/cilastatin may increase risk for seizures. Minimum dilution is 10 mg/ml and should be infused IV over ≥1 h. IM and SC administration are contraindicated because of high pH (pH=11)
Heparin sodium	Heparinization for hemodialysis. Loading dose, 10–30 IU/kg, and maintenance, 10–20 IU/kg/h Maintenance (intermittent): 75–100 U/kg/dose Q4 h IV	1,000, 5,000 IU/ml	Heparin flush: lower doses in younger children to avoid systemic heparinization. Peripheral line: 1–2 ml of 10 U/ml solution Q4 h. Central line: 2–3 ml of 100 U/ml Q24 h. TPN central/arterial line: 0.5–1 U/ml. Heparin effects may be reversed with protamine
Heparin, low molecular weight	0.2–0.4 U/ml	100 mg/ml (3 ml). Prefilled syringe: 100, 150 mg/1 ml	Has more specific anti-Xa activity, longer half-life, and more predictable dose-therapeutic effect relationship. LMWH therapy monitored by following anti-Xa activity checked 4 h after dose. Anticoagulation: 0.5–1.0 U/ml. DVT prophylaxis: age <2 mo, 0.75 mg/kg/dose Q12 h SC; >2 mo, 0.5 mg/kg/dose q12 h SC. Protamine is the antidote
Imipramine	25–50 mg/dose 2 h before bed time	Tabs: 25 mg	Side efffects include constipation, drowsiness, dry mouth, urinary retention, dizziness. Overdose may cause life-threatening arrhythmia

(continued)

Iron parenteral	Iron dextran IV, IM: *Total replacement dose* of iron dextran (ml) = 0.0476 × lean body wt (kg) × (desired Hb [g/dl] – measured Hb [g/dl]) + 1 ml per 5 kg lean body weight (up to max. of 14 ml). *Max. daily (IM) dose*: *<5 kg*, 0.5 ml (25 mg); *5–10 kg*, 1 ml (50 mg); *>10 kg*, 2 ml (100 mg). *IM*: use "Z-track" technique. *Test dose*: 25 mg (12.5 mg for infants) IV over 5 min or IM. May initiate treatment dose 1 h after test dose. *IV*: Dilute in NS at a max. concentration of 50 mg/ml and infuse over 1–6 h at a max. rate of 50 mg/min Iron saccharate: (doses in elemental iron): Usual dose: 3 mg/kg IV thrice a week. Test dose: children<14 kg: 1.5 mg/kg IV, >14kg: 20 mg IV. IV infusion: dilute in NS to a concentration of 1 mg/ml. Infuse 100 mg dose over at least 15 mins Iron sucrose: 20 mg/ml (5 ml) (20 mg elemental Fe, 300 mg sucrose/ml) Iron sucrose: 1 mg/kg/dialysis adequate for correcting ferritin levels and 0.3 mg/kg/dialysis for maintaining ferritin levels between 193 and 250 mcg/l. Should be administered during the last hour of each dialysis at a frequency of three times a week. May administer drug undiluted over 2–5 min; or as an infusion, dilute each 100 mg with a max. of 100 ml NS and infuse over at least 15 min. A 10 mg test dose should be given prior to the actual dose Ferric gluconate IV: Child ≥6 y: 1.5 mg/kg elemental Fe (0.12 ml/kg) IV. Max. dose: 125 mg elemental Fe/dose. Dilute dose in 25 ml NS and infuse over 1 h. Most require eight doses at eight sequential dialysis treatments to achieve a favorable response	Iron dextran: 50 mg elemental Fe/ml) (1, 2 ml); products containing phenol 0.5 % are only for IM administration; products containing sodium chloride 0.9 % via IM or IV route Iron saccharate: 20 mg/ml elemental iron injection Ferric gluconate IV: 62.5 mg/ml (5 ml) (12.5 mg elemental Fe, benzyl alcohol 9 mg/ml and 20 % sucrose)	Adverse effects include hypotension, GI disturbances, fever, rash, myalgias, arthralgia, cramps, and headaches. Hypersensitivity reactions have been reported. IM administration is possible only with iron dextran salt. Follow infusion recommendations for specific products. Monitor vital signs during IV infusion. TIBC levels may not be meaningful within 3 week after dosing

Ketamine	Injection: 10 mg/ml, 50 mg/ml, 100 mg/ml	0.5–1 mg/kg IV with additional boluses of 0.25–0.5 mg/kg to a max. total dose of 2.0 mg over 20 min. Rate of IV infusion should not be >0.5 mg/kg/min and should not be administered in less than 1 min	May cause hypertension, hypotension, emergence reactions, tachycardia, laryngospasm, respiratory depression, and stimulation of salivary secretions. Intravenous use may induce general anesthesia. Benzodiazepine may be added to prevent emergence phenomenon. Give atropine also to decrease secretions
Magnesium (oral)	Treatment of hypomagnesemia: 10–20 mg elemental magnesium/kg/dose PO QID. Supplement: 3–6 mg/kg/d divided TID to QID. Max. 400 mg PO	Oral solution: 100 mg/ml (magnesium glucoheptonate 5.21 mg, 0.21 mmol elemental magnesium/ml). Tabs: 500 mg (magnesium gluconate 29.31 mg, 1.2 mmol elemental magnesium/ml)	May cause hypermagnesemia, hypotension, respiratory depression, and diarrhea. To be taken with food; use with caution in renal failure
Midazolam	Injection: 1, 5 mg/ml Nasal spray: 5 mg/ml (0.5 mg/ actuation {0.1 ml})	0.05–0.1 mg/kg/dose over 2–3 min. May repeat dose PRN in 2–3-min intervals up to a max. total dose of 6 mg in children <5 y and 10 mg in older children Nasal spray: 0.2–0.3 mg/kg	Use with caution in CHF, renal impairment, pulmonary disease, hepatic dysfunction and in neonates. Causes respiratory depression, hypotension, and bradycardia. Use lower doses or reduce dose when given in combination with narcotics or in patients with respiratory compromise
Oxybutynin	<5 y: 0.2 mg/kg/dose PO Q 8 h. >5 y: 2.5–5 mg PO Q 8–12 h	Tabs: 2.5 mg, 5 mg. Syrup 2.5 mg/5 ml	Side effects: dry mouth, blurred vision, tachycardia, constipation
Phenazopyridine	Child >6 y: 12 mg/kg/24 h ÷ TID PO until symptoms of lower urinary tract irritation are controlled or 2 d	Tabs: 100, 150, 200 mg. Syrup: 10 mg/ml	
Phenoxybenzamine	0.3–0.5 mg/kg/24 h PO BID	Caps: 10 mg	
Polyallylamine hydrochloride (Sevelamer)	100–150 mg/kg/dose PO TID	Tabs: 400, 800 mg	Adverse effects: metabolic acidosis, hypertension or hypotension, GI upset. To be taken with meals
Tolterodine	1 mg BID, may increase to 2 mg BID	Tabs: 1.0, 2.0 mg, 2 mg	Side effects: dry mouth, dry eyes, headache, blurred vision, and constipation
Indomethacin	2–5 mg PO TDS. Start at 1–2 mg/kg/24 hr ÷ BID-QID PO; max. dose: the lesser of 4 mg/kg/24 hr or 200 mg/24 hr	Caps: 25 mg. Suspension: 25 mg/ml	Side effects: gastritis, dizziness

(continued)

Rasburicase	0.1–0.2 mg/kg/dose (rounded down to the nearest whole 1.5 mg multiple) IV over 30 min × 1. If needed, dose may be repeated Q24 h for up to 4 additional doses	Injection: 1.5, 7.5 mg	Contraindicated in G6PD deficiency or history of hypersensitivity, hemolytic reactions, or methemoglobinemia with rasburicase. To be used with caution in asthma, allergies, hypersensitivity with other medications, and children <2 y (decreased efficacy and increased risk for rash, vomiting, diarrhea, and fever). Common side effects include nausea, vomiting, abdominal pain, discomfort, diarrhea, constipation, mucositis, fever, and rash. For monitoring, uric acid blood samples must be sent to the laboratory immediately. Blood should be collected in prechilled tubes containing heparin and placed in an ice-water bath to avoid potential falsely low uric acid levels. Centrifugation in a precooled centrifuge (4 °C) is indicated. Plasma samples must be assayed within 4 h of sample collection
Sodium polystyrene sulfonate (Potassium-binding resin)	0.5–1 g/kg/dose Q6 h PO or Q 2–6 h PR	Suspension: 15 g/60 ml	Practical exchange ratio: 1 mEq K per 1 g resin, 1 mEq Na delivered for each mEq K removed. Contraindicated in obstructive bowel disease, neonates with reduced gut motility, and oral administration in neonates. Use cautiously in presence of renal failure, CHF, hypertension, or severe edema. May cause hypokalemia, hypernatremia, hypomagnesemia, and hypocalcemia. Do not administer with antacids or laxatives containing Mg^{2+} or Al^{3+}. Systemic alkalosis may result. Retain enema in colon for at least 30–60 min
Valacyclovir	30 mg/kg/dose PO TID (to mimic an IV acyclovir regimen of 250 mg/m²/dose or 10 mg/kg/dose TID) 20 mg/kg/dose PO TID (to mimic a PO acyclovir regimen of 20 mg/kg/dose four or five times a day)	Tabs: 500, 1,000 mg. Oral suspension: 50 mg/ml	This pro-drug is metabolized to acyclovir with better oral absorption than acyclovir. Use with caution in hepatic or renal insufficiency. Concomitant probenecid or cimetidine can reduce the rate of conversion to acyclovir. Nausea, vomiting, and headache are common. See *acyclovir* for additional drug interactions and adverse effects
Valganciclovir	CMV prophylaxis in kidney transplantation: 900 mg PO QD starting within 10 d of transplantation until 100 d post transplantation	Tabs: 450 mg. Oral suspension: 60 mg/ml	This pro-drug is metabolized to ganciclovir with better oral absorption than ganciclovir. Contraindicated with hypersensitivity to valganciclovir/ganciclovir, ANC <500/mm³, platelets <25,000/mm³, hemoglobin <8 g/dl, and patients on hemodialysis. Use with caution in renal insufficiency, bone marrow suppression, or receiving myelosuppressive drugs or irradiation. May cause headache, insomnia, peripheral neuropathy, diarrhea, vomiting, neutropenia, anemia, and thrombocytopenia. Patient advised to use effective contraception during and for at least 90 d after therapy. See ganciclovir for drug interactions and additional adverse effects. All doses are administered with food and advised to avoid direct contact with broken or crushed tablets with the skin or mucous membranes

CBC complete blood count, *CHF* congestive heart failure, *GI* gastrointestinal

17.4 Drugs Dosages in Renal Failure

Introduction: Alterations in renal functions may have an effect on the absorption, bioavailability, or metabolism of some drugs. In patients with renal insufficiency, the dose of a particular drug may have to be adjusted either by lengthening the interval between doses or by reducing the dose or both, to ensure that adequate blood levels of the drug are achieved without the risk of toxicity. Ideally, the dose or the dose interval of the drug should be adjusted according to plasma levels of the drug, whenever possible. Modifications of the dose or the dose interval may be required in patients undergoing dialysis when >25 % of the drug is removed by the dialysis procedure.

The following table gives a list of commonly used drugs which need to have dose or dose interval modifications based on creatinine clearance (CrCl ml/min) and may require a supplemental dose when the child is subjected to hemodialysis (HD) or peritoneal dialysis (PD) or continuous renal replacement therapy (CRRT).

17.4.1 Antimicrobials Requiring Dosage Adjustments in Renal Failure

Drug	Normal dose	CrCl (ml/min/1.73 m^2)	Drug dose	Supplemental dose for dialysis
Acyclovir (IV)	10 mg/kg/dose q 8 h	30–50	10 mg/kg/dose q 12 h	HD: 5 mg/kg/dose 24 h after dialysis PD: 5 mg/kg dose q 24 h CRRT: 10 mg/kg/dose q12 h
Amikacin	5–7.5 mg/kg/dose q 8 h	30–50 10–30 <10	5–7.5 mg/kg/dose q 12–18 h 5–7.5 mg/kg/dose q 18–24 h 5–7.5 mg/kg/dose q 48–72 h	HD: 5 mg/kg as indicated by serum levels PD: 5 mg/kg as indicated by serum levels IP-LD: 25 mg/l IP-MD: 12 mg/l CRRT: 7.5 mg/kg q 12 h, monitor serum concentrations
Amoxicillin	10–25 mg/kg/dose q 8 h IV, IM, PO	30–50 10–29 <10	100 % 8–20 mg/kg dose q12 h 8–20 mg/kg dose q 24 h	HD: 8–20 mg/kg dose 24 h after dialysis PD: 8–20 mg/kg dose q 24 h CRRT: not applicable

(continued)

Drug	Normal dose	CrCl (ml/min/1.73 m^2)	Drug dose	Supplemental dose for dialysis
Amoxicillin/clavulanate	25–45 mg/kg/24 h ÷ Q12 h PO	30–50	100 %	HD: 8–20 mg/kg dose 24 h after dialysis
		10–29	8–20 mg/kg dose q12 h	PD: 8–20 mg/kg dose q 24 h
		<10	8–20 mg/kg dose q 24 h	CRRT: not applicable
Amphotericin B	0.5–1.5 mg/kg/dose IV over 6–24 h	No dose modification for any GFR		HD, PD, CRRT: 100 %
Amphotericin B, liposomal		No guidelines established		
Ampicillin	35–50 mg/kg/dose q6 h IV, IM, PO	30–50	35–50 mg/kg dose q 6 h	HD: 35–50 mg/kg dose q 12 h
	100 mg/kg/dose q6 h for severe infections	10–29	35–50 mg/kg dose q 8–12 h	PD: 35–50 mg/kg dose q 12 h
		<10	35–50 mg/kg dose q 12 h	CRRT: 35–50 mg/kg dose q 6 h
Ampicillin/sulbactam	Moderate inf. 100-150 mg/kg/24 h q6 h IM, IV.	30–50	35–50 mg/kg dose q 8 h	HD: 35–50 mg/kg dose q 24 h
	Severe inf. 200-400 mg/kg/24 h q 6 h IM, IV	10–29	35–50 mg/kg dose q 12 h	PD: 35–50 mg/kg dose q 24 h
		<10	35–50 mg/kg dose q 24 h	IP-LD: 1 g/l IP-MD: 100 mg/l CRRT: 35–50 mg/kg dose q 8 h
Azithromycin	15 mg/kg/dose on day 1, then 7.5 mg/kg/dose q 24 h on day 2–5 PO	100 %	100 %	HD, PD, CRRT: 100 %
Aztreonam	30–40 mg/kg/dose q8 h IV	30–50	100 %	HD: 7.5–10 mg/kg q 12 h
		10–29	15–20 mg/kg dose q8 h	PD: 7.5–10 mg/kg q 12 h
		<10	7.5–10 mg/kg dose q 12 h	IP-LD: 1 g/l M: 250 mg/l CRRT: 100 %
Cefadroxil	30 mg/kg/24 h q12 h PO	10–30	15 mg/kg/dose q 24 h	HD: 15 mg/kg q 24 h
		<10	15 mg/kg/dose q 36 h	PD: 15 mg/kg q 36 h
Cefazolin	50–100 mg/kg/24 h q 6 h IV, IM	10–30	25 mg/kg/dose q12 h	HD: 25 mg/kg q 24 h
		<10	25 mg/kg/dose q 24 h	PD: same as HD IP-LD: 500 mg/l IP-MD: 125 mg/l CRRT: 25 mg/kg q 48 h
Cefepime	100 mg/kg/24 h q 12 h IV/IM	30–50	50 mg/kg/dose q 24 h	HD: 50 mg/kg q 24 h
		10–50	50 mg/kg/dose q 24 h	PD: same as HD
		<10	50 mg/kg q 48 h	CRRT: 50 mg/kg q 12 h

Drug	Normal dose	CrCl (ml/min/1.73 m^2)	Drug dose	Supplemental dose for dialysis
Cefixime	8 mg/kg/24 h q12–24 h PO	30–50	100 %	HD: supplemental dose required
	Max. dose: 400 mg/24 h	10–29	6 mg/kg dose q 12 h	PD: not required
		<10	4 mg/kg dose q12 h	
Cefotaxime	100–200 mg/kg/24 h q8–12 h IV	30–50	35–70 mg/kg dose q 8–12 h	HD: 35–70 mg/kg dose q 24 h
		10–29	35–70 mg/kg dose q 12 h	PD: same as HD
		<10	35–70 mg/kg dose q 24 h	IP-LD: 500 mg/l MD: 125 mg/l CRRT: 35–70 mg/kg dose q 12 h
Cefoxitin	80–160 mg/kg/24 h q4–8 h IM/IV	30–50	20–40 mg/kg dose q 8 h	HD: 20–40 mg/kg dose q 24 h
		10–29	20–40 mg/kg dose q 12 h	PD: same as HD
		<10	20–40 mg/kg dose q 24 h	CRRT: 20–40 mg/kg dose q 8 h
Ceftazidime	15–25 mg/kg/dose q8 h IV, IM. In severe infections, 50 mg/kg/dose q6 h	30–50	50 mg/kg dose q 12 h	HD: 50 mg/kg dose q 48 h, give on dialysis days after HD
		10–29	50 mg/kg dose q 24 h	PD: 50 mg/kg dose q 48 h
		<10	50 mg/kg dose q 48 h	IP-LD: 250 mg/l MD: 125 mg/l CRRT: 50 mg/kg dose q 12 h
Ceftizoxime	Infant 1–6 mo: 100–200 mg/kg/24 h q 6–8 h IV, IM	30–50	50 mg/kg dose q 8 h	HD: 50 mg/kg dose q 24 h, after HD
	Infant>6 mo and child: 150–200 mg/kg/24 h q6–8 h IV, IM	10–29	50 mg/kg dose q 12 h	PD: 50 mg/kg dose q 24 h
		<10	50 mg/kg dose q 24 h	IP-LD: 250 mg/l, MD: 125 mg/l CRRT: 50 mg/kg dose q 8 h
Cefuroxime sodium (IV)	75–150 mg/kg/24 h ÷ Q8 h	30–50	100 %	HD: 25–50 mg/kg dose q 24 h, after HD
		10–29	25–50 mg/kg dose q 12 h	PD: 25–50 mg/kg dose q 24 h
		<10	25–50 mg/kg dose q 24 h	IP-LD: 500 mg/l MD: 125 mg/l CRRT: 25–50 mg/kg dose q 8 h

(continued)

Drug	Normal dose	CrCl (ml/ min/1.73 m^2)	Drug dose	Supplemental dose for dialysis
Cephalexin	7.5 mg/kg/dose q 6 h PO	30–50	5–10 mg/kg dose q 8 h	HD: 5–10 mg/kg dose q 24 h after HD
		10–29	5–10 mg/kg dose q 12 h	PD: 5–10 mg/kg dose q 24 h
		<10	5–10 mg/kg dose q 24 h	CRRT: not applicable
Chloramphenicol	40 mg/kg/dose stat then 25 mg/kg/ dose q6–24 h IV, IM, PO	100 %	100 %	None
Chloroquine	10 mg/kg/dose q24 h PO for 3 d, or 4 mg/kg/dose q12 h IM for 3 d	30–50	100 %	None
		10–29	100 %	
		<10	50 %	
Ciprofloxacin	4–7 mg/kg/dose q12 h IV	30–50	100 %	HD: 10–15 mg/kg dose q 24 h after dialysis
		10–29	10–15 mg/kg dose q 18 h	PD: 10–15 mg/kg dose q 24 h
		<10	10–15 mg/kg dose q 24 h	IP-LD: 50 mg/l 10–15 mg/kg dose q CRRT: 10–15 mg/ kg dose q 12 h
Clarithromycin	7.5–15 mg/kg/dose q12 h PO	30–50	100 %	HD: 4 mg/kg dose q 24 h
		10–29	4 mg/kg dose q 12 h	PD: 4 mg/kg dose q 24 h
		<10	4 mg/kg dose q 24 h	CRRT: not applicable
Doxycycline	Initial: PO/IV <45 kg: 2.2 mg/kg/dose BID x 1 d to max. dose of 200 mg/24 h >45 kg: 100 mg/dose BID x 1 d Maintenance: PO/IV <45 kg: 2.2–4.4 mg/kg/dose QD–BID >45 kg:100–200 mg/24 h QD–BID	30–50	100 %	HD: 1 mg/kg dose q 12 h
		10–29	100 %	PD: 1 mg/kg dose q 12 h
		<10	1 mg/kg dose q 12 h	CRRT: 100 %
Erythromycin	10 mg/kg/dose q6 h IV, PO	30–50	100 %	HD: 10–17 mg/kg dose q 8 h
		10–29	100 %	PD: 10–17 mg/kg dose q 8 h
		<10	10–17 mg/kg dose q 8 h	CRRT: 100 %
Ethambutol	25 mg/kg/dose q24 h IV, PO	30–50	100 %	HD: 15–25 mg/kg dose 48 h
		10–29	15–25 mg/kg dose 36 h	PD: 15–25 mg/kg dose 48 h
		<10	15–25 mg/kg dose 48 h	CRRT: 100 %

Drug	Normal dose	CrCl (ml/ min/1.73 m^2)	Drug dose	Supplemental dose for dialysis
Fluconazole	6 mg/kg/dose stat, then 3 mg/kg/ dose q24 h IV, PO	30–50	1.5–6 mg/kg/d q 24 h	HD: 1.5–6 mg/kg dose q 48 h
		10–29	1.5–6 mg/kg/d q 24 h	PD: 1.5–6 mg/kg dose q 48 h
		<29	1.5–6 mg/kg/d q 48 h	CRRT: 6 mg/kg dose q 24 h
Flucytosine	400–1,200 mg/m^2/dose q6 h IV, IM	30–50	25–37.5 mg/ kg dose q 8 h	HD: 25–37.5 mg/ kg dose q 24 h
		10–29	25–37.5 mg/ kg dose q 12 h	PD: 25–37.5 mg/ kg dose q 24 h
		<10	25–37.5 mg/ kg dose q 24 h	CRRT: 25–37.5 mg/kg dose q 8 h, monitor serum concentrations
Foscarnet	60–80 mg/kg/24 h q 8 h IV	30–50	60–80 mg/kg dose q 48 h	HD, PD: not recommended
		10–30	50–65 mg/kg q 48 h	CRRT: 60–80 mg/ kg/q 48 h
		<10	Not recommended	
Ganciclovir	20 mg/kg/dose q8 h PO	30–50	IV induction 2.5 mg/kg dose q24 h. MD: 1.25 mg/ kg dose q 24 h. PO 100 %	HD: IV induction 1.25 mg/kg dose 3×/week. MD: 0.625 mg/kg dose 3×/week PO: 30 mg/kg dose 3×/week. All doses after dialysis. PD: same as HD CRRT: IV induction 2.5 mg/ kg dose q24 h. IV maintenance: 1.25 mg/kg dose q 24 h. PO 100 %
		10–30	IV induction 1.25 mg/kg dose q24 h. MD: 0.625 mg/kg dose q 24 h. PO 30 mg/kg dose q 12 h	
		<10	IV induction 1.25 mg/kg dose 3×/week. MD: 0.625 mg/kg dose 3×/week PO: 30 mg/kg dose q24 h	

(continued)

Drug	Normal dose	CrCl (ml/min/1.73 m^2)	Drug dose	Supplemental dose for dialysis
Gentamicin	2–2.5 mg/kg/dose q 8 h IV	30–50	2.5 mg/kg dose q 12–18 h	HD: 2 mg/kg as indicated by serum concentrations
		10–29	2.5 mg/kg dose q 1–24 h	PD: same as HD
		<10	2.5 mg/kg dose q48–72 h	IP-LD: 8 mg/l, MD: 4 mg/l CRRT: 2–2.5 mg/kg q 12–24 h, monitor serum concentrations
Griseofulvin	<2 y:20–25 mg/kg/dose/24 h PO QD or BID; give with milk, eggs, fatty foods		100 % dose for any GFR	None
Imipenem/cilastatin	25 mg/kg/dose q6 h IV	30–50	7.5–12.5 mg/kg dose q 8 h	HD: 7.5–12.5 mg/kg dose q 24 h after dialysis
		10–29	7.5–12.5 mg/kg dose q 12 h	PD: 7.5–12.5 mg/kg dose q 24 h IV
		<10	7.5–12.5 mg/kg dose q 24 h	IP-LD: 500 mg/l IP-MD:200 mg/l CRRT:7.5 mg/kg dose Q8 h
Isoniazid	10 mg/kg/dose q 24 h IV, IM, PO	100 % for any GFR		HD: 100 % dose after dialysis PD, CRRT: 100 % dose
Lamivudine	4 mg/kg/dose q12 h	30–50	4 mg/kg dose q 24 h	HD: 1 mg/kg dose q24 h
		10–29	2 mg/kg dose q 24 h	PD: same as HD
		<10	1 mg/kg dose q 24 h	CRRT: 4 mg/kg dose q 24 h
Levofloxacin	5–10 mg/kg/dose q12–24 h IV, PO	30–50	100 %	HD: 5–10 mg/kg dose q 48 h
		10–29	5–10 mg/kg dose q 24 h	PD: 5–10 mg/kg dose q 48 h
		<10	5–10 mg/kg dose q 48 h	CRRT: 10 mg/kg dose q 24 h
Linezolid	10 mg/kg/dose Q8 h IV/PO	Any GFR	100 %	HD: 10 mg/kg dose 12 h PD: as for HD CRRT:100 %

Drug	Normal dose	CrCl (ml/min/1.73 m^2)	Drug dose	Supplemental dose for dialysis
Meropenem	10–20 mg/kg/dose q8 h IV	30–50	20–40 mg/kg dose q 12 h	HD: 10–20 mg/kg dose q 24 h after dialysis
		10–29	10–20 mg/kg dose q 12 h	PD: 10–20 mg/kg dose q 24
		<10	10–20 mg/kg dose q 24 h	CRRT: 20–40 mg/kg dose q 12 h after
Metronidazole	15 mg/kg/dose stat then 7.5 mg/kg/dose q8–12 h r IV, PO, PR	30–50	100 %	HD: 4 mg/kg dose q 6 h
		10–29	100 %	PD: 4 mg/kg dose q 6 h
		<10	4 mg/kg dose q 6 h	CRRT: 100 %
Nalidixic acid	15 mg/kg/dose q 6 h PO	>50 <50	100 % Avoid use	HD, PD, CRRT: avoid use
Netilmicin	2.25 mg/kg/dose q8 h IV	>50 10–50 <10	50–90 % 20–60 % 10–20 %	HD: give ½ dose after dialysis PD: 3–4 mg/l/d CRRT: dose for GFR 10–50, measure plasma levels
Ofloxacin	5 mg/kg/dose q 8 h PO, IV.	30–50	7.5 mg/kg dose q 24 h	HD: 7.5 mg/kg dose q 48 h
		10–29	7.5 mg/kg dose q 24 h	PD: 7.5 mg/kg dose q 48 h
		<10	7.5 mg/kg dose q 48 h	CRRT: 7.5 mg/kg dose q 24 h
Oseltamivir	*Treatment of influenza (H_1N_1)* 6 mo to 1 y of age 3 mg/kg given twice a day for 5 d	10–30	75 mg PO QD × 5 d	No data
	In older children Weight (kg) / Dosage for 5 d (mg PO BID) / Volume of Oral Suspension (ml) ≤15 / 30 / 2.5 >15–23 / 45 / 3.75 >23–40 / 60 / 5 >40 / 75 / Children > 13 y of age: 75 mg twice daily for 5 d	<10	No recommended dosage regimen	
Penicillin G aqueous K$^+$ and Na$^+$ (IV)	450,000–500,000 U/kg/24 h q 4–6 h	>50	100 %	HD: dose after dialysis
		10–50	75 %	PD: dose for GFR < 10
		<10	25–50 %	Dose for GFR 10–50

(continued)

Drug	Normal dose	CrCl (ml/ min/1.73 m²)	Drug dose	Supplemental dose for dialysis
Penicillin V K⁺ (PO)	25–50 mg/kg/24 h q6–8 h PO. Max. dose: 3 g/24 h 250 mg PO BID, TID	100 % dose for any GFR		HD: Dose after dialysis PD: Dose if GFR < 10 CRRT: not applicable
Pentamidine	4 mg/kg/24 h IM/IV QD	30–50 10–29 <10	100 % 4 mg/kg dose q 36 h 4 mg/kg dose q 48 h	HD: 4 mg/kg dose q 48 h after dialysis on dialysis days PD: 4 mg/kg dose q 48 h CRRT: 100 %
Piperacillin	50 mg/kg/dose q 6–8 h IV	30–50 10–29	50–75 mg/kg dose q 8 h 50–75 mg/kg dose q 12 h 50–75 mg/kg dose q 12 h	HD: 50–75 mg/kg dose q 12 h PD: 50–75 mg/kg dose q 12 h, IP, no LD, MD: 250 mg/l CRRT: 50–75 mg/kg dose q 8 h
Piperacillin/ tazobactam	Piperacillin 300–400 mg/kg/24 h IV Q6–8 h	30–50 10–29 <10	35–50 mg/kg dose q 6 h 35–50 mg/kg dose q 8 h 35–50 mg/kg dose q 8 h	HD: 50–75 mg/kg dose q 12 h PD: 50–75 mg/kg dose q 12 h CRRT: 35–50 mg/kg dose q 12 h
Primaquine	0.3 mg/kg/dose q 24 h PO for 14–21 d	100 % dose for any GFR		HD, PD: no data CRRT: dose for GFR 10–50 %
Pyrazinamide	25–35 mg/kg/dose q 24 h PO	30–50 10–29 <10	100 % 40 mg 3×/ week 40 mg 3×/ week	HD: 40 mg 3×/ week PD: 40 mg 3×/ week CRRT: not to be given if CrCl <30 ml/ min/1.73 m²
Ribavirin	20 mg/ml at 25 ml/h for 12–18 h/d for 3–7 d, or 5–15 mg/kg/dose q8–12 h PO	>50 10–50 <10	100 % 100 % 50 %	HD: dose after dialysis PD: dose for GFR < 10 CRRT: dose for GFR < 10
Rifampicin	10–15 mg/kg/dose q 24 h IV, PO	Any GFR	100 %	HD, PD, CRRT: 100 %

Drug	Normal dose	CrCl (ml/ min/1.73 m²)	Drug dose	Supplemental dose for dialysis
Streptomycin sulfate	20–40 mg/kg/24 h IM QD. Max. daily dose: 1 g/24 h	>50	q 24 h	HD: 50 % dose after dialysis
	Twice weekly: 20–40 mg/kg/dose IM twice weekly. Max. daily dose: 1.5 g/24 h	10–50	q 24–72 h	PD: 20–40 mg/l
		<10	q 72–96 h	CRRT: dose for GFR 10–50
Trimethoprim-sulfamethoxazole (cotrimoxazole)	8–12 mg/kg/24 h ÷ BID	30–50	5–7.5 mg/kg dose q 8 h	HD, PD: not recommended
		10–29	5–10 mg/kg dose q 12 h	CRRT: 5 mg/kg dose q 8 h
		<10	Not recommended	
Ticarcillin	200–300 mg/kg/24 h q 4–6 h. Max. dose: 18–24 mg/24 h	30–50	100 %	HD: 50–70 mg/kg dose q 12 h
		10–29	50–70 mg/kg dose q 8 h	PD: 50–70 mg/kg dose q 12 h
		<10	50–70 mg/kg dose q 12 h	CRRT: 50–70 mg/kg dose q 8 h
Ticarcillin/clavulanate	200–300 mg/kg/24 h q 4–6 h. Max. dose: 18–24 mg/24 h	30–50	100 %	HD: 50–70 mg/kg dose q 12 h. Give q24 h if there is liver failure also.
		10–29	50–70 mg/kg dose q 8 h	PD: same as HD.
		<10	50–70 mg/kg dose q 12 h. Give q24 h if there is liver failure also	CRRT: 50–70 mg/kg dose q 8 h
Tobramycin	2–2.5 mg/kg/dose q6–8 h IV, IM	Any degree of renal insufficiency	2.5 mg/kg; subsequent doses determined by levels	HD: 2 mg/kg; subsequent doses determined by levels PD: same as HD IP-LD: 8 mg/l IP-MD: 4 mg/l CRRT: 2–2.5 mg/kg every 12–24 h, monitor serum levels
Valacyclovir	20 mg/kg/dose q 8 h PO	30–50	20 mg/kg dose q 12 h	HD: 10 mg/kg dose q 24 h, give after dialysis
		10–29	20 mg/kg dose q 24 h	PD: 10 mg/kg dose q 24 h
		<10	10 mg/kg dose q 24 h	CRRT: N/A

(continued)

Drug	Normal dose	CrCl (ml/ min/1.73 m^2)	Drug dose	Supplemental dose for dialysis
Valganciclovir (see ganciclovir)		Not available		
Vancomycin	10 mg/kg/dose q6 h IV	30–50	10 mg/kg dose q 12 h	HD: 10 mg/kg dose as needed per serum concentration monitoring
		10–29	10 mg/kg dose q 18–24 h	PD: 10 mg/kg dose as needed per serum concentration monitoring or IP- LD and IP-MD:500 mg/l
		<10	10 mg/kg dose as needed per serum concentration monitoring	CRRT: 10 mg/kg dose q 12–24 h, monitor serum concentrations
Zidovudine	120 mg/m^2/dose IV q 6 h or continuous IV infusion 20 mg/m^2/ hror 160 mg/m^2/dose PO q 8 h	30–50	100 %	HD: 50 % Q 8 h, unless continuous
		10–29	100 %	PD: 50 % Q 8 h, unless continuous
		<10	50 % q 8 h	CRRT: 100 %

17.4.2 Non-antimicrobials requiring adjustments in renal failure

Drug	Normal dose	CrCl (ml/min)	Dose in renal failure	Supplemental dose for dialysis
Acetaminophen	10–15 mg/kg/ dose q 4–6 h PO	>50	q 4 h	HD, PD: Q 8 h
		10–50	q 6 h	CRRT: 100 %
		<10	q 8 h	
Acetazolamide	5–10 mg/kg/ dose q 6–8 h PO	>50	q 6 h	No data
		10–50	Q 12 h	
		<10	Avoid use	
Acetylsalicylic acid	10–15 mg/kg q 6 h PO	30–50	100 %	HD: give after dialysis
		10–29	100 %	PD: avoid use
		<10	Avoid	CRRT: 100 %, monitor levels.
Allopurinol	10 mg/kg/dose q 12 –24 h	>50	50 %	HD, PD: 30 %
		10–50	50 %	CRRT: 50 %
		<10	30 %	
Amlodipine	0.05–0.2 mg/kg q 24 h PO	100 % for any GFR		HD, PD: 100 % CRRT: 100 %, titrate to effect

Drug	Normal dose	CrCl (ml/min)	Dose in renal failure	Supplemental dose for dialysis
Aminophylline (doses based on theophylline)	Loading dose: 6 mg/kg IV. Maintenance dose 1–12 y.: 0.8 mg/kg/h. IV 12–16 y.: 0.7 mg/kg/h. IV	100 % for any GFR		HD, PD, CRRT: 100 %
Atenolol	1–2 mg/kg/dose PO. Q 12–24 h	30–50	1 mg/kg q 24 h	HD: 1 mg/kg q 48 h, give on HD days, after dialysis
		10–29	1 mg/kg q 48 h	PD: 1 mg/kg q 48 h
		<10	1 mg/kg q 48 h	CRRT: 1 mg/kg q 24 h
Azathioprine	1–3 mg/kg/dose q 24 h IV, PO	30–50	75 % q 24 h	HD: 50 % q 24 h
		10–29	75 % q 24 h	PD: 50 % q 24 h
		<10	50 % q 24 h	CRRT: 75 % q 24 h
Captopril	0.1–1 mg/kg/dose q 8 h PO	30–50	75 %	HD, PD: 50 %
		10–29	75 %	CRRT: 75 %
		<10	50 %	
Carbamazepine	5–10 mg/kg/dose q 8 h PO	30–50	100 %	HD, PD: 75 %
		10–29	100 %	CRRT: monitor levels
		<10	75 %	
Cetirizine	0.25 mg/kg/dose q 12–24 h PO	30–50	100 %	HD, PD: 50 %
		10–29	50 %	CRRT: NA
		<10	Not recommended	
Chloral hydrate	50–75 mg/kg/dose	<50	Avoid use	NA
Chlorothiazide	2–20 mg/kg/dose IV q 12–24 h.	<50	May be ineffective	NA
Cimetidine	5–10 mg/kg/dose q 6 h PO	>50	100 %	HD: none
		10–50	50 %	PD: none
		<10	25 %	
Clonidine	3–5 mcg/kg q 8–12 h PO, IV	100 % for any GFR		HD, PD: none
Daunorubicin	30 mg/m2/dose weekly IV	100 % for any GFR		No data
Diazepam	0.1–0.4 mg/kg/dose IV, PR	100 % for any GFR		HD, HD, CRRT: 100 %
Diclofenac	1 mg/kg/dose q 8–12 h PO	>50	50–100 %	HD, PD: none
		10–50	25–50 %	
		<10	25 %	

(continued)

Drug	Normal dose	CrCl (ml/min)	Dose in renal failure	Supplemental dose for dialysis
Digoxin	15 mcg/kg/dose stat, then 5 mcg/kg/dose 6 h later, then 3–5 mcg/kg/dose q 12 h. PO	30–50 10–30 <10	75 % 50 % or q 36 h 25 % or q 48 h	HD: 25 % or q 48 h PD: 25 % or q 48 h CRRT: 75 % titrate to desired effect. Monitor serum concentration
Diphenhydramine	5 mg/kg/d q 6–8 h PO, IV, IM	100 % for any GFR		HD, PD, CRRT: 100 %
Dipyridamole	1–2 mg/kg/dose q 6–8 h PO	100 % for any GFR		HD, PD, CRRT: no data
Enalapril Use not recommended in infants and children with GFR <30 ml/min/1.73 m^2	0.1 mg/kg q 24 h PO	30–50 10–29 <10	75 % 75 % 50 %	HD: 50 % PD: 50 % CRRT: 75 %
Enoxaparin	1 mg/kg 8–12 h SC	30–50 10–30 <10	100 % 70 % 50 % q 24 h	HD, PD: 50 % Monitor PTT or ACT and adjust dose
Felodipine	0.1 mg/kg/dose q 24 h PO	100 % for any GFR		HD, PD: none. Dose for GFR 10–50
Fentanyl	1–2 mcg/kg/dose IV	30–50 10–29 <10	75 % 75 % 50 %	HD, PD: 50 % CRRT: 75 %
Gabapentin	8–50 mg/kg/d PO q 8 h	30–50 15–29 <15	75 % q 12 h 75 % q 24 h 75 % q 48 h	HD: 75 % q 48 h and extra dose after each 4 h dialysis. PD: 75 % q 48 h CRRT: not known
Haloperidol	0.01 mg/kg/dose q 12 h PO	100 % for any GFR		HD, PD: none CRRT: dose for GFR 10–50
Heparin	75 IU/kg/dose stat then 10–15 IU/kg/h IV	30–50 10–29 <10	100 % 100 % 50 %	HD: 50 % PD: 50 % CRRT: monitor PT or ACT and adjust dose
Hydralazine	0.4 mg/kg/dose 12 h PO	30–50 10–29 <10	q 8 h q 8 h q 12–24 h	HD: q 12–24 h PD: q 12–24 h CRRT: q 8 h

Drug	Normal dose	CrCl (ml/min)	Dose in renal failure	Supplemental dose for dialysis
Hydrochlorothiazide	1–1.5 mg/kg/dose q 12–24 h PO	30–50 10–29 <10	100 % Not recommended Not recommended	HD, PD: not recommended CRRT: 100 %
Ibuprofen	5–10 mg/kg/dose q4–8 h PO	100 % for any GFR		HD, PD, CRRT: 100 %
Indomethacin	0.5–1.0 mg/kg/dose q 8 h PO	100 % for any GFR		HD, PD, CRRT: 100 %
Insulin (regular)	0.05–0.2 IU/kg/dose SC PRN	>50 10–50 <10	100 % 75 % 50 %	HD, PD: none CRRT: dose for GFR 10–50
Labetalol	1–2 mg/kg q 12 PO	100 % dose for any GFR		PD, HD: 100 % CRRT: 100 % and titrate to effect
Lamotrigine	0.2–4.0 mg/kg/dose q 12–24 h PO	30–50 15–29 <15	100 % 100 % 50 %	HD, PD: 50 % CRRT: NA
Levetiracetam	20–60 mg/kg/d q 12 h	50 % for any GFR	50 %	HD, PD: 50 % CRRT: NA
Lisinopril	0.1–1.0 mg/kg q 24 h PO	30–50 15–29 <15	50 % 50 % 25 %	HD: 50 % PD: 25 % CRRT: 50 %
Lithium	5–20 mg/kg/dose q 8–24 h PO	>50 10–50 <10	100 % 50–75 % 25–50 %	HD: dose after dialysis PD: none CRRT: dose for GFR 10–50
Lorazepam	0.02–0.06 mg/kg/dose q 8–24 h. PO	100 % for any GFR		HD, PD: 100 % CRRT: 100 %. Titrate to effect; propylene glycol as vehicle may cause toxicity
Losartan	0.5–2.0 mg/kg/dose q 24 h PO	100 % for any GFR		HD, PD: none Dose for GFR 10–50
Methotrexate	10–20 mg/m2/dose weekly for arthritis	>50 10–50 <10	50 % 50 % 30 %	HD, PD: 30 % CRRT: 50 %, monitor serum concentrations

(continued)

Drug	Normal dose	CrCl (ml/min)	Dose in renal failure	Supplemental dose for dialysis
Methyldopa	3 mg/kg/dose q 8 h PO	>50 10–50 <10	q 8 h q 8–12 h q 12–24 h	HD: dose after dialysis PD: none CRRT: dose for GFR 10–50
MESNA	IV: 20 % w/w of ifosfamide or cyclophosph-amide PO: 40 % w/w of alkylating agent in three doses 4 h apart	100 % for any GFR		HD, PD, CRRT: 100 %
Metoclopramide	0.15–0.3 mg/kg/dose q 6 h IV, IM, PO	30–50 10–29	75 % 50 %	HD, PD: 25 % CRRT: 50 %
Midazolam	0.1–0.2 mg/kg/dose IV, IM	30–50 10–29 <10	100 % 75 % 50 %	Not applicable
Milrinone	50–75 mcg/kg IV over 15 min. maintenance 0.25–0.75 mcg/kg/min	30–50 10–29 <10	0.33–0.43 mcg/kg/min 0.23–0.33 mcg/kg/min 0.2 mcg/kg/min	HD: 0.2 mcg/kg/min PD: same as HD CRRT: 0.33–0.43 mcg/kg/min, titrate to effect
Morphine	0.1–0.2 mg/kg/dose q 4 h IV	10–50 <10	75 % 50 %	HD, PD, CRRT: 50 %
Naproxen	5–10 mg/kg/dose q 8–12 h PO	100 % for any GFR		HD, PD: none CRRT: dose for GFR 10–50
Omeprazole	0.4–0.8 mg/kg/dose q 12–24 h PO	100 % for any GFR		No data
Oxcarbazepine	10–40 mg/kg/d q 12 h	30–50 10–29 <10	100 % 50 % 50 %	Data not available
Pentobarbital	0.5–1 mg/kg/dose q 6–8 h IV, IM, PO	100 % for any GFR		HD, PD: 100 %. CRRT: 100 % and titrate to effect. Solution contains alcohol and propylene glycol which are not dialyzable and may cause toxicity

Drug	Normal dose	CrCl (ml/min)	Dose in renal failure	Supplemental dose for dialysis
Phenazopyridine	12 mg/kg/d q 8 h	50–80 <50	Normal Avoid use	Not available
Phenobarbital	5 mg/kg/dose q 24 h. IV, IM, PO	30–50 10–29 <10	100 % 100 % 50 % q 24 h	HD: 100 % and monitor levels PD: 50 % and monitor CRRT: 10 mg/kg dose q 8 h, monitor levels
Phenytoin	2–3 mg/dose q 8–12 h	100 % for any GFR		100 % for PD, HD. CRRT: monitor levels
Rasburicase	0.1–0.2 mg/kg/ dose IV over 30 min × 1. May be repeated Q24 h for up to 4 additional doses	100 % for any GFR		HD, PD, CRRT: 100 %
Ranitidine	2–4 mg/kg/ dose q 8–12 h PO	30–50 10–29 <10	PO: 2 mg/kg dose q 12 h IV: 1 mg/kg dose q 12 h PO: 1 mg/kg dose q 12 h IV: 0.5 mg/kg dose q 12 h PO: 1 mg/kg dose q 24 h IV: 0.5 mg/kg dose q 24 h	HD: PO, 1 mg/kg dose q 24 h; IV, 0.5 mg/kg dose q 24 h PD: same as HD CRRT: PO, 2 mg/ kg q 12 h; IV, 1 mg/kg q 12 h
Spironolactone	6.25–25 mg/ dose q 12 h PO	>50 10–50 <10	Q 6–12 h Q 6–12 h Avoid use	HD, PD: not applicable CRRT: avoid use
Terbutaline	0.05–0.1 mg/ kg/dose q 6 h	GFR: 10–50 ml/min GFR <10 ml/ min	100 % for any GFR Avoid use	HD, PD, CRRT: 100 %
Thiopental	1.5–5.0 mg/kg IV, repeat PRN or 1–12 mg/ kg/h at concentration 2–4 mg/ml in D5W or NS	<10	75 %	NA

(continued)

Drug	Normal dose	CrCl (ml/min)	Dose in renal failure	Supplemental dose for dialysis
Topiramate	1–10 mg/kg/dose q 12–24 h PO	30–50 10–29 <10	50 % 50 % 25 %	HD: 25 % and supplemental dose post dialysis PD: 25 % CRRT: 50 %
Triamterene	2 mg/kg/dose q 8–24 h PO	>50 10–50 <10	q 12 h q 12 h Avoid use	HD, PD, CRRT: avoid use
Valproate	6–20 mg/kg/dose q 8 h	100 % for any GFR		HD, PD, CRRT: 100 %
Verapamil	1–3 mg/kg/dose q 8–12 h PO	100 % for any GFR		HD, PD: none CRRT: dose for GFR 10–50
Vigabatrin	40–150 mg/kg/dose q 24 h PO	>50 10–50 <10	100 % 50 % 25 %	HD, PD: no data CRRT: dose for GFR 10–50
Warfarin	0.05–0.2 mg/kg/dose q 24 h PO	100 % for any GFR		100 % for HD and PD. CRRT: monitor PT/INR

CrCl creatinine clearance, *GFR* glomerular filtration rate, *HD* hemodialysis, *K+* potassium, *Na+* sodium, *PD* peritoneal dialysis, *CRRT* continuous renal replacement therapies, *IP-LD* intraperitoneal loading, *IP-MD* intraperitoneal maintenance

17.5 Diagnostic Protocols

17.5.1 Midstream Urine Collection

This method is used for collection of urine for culture in children who are toilet trained. Cleansing the perineum with plain water prior to urine collection decreases the rate of contamination. Avoid use of antiseptics and disinfectants. For girls, the labia should be spread and the perineum cleansed two to three times. For boys, the foreskin should be retracted before cleansing, and the meatus should be cleansed in a similar fashion. Contact of the urinary stream with the mucosa can be minimized by pulling back the foreskin in boys and by spreading the labia in girls during urination. The child should urinate into a toilet, and midway through urination, a specimen should be collected in a sterile container.

17.5.2 Suprapubic Aspiration (SPA)

It is a safe and effective method for obtaining uncontaminated urine specimens for urine culture in infants and young children. The sensitivity of the aspirated urine for bacteriuria on urinalysis approaches 100 %. As the distended bladder extends above the level of the pubic symphysis, it is easy to access percutaneously. Ensure that the baby has not passed urine for an hour before the procedure.

17.5.2.1 Materials Required

Sterile gloves, sterile drape, povidone-iodine solution, local anesthetic (1 or 2 % lidocaine injection) with syringe and needle, sterile syringe (2 or 5 ml), 22-gauge needle, sterile urine specimen container, sterile dressing material, sterile gauze.

17.5.2.2 Procedure

The child is restrained in the supine and frog leg position to stabilize the pelvis. The site for needle insertion, in the midline, approximately 1–2 cm above the pubic symphysis, is cleaned with povidone-iodine solution and draped. The planned puncture site may be locally anesthetized with lidocaine. A 1.5 in., 22-gauge needle attached to a 2- or 5-ml syringe is inserted at the pre-identified site. The needle should be angled 10–20° cephalad and advanced under negative pressure until urine returns. The needle should be partially withdrawn and redirected at an angle more perpendicular to the frontal plane if the initial attempt is unsuccessful. Seal site with tincture benzoin or a sterile gauze. The success rate of obtaining urine with SPA improves if performed under ultrasound guidance. Keep a sample collection bottle ready to collect in case urine is voided while attempting SPA.

17.5.3 Per-Urethral Catheterization (PUC)

17.5.3.1 Indications

1. Relief from acute or chronic urinary retention
2. For monitoring of urine output in a critical care setting
3. Prior to some imaging procedures, e.g., voiding cystourethrogram
4. Collection of urine for urine culture
5. Bladder trauma

17.5.3.2 Materials Required

Sterile gloves, gauze and drape, povidone-iodine solution, 2 % lidocaine jelly, catheter of appropriate type and size (up to 6 months, 6 F; 1–3 y, 8 F; 4–6 y, 10 F; 11–12 y, 12 F), gauze and sterile urine specimen container. For temporary catheterization for a few days or for radiological studies, an infant feeding tube may be used. Foley catheters are available as latex/silicone catheters; the latter are recommended for a longer period because of the relatively inert nature of silicone. A smaller catheter is preferred in all situations to obviate chances of injury and infection except in specific situations (hematuria, pyuria, graveluria) where blockages are frequent.

17.5.3.3 Procedure

1. With adequate preparation and explanation regarding the procedure to child or caretaker, discomfort and anxiety regarding the procedure can be minimized.
2. Provide privacy for the patient, then position and drape appropriately.
3. Open a catheter tray, maintaining sterile technique, and put on sterile gloves.
4. If inserting a Foley catheter, test-inflate the balloon with normal saline to ensure it works properly; if a urine specimen is required, make sure you have the appropriate container.
5. For catheterization of a female: hold labia open with nondominant hand throughout cleaning (nondominant hand becomes contaminated).
6. Use forceps to hold cotton swabs soaked in an antiseptic (e.g., povidone-iodine) solution, stroking from the front to the back (the dominant hand uses forceps for cleaning, so it remains sterile).
7. For catheterization of a male: hold shaft of penis with nondominant hand throughout cleaning (nondominant hand becomes contaminated), and gently retract the prepuce to clean the smegma, except in infants when the prepuce may be physiologically adherent to the glans. Use forceps to hold cotton swabs soaked in an antiseptic solution.
8. Cleanse in a circular motion, starting at the urinary meatus and working outward.
9. Use adequate lubrication: coat the catheter tip and meatus with lubricant containing 2 % lidocaine jelly or inject into the urethra using a 2-ml syringe without a needle.
10. The catheter is inserted into the urethra with the dominant hand while continuing to hold labia/penis with nondominant hand. Entry of catheter into the bladder is confirmed by free flow of urine via the catheter. (In a female: if catheter is inadvertently inserted into the vagina instead of the urethra, leave the catheter in place as a marker and attempt catheterizing the urethra with a new sterile catheter.)
11. Drain urine from the bladder, and remove catheter, or inflate catheter balloon with 3–5 ml of sterile water and withdraw till the balloon fixes at the internal meatus. Outlet port is connected to a closed sterile drainage bag and the catheter is fixed securely with adhesive tapes to the lower anterior abdominal wall/thigh. A small loop of catheter is left free between the meatus and the site at which the tape is fixed to prevent undue traction and injury.
12. In males, the retracted prepuce is repositioned at the conclusion of the catheterization.

17.5.3.4 Urinary Catheter Care

The urethral orifice, catheter, and genital areas are to be washed daily with soap and water. The efficacy of chemical antisepsis is unproven. Prophylactic antibiotics are not necessary as the drainage system may only be opened under aseptic conditions. Routine bladder irrigation should be avoided since it would increase the risk of infection.

17.5.3.5 Complications

They are related to improper placement or prolonged use of per-urethral bladder drainage. They include acute urethral injury, urethritis, periurethritis, cystitis, ascending urinary tract infection, meatitis, meatal stenosis, urethral stricture, and bladder calculi. Extreme care should be exercised when catheterizing a child with suspected posterior urethral valves since there is a risk of creating a false passage. Intravesicular catheter knotting is a rare complication. It can be avoided by limiting the length of inserted catheter by using short catheters, premeasuring an estimated length, and inserting the catheter only as far as necessary to obtain urine flow.

17.5.4 Clean Intermittent Catheterization (CIC)

It involves periodic insertion of a catheter into the bladder to evacuate urine and is an accepted method of management for individuals with neurogenic bladder. The procedure should be explained to the caretaker and to the child.

1. Wash hands well. Gloves are not needed.
2. Assemble materials required: catheter (infant feeding tube, a rubber, or steel catheter), water-soluble lubricant, and hand wipes or cloth soaked with soap and water.
3. If it is an infant, a protective pad may be kept below the child.
4. Cleanse the perineum or penis with mild soap and water, or with a hand wipe. For girls, spread labia and clean front to back. For boys, if uncircumcised, pull back foreskin and clean head of penis.
5. Lubricate catheter tip, hold the catheter near the tip and insert it into the urethra until urine flows. Do not use force; if slight resistance is felt, it may help to twist the catheter.
6. Place the other end of the catheter in the toilet or collection container before urine flows out of the catheter; hold the catheter in place until urine ceases to flow.
7. Withdraw the catheter gently and slowly; there is often an additional gush of urine.
8. Measure the urine and record if required; discard the urine and rinse the container.
9. Clean the catheter and store in a clean container.
10. Wash hands thoroughly.

Catheterization schedule should be individualized based on the bladder capacity and fluid intake, usually 2–3 hourly throughout the day. Depending on the child's condition, nighttime indwelling catheter for continuous drainage may be opted for. The child can be taught to perform self CIC when feasible; this shift of responsibility is a gradual process, initiated by allowing the child to assist the parents and later do CIC independently.

The commonest complication is urinary tract infections (UTI). Strategies for reducing UTI include thorough hand washing, rinsing the catheter immediately before and after use, minimizing the number of people catheterizing an individual, use of adequate amounts of lubricant to minimize urethral trauma, and strict adherence to the established individualized catheterization schedule, to prevent excess bladder distention and/or reflex bladder contractions. Adequate fluid intake, meticulous bowel management to prevent constipation, and prompt thorough cleansing after defecation decrease the risk of UTI.

Catheter care involves washing catheters with soap and water. A water-filled syringe may be used to flush the catheter. After use the catheter is placed on a towel or hung to dry in a clean, appropriate, and designated area. Catheters may be reused multiple times; discard if the catheter appears cloudy after washing or becomes too soft to insert.

17.5.5 Instructions for 24-h or a "Timed Urine Collection"

The collection should be started after waking up in the morning after the bladder has been emptied for the first time, i.e., first void is to be discarded. The exact time should be noted. The urine should be collected during the day and night in an empty collection bottle and may be stored at room temperature; refrigerate if possible. Any urine passed with a bowel movement should be collected, if possible without including feces with the urine collection. The collection is completed by collecting the first urine passed the next morning (within approximately 10 min before or after the time of the first morning void on the first day). The exact time of the final collection is to be noted, even if it is not the same time as when collection began on day one.

17.5.6 Instructions for a Split Urine Collection

This is done to determine whether the patient has orthostatic proteinuria. Discard first morning void and collect all daytime urine samples in the "daytime urine jug." Normal daily activities are permitted. In the evening, the patient lies down 2 h before going to bed. Just before sleeping, patient goes to the bathroom; this urine is added to the daytime jug. Lying down for 2 h helps to avoid mixing urine made at night, with urine made during the day. Urine samples, if any, are collected in the "nighttime urine jug." The first morning urine sample next morning is added to the nighttime urine jug.

17.6 Procedures

17.6.1 Voiding/Micturating Cystourethrogram (VCUG, MCUG)

It is a procedure for visualization of the urinary bladder and the lower urinary tract with the help of a low iodine concentration contrast dye which is instilled into the bladder by a per-urethral catheter or through a suprapubic needle. It has 2 phases: a filling phase and a voiding phase. The bladder capacity and contour are noted during the filling and the filled phase while VUR and urethra and the bladder emptying are noted during the voiding phase. VUR can be detected during both phases. The voiding phase is best visualized after removing the catheter in the bladder. It is important to counsel the parents and the older child to decrease their apprehension and ensure their cooperation during the procedure.

17.6.1.1 Indications

1. Evaluation of antenatally diagnosed hydronephrosis
2. Evaluation of UTI
3. Evaluation of anatomic urinary tract anomalies, e.g., posterior urethral valves, solitary functioning kidney, reno-ureteric duplications, and ureteroceles
4. When vesicoureteric reflux is suspected
5. Neurogenic bladder

17.6.1.2 Technique

1. Sterile per-urethral bladder catheterization is performed with an infant feeding tube or a catheter which is preferably a smaller size for age, to allow easy urethral voiding. A warm radiology procedure room and gradual instillation of intravesical contrast at body temperature facilitates a near physiologic voiding. A scout film of the abdomen is obtained prior to instillation of the radiocontrast dye. The bladder is filled, via an indwelling catheter/suprapubic cystostomy catheter/vesicostomy (with a Foley catheter, balloon inflated to occlude the stoma), to a calculated capacity for age [<2 y: weight × 7 ml, >2 y (age +2) × 30 ml)] or until periurethral leak occurs, with 1:1 contrast dilution with isotonic saline. Intermittent fluoroscopic exam of bladder is performed during the filling phase, and the catheter is removed just prior to voiding in older communicative children or when a pericatheter leak is seen in the younger child.
2. Anteroposterior and oblique visualization of the kidneys, ureters, and bladder regions during filling and additional oblique images of the urethra during voiding phase are obtained.
3. Information about post-void residue in the bladder is obtained prior to the termination of the procedure.

17.6.2 Renal Biopsy

The histopathological evaluation of renal tissue is required to diagnose, prognosticate, and guide the treatment of primary and secondary renal diseases. In neonates an open biopsy may be performed under general anesthesia. A single kidney is no longer considered a contraindication to a kidney biopsy; the procedure has become safer. Severe hydronephrosis is a contraindication to the procedure.

17.6.2.1 Prerequisites

1. Obtain informed consent.
2. Hemoglobin/packed cell volume should be checked, platelet count should be >50,000/mm^3, PT INR (≤1.3), and APTT should be normal. Drugs such as NSAIDs and warfarin should be stopped at least 1 week prior to the biopsy, and heparin should be withheld for a minimum of 12 h before the procedure. Bleeding time

(BT) should be checked in case of azotemia; if BT≥8 min, give desmopressin (intranasal, 2–4 mcg/kg/dose 2 h before procedure; intravenous, 0.2–0.4 mcg/kg/dose over 20 min). In case the biopsy is required urgently, platelet transfusion, vitamin K, or fresh frozen plasma may be given as indicated prior to the procedure.
3. Blood should be typed.
4. Secure intravenous access.
5. Keep patient nil orally 4–6 h prior to the procedure.
6. Deep sedation is not required if cooperation of the patient with regard to breath holding is possible.
7. Blood pressure should be well controlled.
8. Hospitalization; observation for at least 6 h post procedure.

17.6.2.2 Materials Required

Biopsy needle (automatic spring loaded biopsy device), sizes 18 G (<8 y) and 16 G (>8 y); a dissecting microscope or a high-resolution lens to confirm adequacy of sample; and a collection/transport medium in containers (containing isotonic saline, 20 % formaldehyde, glutaraldehyde).

17.6.2.3 Sedation

Midazolam injection 0.02–0.1 mg/kg IV slowly over 2–3 min (max. total dose of 10 mg) followed by fentanyl injection 1.0 mcg/kg/dose over 2–3 min and repeat every 5 min, max. four doses, or ketamine injection 1 mg/kg/dose IV initial dose can be repeated at 0.25 mg/kg as required. Use of ketamine should preferably be combined with atropine and midazolam. Ketamine should be avoided if hypertension is not well controlled. Monitoring of vital parameters and pulse oximetry should be done throughout the procedure and equipment for resuscitation should be readily available.

17.6.2.4 Procedure

1. Imaging guidance by ultrasound is used in most instances. Usually the left kidney is biopsied. Biopsies should be obtained as close to the periphery of the kidney as possible, to minimize bleeding and maximize the amount of cortex in the specimen (at least 1 cm thick and should not contain cysts, masses, calculi, or arteriovenous fistulae).
2. For native kidneys, the patient is positioned prone, with arms and forearms abducted on the side of the head, and a rolled towel or a wedge may be placed under the abdomen to eliminate the lumbar lordosis. The lower pole is the optimal site and the route chosen should be the shortest one possible without passing through bowel, ribs, or large vessels.
3. Once the target is identified by ultrasonography, the distance from the skin is measured and the point for biopsy is marked on the skin.
4. The native kidney moves inferiorly with inspiration and biopsies may be performed in suspended respiration in older children. Practicing breath holds should be performed with the patient during the pre-biopsy ultrasound.

5. For transplanted kidneys, the patient is placed in the supine or left lateral decubitus position if the kidney is in the right lower quadrant and in the right lateral decubitus if the kidney is in the left lower quadrant, if there is overlying bowel gas in the supine position. The upper or lower pole may be used. Since transplant kidneys usually do not move during respiration, suspended respiration is not necessary.
6. The skin site is prepared in a sterile manner and is then appropriately draped.
7. Strict asepsis should be maintained and vital signs monitored throughout the procedure.
8. Local anesthetic infiltration with 2 % lidocaine injection may be used to minimize discomfort at the site and the soft tissues along the intended biopsy tract.
9. A small stab incision is given at the intended skin entrance site to allow ready passage of the biopsy needle.
10. The needle is inserted at the planned site till the feeling of resistance (renal capsule). If feasible ask the patient to hold the breath then advance the gun slightly and fire it. Withdraw the gun immediately.
11. At some centers real-time ultrasonographic guidance is preferred using a built-in guide to improve accuracy. The biopsy needle is placed into the guide, and the needle tip is inserted into the skin incision. The transducer is moved down the needle and placed on the skin. The needle is then advanced toward the kidney under real-time ultrasonographic guidance.
12. 2–3 cores of tissues can be obtained and the adequacy of sample can be tested under a lens (glomeruli seen as small red dots). A biopsy sample is considered adequate when a specimen contains ten or more glomeruli and two small arteries. Corticomedullary junction tissue is required when evaluating transplant kidneys or when evaluating for FSGS.
13. Post-biopsy ultrasound should be performed to exclude a perinephric hematoma and a pressure dressing should be applied over the biopsy site.

17.6.2.5 Post-procedure Care

1. The patient remains supine for 6 h after biopsy and should have vital signs closely monitored.
2. Encourage adequate fluid intake to maintain hydration.
3. Watch for abdominal pain, fever, vomiting, persistent gross hematuria, hypotension, and pallor.
4. Avoid contact sports for 2–3 weeks.
5. A sample of each void is racked to evaluate for clots or gross hematuria.
6. A repeat renal ultrasound scan and hemoglobin may be assessed every 6 h if bleeding is suspected. If the 6-h ultrasound scan demonstrates no complications, the patient is discharged. If there is evidence of active bleeding, such as a hematoma which is increasing in size or gross hematuria, the patient is hospitalized for monitoring.

17.6.2.6 Complications

1. Complications of analgesia and anesthesia.
2. Hemorrhage: Perirenal hemorrhage presents with loin pain, sometimes with palpable mass and signs of blood loss. Hemorrhage into renal pelvis presents with persistent gross hematuria and sometimes clot retention.

3. Arteriovenous fistula: Fortunately rare and most of them resolve spontaneously. Few patients develop symptoms like persistent hematuria, hypertension, and high-output cardiac failure necessitating endovascular embolization or partial nephrectomy.

17.6.2.7 Contraindications

Bleeding diathesis, horseshoe or other anatomically abnormal kidneys, severe hydronephrosis, polycystic kidneys, uncontrolled hypertension, and small contracted kidneys (high risk of bleeding and may not yield useful information). An open biopsy can be considered in some situations, to reduce the risk of complications.

17.6.3 Plasma Exchange

Plasmapheresis is an extracorporeal therapy which involves the removal, treatment, and return of (components of) plasma from the circulation. When, additionally, replacement solutions like albumin or frozen plasma are prescribed to the patient, it is referred to as “plasma exchange.” These terms are often used interchangeably. Serial sessions with concomitant immunosuppressive therapy are often required.

17.6.3.1 Indications

1. Atypical hemolytic uremic syndrome
2. Anti-glomerular basement disease membrane disease
3. Anti-neutrophil cytoplasmic antibody (ANCA)-associated vasculitis, when patient has severe renal failure or pulmonary hemorrhage
4. FSGS recurrence in transplant kidney
5. Acute vascular allograft rejection
6. Crescentic glomerulonephritis
7. Systemic lupus erythematosus: in lupus cerebritis and in very severe disease
8. Guillain-Barré syndrome – along with IV immunoglobulin (IVIG) infusions
9. Acute crisis of myasthenia gravis

17.6.3.2 Materials Required

1. Plasma filter: allows passage of immunoglobulins and complexes and holds back formed cellular elements. (i) Surface area, 0.15 m^2; extracorporeal volume, 23 ml; and minimum blood flow rate, 50 ml/min. (ii) Surface area, 0.35 m^2; extracorporeal volume, 41 ml; and minimum blood flow rate, 100 ml/min).

Table 17.1 Blood flow rates and plasma filtration rates with different filters

Blood flow rate (Qb ml/min)	Plasma filtration rate (ml/min)	
	Surface area: 0.15 m^2	Surface area: 0.35 m^2
50	15–19	–
100	29–36	39–48
150	43–53	57–69
200	54–67	74–91

2. Blood lines – 61 ml (pediatric), 167 ml (adult)
3. Replacement solutions:
   - Frozen plasma (FP) provides coagulation factors and immunoglobulins. It needs to be cross matched with recipient's blood group. Since it contains citrate, calcium replacement is advisable. Specific indications for the use of FP are HUS/thrombotic thrombocytopenic purpura (TTP), liver failure, and coagulopathy with inhibitors.
   - 5 % albumin lacks coagulation factors and is expensive in developing countries. An alternative is to infuse 1/3 replacement with crystalloid such as isotonic saline (NS) or Ringer's lactate (RL) and the remaining 2/3 with 5 % albumin.

17.6.3.3 Vascular Access

- Long-term access: A permanent catheter (permcath) in the internal jugular (IJV) or subclavian vein or an arteriovenous fistula
- Acute short-term access obtained by a dual-lumen central venous catheter in the internal jugular, femoral, or subclavian vein

17.6.3.4 Procedure

- Exchange volume: single plasma volume exchange removes 63 % fraction, after second volume exchange in the same session increases it by 85 %. Exchanging more than two volumes in one session is not recommended. Estimated plasma volume in ml is $\{0.0\,65 \times \text{weight (kg)}\} \times \{1\text{-hematocrit}\} \times 1{,}000$.
- Blood flow rate: 5 ml/kg/min; rate of plasma removal should be less than 50 ml/kg/h.
- Duration of therapy (min.) can be calculated as follows: plasma volume x exchange (1–1.5)/plasma filtration rate.
- Anticoagulation with heparin: loading dose of 50 IU/kg, followed by infusion rate of 15–20 IU/kg/h (max. 1,000 U/h.); half-hourly monitoring of activated clotting time should be done with a target of 180–220 s (1.5–2 times of normal).
- Anticoagulation with acid citrate dextrose (29.3 g citrate/l) dextrose solution in ml/h = 1.5 times blood flow in ml/min and calcium chloride (8 g/l or 72 mmol/l) at a rate of 0.4 times rate of acid citrate dextrose. Watch for hypocalcaemia. Replacement fluid and calcium chloride infusion should always be given post filter.
- When using albumin as a replacement fluid, monitor PT/PTT before third and subsequent procedures. If it is more than 1.5 times greater than normal, FP should be used as a replacement fluid.
- Potassium can be added to prevent hypokalemia (4 mmol K = 2 ml KCl for each liter of albumin).

17.6.3.5 Complications

- Hypotension due to excessive extracorporeal volume, decreased oncotic pressure, delayed or inadequate fluid replacement, and anaphylaxis.
- Hypocalcemia and metabolic alkalosis may occur due to excess citrate.

- Thrombocytopenia.
- Hypokalemia.
- Allergic reaction to replacement fluid: Sensitivity to replacement fluid can be prevented by using premedication with intravenous hydrocortisone 2–4 mg/kg/dose (up to 100 mg) along with intravenous chlorpheniramine maleate (0.1 mg/kg).
- Excess anticoagulation with heparin may result in bleeding complications.

17.6.4 Central Venous Access

Central venous access may be obtained using temporary or permanent catheters. The permanent catheters are usually inserted by surgeons in the operating room; techniques of bedside insertion of temporary catheters are given in this section.

17.6.4.1 Prerequisites

The same as given above (see "Prerequisites for Renal Biopsy").

17.6.4.2 Equipment

Hemodialysis catheter kit, two syringes 5 cm^3 each, dilute heparin to 10 IU/ml (flush both ports of the catheter), lidocaine injection for local anesthesia (use 24, 26 G needles), isotonic saline, suture material (3.0 silk)

Table 17.2 Central venous access: recommended catheter size as per weight of the child

Patient weight	Catheter size
Neonate	Single-lumen 5 F in 2 different veins
3–6 kg	Dual-lumen 7.0 F
6–25 kg	Dual-lumen 8.0 F
25–40 kg	Dual-lumen 10.0 F
>40 kg	Dual-lumen 12.0 F

17.6.4.3 Procedure (Seldinger Technique)

1. Prepare the site and drape in sterile fashion. Use lidocaine for infiltration at local site.
2. Insert cannula attached to a syringe partially filled with saline, applying negative pressure. When there is blood return, disconnect the syringe from cannula, remove the needle, and insert a guide wire through the cannula into the vein. For a physician with limited experience, these steps should be first carried out using a small (21G) cannula to locate the vein before proceeding with large-bore cannula. If an artery is punctured, remove the cannula and use firm compression for 5 min.
3. Thread the dilator over the guide wire and dilate entry point into vessel by a twisting movement.
4. Pass the entire catheter over the wire until the hub is at the skin surface.
5. Slowly remove the guide wire; confirm free flow of blood from both ports of HD catheter.

6. Secure the catheter by sutures and flush with saline. Leave heparinized saline in the ports as per instructions on the catheter.
7. Apply a sterile dressing over the site.
8. For neck vessels obtain a chest radiograph to rule out pneumothorax or hemothorax and to check the catheter position (confirm at superior vena cava-right atrium junction, i.e., catheter tip should lie at the anterior end of the second rib).

17.6.4.4 Insertion Site

Femoral catheters are preferred in patients with acute pulmonary edema (as head high position can be given during the procedure) or when coagulation parameters are altered, since pressure can be applied directly against a bone, over the insertion site. The site is not recommended in ambulatory patients. IJV (internal jugular vein) is the preferred site for the insertion of temporary access. The straight course of right IJV to the right atrium, absence of thoracic duct on the right side, and lower pleural dome on the right side makes right side preferable compared to left IJV. Subclavian vein has higher insertion-related complications like pneumothorax, hemothorax, subclavian artery injury, brachial plexus injury, and a higher risk of developing subclavian vein stenosis.

Femoral Vein

- The child should lie supine with the hip flexed and abducted.
- Place a pad of bed linen under the hips.
- Locate the femoral artery just distal to the inguinal crease. Femoral vein lies medial to artery (5 mm in infants and toddler, 10 mm in adolescents and adults). Place the thumb of the nondominant hand on the femoral artery. Insert the needle medial to the thumb.
- The needle should enter the skin 2–3 cm distal to the inguinal ligament at a 30° angle to avoid entering the abdomen. Keep the axis of the cannula parallel to axis of thigh. When blood flow is obtained, continue with Seldinger technique.

Internal Jugular Vein (IJV)

IJV runs behind the sternocleidomastoid muscle close to lateral border of the carotid artery.

- Place patient in 15–20° Trendelenburg position (head down).
- Hyperextend the neck, using a roll of bed linen under shoulders, to tense the sternocleidomastoid muscle, and turn the head away from the site of line placement.
- Standing at the head end of patient, palpate the sternal and clavicular heads of the muscle and enter at the apex of the triangle formed. An alternative landmark for puncture is halfway between the sternal notch and tip of the mastoid process.
- Palpate carotid artery and protect it by pushing it medially. Insert the needle at a 30° angle to the skin, and aim toward the ipsilateral nipple. When blood flow is obtained, continue with Seldinger technique.

Subclavian Vein

- Subclavian vein lies in the angle formed by medial 1/3 of clavicle and the first rib in which the subclavian vein crosses over the first rib to enter thoracic cavity.
- Position the child in the 20° Trendelenburg position with head turned to side opposite to that of insertion, and place a narrow roll of linen between the shoulder blades to hyperextend the back.
- Identify the midpoint of the clavicle and the suprasternal notch. Insert cannula attached with saline-filled syringe from midpoint of clavicle. Advance needle toward middle 1/3rd and outer 2/3rd of clavicle. After hitting the clavicle, glide the cannula close to under surface of the clavicle. After entering space between clavicle and first rib, advance cannula directed aiming at the suprasternal notch. While needle is advanced, gentle aspiration is maintained. When blood flow is obtained, continue with Seldinger technique.

17.6.4.5 Complications of Central Venous Catheter Insertion

- Insertion related (immediate): arterial puncture, pneumothorax, hemothorax, arrhythmia, air embolism, perforation of vein or cardiac chamber, and pericardial tamponade. Injury to adjacent structures like brachial plexus, trachea, and recurrent laryngeal nerve. Delayed complications include thrombosis, infection, vascular stricture, and A-V fistula.
- Catheter dysfunction, if occurs soon after insertion, may be due to improper placement or due to an intracatheter thrombus. Late catheter dysfunction may occur due to fibrin sleeves, mural thrombosis, central vein stenosis, thrombosis, or stricture and due to catheter fragment in circulation.
- Infection which may be local site infection or catheter-related blood stream infection (CRBSI).

17.6.5 Acute Peritoneal dialysis

Acute peritoneal dialysis (PD), using a "temporary rigid catheter with a metal stylet," is a lifesaving procedure in patients with AKI, especially in regions with limited resources. The technique of insertion of the temporary rigid catheter, the procedure, monitoring, complications, and troubleshooting for acute PD are given below. Contraindications to this procedure include recent abdominal surgery or trauma, extensive intra-abdominal adhesions, necrotizing enterocolitis, a large intra-abdominal mass, diaphragmatic hernia, ventriculoperitoneal shunt, and prune belly syndrome.

A "permanent soft catheter" may be used when it is anticipated that the need for PD will be longer than a few days. Insertion of this catheter (percutaneously with the help of a guide wire and a peel-away sheath) may be done at the bedside. This technique is also described at the end of this chapter. The catheter insertion can also be done by a surgeon in the operating room (peritoneoscopic/laparoscopic/open method).

17.6.5.1 Materials Required

1. A PD catheter kit has a straight, rigid PD catheter with numerous side holes at the end and a metal stylet that is used to guide insertion. A 10 F neonatal chest drain tube may be used instead of a PD catheter in newborns. PD catheter sizes available are neonatal size, pediatric size for a child <20 kg, and adult size for children >20 kg.
2. PD fluid: Lactate buffered electrolyte balanced dextrose solution is most often used. (Constituents of a standard PD solution are dextrose 1.7 g/dl (0.094 mmol/l), sodium 130 mmol/l, chloride 100 mmol/l, acetate/lactate 3.88 mmol/l, magnesium 1.23 mmol/l, calcium 1.5 mmol/l, and osmolality 355 mOsm/kg.) Special PD fluids (bicarbonate-based and chloride-based) may be needed in special situations.
3. Others Sterile dressing tray with suture materials, sterile surgical blade no. 11, hypodermic sterile needle 18 G, urobag, IV sets, 2- and 3-way connectors, a Y connector set, 2 % lidocaine injection, and dressing adhesive.

Peritoneal Dialysis Using Bicarbonate-Based PD Fluid

Indications

Children with severely compromised liver functions and AKI may need PD using bicarbonate-based PD fluid. The use of bicarbonate as a buffer in the dialysate results in better correction of acidosis, lower lactate levels, and improved hemodynamic stability. Lactic acidosis may be profound in low birth weight newborns with sepsis. Bicarbonate-based peritoneal dialysis may be beneficial in this situation.

Composition and Preparation

Bicarbonate-based peritoneal fluid is prepared as follows:

Prepare solution A: 440 ml of 5 % dextrose + 60 ml of $NaHCO_3$
Prepare solution B: 500 ml of normal saline

Solution A 250 ml + solution B 500 ml gives Na140 mEq/l, HCO_3 30 mEq/l, and dextrose 1.5 g/dl. Heparin, insulin, and potassium can be added to bicarbonate-based fluid, if required. However, calcium if indicated should be given intravenously as calcium gets precipitated with bicarbonate, if added to the PD fluid.

Peritoneal Dialysis Using Chloride-Based PD Fluid

Indications

Children with severe metabolic alkalosis associated with a chloride depleted state may need PD using chloride-based (instead of lactate-based) PD fluid.

Composition

0.9 % NaCl (150 mmol/l of Na instead of 130 mmol/l in PD fluid)-based PD fluid is used to counteract metabolic alkalosis.

Dialysis

Maintenance doses of potassium, calcium, and magnesium can be infused intravenously. Inadequate ultrafiltration is a concern as the PD fluid is isotonic. In the event of poor ultrafiltration, hyperosmolar dextrose can be added to the PD fluid to facilitate ultrafiltration.

17.6.5.2 Procedure

1. Catheterize the bladder.
2. Ensure that the dialysis fluid is warmed to the body temperature.
3. Prepare and drape abdomen with the patient in supine position.
4. Identify the midpoint of the line joining the umbilicus to the pubic symphysis or in a neonate on a paramedian line a little lateral to rectus sheath. Give local anesthesia down to the peritoneum. Insert an 18-gauge needle at the planned site and infuse 20–30 ml/kg of dialysate fluid to create a fluid cushion.
5. Make a stab skin incision and insert the catheter with stylet perpendicular to the abdominal wall with a twisting motion. Penetration of peritoneum will be indicated by sudden feeling of "give way" and gush of dialysate fluid out via the catheter. Withdraw the stylet gradually, simultaneously advancing the catheter toward the opposite pelvic cavity. Attach the connecting set to the catheter and run in dialysate fluid to confirm free flow. Allow about half of dialysate fluid to drain out by gravity. Start the next inflow. The initial 2–3 cycles can be rapid without a dwell time.
6. Secure the catheter in place, if required with a purse string suture.

17.6.5.3 Peritoneal Dialysis Prescription and Monitoring for Acute PD

Acute peritoneal dialysis may be done by performing exchanges manually or with the use of an automated cycler.

1. Fill volume 30–50 ml/kg, run-in time 5–10 min, dwell time 20–30 min, and outflow time 10–20 min constitute the usual dialysis prescription. Each cycle usually lasts for 1 h. Avoid excessive abdominal distention and respiratory compromise.
2. Addition of potassium to the dialysis fluid may be withheld for initial 8–10 cycles. Subsequently 2–4 mmol/l of KCl can be added depending on the serum potassium level.
3. Heparin (500 IU/l) may be added to prevent clot formation particularly to the first liter of fluid and when outflow contains blood and fibrinous material.
4. Dialysis can be continued for 48–72 h (total treatment time). It is preferable to remove the acute PD catheter after 72 h (risk of infection if the catheter is left in place for a longer period) and reinsert later if required. Before removing the catheter, drain out dialysate fluid completely.
5. Modifications: In patients with pulmonary edema, dwell time can be shortened to 15–20 min and 2.5 % dextrose containing PD fluid can be used to remove fluid rapidly.
6. Monitoring: Maintain pulse, blood pressure, and intake/output hourly charts; serum electrolytes and blood sugar every 8 h and blood urea and creatinine every 24 h. Watch changes in appearance of returning peritoneal fluid (infection, blood, fibrin threads). Send PD fluid for analysis: cell count, gram stain, culture, and antibiotic sensitivity if patient is febrile or drained PD fluid color transparency is altered.

Complications and troubleshooting

Blood-stained effluent	Add heparin to dialysate fluid to prevent catheter blockage. Usually diminishes with subsequent cycles
Poor drainage	Ensure adequate fill. Catheter may be blocked with fibrin or omentum plug. Flush, reposition, or remove and reinsert catheter
Pericatheter leak	During insertion of catheter ensure that all holes are intraperitoneal.
	Purse string suture at base prevents a leak.
	Try small fill volumes
Abdominal pain during inflow	May be because of peritonitis, cold dialysate fluid, hypertonic solution, or excessive fill volume
Hypokalemia, hypernatremia, hyperglycemia	Regular monitoring and appropriate correction
Respiratory embarrassment	Because of overdistention of abdomen or pleural effusion. Decrease dwell volumes
Peritonitis	Manifests as abdominal pain and cloudy peritoneal fluid containing more than 100 cells/mm^3, predominantly neutrophils (>50 %). Usual organisms are gram-positive bacteria (size of S. epidermidis, S. aureus). Start initial treatment with broad-spectrum antibiotics covering both gram-positive and gram-negative organisms until availability of gram stain or culture report
Bowel perforation	Manifests with watery diarrhea and fecal material in dialysate effluent. Remove catheter and administer antibiotics; may require surgical exploration

17.6.5.4 Percutaneous Insertion of a Permanent Soft Catheter

Seldinger Technique

- Tenckhoff PD catheters (single cuff) are used (choose the size depending on the age and size of the child).
- The procedure is performed under local anesthesia. Prophylactic antibiotics (e.g., cefazolin) may be given intravenously 1 h before the procedure.
- A small incision is made above the entrance site, usually in the midline with blunt dissection of the abdominal rectus sheath.
- The peritoneal cavity is entered through the incision with an 18-gauge needle and filled with 20 ml/kg of isotonic saline. With proper needle placement, the patient should not experience pain or resistance to filling the cavity with fluid.
- A 0.035-in. guide wire is advanced into the abdomen and the introduction needle is removed.
- A dilator and the peel-away sheath are advanced over the wire into the abdominal cavity.
- The wire and the dilator are removed and the catheter is placed on the stylet and is advanced through the sheath.
- The intraperitoneal segment is advanced until the proximal cuff is located in the preperitoneal space.
- The peel-away sheath and stylet are removed and the catheter position is checked.

- A tunnel is created to the selected exit site (paramedian or lateral abdominal location rather than in the midline) with the placement of the distal cuff subcutaneously, 2 cm from the exit site.
- The entrance site is closed.
- Catheter patency is assured by infusing 20–30 ml/kg of peritoneal dialysate over 5 min and allowing its drainage for an additional 5 min.

17.7 Nutritional Aspects

17.7.1 Maintenance Fluid Calculations by Body Weight

<10 kg	100 ml/kg/d
11–20 kg	1,000 ml + 50 ml/kg (for each kg >10 kg)
>20 kg	1,500 ml + 20 ml/kg (for each kg >20 kg)

17.7.2 Recommended Calorie, Protein, Calcium, and Phosphorous Intake

	Recommended daily Allowance		Hemodialysis	Peritoneal dialysis[a]		
	Calories (Kcal/kg)	Proteins g/kg	Proteins g/kg	Proteins g/kg	Calcium mg/d	Phosphorous mg/d
0–6 mo	100–110	2.2	2.6	3.0	400	300
6–12 mo	95–105	1.5	2.0	2.4	600	500
1–3 y	90	1.1	1.6	2.0	800	800
4–10 y	70	0.95	1.6	2.0	800	800
11–14 y (boys)	55	0.95	1.4	1.8	1,200	1,200
11–14 y (girls)	47	0.95	1.4	1.8	1,200	1,200
15–18 y (boys)	45	0.85	1.3	1.5	1,200	1,200
15–18 y (girls)	40	0.85	1.2	1.5	1,200	1,200

[a]In patients on PD, 10 % of total calorie intake can be absorbed via dextrose from the dialysate

17.7.3 Foods High in Sodium Content

Salt
Baking soda
Salted wafers, popcorns, salted biscuits
Papads (Asian preparation)

Salted pickles, chutneys, curry powder (Asian preparation)
Commercial salad dressings and sauces
Soup cubes/powder
Soft drinks containing sodium benzoate
Bakery products, bread, biscuits
Nuts such as salted cashew nuts, pistachio, walnuts, peanuts
Commercial cheese
Preservative-containing foods
Canned and tinned foods
Seafood, chicken, dried fish, bacon, ham
Meat, yeast extracts like marmite
Proprietary drinks – Bournvita, chocolate drinks, Horlicks
Milk and curds
Pulses and legumes – all varieties
Vegetables such as cauliflower, snakegourd, beetroot, carrot, coriander leaves, fenugreek (methi) leaves, lettuce, spinach (palak), amaranth, radish

17.7.4 Foods with High Levels of Potassium Content

Unless noted, one serving is ½ cup (120 ml or 4 oz). These foods have greater than 250 mg of potassium per serving and should be avoided or eaten in very small portions if a low-potassium diet is prescribed

Grains	Whole-grain breads, wheat bran, granola and granola bars, barley, ragi, wheat flour All pulses All leafy vegetables such as amaranth, coriander leaves, drumstick leaves, spinach, potato, sweet potato, yam, drumstick, green papaya, sword beans Milk, fish especially sardines Nuts such as cashew nuts, almonds; oilseeds such as peanuts Condiments and spices, jaggery Fruits such as sweet lime, mango, banana, chikoo, apricots, dates, figs, melons, oranges, pears Brown sugar, coffee, cocoa powder, chocolate
Beverages	Sports drinks, instant breakfast mix, soy milk
Snack foods/sweets	Peanut butter (2 tablespoons), nuts or seeds (1 oz), fig cookies, chocolate (1.5–2 oz), molasses (1 tablespoon)
Fruits	Apricots, avocado (¼ whole), bananas (½ whole), coconut, melon (cantaloupe and honeydew), kiwi, mango, nectarines, oranges, orange juice, papaya, pears (fresh), plantains, pomegranate (and juice), dried fruits (apricots 5 halves), dates (5), figs, prunes, raisins, prune juice, yams
Vegetables	Bamboo shoots, baked or refried beans, beets, broccoli (cooked), brussels sprouts, cabbage (raw), carrots (raw), chard, greens (except kale), kohlrabi, olives, mushrooms (canned), potatoes (white and sweet), parsnips, pickles, pumpkin, rutabaga, sauerkraut, spinach (cooked), squash (acorn, butternut, hubbard), tomato, tomato sauce, tomato juice, and vegetable juice cocktail

(continued)

Dairy products	Milk and milk products, buttermilk, yogurt
Proteins	(3-oz serving) clams, sardines, scallops, lobster, whitefish, salmon (and most other fish), ground beef, sirloin steak (and most other beef products), pinto beans, kidney beans, black beans, navy beans (and most other peas and beans, serving size ½ cup)
Soups	Salt-free soups and low-sodium bouillon cubes, unsalted broth
Condiments	Imitation bacon bits, salt, or salt substitutes (avoid completely)

17.7.5 Foods with Low Levels of Potassium Content

(Less than 250 mg potassium per serving, one serving is ½ cup (4 oz, 120 ml)

Grains	Foods prepared with white flour (e.g., pasta, bread), white rice, semolina
Beverages	Nondairy creamer, fruit punch, drink mixes, tea (<2 cups or 16 oz/day), coffee (<1 cup or 8 oz/day)
Sweets	Angel or yellow cake, pies without chocolate or high-potassium fruits, cookies without nuts, or chocolate
Fruits	Apples (1), apple juice, applesauce, apricots (canned), blackberries, blueberries, cherries, cranberries, fruit cocktail (drained), grapes, grape juice, grapefruit (½), mandarin oranges, papaya, peaches (½ fresh or ½ cup canned), pears (1 small fresh or ½ cup canned), pineapple (1/4) and juice, plums (1 whole), raspberries, strawberries, tangerine (1 whole), watermelon (1 cup)
Vegetables	Alfalfa sprouts, asparagus (6 spears), green or wax beans, broadbeans, cabbage (cooked), carrots (cooked), cauliflower, celery (1 stalk), corn (½ fresh ear or ½ cup), cucumber, eggplant, kale, lettuce, mushrooms (fresh), okra, onions, parsley, green peas, green peppers, radish, rhubarb, water chestnuts (canned, drained), watercress, spinach (raw, 1 cup), squash (yellow), zucchini, ridgegourd, snakegourd, bottlegourd, beetroot, fenugreek leaves (methi), green mango
Proteins	Chicken and meat boiled in excess water twice and drained turkey (3 oz), tuna, eggs (white), baloney, shrimp, sunflower or pumpkin seeds (1 oz), raw walnuts, almonds, cashews, peanuts (all 1 oz), flax seeds (2 tablespoons ground), unsalted peanut butter (1 tablespoon)
Dairy products	Cheddar or swiss cheese (1 oz), cottage cheese (½ cup)

17.7.5.1 Reducing Potassium Levels in Vegetables

Leaching is a process of soaking raw or frozen vegetables in water for at least 2 h before cooking to "pull" some of the potassium out of the food and into the water. Wash and then cut the raw vegetable into thin slices. Vegetables with a skin (e.g., potatoes, carrots, beets, rutabagas) should be peeled before slicing. Rinse the cut vegetables in warm water. Soak the vegetables for at least 2 h in unsalted warm water (approximately 10 parts water to 1 part vegetables). If possible, change the water every 4 h. Drain the soaking water. Rinse the vegetables again with warm water. Cook vegetables as desired, using a large amount of unsalted water (approximately 5 parts water to 1 part vegetables). Drain the cooking water.

17.7.6 Foods High in Calcium Content

1. Cereals such as ragi, whole bengal, gram (chana), moth beans (matki), red beans, soybeans, horse gram
2. All green leafy vegetables
3. Oilseeds such as dry coconut, sesame seeds, mustard seeds, asafoetida, dry cloves, coriander and cumin seeds, poppy seeds
4. Figs and all dry fruits such as cashew nuts, almonds
5. Fish, mussels, red meat
6. Milk and milk products

17.7.7 Foods High in Phosphate Content

1. Cereals
2. Soybean. Moderate sources of phosphorus are bengal gram, chick pea, cowpea, and red beans
3. Almond, cashew nuts, sesame seeds, mustard seeds, pistachio, cumin seeds, poppy seeds
4. Dry fishes
5. Milk powder, milk

17.7.8 Foods High in Oxalate Content

Almonds, cashew nuts, sesame seeds
Cocoa, coffee, tea, chocolate
Green leafy vegetables such as spinach, amaranth, curry leaves, drumstick leaves, mustard leaves, neem leaves, colocasia leaves, dry lotus stem, green plantain, and goose berries

17.7.9 Dietary Guidelines for Obesity and Dyslipidemia

1. Reduce added sugars, including sugar-sweetened drinks and juices.
2. Use canola, soybean, or safflower oils or other unsaturated oils, in place of solid fats during food preparation.
3. Use fresh vegetables and fruits and serve at every meal; be careful with added sugar and sauces.
4. Limit high-calorie sauces such as Alfredo, cream sauces, and cheese sauces.
5. Eat whole-grain breads and cereals rather than refined products.
6. Eat more legumes (beans) and tofu in place of meat.

7. Read food labels – especially for breads, breakfast cereals, and prepared foods – for content, and choose high fiber, low salt, and low sugar alternatives.
8. If nonvegetarian, introduce and regularly serve fish. Remove the skin from poultry before eating; use only lean cuts of meat and reduced-fat meat products.

17.7.10 Total Parenteral Nutrition

Nutrient	Initial dose	Advancement	Maximum
Glucose	5–10 %	2.5–5 %/d	12.5 % in peripheral vein 18 mg/kg/min (maximum rate of infusion)
Protein	1 g/kg/d	0.5–1 g/kg/d	3 g/kg/d 10–16 % of calories
Fat	0.5–1 g/kg/d	1 g/kg/d	4 g/kg/d 0.17 g/kg/h (maximum rate of infusion)

Parenteral nutrition formulation recommendations

Component	Preterm	Term infants	1–3 y	4–6 y	7–10 y	11–18 y
Energy (kcal/kg/d)	85–105	90–108	75–90	65–80	55–70	30–55
Protein (gm/kg/d)	2.5–4	2.5–3.5	1.5–2.5	1.5–2.5	1.5–2.5	0.8–3
Sodium (mEq/kg/d)	2–4	2–4	2–4	2–4	2–4	60–150 mEq/d
Potassium (mEq/kg/d)	2–4	2–4	2–4	2–4	2–4	70–180 mEq/d
Calcium (mg/kg/d)	50–60	20–40	10–20	10–20	10–20	200–800 mg/d
Phosphorus (mg/kg/d)	30–45	30–45	15–40	15–40	15–40	280–900 mg/d
Magnesium (mEq/kg/d)	0.5–1	0.25–1	0.25–0.5	0.25–0.5	0.25–0.5	8–24 mEq/d
Zinc (mcg/kg/d)	325–400	100–250	100	100	50	2–5 mg/d
Copper (mcg/kg/d)	20	20	20	20	5–20	200–300 mcg/d
Manganese (mcg/kg/d)	1	1	1	1	1	40–50 mcg/d
Selenium (mcg/kg/d)	2	2	2	2	1–2	40–60 mcg/d

17.8 Tools

17.8.1 Growth Charts: Weight, Height, BMI

17.8.1.1 CDC Charts

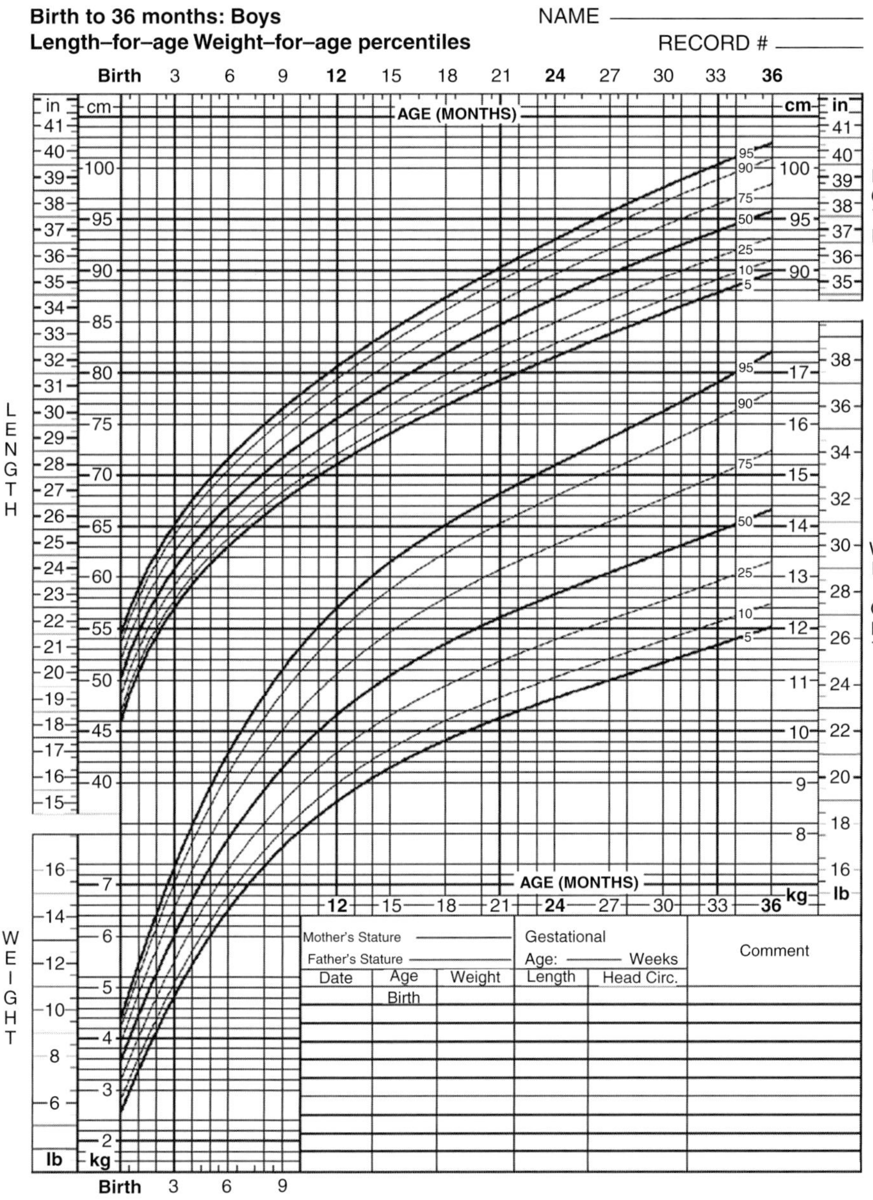

Birth to 36 months: Girls
Length–for–age and Weight–for–age percentiles

NAME ______________________

RECORD# ____________

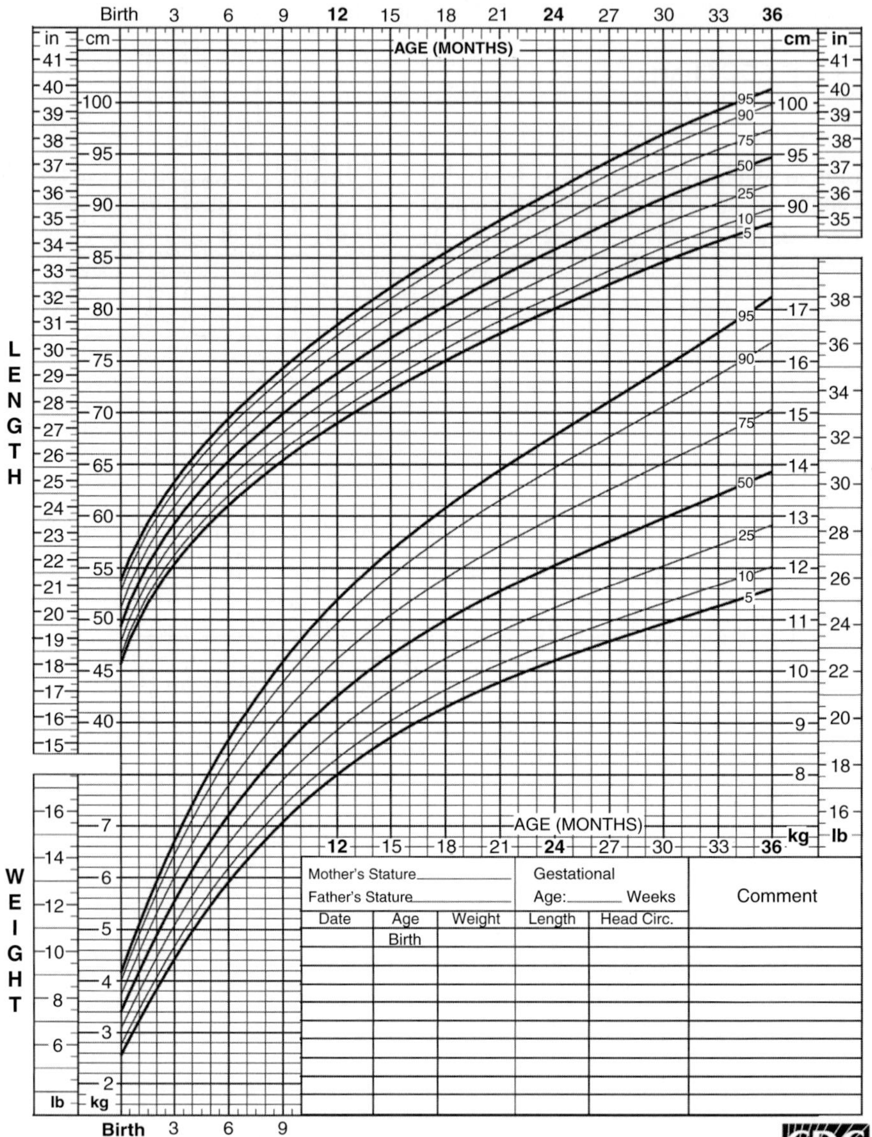

Published May 30, 2000 (modified 4/20//01.
SOURCE: Developed by the National Center for Health Statistics in collaboration with the National Center for Chronic Disease Prevention and Health Promition (2000).
http://www.cdc.gov/growthcharts

SAFER · HEALTHIER · PEOPLE™

2 to 20 years: Boys
Stature–for–age and Weight–for–age percentiles

NAME ____________________

RECORD # ____________

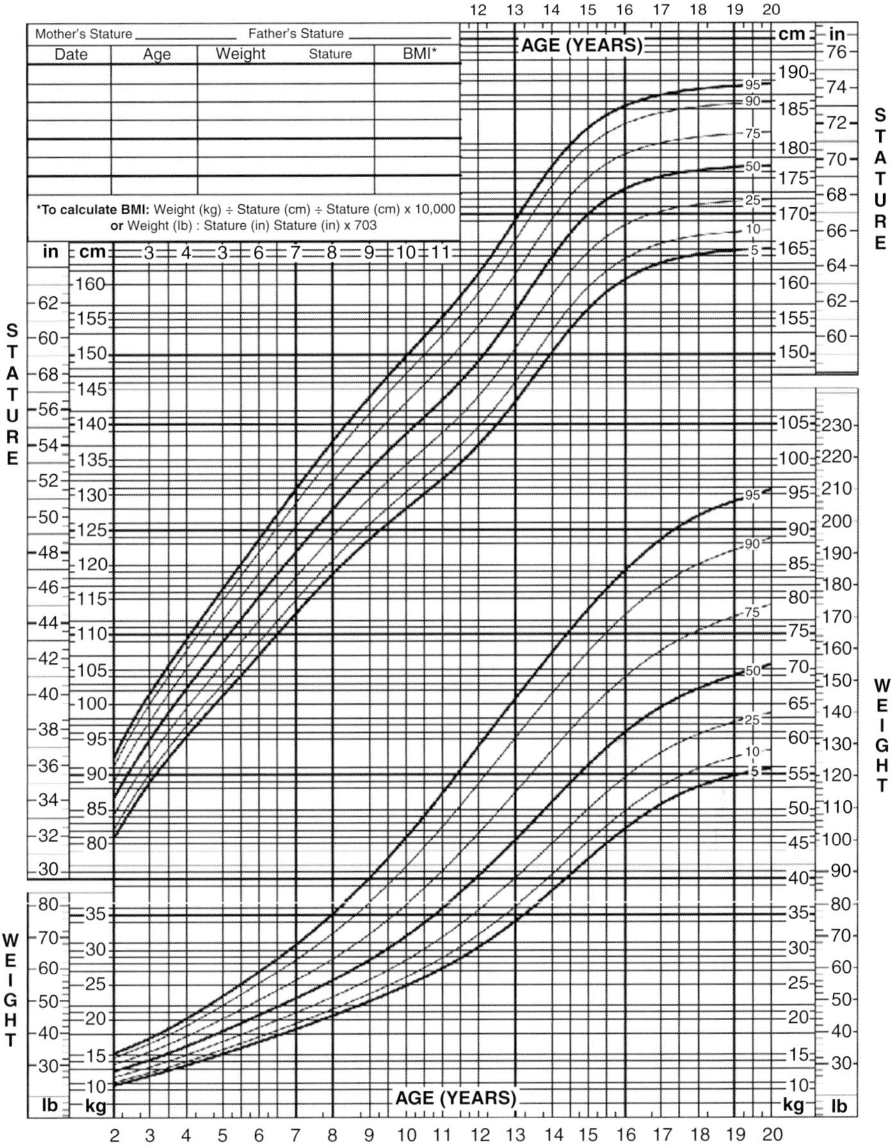

Published May 30,2000 (modified 11/21/00).

SOURCE: Developed by the National center for Health Statistics in collaboration with the National Center for Chronic Disease Prevention and Health Promotion (2000)
http://www.cdc.gov/growthcharts

SAFER•HEALTHIER• PEOPLE™

2 to 20 years: Girls
Stature–for–age and Weight–for–age percentiles

NAME

RECORD # ____________

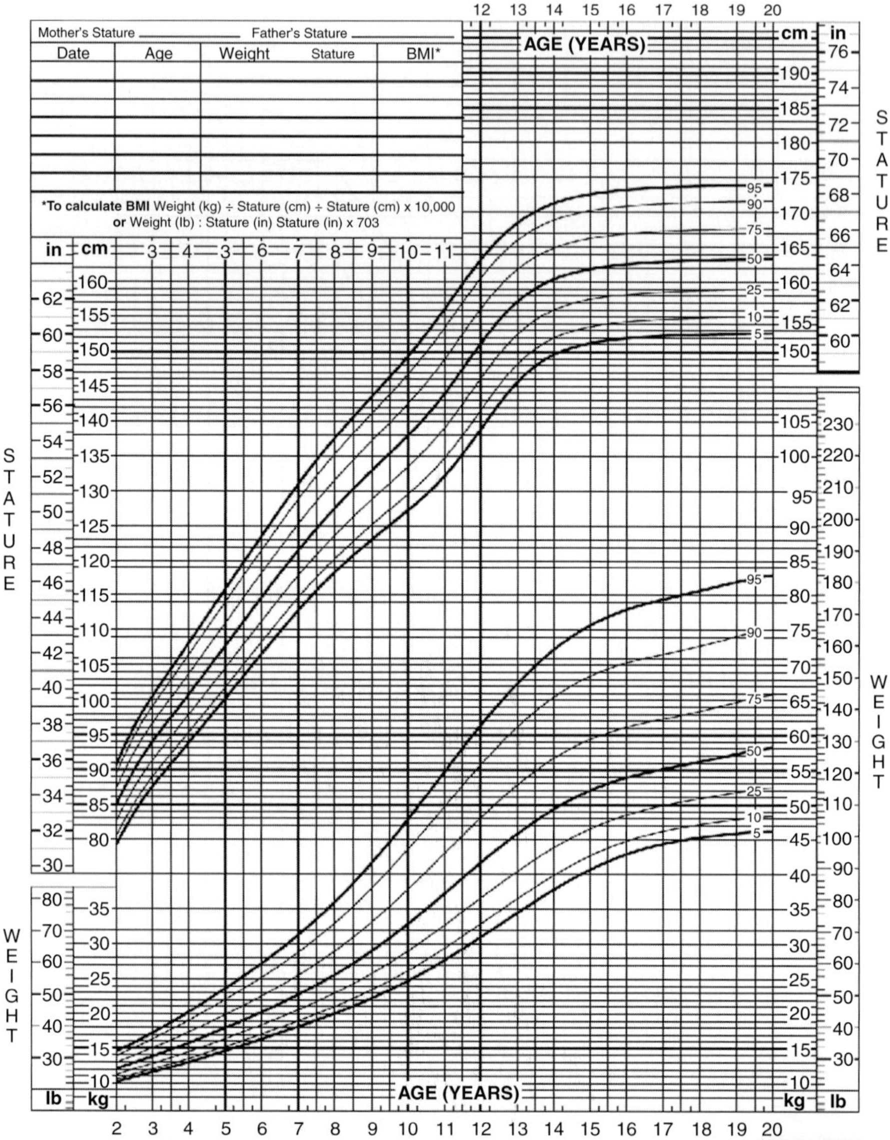

Published May 30,2000 (modified 11/21/00).
SOURCE: **Developed by the National center for Health Statistics in collaboration with the National Center for Chronic Disease Prevention and Health Promotion (2000)**
http://www.cdc.gov/growthcharts

SAFER•HEALTHIER• PEOPLE™

17.8.2 WHO Standards

17.8.2.1 Weight

Weight-for-age BOYS

Birth to 5 years (z-scores)

World Health Organization

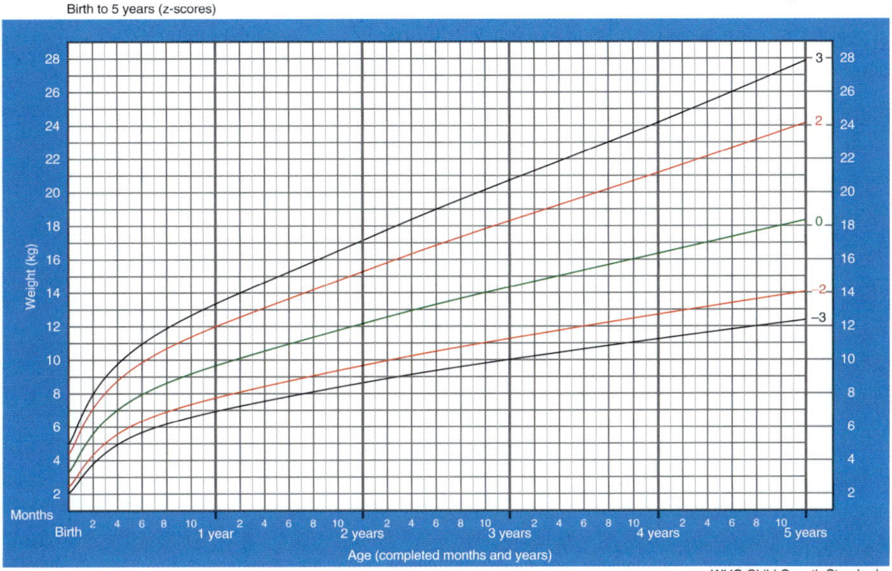

WHO Child Growth Standards

Weight-for-age BOYS

5 to 10 years (z-scores)

World Health Organization

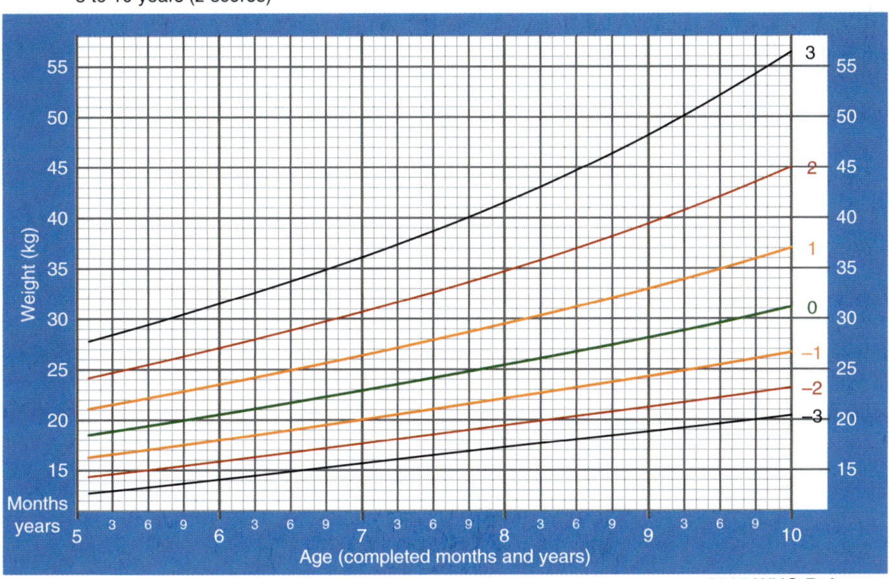

2007 WHO Reference

Weight-for-age GIRLS

Birth to 5 years (z-scores)

World Health Organization

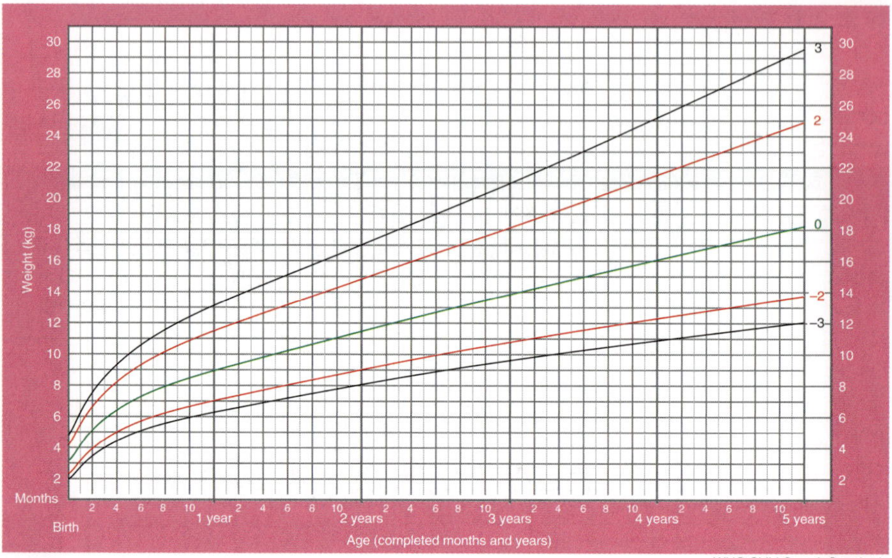

WHO Child Growth Standards

Weight-for-age GIRLS

5 to 10 years (z-scores)

World Health Organization

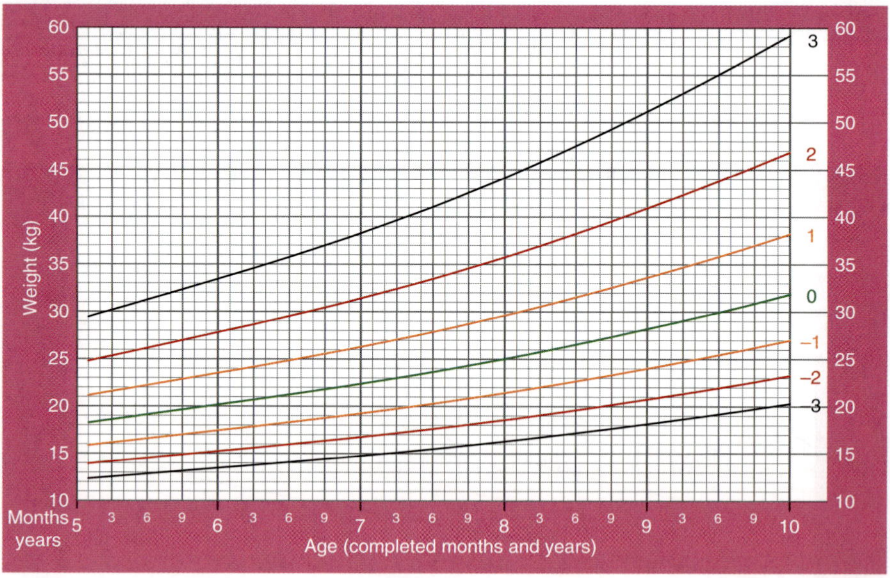

2007 WHO Reference

17.8.2.2 Height

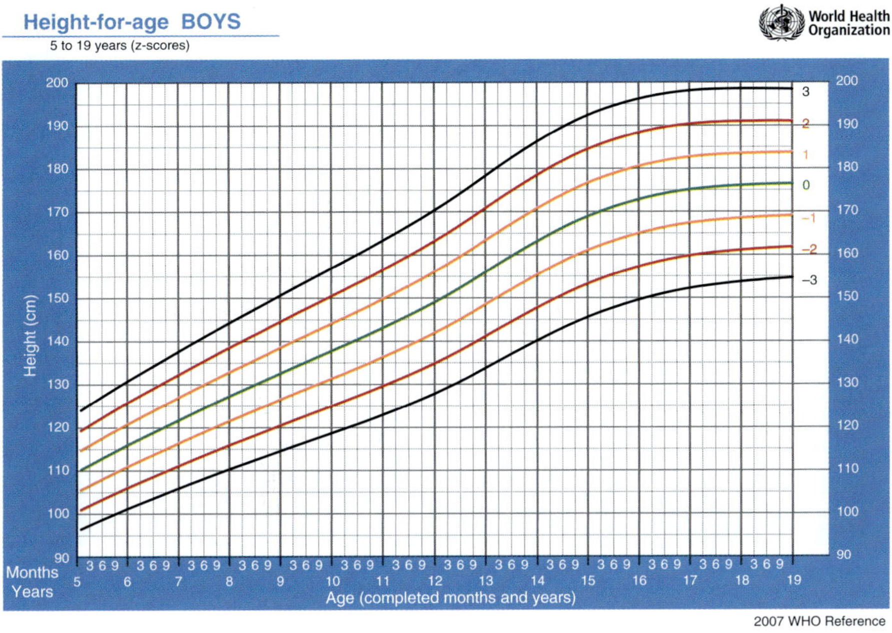

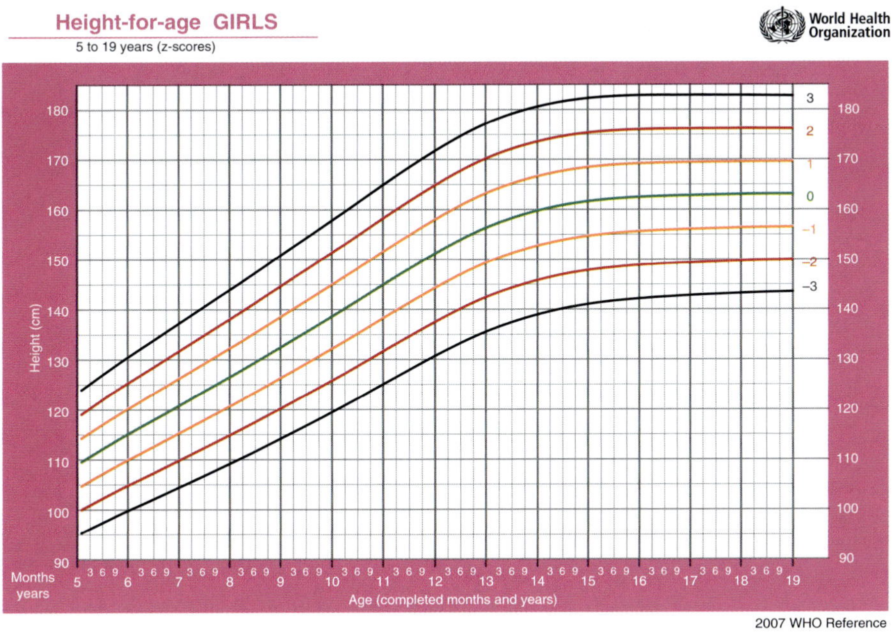

Length/height-for-age BOYS

World Health Organization

Birth to 5 years (z-scores)

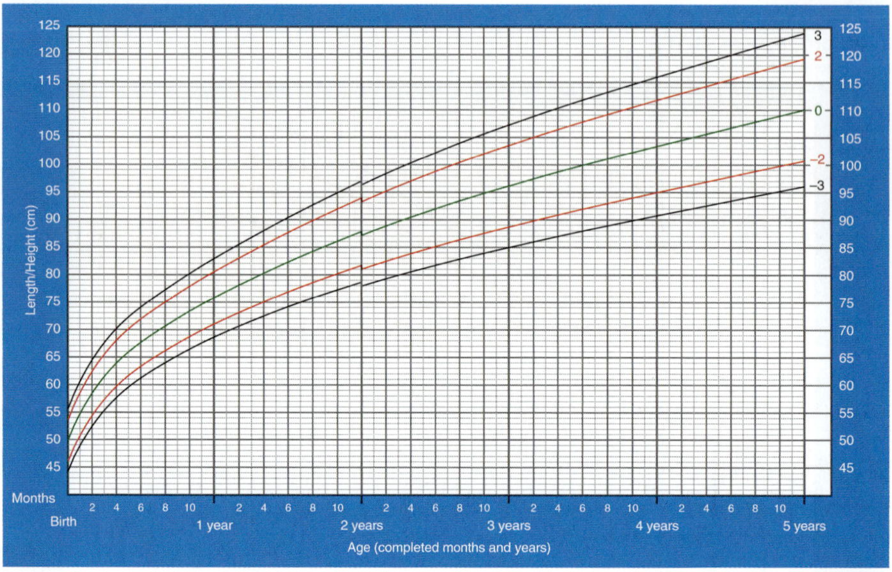

WHO Child Growth Standards

Length/height-for-age GIRLS

World Health Organization

Birth to 5 years (z-scores)

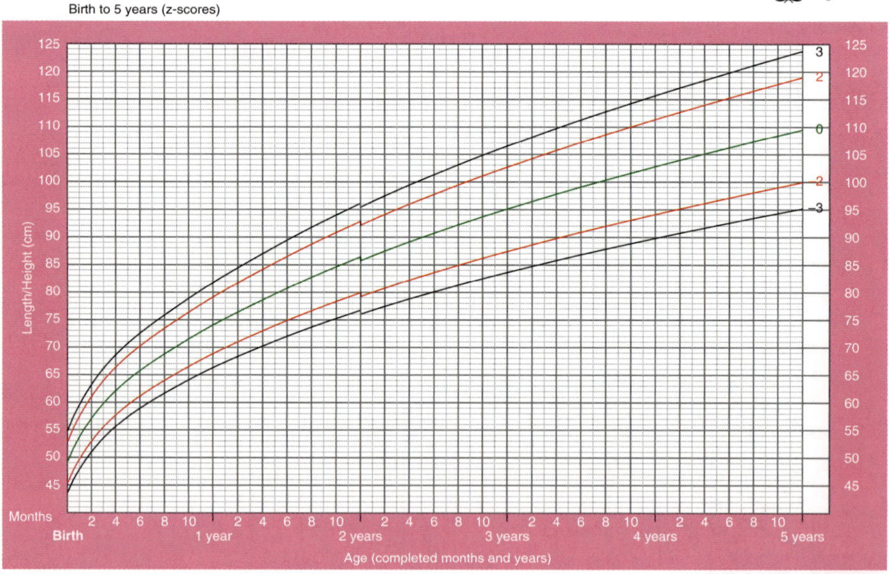

WHO Child Growth Standards

17.8.2.3 BMI

BMI-for-age BOYS

5 to 19 years (z-scores)

World Health Organization

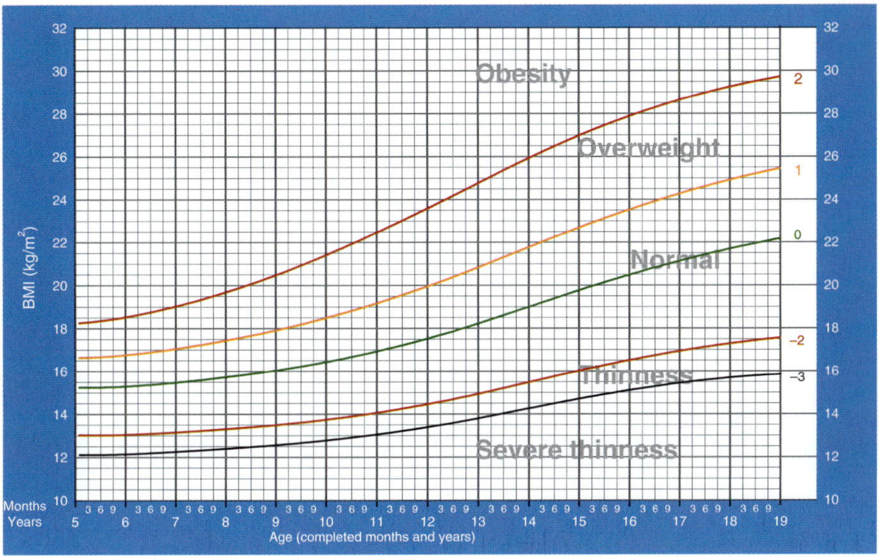

BMI-for-age GIRLS

5 to 19 years (z-scores)

World Health Organization

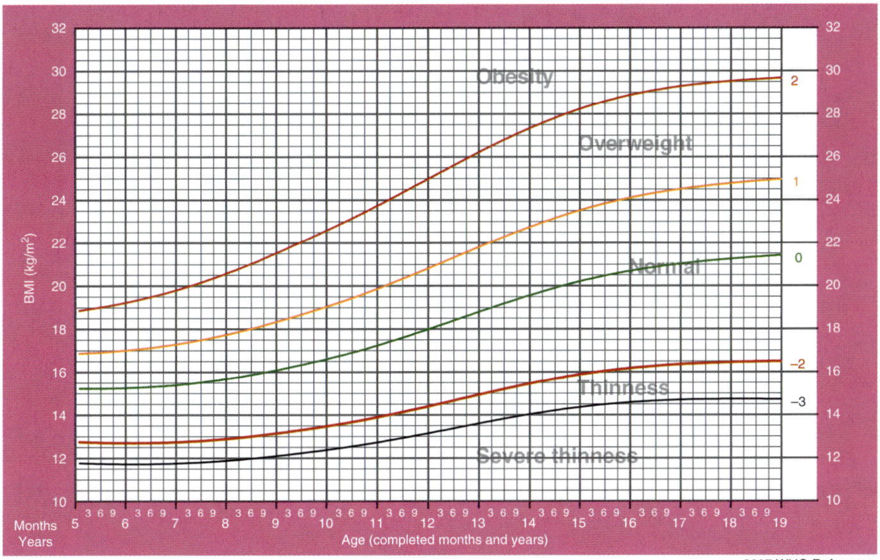

2007 WHO Reference

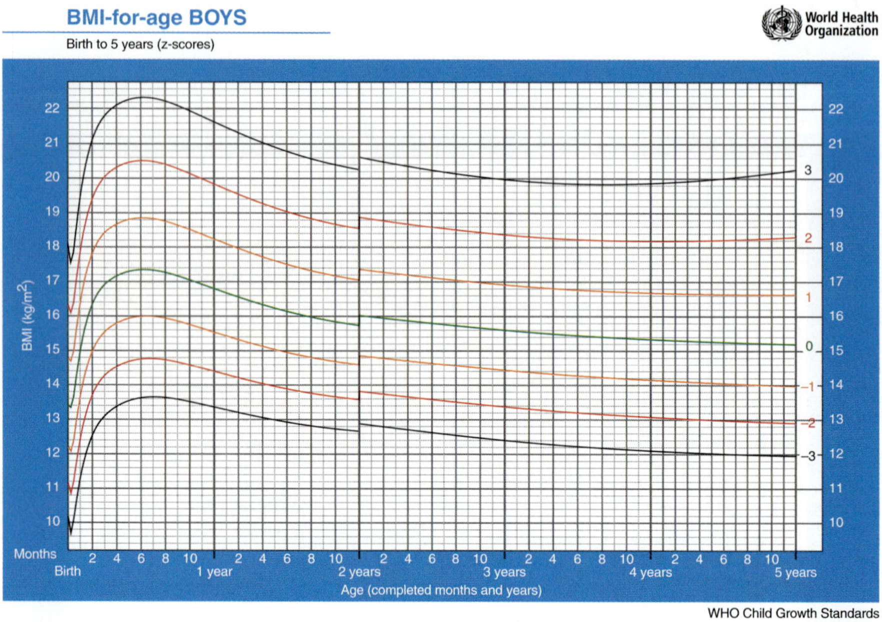
BMI-for-age BOYS
Birth to 5 years (z-scores)
World Health Organization
BMI (kg/m²)
22
21
20
19
18
17
16
15
14
13
12
11
10
3
2
1
0
−1
−2
−3
Months
2 4 6 8 10 2 4 6 8 10 2 4 6 8 10 2 4 6 8 10 2 4 6 8 10
Birth
1 year
2 years
3 years
4 years
5 years
Age (completed months and years)
WHO Child Growth Standards

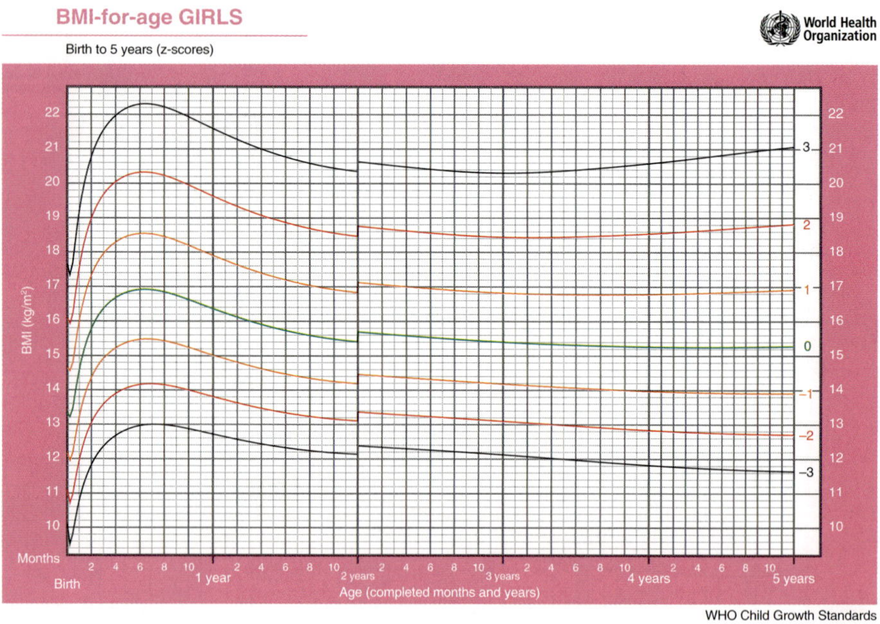
BMI-for-age GIRLS
Birth to 5 years (z-scores)
World Health Organization
BMI (kg/m²)
22
21
20
19
18
17
16
15
14
13
12
11
10
3
2
1
0
−1
−2
−3
Months
2 4 6 8 10 2 4 6 8 10 2 4 6 8 10 2 4 6 8 10 2 4 6 8 10
Birth
1 year
2 years
3 years
4 years
5 years
Age (completed months and years)
WHO Child Growth Standards

17.8.3 Surface Area Nomograms

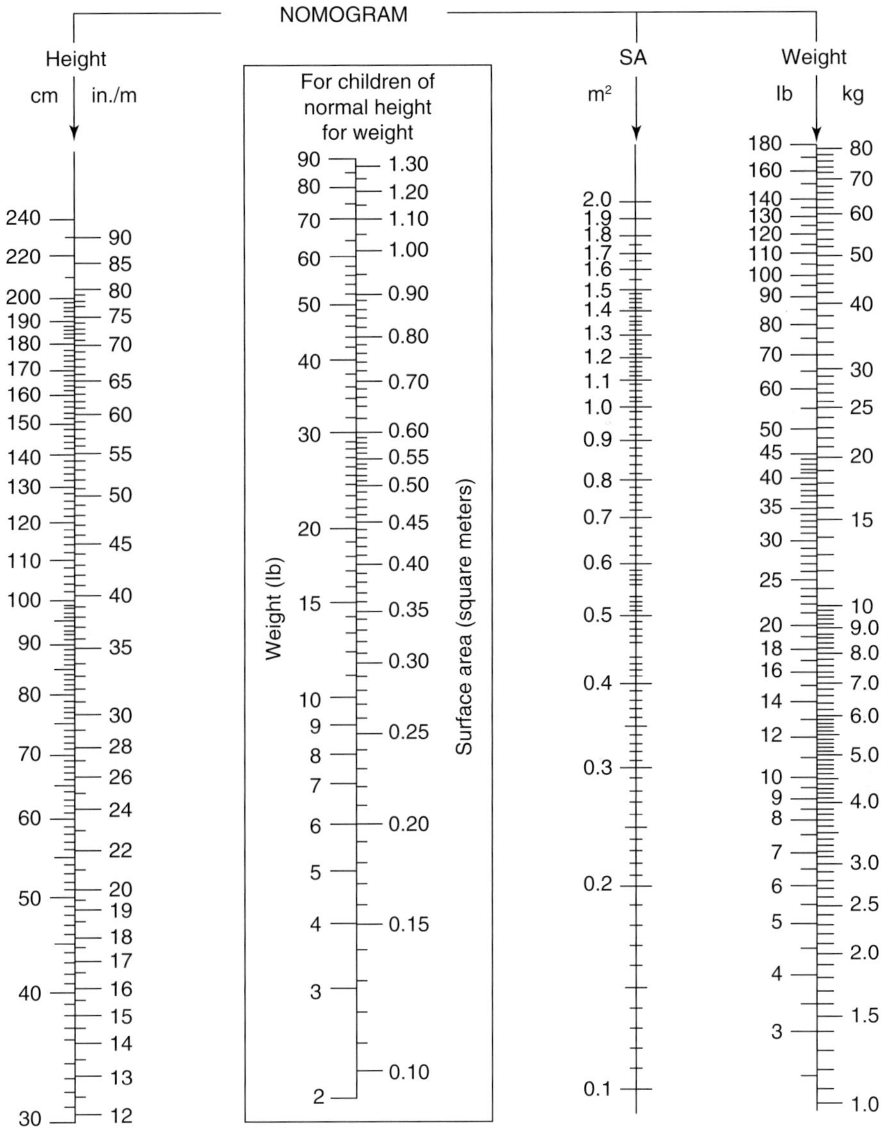

17.8.4 Percentiles for Blood Pressure

BP Levels for Boys by Age and Height Percentile

Updated: January, 2012

Age yrs	BP Percentile	Systolic BP (mmHg)							Diastolic BP (mmHg)						
		5th	10th	25th	50th	75th	90th	95th	5th	10th	25th	50th	75th	90th	95th
2	Height - *inches*	31.9	32.4	33.3	34.2	35.1	36.0	36.5	31.9	32.4	33.3	34.2	35.1	36.0	36.5
	Height - *cm*	81.1	82.4	84.5	86.9	89.2	91.4	92.6	81.1	82.4	84.5	86.9	89.2	94.4	92.6
	NT	84	85	87	88	90	92	92	39	40	41	42	43	44	44
	PreHT	97	99	100	102	104	105	106	54	55	56	57	58	58	59
	Stage 1 HT	101	102	104	106	108	109	110	59	59	60	61	62	63	63
	Stage 2 HT	114	115	116	118	120	122	122	71	72	73	74	75	76	76
3	Height - *inches*	35.1	35.6	36.5	37.5	38.6	39.5	40.1	35.1	35.6	36.5	37.5	38.6	39.5	40.1
	Height - *cm*	89.2	90.5	92.7	95.3	97.9	100.4	101.9	89.2	90.5	92.7	95.3	97.9	100.4	101.9
	NT	86	87	89	91	93	94	95	44	44	45	46	47	48	48
	PreHT	100	101	103	105	107	108	109	59	59	60	61	62	63	63
	Stage 1 HT	104	105	107	109	110	112	113	63	63	64	65	66	67	67
	Stage 2 HT	116	117	119	121	123	124	125	76	76	77	78	79	80	80
4	Height - *inches*	37.6	38.2	39.3	40.4	41.5	42.5	43.1	37.6	38.2	39.3	40.4	41.5	42.5	43.1
	Height - *cm*	96.5	97.1	99.7	102.5	105.4	108.0	109.5	96.5	97.1	99.7	102.5	105.4	108.0	109.5
	NT	88	89	91	93	95	96	97	47	48	49	50	51	51	52
	PreHT	102	103	105	107	109	110	111	62	63	64	65	66	66	67
	Stage 1 HT	106	107	109	111	112	114	115	66	67	68	69	70	71	71
	Stage 2 HT	118	119	121	123	125	126	127	79	80	81	82	83	83	84
5	Height - *inches*	39.9	40.6	41.7	43.0	44.2	45.3	46.0	39.9	40.6	41.7	43.0	44.2	45.3	46.0
	Height - *cm*	101.5	103.2	106.0	109.2	112.3	115.1	116.8	101.5	103.2	106.0	109.2	112.3	115.1	116.8
	NT	90	91	93	95	96	98	98	50	51	52	53	54	55	55
	PreHT	104	105	106	108	110	111	112	65	66	67	68	69	69	70
	Stage 1 HT	108	109	110	112	114	115	116	69	70	71	72	73	74	74
	Stage 2 HT	120	121	123	125	126	128	128	82	83	84	85	86	86	87
6	Height - *inches*	42.2	43.0	44.2	45.5	46.9	48.1	48.8	42.2	43.0	44.2	45.5	46.9	48.1	48.8
	Height - *cm*	107.3	109.2	112.2	115.7	119.1	122.1	123.9	107.3	109.2	112.2	115.7	119.1	122.1	123.9
	NT	91	92	94	96	98	99	100	53	53	54	55	56	57	57
	PreHT	105	106	108	110	111	113	113	68	68	69	70	71	72	72
	Stage 1 HT	109	110	112	114	115	117	117	72	72	73	74	75	76	76
	Stage 2 HT	121	122	124	126	128	129	130	85	85	86	87	88	89	89
7	Height - *inches*	44.6	45.3	46.6	48.0	49.5	50.8	51.6	44.6	45.3	46.6	48.0	49.5	50.8	51.6
	Height - *cm*	113.2	115.1	118.4	122.0	125.7	129.0	131.0	113.2	115.1	118.4	122.0	125.7	129.0	131.0
	NT	92	94	95	97	99	100	101	55	55	56	57	58	59	59
	PreHT	106	107	109	111	113	114	115	70	70	71	72	73	74	74
	Stage 1 HT	110	111	113	115	117	118	119	74	74	75	76	77	78	78
	Stage 2 HT	122	123	125	127	129	130	131	87	87	88	89	90	91	91
8	Height - *inches*	46.8	47.6	48.9	50.4	52.0	53.4	54.3	46.8	47.6	48.9	50.4	52.0	53.4	54.3
	Height - *cm*	118.8	120.8	124.3	128.1	132.1	135.7	137.8	118.8	120.8	124.3	128.1	132.1	135.7	137.8
	NT	94	95	97	99	100	102	102	56	57	58	59	60	60	61
	PreHT	107	109	110	112	114	115	116	71	72	72	73	74	75	76
	Stage 1 HT	111	112	114	116	118	119	120	75	76	77	78	79	79	80
	Stage 2 HT	124	125	127	128	130	132	132	88	89	90	91	92	92	93
9	Height - *inches*	48.7	49.6	51.0	52.7	54.3	55.8	56.7	48.7	49.6	51.0	52.7	54.3	55.8	56.7
	Height - *cm*	123.8	126.0	129.6	133.7	137.9	141.8	144.1	123.8	126.0	129.6	133.7	137.9	141.8	144.1
	NT	95	96	98	100	102	103	104	57	58	59	60	61	61	62
	PreHT	109	110	112	114	115	117	118	72	73	74	75	76	76	77
	Stage 1 HT	113	114	116	118	119	121	121	76	77	78	79	80	81	81
	Stage 2 HT	125	126	128	130	132	133	134	89	90	91	92	93	93	94

BP Levels for Boys by Age and Height Percentile (Cont'd)

IPHA

Updated: January, 2012

Age yrs	BP Percentile	Systolic BP (mmHg)							Diastolic BP (mmHg)						
		5th	10th	25th	50th	75th	90th	95th	5th	10th	25th	50th	75th	90th	95th
10	Height - *inches*	50.5	51.4	52.9	54.7	56.4	58.0	59.0	50.5	51.4	52.9	54.7	56.4	58.0	59.0
	Height - *cm*	128.2	130.5	134.4	138.8	143.3	147.4	149.0	128.2	130.5	134.4	138.8	143.3	147.4	149.0
	NT	97	98	100	102	103	105	106	58	59	60	61	61	62	63
	PreHT	111	112	114	115	117	119	119	73	73	74	75	76	77	78
	Stage 1 HT	115	116	117	119	121	122	123	77	78	79	80	81	81	82
	Stage 2 HT	127	128	130	132	133	135	135	90	91	91	93	93	94	95
11	Height - *inches*	52.1	53.1	54.7	56.6	58.5	60.2	61.2	52.1	53.1	54.7	56.6	58.5	60.2	61.2
	Height - *cm*	132.4	134.9	139.0	143.7	148.5	152.9	155.6	132.4	134.9	139.0	143.7	148.5	152.9	155.6
	NT	99	100	102	104	105	107	107	59	59	60	61	62	63	63
	PreHT	113	114	115	117	119	120	121	74	74	75	76	77	78	78
	Stage 1 HT	117	118	119	121	123	124	125	78	78	79	80	81	82	82
	Stage 2 HT	129	130	132	134	135	137	137	91	91	92	93	94	95	95
12	Height - *inches*	54.1	55.1	56.8	58.8	60.8	62.6	63.7	54.1	55.1	56.8	58.8	60.8	62.6	63.7
	Height - *cm*	137.3	139.9	144.3	149.3	154.4	159.0	161.9	137.3	139.9	144.3	149.3	154.4	159.0	161.9
	NT	101	102	104	106	108	109	110	59	60	61	62	63	63	64
	PreHT	115	116	118	120	121	123	123	74	75	75	76	77	78	79
	Stage 1 HT	119	120	122	123	125	127	127	78	79	80	81	82	82	83
	Stage 2 HT	131	132	134	136	138	139	140	91	92	93	94	95	95	96
13	Height - *inches*	56.5	57.6	59.5	61.6	63.7	65.6	66.7	56.5	57.6	59.5	61.6	63.7	65.6	66.7
	Height - *cm*	143.6	146.4	151.1	156.4	161.7	166.6	169.5	143.6	146.4	151.1	156.4	161.7	166.6	169.5
	NT	104	105	106	108	110	111	112	60	60	61	62	63	64	64
	PreHT	117	118	120	122	124	125	126	75	75	76	77	78	79	79
	Stage 1 HT	121	122	124	126	128	129	130	79	79	80	81	82	83	83
	Stage 2 HT	133	135	136	138	140	141	142	92	92	93	94	95	96	96
14	Height - *inches*	59.3	60.5	62.5	64.6	66.7	68.6	69.7	59.3	60.5	62.5	64.6	66.7	68.6	69.7
	Height - *cm*	150.5	153.6	158.7	164.1	169.5	174.2	177.0	150.5	153.6	158.7	164.1	169.5	174.2	177.0
	NT	106	107	109	111	113	114	115	60	61	62	63	64	65	65
	PreHT	120	121	123	125	126	128	128	75	76	77	78	79	79	80
	Stage 1 HT	124	125	127	128	130	132	132	80	80	81	82	83	84	84
	Stage 2 HT	136	137	139	141	143	144	145	92	93	94	95	96	97	97
15	Height - *inches*	61.7	62.9	64.9	67.0	69.0	70.8	71.8	61.7	62.9	64.9	67.0	69.0	70.8	71.8
	Height - *cm*	156.7	159.8	164.8	170.1	175.3	179.8	182.4	156.7	159.8	164.8	170.1	175.3	179.8	182.4
	NT	109	110	112	113	115	117	117	61	62	63	64	65	66	66
	PreHT	122	124	125	127	129	130	131	76	77	78	79	80	80	81
	Stage 1 HT	126	127	129	131	133	134	135	81	81	82	83	84	85	85
	Stage 2 HT	139	140	141	143	145	147	147	93	94	95	96	97	98	98
16	Height - *inches*	63.3	64.5	66.3	68.4	70.3	72.0	73.0	63.3	64.5	66.3	68.4	70.3	72.0	73.0
	Height - *cm*	160.8	163.7	168.5	173.6	178.6	182.9	185.5	160.8	163.7	168.5	173.6	178.6	182.9	185.5
	NT	111	112	114	116	118	119	120	63	63	64	65	66	67	67
	PreHT	125	126	128	130	131	133	134	78	78	79	80	81	82	82
	Stage 1 HT	129	130	132	134	135	137	137	82	83	83	84	85	86	87
	Stage 2 HT	141	142	144	146	148	149	150	95	95	96	97	98	99	99
17	Height - *inches*	64.2	65.3	67.1	69.0	70.9	72.6	73.6	64.2	65.3	67.1	69.0	70.9	72.6	73.6
	Height - *cm*	163.1	165.8	170.4	175.3	180.2	184.5	187.0	163.1	165.8	170.4	175.3	180.2	184.5	187.0
	NT	114	115	116	118	120	121	122	65	66	66	67	68	69	70
	PreHT	127	128	130	132	134	135	136	80	80	81	82	83	84	84
	Stage 1 HT	131	132	134	136	138	139	140	84	85	86	87	87	88	89
	Stage 2 HT	144	145	146	148	150	151	152	97	98	98	99	100	101	102

The 90th percentile is 1.28 SD, the 95th percentile is 1.645 SD, and the 99th percentile is 2.326 SD over the mean.

NT = normotensive (50th percentile **PreHT** = pre-hypertensive (90th percentile) **HT** = hypertensive (95th percentile for stage 1 and 99th% + 5 mmHg for stage 2)

BP Levels for Girls by Age and Height Percentile

Updated: January, 2012

 IPHA

Age yrs	BP Percentile	Systolic BP (mmHg)							Diastolic BP (mmHg)						
		5th	10th	25th	50th	75th	90th	95th	5th	10th	25th	50th	75th	90th	95th
2	Height - inches	31.4	31.9	32.7	33.6	34.5	35.4	35.9	31.4	31.9	32.7	33.6	34.5	35.4	35.9
	Height - cm	79.6	80.9	83.0	85.4	87.7	89.9	91.1	79.6	80.9	83.0	85.4	87.7	89.9	91.1
	NT	85	85	87	88	89	91	91	43	44	44	45	46	46	47
	PreHT	98	99	100	101	103	104	105	57	58	58	59	60	61	61
	Stage 1 HT	102	103	104	105	107	108	109	61	62	62	63	64	65	65
	Stage 2 HT	114	115	116	117	119	120	121	74	74	75	75	76	77	77
3	Height - inches	34.6	35.1	36.0	37.1	38.1	39.1	39.7	34.6	35.1	36.0	37.1	38.1	39.1	39.7
	Height - cm	87.8	89.2	91.6	94.2	96.9	99.3	100.8	87.8	89.2	91.6	94.2	96.9	99.3	100.8
	NT	86	87	88	89	91	92	93	47	48	48	49	50	50	51
	PreHT	100	100	102	103	104	106	106	61	62	62	63	64	64	65
	Stage 1 HT	104	104	105	107	108	109	110	65	66	66	67	68	68	69
	Stage 2 HT	116	116	118	119	120	121	122	78	78	79	79	80	81	81
4	Height - inches	37.0	37.6	38.6	39.8	40.9	42.0	42.7	37.0	37.6	38.6	39.8	40.9	42.0	42.7
	Height - cm	94.0	95.6	98.1	101.0	104.0	106.8	108.4	94.0	95.6	98.1	101.0	104.0	106.8	108.4
	NT	88	88	90	91	92	94	94	50	50	51	52	52	53	54
	PreHT	101	102	103	104	106	107	108	64	64	65	66	67	67	68
	Stage 1 HT	105	106	107	108	110	111	112	68	68	69	70	71	71	72
	Stage 2 HT	117	118	119	120	122	123	124	81	81	81	82	83	84	84
5	Height - inches	39.5	40.2	41.3	42.5	43.8	45.0	45.7	39.5	40.2	41.3	42.5	43.8	45.0	45.7
	Height - cm	100.4	102.0	104.8	108.0	111.2	114.3	116.1	100.4	102.0	104.8	108.0	111.2	114.3	116.1
	NT	89	90	91	93	94	95	96	52	53	53	54	55	55	56
	PreHT	103	103	105	106	107	109	109	66	67	67	68	69	69	70
	Stage 1 HT	107	107	108	110	111	112	113	70	71	71	72	73	73	74
	Stage 2 HT	119	119	121	122	123	125	125	83	83	84	84	85	86	86
6	Height - inches	42.1	42.8	43.9	45.3	46.7	48.0	48.8	42.1	42.8	43.9	45.3	46.7	48.0	48.8
	Height - cm	106.9	108.6	111.6	115.0	118.6	121.9	123.9	106.9	108.6	111.6	115.0	118.6	121.9	123.9
	NT	91	92	93	94	96	97	98	54	54	55	56	56	57	58
	PreHT	104	105	106	108	109	110	111	68	68	69	70	70	71	72
	Stage 1 HT	108	109	110	111	113	114	115	72	72	73	74	74	75	76
	Stage 2 HT	120	121	122	124	125	126	127	85	85	85	86	87	88	88
7	Height - inches	44.5	45.2	46.5	47.9	49.4	50.8	51.7	44.5	45.2	46.5	47.9	49.4	50.8	51.7
	Height - cm	113.1	114.9	118.1	121.8	125.6	129.1	131.3	113.1	114.9	118.1	121.8	125.6	129.1	131.3
	NT	93	93	95	96	97	99	99	55	56	56	57	58	58	59
	PreHT	106	107	108	109	111	112	113	69	70	70	71	72	72	73
	Stage 1 HT	110	111	112	113	115	116	116	73	74	74	75	76	76	77
	Stage 2 HT	122	123	124	125	127	128	129	86	86	87	87	88	89	89
8	Height - inches	46.7	47.5	48.8	50.3	51.9	53.4	54.3	46.7	47.5	48.8	50.3	51.9	53.4	54.3
	Height -cm	118.5	120.5	123.9	127.8	131.9	135.6	137.9	118.5	120.5	123.9	127.8	131.9	135.6	137.9
	NT	95	95	96	98	99	100	101	57	57	57	58	59	60	60
	PreHT	108	109	110	111	113	114	114	71	71	71	72	73	74	74
	Stage 1 HT	112	112	114	115	116	118	118	75	75	75	76	77	78	78
	Stage 2 HT	124	125	126	127	128	130	130	87	87	88	88	89	90	91
9	Height - inches	48.5	19.3	50.8	52.4	54.1	55.7	56.6	48.5	19.3	50.8	52.4	54.1	55.7	56.6
	Height - cm	123.2	125.3	129.0	133.1	137.4	141.4	143.8	123.2	125.3	129.0	133.1	137.4	141.4	143.8
	NT	96	97	98	100	101	102	103	58	58	58	59	60	61	61
	PreHT	110	110	112	113	114	116	116	72	72	72	73	74	75	75
	Stage 1 HT	114	114	115	117	118	119	120	76	76	76	77	78	79	79
	Stage 2 HT	126	126	128	129	130	132	132	88	88	89	89	90	91	92

BP Levels for Girls by Age and Height Percentile *(Cont'd)*

Updated: January, 2012

Age yrs	BP Percentile	Systolic BP (mmHg)							Diastolic BP (mmHg)						
		5th	10th	25th	50th	75th	90th	95th	5th	10th	25th	50th	75th	90th	95th
10	Height - *inches*	50.2	51.1	52.6	54.4	56.2	57.9	58.9	50.2	51.1	52.6	54.4	56.2	57.9	58.9
	Height - *cm*	127.5	129.8	133.7	138.2	142.8	147.0	149.6	127.5	129.8	133.7	138.2	142.8	147.0	149.6
	NT	98	99	100	102	103	104	105	59	59	59	60	61	62	62
	PreHT	112	112	114	115	116	118	118	73	73	73	74	75	76	76
	Stage 1 HT	116	116	117	119	120	121	122	77	77	77	78	79	80	80
	Stage 2 HT	128	128	130	131	132	134	134	89	89	90	91	91	92	93
11	Height - *inches*	52.1	53.1	54.9	56.8	58.7	60.5	61.6	52.1	53.1	54.9	56.8	58.7.	60.5	61.6
	Height - *cm*	132.4	135.0	139.4	144.3	149.2	153.7	156.4	132.4	135.0	139.4	144.3	149.2	153.7	156.4
	NT	100	101	102	103	105	106	107	60	60	60	61	62	63	63
	PreHT	114	114	116	117	118	119	120	74	74	74	75	76	77	77
	Stage 1 HT	118	118	119	121	122	123	124	78	78	78	79	80	81	81
	Stage 2 HT	130	130	131	133	134	135	136	90	90	91	92	92	93	94
12	Height - *inches*	54.8	55.9	57.7	59.6	61.6	63.3	64.4	54.8	55.9	57.7	59.6	61.6	63.3	64.4
	Height - *cm*	139.2	142.0	146.5	151.5	156.4	160.8	163.5	139.2	142.0	146.5	151.5	156.4	160.8	163.5
	NT	102	103	104	105	107	108	109	61	61	61	62	63	64	64
	PreHT	116	116	117	119	120	121	122	75	75	75	76	77	78	78
	Stage 1 HT	119	120	121	123	124	125	126	79	79	79	80	81	82	82
	Stage 2 HT	132	132	133	135	136	137	138	91	91	92	93	93	94	95
13	Height - *inches*	57.4	58.4	60.1	61.9	63.8	65.4	66.4	57.4	58.4	60.1	61.9	63.8	65.4	66.4
	Height - *cm*	145.9	148.4	152.7	157.3	162.0	166.1	168.6	145.9	148.4	152.7	157.3	162.0	166.1	168.6
	NT	104	105	106	107	109	110	110	62	62	62	63	64	65	65
	PreHT	117	118	119	121	122	123	124	76	76	76	77	78	79	79
	Stage 1 HT	121	122	123	124	126	127	128	80	80	80	81	82	83	83
	Stage 2 HT	133	134	135	137	138	139	140	92	92	93	94	94	95	96
14	Height - *inches*	58.9	59.9	61.4	63.2	64.9	66.5	67.4	58.9	59.9	61.4	63.2	64.9	66.5	67.4
	Height - *cm*	149.7	152.1	156.0	160.5	164.9	168.9	171.3	149.7	152.1	156.0	160.5	164.9	168.9	171.3
	NT	106	106	107	109	110	111	112	63	63	63	64	65	66	66
	PreHT	119	120	121	122	124	125	125	77	77	77	78	79	80	80
	Stage 1 HT	123	123	125	126	127	129	129	81	81	81	82	83	84	84
	Stage 2 HT	135	136	137	138	140	141	141	93	93	94	95	95	96	97
15	Height - *inches*	59.6	60.5	62.0	63.7	65.5	67.0	68.0	59.6	60.5	62.0	63.7	65.5	67.0	68.0
	Height - *cm*	151.3	153.6	157.5	161.9	166.3	170.2	172.6	151.3	153.6	157.5	161.9	166.3	170.2	172.6
	NT	107	108	109	110	111	113	113	64	64	64	65	66	67	67
	PreHT	120	121	122	123	125	126	127	78	78	78	79	80	81	81
	Stage 1 HT	124	125	126	127	129	130	131	82	82	82	83	84	85	85
	Stage 2 HT	136	137	138	139	141	142	143	94	94	95	96	96	97	98
16	Height - *inches*	59.8	60.7	62.3	64.0	65.7	67.3	68.2	59.8	60.7	62.3	64.0	65.7	67.3	68.2
	Height - *cm*	151.9	154.3	158.2	162.6	166.9	170.9	173.2	151.9	154.3	158.2	162.6	166.9	170.9	173.2
	NT	108	108	110	111	112	114	114	64	64	65	66	66	67	68
	PreHT	121	122	123	124	126	127	128	78	78	79	80	81	81	82
	Stage 1 HT	125	126	127	128	130	131	132	82	82	83	84	85	85	86
	Stage 2 HT	137	138	139	140	142	143	144	95	95	95	96	97	98	98
17	Height - *inches*	60.0	60.9	62.4	64.1	65.9	67.4	68.3	60.0	60.9	62.4	64.1	65.9	67.4	68.3
	Height - *cm*	152.3	154.6	158.6	162.9	167.3	171.2	173.6	152.3	154.6	158.6	162.9	167.3	171.2	173.6
	NT	108	109	110	111	113	114	115	64	65	65	66	67	67	68
	PreHT	122	122	123	125	126	127	128	78	79	79	80	81	81	82
	Stage 1 HT	125	126	127	129	130	131	132	82	83	83	84	85	85	86
	Stage 2 HT	138	138	139	141	142	143	144	95	95	96	96	97	98	98

The 90th percentile is 1.28 SD, the 95th percentile is 1.645 SD, and the 99th percentile is 2.326 SD over the mean.

NT = normotensive (50th percentile **PreHT** = pre-hypertensive (90th percentile) **HT** = hypertensive (95th percentile for stage 1 and 99th% + 5 mmHg for stage 2)

17.8.5 Nomogram for Renal Length

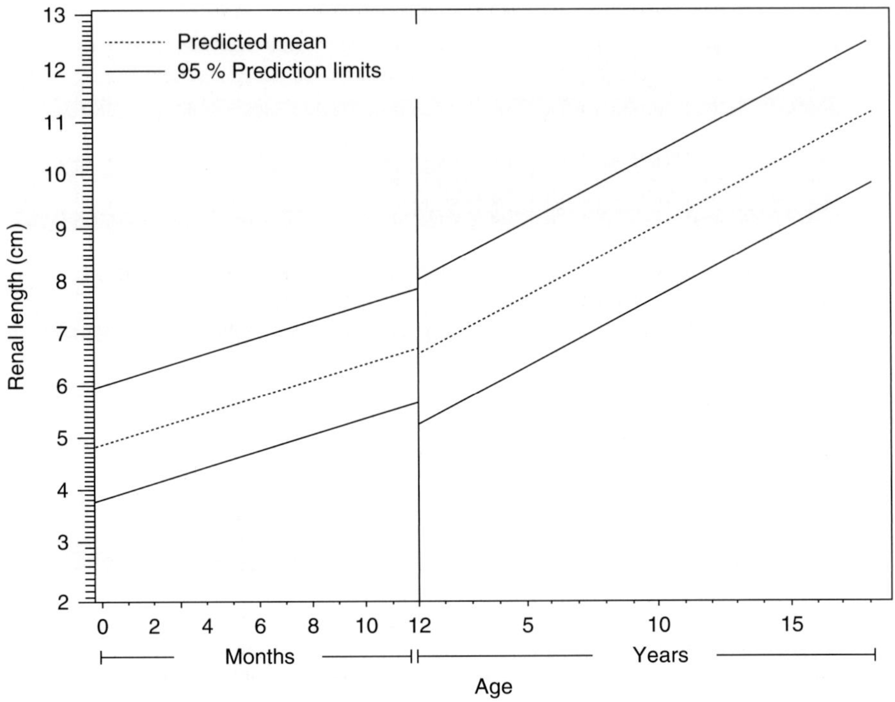

Index

K. Phadke et al. (eds.), *Manual of Pediatric Nephrology*,
DOI 10.1007/978-3-642-12483-9, © Springer-Verlag Berlin Heidelberg 2014

I

K

O

S

T

Printing and Binding: Stürtz GmbH, Würzburg